To George & Judy

c Love,

Martin 8/29/93.

EFFECTIVE

Medical Imaging

A Signs and Symptoms Approach

EFFECTIVE

Medical Imaging

A Signs and Symptoms Approach

Martin F. Sturman, M.D., F.A.C.P.

Director of Nuclear Medicine
and Ultrasonography
St. Michael's Medical Center
Newark, New Jersey

Consultant in Radiology
St. Vincent's Hospital and Medical Center
New York, New York

with contributions from

Paul J. Rosch, M.D., F.A.C.P., Medical Editor
Patrick J. Conte, Jr., M.D., Radiological Editor

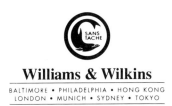

Williams & Wilkins

BALTIMORE • PHILADELPHIA • HONG KONG
LONDON • MUNICH • SYDNEY • TOKYO

A WAVERLY COMPANY

Editor: David C. Retford
Managing Editor: Marjorie Kidd Keating
Copy Editor: Bruce Totaro
Designer: Norman W. Och
Illustration Planner: Ray Lowman
Production Coordinator: Kimberly Nawrozki
Cover Designer: Norman W. Och

Copyright © 1993
Williams & Wilkins
428 East Preston Street
Baltimore, Maryland 21202, USA

Printed in the United States of America

Library of Congress Cataloging in Publication Data

Sturman, Martin F.
    Effective medical imaging : a signs and symptoms approach / Martin
  F. Sturman ; with contributions from Paul J. Rosch, Patrick
  J. Conte, Jr.
     p. cm.
    Includes index.
    ISBN 0-683-07934-4
    1. Diagnostic imaging.   2. Symptomatology.   I. Rosch, Paul J.
  II. Conte, Patrick J.   III. Title.
    [DNLM: 1. Diagnostic Imaging.   WN 200 S936a]
  RC78.7.D53S78   1993
  616.07′54—dc20
  DNLM/DLC
  for Library of Congress   92-48197
                                           CIP

93 94 95 96 97
1 2 3 4 5 6 7 8 9 10

To my wife, Julie,
and
to the memory of my parents

Foreword

In the last two decades, medical imaging has grown faster than the overall growth in health care in the United States. From Medicare data, the average annual growth of all medical services in the mid-1980s was 12% per year. The compounded growth rate for imaging was 18%, and for high-technology or "advanced" imaging services the growth was 32% per year. These numbers are astonishing in one sense but are reflections of the new technology that has become available to perform medical imaging and the recognition of value added from imaging in the care of patients.

There are several important implications of the rapid growth in delivery of imaging services. First, the addition of new imaging modalities such as ultrasonography, computed tomography, and magnetic resonance imaging make selection of the appropriate test by clinicians far more challenging than before. The knowledge base necessary to make informed decisions is vastly greater. Each modality has different strengths and weaknesses. Even when imaging the same organ, such as the brain or liver, selection of modality is heavily influenced by the disease process under investigation. It is possible to select a modality based on the most likely clinical diagnosis, only to realize in retrospect that a different modality would have been preferable based on the final diagnosis.

Dr. Sturman's book takes on the daunting task of trying to sort out these issues. He starts by providing the reader with general principles and background material on the various modalities as a basis for their application.

But, the unique aspect of *Effective Medical Imaging* is the presentation of imaging approaches by chief complaints, signs, symptoms, or conditions. Dr. Sturman's description begins in each case in the manner that the patient actually presents to his or her physician. In the classic textbook approach, disease taxonomy is used as the basis of organization and presentation. That is, the discussion begins with the diagnosis and proceeds to the clinical findings. This is backwards. In practice, the work-up does not begin with the diagnosis but culminates with it, and the physician is challenged to synthesize clinical, laboratory, and imaging data. Thus, Dr. Sturman's approach corresponds to the process as we actually encounter it in everyday practice.

By logical extension, the *Effective Medical Imaging* addresses another important implication of the growth in imaging in today's health care climate. Payers and government agencies are challenging physicians to demonstrate as never before the value of their services, largely to justify their high and increasing costs. Unnecessary use of diagnostic imaging services due to lack of understanding of efficacy or appropriate application is a definite factor in the cost of health care. Although it is not possible to place an exact dollar value on the cost of unnecessary use, it is still highly worthwhile to seek better approaches to test selection. Dr. Sturman's work is aimed directly at this question.

Although most physicians probably feel comfortable ordering diagnostic tests in their areas of special expertise, the explosion of technology and the rapidity of clinical development make it challenging to keep up. In particular, the predictive value of positive and negative results is not intuitive and is very difficult to keep in context. *Effective Medical Imaging* should provide a firm foundation and point of reference for the practicing physician in this regard.

Probably the most important aspect of this book is that it will stimulate the reader to think more critically about the diagnostic imaging process, both in the application of tests and in the assessment of their results. Dr. Sturman has taken an unconventional approach to this process—but one that should prove very worthwhile.

James H. Thrall, M.D.
Radiologist-in-Chief
Massachusetts General Hospital
and Juan M. Taveras
Professor of Radiology
Harvard Medical School
Boston, Massachusetts

Preface

From inability to let well alone; from too much zeal for the new and contempt for what is old; from putting knowledge before wisdom, science before art and cleverness before common sense; from treating patients as cases; and from making the cure of the disease more grievous than the endurance of the same, Good Lord, deliver us.

Sir Robert Hutchison

I have seen so many inappropriate and unnecessary studies ordered by so many good physicians during my years in practice, I felt a "guide for the perplexed" was sorely needed. The format and style of this book is intended to reflect my conviction that only signs and symptoms, and therefore a careful history and physical, provide the major clues to correct diagnosis. All too often this time-tested but sadly neglected approach has been subordinated to the pressures of time and the indiscriminate ordering of various testing procedures in a misguided search for some shortcut. Diagnosis should be approached as a *hierarchical order* of limited probabilities rather than an unabridged list of potential possibilities. This represents a deviation from classical medical teaching (1).

Hence, I have made no attempt to be exhaustive, because, by deemphasizing or omitting rare conditions, we may more appropriately concentrate on those disorders that are most frequently encountered. Certain discussions may reveal a tendency toward condensation and repetition and at times may appear unduly dogmatic or speculative. Perhaps making broad generalizations expressing a strong point of view in an authoritarian fashion may displease some readers, but for others I hope it will provide a refreshing change for medical texts, which traditionally have tended toward the bland.

This book is about the survival of common-sense medicine and the preservation of clinical judgment in an age of exploding technology. Physicians are overwhelmed by the sheer proliferation of newer modalities and techniques in the field of diagnostic imaging, many of which were unavailable or unheard of only a few years ago. We have seen such "hi-tech" procedures more and more misunderstood and overused because of the sheer confusion brought about by increasing numbers of competing and overlapping imaging procedures. There appears to be a widespread assumption that the latest enhancement automatically will become the procedure of choice for all diagnostic imaging procedures. Moreover, there is a widespread and uncritical acceptance of the novel in the misguided belief that the new is necessarily better than the old, and time-tested aproaches are somehow quaint and should be regarded with deep skepticism.

In magnetic resonance imaging (MRI) of the brain 20 or more lesions may be disclosed in patients with multiple sclerosis, where computed tomography (CT) discloses only a few, though clearly CT is indeed superior to MRI in other situations. Yet in the management and prognosis of multiple sclerosis, very little has changed since the early days when the diagnosis was largely made by neurological history and examination.

Perhaps this is the price we must pay for specialization. Hematologists, oncologists, angiographers, endoscopists, and pediatric neurologists, like some modern composers, are busy writing music for each other. Though *they* may share some common language, it is frequently a foreign tongue for the family practitioner or primary care internist, who must make prompt but practical decisions that could involve life-and-death situations.

Although sincerity is not lacking in medical specialists, one cannot escape the suspicion that a few may be unconsciously self-serving. It is a platitude that specialization is the greatest problem in medicine today, that medicine, though it purports to be "holistic" in treating the entire patient, fragments him into a collection of organ systems, a form of reductionism run rampant. The narrow viewpoint of the imaging specialist was brought home to me recently when I was asked to contribute, along with experts in MRI and CT scanning, to an article on imaging in acute abdominal pain, but ultimately had to withdraw because of irreconcilable viewpoints. Clearly, my colleagues had seen many cases of intraabdominal collections (a very rare cause of acute pain) and few cases of intestinal obstruction and appendicitis. From this, the entire orientation was directed—not toward the common causes of abdominal pain, *but toward the rare conditions for which MRI and CT might be appropriate.*

This experience points out another problem arising from the steady replacement of traditional imaging, specifically plain radiography, by the newer procedures. Radiologists coming out of residency over the past 15–20 years find themselves spending an increasing proportion of their training in CT, MRI, and invasive procedures, leaving far less time for reading plain films and performing barium studies. This problem is compounded by the alarming decline in demand for routine basic procedures, particularly barium contrast studies, a result of competition by endoscopists. Ask any radiologist over the age of 40–45 about the skills of younger colleagues in reading chest radiographs, gastrointestinal series, and bone films compared to the older generation.

Emerson (2) saw the dangers of specialization more than 150 years ago when he wrote of the "amputation" of society, each trade and profession "ridden by the routine of his craft.... The priest becomes a form; the attorney a statute-book; the mechanic a machine; the sailor a rope of the ship" (2). (And the doctor an MRI scan?)

The deemphasis of the clinical approach results clearly from our love affair with any form of novelty. To paraphrase Andy Worhol, at the present rate, in the future, every new test and therapy will be famous for 15 minutes. Aldous Huxley once defined progress as "better toys." It also has been observed that for Americans, anything new is good; to the British, anything new is bad. Certainly, it seems that physicians, like most other professionals, are increasingly becoming subservient to the 20th century god of technology, either because of seduction or surrender. In contemporary society the sheer power of peer pressure generated by institutions, organizations, and especially commercial interests tends to dictate how we act as physicians both in ordering tests and even prescribing therapy. In becoming part of a collective will that acquiesces to perceived wisdom, we have surrendered our individuality and our very power to think for ourselves. This may be the primary reason that we defer to the test rather than rely on our clinical judgment. We learn early on to trust that Big Mother, whether She is the government, the company, the laboratory, or the imaging department, will take care of us. No need to worry, just get on with the establishment work-up. As Walter Lipmann remarked, "When we all think alike, then no one is thinking."

Thus, it is not surprising that the clinical approach to many sick patients has often evolved into investigative anarchy, a kind of scattershot process in which every conceivable relevant or irrelevant diagnostic study is ordered as soon as possible. "Plugging the patient into the laboratory" accurately describes this type of mindless medicine. It represents the search for a quick diagnosis that is directed not by intellect, experience, or any orderly thought process, but rather driven by a perceived need to make a diagnosis or "do something" as fast as possible. This trend has accelerated in recent years because of cost containment pressures and closer scrutiny of hospital admission and stays by utilization review committees, peer review organizations, and other monitoring and regulatory agencies as well as fiscal intermediaries.

Another cause of excessive and unnecessary testing is the pervasive fear of malpractice litigation. This is often used to justify needless procedures because of the entrenched belief that the more tests ordered, the less the likelihood of being sued. All too frequently, this proves to be a fallacy that can backfire, especially when such extraneous tests disclose some irrelevant finding that now mandates the need for still further procedures that are not pertinent, and in turn may lead to various types of clinical disasters, the so-called "cascade effect."

Today, so many diagnostic procedures are being indiscriminately ordered without clinical justification that our health care system is in jeopardy of bankruptcy. A national health bill of $840 billion has been estimated for 1992 by the Commerce Department, of which perhaps $60–70 billion was expended for clinical testing. Most of this cost is accounted for by various types of imaging (including invasive) procedures. How much medical investigation is unnecessary and therefore a needless economic and social waste is speculative, but I speculate it could well be in excess of $75 billion a year.

After a total of 35 years in medical practice, including family practice, internal medicine, endocrinology, nuclear medicine, and ultrasonography, I have become increasingly impressed with the need to demythologize the hype of constantly inflated imaging claims. What practicing physicians sorely need are guidelines that not only to identify the relative merits and indications for various imaging procedures but also put them in perspective as to priority and cost effectiveness. Despite the recent popularity of cook book-type, rule-based, diagnostic algorithms, deciding which imaging procedure is best for a given situation is a constantly recurring problem. Such information is not readily available, and it became obvious to me that such assistance could best be provided by developing a text that emphasized the clinical approach to diagnosis. My orientation, therefore, will be directed to signs and symptoms rather than diseases or procedures. I hope to illustrate the prime importance of information gleaned from the patient with a thorough history and a careful physical examination, a notion regarded today as an empty platitude more often than a clinical dictum. There is nothing wrong with restating the obvious. Goethe once remarked, "Everything has already been thought of. The only problem is thinking of it again." Put in current terms, diagnosis is "hypothesis driven"; it springs from the synthesis of ideas evoked by a set of clinical findings.

If diagnosis requires any laboratory or imaging corroboration (and it should be emphasized that most office and many hospital patients do not require any more than routine medical testing), the choice of such investigation must be founded on principles long ago enunciated in the teaching and practice of medicine. The keystone remains the time-honored clinical assessment of the sick patient, provided it is conducted in a thorough and thoughtful fashion.

A recent case history is illustrative. Not long ago we received a frantic call in the ultrasound department for "immediate abdominal and pelvic ultrasound" on a patient with "acute left abdominal pain and tenderness" thought by the house staff to be a ruptured diverticulum. "Why not get an upright radiograph of the abdomen, followed by a careful barium enema?" we suggested, but to no avail. When the patient arrived it was obvious his pain was in the left *flank* and not the left abdomen. In fact, the abdomen was soft, though there was tenderness and guarding over the left hypochondrium. A simple urinalysis had not yet been done (though microscopic hematuria was subsequently found). Sonography of the kidneys promptly confined calcification in the collecting system on the left, with minimal pelviectasis, consistent with a renal calculus. Clinically, it seems likely that the physicians and students involved were uncertain about the most likely diagnosis. For them, the easiest way out was to order tests that might "cover the waterfront," rather than a simple procedure, which would have confirmed or ruled out their clinical impression. Increasing in frequency are requests for sonographic examinations of the soft tissues for abscess or of the scrotum for vague testicular pain or obvious hydrocoele. In these instances, just as in the patient with congestive failure when an intern requests that pulmonary embolism be ruled out, common sense or inability to perform the clinical examination has given way to hysteria.

Endless examples of this come to mind. They all result from a growing failure to develop clinical acumen during medical school training, as well as the tendency to substitute such skills for testing procedures that do not require personal time with the patient or thinking about the problem in a careful and logical manner.

This need not be a routine consequence of scientific progress. Every new technology brings with it the peril of being misapplied or abused when it is not viewed in proper perspective. This is certainly not the fault of technology. Even though physicists invent spectacular new devices such as magnetic resonance imagers, we are not thereby excused from asking the patient where it hurts.

REFERENCES

1. Fulop M. Teaching differential diagnosis to beginning clinical students. Am J Med 1985;79(6):745–759.
2. Emerson RW. *The American scholar*, an oration delivered before the Phi Beta Kappa Society at Cambridge, August 31, 1837. Quoted by Cynthia Ozick. *The moral necessity of metaphor*. Harpers May 1988: 62–68.

Acknowledgments

To describe a medical textbook as "single-authored" edges toward an oxymoron. Without the forbearance, encouragement, and many creative suggestions of my wife, Julie Sturman, B.F.A., R.N., the guidance of my editors, and the generous help and advice of numerous friends and colleagues, this project would never have reached completion. Among others, my profound gratitude goes to: my son, Henry R. Sturman, M.Sc. (Eng., Delft), who with enormous patience, guided me through the perils and profundities of conditional probability and Bayes' Theorem, helped enormously with Chapter 2, wrote the programs, designed the tables for predictive values, and wrote the mathematical sections, Appendixes A and B.

Special thanks to my stepson, Steven J. Brown, M.D., Assistant Professor, Division of Nuclear Medicine, Hahnemann University Medical School, for his invaluable help in preparing the graphs, and for the endlessly intriguing discussions about diagnostic practice and malpractice.

Deep gratitude to my dear friend and esteemed teacher, Professor John M. Ledingham, former Director of the Medical Unit, The London Hospital for his outcoming help in general medicine and hypertension, and my other dear friends and colleagues, in particular, Dr. Stanley E. Goodman, M.D., for his enormous contribution in general surgery, and my superb medical editor, Paul J. Rosch, M.D., Masters in English both in fact and in practice. I express gratitude to my friend, Professor Milton G. Gross, for his invaluable assistance on the adrenal and thyroid sections and to my other friends, former colleagues, and mentors at the University of Michigan Medical Center, for their help in general medicine and endocrinology, Professors of Medicine, Brahm Shapiro, M.D., James C. Sisson, M.D., and William H. Beierwaltes, M.D.

I thank Chuck Denison, M.S., statistician, and many other statisticians and epidemiologists of the National Center For Health Statistics (NCHS) for supplying invaluable statistical data, including data tapes and disks from the National Hospital Discharge Survey (NHDS) and the National Ambulatory Medical Care Survey (NAMCS). In addition to Chuck, others at the NCHS giving generously of their time included: Jacob J. Feldman, Ph.D., Associate Director for Analysis, Tommy McLemore, M.S.P.H., James E. DeLozier, M.S. and Raymond O. Gagnon, M.S.

Thanks to the National Library of Medicine and *Grateful Med* and especially the indefatigable ladies of the Aquinas Medical Library, St. Michael's Medical Center, Manager Joann V. Mehalick, whose searching ability rivals that of Sherlock Holmes, Pauline F. Willis and the late Jean L. Bernard who labored endlessly in tracking and copying more than 1600 references.

In general radiology, I am indebted to my radiological editor, Patrick, J. Conte, M.D., Senior Attending in Radiology and Medicine, St. Michael's Medical Center; to Roger C. Sanders, M.D., Clinical Professor of Radiology and Obstetrics, University of Maryland; and to David J. Ott, M.D., and David W. Gelfand, M.D., Professors of Radiology at Bowman Gray School of Medicine.

Grateful thanks to my friend and mentor, James E. Carey, M.S., Assistant Professor of Radiation Physics and Medical Nuclear Physicist, University of Michigan Center and to the Society of Nuclear Medicine, and the Subcommittee on Risks of Low-Level Ionizing Radiation who prepared the outstanding book, *Low Level Radiation Effects: A Fact Book*, from which I obtained secondary references of the tables for Chapter 4.

In the fields of probability and statistics, I am indebted to two Professors of Mathematics, my dear friend Manuel Perez, Ph.D., of the New Jersey Institute of Technology, and Robert van Glabbeek, Ph.D., of Stanford University, as well as my close friend, Mark Pilipski, B.A., of Hoffmann-LaRoche Laboratories.

Edward S. Johnson, M.D., Program Director Infectious Diseases, St. Michael's Medical Center, and Chairman, Infectious Diseases, Seton Hall School of Graduate Medical Education, and members of The Centers for Disease Control (CDC) made invaluable contributions to the chapter on AIDS.

Philip S. Brachman, M.D., Professor, Center for International Health and School of Public Health, Emory University School of Medicine, and Debra Mayer Quesada, M.D., Hospital Epidemiologist, University Hospital, New Jersey College of Medicine and Dentistry gave important additional assistance in epidemiology.

I appreciate the invaluable help given me by my colleagues:

Irvin D. Goldfarb, M.D. (cardiology), William R. Chenitz, M.D. (nephrology), Marc Adelman, M.D. (critical care, pulmonary), Frederic F. Flach, M.D. (psychiatry), Nicholas G. Barenetsky, M.D. (endocrinology), Diana Lake, M.D. (oncology), Jacob I. Haft, M.D. (cardiology), Raymond E. Carnes, M.D. and Elizabeth Dawson, M.D. (pathology), Henry Green, M.D. (pulmonary), Humbert L. Riva, M.D. (obstetrics/gynecology), Robin Rosenberg, M.D. (colon/rectal surgery), Jane C. Orient, M.D. (medicine), Donald L. Levine, M.D. (medicine/cardiology), Frank McGeehan, M.D. (cardiology), Michael Gratch, M.D. (orthopedic surgery), Raymon S. Silen, M.D. (general surgery), Roger W. Cooper, M.D. (pediatrics), Robert Soufer, M.D. (cardiology), Ira M. Rutkow, M.D., (surgery), and Marvin Burns, Biotech, Inc. (health statistics).

A Parable From Futureland

Once upon a time when the talk shows and the sitcoms no longer satisfied popular taste, giant colloquia were held to discuss various philosophical issues. These were available on world-wide television to hundreds of millions of viewers. One such seminar originating on a Swiss mountaintop dealt with the question, "What is two plus two?" Present were several important world class experts from diverse disciplines.

The mathematician quickly answered, "four," when first asked, "What is two plus two?"

Next in turn was the physicist who replied, "in the neighborhood of four."

The engineer responded with, "four point zero, zero, zero, zero plus or minus zero."

The economist without hesitation said, "two plus two is seven."

Next, it was the lawyer's turn. He looked at the host and asked, "Could you repeat the question?" After it was again posed, the lawyer pondered a moment, shrugged his shoulders and inquired, "What would you like?"

Finally it was the physician's opportunity. He slowly repeated the question over and over again. Finally his eyes brightened, he smiled and announced, "Let's order a test."

Contents

1

The Problems of Certainty
and Naming

When I say that a thing is true, I mean that I cannot help believing it. . . . But . . . I do not venture to assume that my inabilities in the way of thought are inabilities of the universe. I therefore define truth as the system of my limitations, and leave absolute truth for those who are better equipped. . . . Certitude is not the test of certainty. We have been cock-sure of many things that were not so.

Justice Holmes

The Problem of Certainty

The triumphs of 20th century science and technology have occurred during a period of savagery almost unparalleled in human history. These ideological storms, violent social upheavals, wars, totalitarianisms of both the right and the left, Nazism, and the Russian and Chinese Revolutions have shaken our belief in the perfectibility of human society. Modern science in the personae of relativity, quantum physics, and mathematical logic have shattered other cherished faiths—namely our beliefs in certainty, determinism, provability, the absolute, perhaps even causality.

It is altogether appropriate to mention these social and scientific cataclysms from the perspective of intellectual history, because they shed light on the changing nature of civilization and society and what this may portend for the future of the medical sciences. The developments of 20th century mathematics and physics have great relevance for us as practicing physicians.

The great contemporary thinker, Sir Isaiah Berlin, in seeking to resolve the problems of moral relativism and the conflicts and incoherencies of human values, returns to the historical concept of certainty (1). He reminds us that our rational world view was first fashioned by Plato and is still the dominant tradition in Western political thought. Briefly touched upon is the kindred scientific tradition that arose out of the same Greek philosophic source. Socrates thought that certainty of the external physical world as well as the world of human behavior could be arrived at by rational means. The Platonic ideal which forms the bedrock of our intellectual, scientific, and political tradition consists of three premises: in the first place, all genuine questions have one and only one true answer; in the second place, there must be a dependable path toward discovery of those answers, in other words, these answers are *knowable*; and in the third place, these true answers, when found, are all compatible with one another (for one truth cannot be incompatible with another) and together form a single coherent whole.

We find these notions prefiguring all the major religions and political systems—even the sciences. Do not Jews, Christians, and Muslims believe the final answers to all human questions have been revealed by God to his chosen prophets and saints? Do not Communists, Fascists, Socialists, and Democrats hold their own creed to be the only true path? Less obvious to the unwary is that even traditional science can be reduced to a kind of dogmatism, a belief that science itself can provide us with all the ultimate answers. The rationalists of the 17th century and the empiricists of the 18th, after all, thought the answers to all human and scientific questions could be discovered by the light of reason. These beliefs lay behind all progressive thought in the 19th century and to a great extent created the foundation of our own faith in the ability of logic and reason to banish stupidity, error, nonsense and superstition (1).

Berlin (1) reminds us that no more rigorous moralist than Kant ever lived, but quotes him as saying: "Out of the crooked timber of humanity no straight thing was ever made." He takes this to be an admonition against dogmatism, against utopianism, against any rationalistic system of thought that issues in "the pursuit of the ideal." Ever since Immanuel Kant took on the empiricists, philosophers have made the case that science is not a purely objective affair. It took the revolutions of 20th century mathematics and physics to shatter our belief in the scientific ideal, the pursuit of universal certainty.

The Strange World of Quantum Theory

> *Eventually, we reach the dim boundary—the utmost limits of our telescopes. There we measure shadows, and we search among ghostly errors of measurement for landmarks that are scarcely more substantial.*
>
> *Edwin Hubble*

We are hardly qualified to delve into the philosophical implications raised by the findings of 20th century mathematics and physics, nor do we claim quantum mechanics is a useful description of our real world. We merely mention some of its implications in an attempt to discover some similarities between the insights of modern physics and the bizarre yet common clinical phenomena seen in medical practice.

The age of absolutes, and with it, the age of certainty, has passed. We know from Einstein's work in special relativity that there is no absolute space and time. Quantum physics demonstrates that the cosmos, the solid state, the atom, all the elementary particles, the very "building blocks of matter," electromagnetic radiation, light, radio, X-rays, and other physical phenomena do not in actuality follow the deterministic physical laws enunciated by classical physics. In fact, quantum physicists have proof that both elementary particles and electromagnetic radiation exist as both waves and particles, simultaneous and dualistic manifestations of a kind of weird probabilistic reality. From Werner Heisenberg's uncertainty principle we learn that it is not possible simultaneously to measure the exact position and momentum of any elementary particle. These examples of uncertainty, in fact, underlie the probabilistic basis of quantum physics. Later, we shall examine the mathematical foundations of medical diagnosis in reference to these same concepts, in particular the probabilistic nature of disease and symptom occurrence and the problem of reducing uncertainty by the strategic use of medical testing.

In certain cleverly designed experiments measuring the polarization of pairs of photons, the French physicist Alain Aspect and his collaborators proved in 1981 that events in one place can be mysteriously correlated with events in a second region far removed from the first, in such a way that instantaneous (and therefore inexplicable) communication over large distances seems to occur. These findings have deep implications for our ideas of causality—and therefore of reality itself. Einstein and many other physicists always have had problems with the consequences of relativity and quantum mechanics for our common-sense view of reality. When quantum theory predicted the results of the Aspect experiments 46 years before they occurred, Einstein called it *"spukhafte fernwirkung"* (spooky actions at a distance) and insisted that no self-respecting universe would permit such behavior. In Einstein's famous letter to Max Born in 1926, in commenting on quantum mechanics and its probabilistic implications for the interpretation of reality, he states, "The theory says a lot, but does not really bring us any closer to the secret of the 'old one' [Einstein's affectionate term for God]. I, at any rate, am convinced that *He* is not playing at dice." (2).

If modern physics were not problem enough for the believers in determinism or even the rules of causality, we find the sociobiologists struggling to abolish what they suggest are the quaint notions of absolute free will. (One is reminded of the story told about Isaac Bashevis Singer, who, when asked what he thought about free will, answered without hesitation, "We must believe in free will; we have no choice.") The consequences for medicine of excessive emphasis on causality lie in the widely held beliefs in disease etiology, that indeed all diseases—and, more broadly, all symptoms—are explainable because they result universally from discoverable causes. We shall attempt throughout this book to question this fundamental paradigm of medical science. We hope to show that, for a large number of clinical presentations, the search for diagnosis, that is, the explainable or the knowable, may well be an idiot's chimera, the perennial cause of untold mischief and economic waste.

The World According to Turing and Gödel

> *Pure mathematics is the subject in which we do not know what we*
> *are talking about, or whether what we are saying is true.*
> *Bertrand Russell*

Other implications for our "modern" beliefs about illness stem from the latest arrivals on the scientific scene, the digital computer and modern scientific logic. Giants in these fields include the late great mathematical figures Alan Turing and Kurt Gödel, who, along with Rene Thom and others, seem to have finished the job of rewriting the map of human knowledge, "so that it now shows potholes and detours not only along every side street and back alley, but on all the major highways and byways as well" (3).

In 1928 in Bologna during the International Congress of Mathematicians, David Hilbert hurled a challenge he first proposed in 1900, a challenge that would ultimately and permanently alter the way we conceive the relationship between provability and actual truth. The fundamental issue he proposed was whether or not it is possible to prove every true mathematical assertion. Was there, in fact, some sort of mathematical truth machine that could *decide* whether any mathematical statement in a formal logical system was true or false? Hilbert himself had absolute faith such a machine or logical method would eventually be found. But less than 3 years after Hilbert's Bologna address, the young Austrian logician Kurt Gödel published a revolutionary paper that rocked the world of mathematics, "turning Hilbert's fondest dream into his greatest nightmare" (3).

Without attempting to delve into mathematical proofs, we will mention some conclusions of Gödel's monumental work. First, it is useful to consider some well-known examples, which may be classified either as logical paradoxes or self-contradictory statements, the "referential tangle." Typical ones include, "I'm an atheist, so help me God"; "What do you think of ignorance?", "I don't know"; a sign stating: "Want to learn to read? Call this number . . ."; and "Are you dead?" "Yes." Furthermore, we have in this very section our very own example: are we indeed certain there is no certainty? The oldest and most classic of all such contradictions is the Epimenides Paradox, one version of which is, "This statement is false."

What Gödel was looking for was a way to express such self-referential statements in the framework of arithmetic, and by extension, to any nontrivial mathematical system. The Gödel equivalent of the above sentence becomes, "This statement is not provable."

Gödel concludes by saying if the statement is provable, then it's true; hence, what it says must be true and it's *not* provable. The converse, of course, also implies an inconsistency, i.e. What Gödel was able to show was that for *any* consistent formal, nontrivial system such as arithmetic, the formalization must be incomplete. That is, there always exist statements that are unprovable; there will always be questions that can be asked but not answered. This has broad logical implications for any similar formal system. In medicine, as in mathematics, it turns out to be worse than useless to search for the holy grail of absolute provability. This is reflected in the present need to pursue diagnostic certainty at all cost and with unproven benefit.

The parallel concepts of provability and decidability have their analog in the idea of computability based on the work of the British mathematician Alan Turing and, later, Turing and Church. They showed that anything which could be described in a rule-based language could be obtained as the result of carrying out a series of computations on a primitive but basic computer called a Universal Turing Machine. It turns out, however, that noncomputable quantities exist that can never be described by a set of rules, (i.e. an algorithm, loosely, a program). This is the equivalent of saying that non- or incomputable means "not governed by rules," examples of which would include "complex, patternless, or even, in the vernacular, random" (4). Again, the reader is entitled to ask what relevance that has for physicians and patients. Our answer is that medical diagnosis, to the extent that we insist on making it rule-based, suffers from the same limitations as the digital computer or any mathematical system. So long as we adhere to a simple unitary concept of *disease*, the formalization will, like arithmetic, always be incomplete. There will often be unprovable assertions as in the Epimenides Paradox. In other words, there will always be questions that can be asked, but some of which can never be answered. For example, if we insist on the concrete concept of disease-as-etiology-and-entity, we frequently end up in serious difficulty as will be demonstrated below.

Probability and Determinism in Medicine

> *We can never finally know. I simply believe that some part of the*
> *human Self or Soul is not subject to the laws of space and time.*
> *Carl Gustav Jung*

In the last two decades we have encountered Rene Thom, Joseph Ford, Jim Yorke, and chaos theory—called by some, Gödel's child. The essence of chaos theory is that some deterministic systems can only be described statistically, that these systems may act in such complicated ways that they behave unpredictably. The best one can do is make probabilistic statements about them. Meteorologists knew about chaos theory long before the mathematicians discovered it. Other related systems called *fractals* are quite common in our universe: the forms of coastlines, the meanderings of rivers, the branchings of trees, and snowflakes. Fractals and chaos theory also have been used to describe our human world of politics, economics and the stock market, and, finally, medicine. For example, the arborizations of bronchi and blood vessels are now being described by fractal geometry, and fractal dynamics have been applied to the study of arrhythmias and congestive heart failure (4, 5).

The relation of chaos to quantum theory, indeterminacy, and provability to medicine lies in the probabilistic nature of both symptom occurrence and disease. There is no way to avoid some degree of diagnostic uncertainty in clinical practice. The sometimes fuzzy nature of clinical hypotheses, even the chaotic and the unexpected, are as much a part of medicine as they are of the physical world and therefore life itself.

There are ultimate limits to the world and to human knowledge. Perhaps our greatest sins as physicians are committed in the name of certainty, in pursuit of the ideal, when we continue to insist on a diagnosis or an explanation at any cost, when we are unable to declare to the patient or his family some simple phrases such as, "we don't know"; "this is not diagnosable, but we see it"; "we don't know what this is, but it's not serious." Perhaps this concept should be reified as a diagnostic entity, the "we see this syndrome." This is among the most common conditions we encounter in the practice of medicine. It may well be that the best clinicians are those who can say, "we see this," with unmistakable and honest conviction.

Clinical Examples of the Unprovable or the Indeterminate

What physician has not seen a patient with unexplained acute abdominal pain? We will learn in the chapters that follow that about 50% of patients seen in emergency rooms with acute abdominal pain have what is called nonspecific abdominal pain (NSAP), that is, pain without cause which subsides with no treatment within a short time. The percentage of NSAP among acute abdominal pain presentations seen in physician's offices may be even higher. How many of these patients are ultimately subjected to radiographs, ultrasound, CT, hospitalization, even endoscopy, laparoscopy, and surgery we may never know. But the pressures to make a diagnosis, to do something, even when something need not be done, are overwhelming. This overpowering need to be certain arises from a fundamental misconception of medical reality: most of these patients can be described, but few can be diagnosed.

Nonanginal chest pain is among the three most common complaints seen in emergency rooms. Perhaps 80–90% of such patients seen in the office also have this thoracic equivalent of nonspecific abdominal pain. How many unnecessary ECGs, stress

Table 1.1.   Percentage of Patients Reporting Each Symptom

Symptom	Medical Group	Nonmedical Group
Skin rash	8	3
Urticaria	5	1
Bad dreams	8	3
Excessive sleepiness	23	23
Fatigue	41	37
Inability to concentrate	25	27
Irritability	20	17
Insomnia	7	10
Loss of appetite	3	6
Dry mouth	5	3
Nausea	3	2
Vomiting	0	0
Diarrhea	5	2
Constipation	4	3
Palpitations	3	3
Giddiness or weakness	2	3
Faintness or dizziness on first standing up	5	5
Headaches	15	13
Fever	3	1
Pain in joints	9	5
Pain in muscles	10	11
Nasal congestion	31	13
Bleeding or bruising	3	3
Bleeding from gums after brushing teeth	21	20
Excessive bleeding from gums after brushing teeth	1	1

Reprinted by permission of the *New England Journal of Medicine* (1968;279:678).

tests, hospitalizations, and even cardiac catheterizations do we perform on such patients? Other common examples of clinical uncertainty or undecidability come to mind: bizarre, transient pains in the extremities, the joints, or just about any locale in the body, weird, atypical headaches, brief tinnitus, feelings of lightheadedness, unexplained attacks of itching, insomnia, fatigue, lassitude, fainting spells, transient weight loss, dizziness, nausea, constipation, diarrhea, sweating, etc. The list is endless.

There is ample literature dealing with this multifaceted problem, a problem that has long plagued us in defining a unitary model of disease. Engel (6) has dealt with this brilliantly and at length. In some studies "hypochondriasis and somatization" are emphasized, as in one report in which between 60–80% of healthy individuals were quoted to have somatic symptoms (7). Other studies have dealt with the ubiquitous complaint of chronic fatigue. In a primary care practice 24% of 1159 consecutive patients complained of this symptom (8). Other reports deal with multiple unexplained symptoms (9, 10), somatization (11), and "psychological distress" (12). In one interesting study, 81% of more than 400 healthy patients on no medications had one or more of the symptoms listed in Table 1.1 (13). An important group includes patients who amplify normal and abnormal body sensations (14). Rosch (15) has made significant contributions to this field by drawing attention to the unifying concept of *stress*. It may seem impossible to subsume all these descriptions under a single heading, but it is certainly useful to conceptualize them as some type of universal clinical archetype. What most of these patients' complaints have in common is their strange,

Table 1.2. Three-Year Incidence and Probable Etiology of 14 Common Symptoms in 1,000 Internal Medicine Outpatients

Symptom	Number of Symptoms	Probable Etiology (percent)		
		Organic	Psychologic	Unknown
Chest pain	96	11	6	83
Fatigue	82	13	21	66
Dizziness	55	18	2	80
Headache	52	10	15	75
Edema	45	36	0	64
Back pain	41	10	0	90
Dyspnea	37	24	3	73
Insomnia	34	3	50	47
Abdominal pain	30	10	0	90
Numbness	26	19	4	77
Impotence	24	21	4	75
Weight loss	18	5	28	67
Cough	15	40	0	60
Constipation	12	0	0	100
Total	567	16	10	74

Reprinted by permission of the *American Journal of Medicine* (1989;86:263).

unprovoked, and often short-lived appearance, their physiologic and anatomic inconsistencies, their failure to conform to any well-defined syndromes or disease entities, and most important of all, their usually benign clinical course. For an even larger group of patients, these symptoms are not transient but recurrent and resistant to therapy. A higher percentage of these individuals would be classified as "functional," even "psychiatric," but increasingly the opinion is being expressed that most of these syndromes or complaints belong in the category of "somatization." As we shall see, it is as much a problem of verifiability as of semantics. The fact remains that for the large majority of such patients we cannot offer a diagnosis in the nosologic sense. It may be, as some psychiatrists say, that neurotics more often tend to feel problems in their bodies rather than in their psyches, but in the broad view, we are all susceptible to unexplained somatic complaints. As clinicians we quickly learn not to take everything too seriously too soon. The most important qualification of a good doctor is a sixth sense for the significant.

One outstanding study has profound implications for the "we-see-this" syndrome and validates its importance with convincing statistical data. Kroenke and Mangelsdorff (16) studied the incidence, diagnostic findings, and outcome of 14 common symptoms in 1000 patients attending the Brooke Army Medical Center medical clinic over a 3-year period. They encountered 567 new complaints with 40% of all 1000 patients reporting at least one new symptom. Although diagnostic testing was performed in more than two-thirds of the cases, an "organic" etiology was demonstrated in only 16%. Table 1.2 (16) shows the incidence and etiology of these 14 common symptoms. Note that the last column under probable etiology is labeled *unknown*, accounting for 74% of diagnoses. Only 10% of all diagnoses were suspected to be psychological. Figure 1.1 shows graphically the extremely low percentage of suspected organic etiologies among 10 common symptoms. Tables 1.3 and 1.4, also from the same article, show other important findings (16). The authors found the cost of discovering an organic diagnosis enormous. Table 1.3 shows, for example, that out of 80 patients with chest pain, only five had organic diagnoses

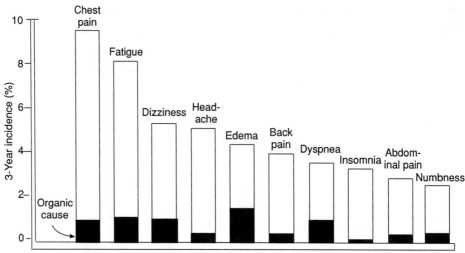

Figure 1.1. Three-year incidence of 10 common symptoms and proportion of symptoms with a suspected organic cause. Reprinted by permission from the *American Journal of Medicine* (1989;86:263).

discovered by testing, a cost of $4354 per diagnosis of organic chest pain (1989 dollars). Headache and back pain were the highest in cost for an "organic" diagnosis, $7778 and $7263, respectively. What the authors have shown convincingly in their series is that blind or undirected testing was of virtually no benefit in establishing an etiology for the listed complaints. Treatment was given for over half the symptoms and was often ineffective. In the total series, where the outcome was documented, half of almost 400 symptoms improved. The authors concluded: "The classification, evaluation, and management of common symptoms need to be redefined. *Diagnostic strategies emphasizing organic causes may be inadequate*" (emphasis added).

We already know what mathematics, physics, and the other hard sciences tell us about provability, the difficulty of certainty, and the necessity of doubt. In the soft sciences, when we continue to be committed to the pursuit of perfection, we embrace a distinctly old-fashioned theology, the Platonic fiction that all our human universe is ultimately understandable. This is not to deny the reality and importance of certainty, but only to stress that clinical knowledge is often incomplete, even tentative. In the clinical sciences we must adopt a healthy skepticism toward diagnostic certainty and its stepchild, therapeutic dogmatism. Only in this way will medicine become scientific, rational, and truly humane.

Naming, Nosology, Medical Descriptions, and the Definition of Disease

> *Just because your doctor has a name for your condition doesn't mean he knows what it is.*
>
> Six Principles for Patients
> Murphy's Law, *Book 2*

Several classification schemes for diseases have been invented over the years. These have been nicely summarized by Bishop (17). In 1928 the National Conference on Disease convened to develop a logical clinical nosology. In 1937 the Ameri-

Table 1.3. Diagnostic Evaluation of 14 Common Symptoms

Symptom	Number (percent) Evaluated	Number of Organic Diagnoses Discovered by Testing*	Estimated Cost (dollars)	
			Per Evaluation	Per Organic Diagnosis[a]
Chest pain	80(83)	5	272	4,354
Fatigue	57(70)	5	130	1,486
Dizziness	34(62)	3	223	2,532[a]
Headache	20(38)	1	389	7,778
Edema	26(58)	4	122	,793
Back pain	31(76)	1	234	7,263
Dyspnea	31(84)	9	209	,720
Insomnia	6(18)	0	110	[b]
Abdominal pain	27(90)	3	202	1,816
Numbness	17(65)	2	160	1,364
Impotence	13(54)	2	161	1,046
Weight loss	18(100)	0	325	[b]
Cough	15(100)	2	147	1,104
Constipation	7(58)	0	409	[b]
Total	382(67)	37	218	2,252

Reprinted by permission of the *American Journal of Medicine* (1989;86:264).
[a]Includes only those diagnoses not apparent after initial interview and physical examination.
[b]Indeterminate since no organic diagnoses discovered by testing.

Table 1.4. Outcome of 14 Common Symptoms

Symptom	Number of Symptoms for Which Outcome Is Known	Number (percent) Improved
Chest pain	57	37(65)
Fatigue	43	20(47)
Dizziness	27	16(59)
Headache	26	10(38)
Edema	25	16(64)
Back pain	21	13(62)
Dyspnea	23	9(39)
Insomnia	10	5(50)
Abdominal pain	16	7(44)
Numbness	17	9(53)
Impotence	11	6(56)
Weight loss	15	6(40)
Cough	10	8(80)
Constipation	6	2(33)
Total	307	164(53)

Reprinted by permission of the *American Journal of Medicine* (1989;86:264).

can Medical Association took over the project and periodically continues to issue editions of *Standard Nomenclature of Diseases and Operations* (18). This system uses an unbelievably complicated dual topographic-etiologic scheme which presents endless problems in the hospital record room.

In 1965, the American College of Pathologists proposed their Standardized Nomenclature of Pathology (SNOP) using a system of coding embodying four elements: topography, morphology, etiology, and function (19). This evolved into an even more convoluted scheme, Systematized Nomenclature of Medicine (SNOMED) using seven indices (20). Significantly, the published material includes a manual with exercises to help train code clerks in its use. According to the preface to the 1984 edition, "These two volumes of the second edition of

Table 1.5. The Major Categories in the ICD-9-CM (*International Classification of Diseases*, 9th revision, clinical modification)

1. Infectious and parasitic diseases	001–139
2. Neoplasms	140–239
3. Endocrine, nutritional, and metabolic diseases and immunologic disorders	240–279
4. Diseases of the blood and blood-forming organs	280–289
5. Mental disorders	290–319
6. Diseases of the nervous system and sense organs	320–389
7. Diseases of the circulatory system	390–459
8. Diseases of the respiratory system	460–519
9. Diseases of the digestive system	520–579
10. Diseases of the genitourinary system	580–629
11. Complications of pregnancy, childbirth, and the puerperium	630–676
12. Diseases of the skin and subcutaneous tissue	680–709
13. Diseases of the musculoskeletal system and connective tissue	710–739
14. Congenital anomalies	740–759
15. Certain conditions originating in the perinatal period	760–779
16. Symptoms, signs, and ill-defined conditions	780–799
17. Injury and poisoning	800–999

SNOMED contain more than 50,000 coded terms and represent the greater majority of all diagnoses and procedures needed for health care data handling." Today few, if any, institutions use SNOMED routinely.

Meanwhile, the World Health Organization (WHO) had been developing the *International Classification of Disease* (ICD). After some revisions the U.S. Government published ICD-9-CM, *International Classification of Disease*, ninth revision, Clinical Modification, as a cause-of-death coding for this country (21). From Table 1.5 (17) one can see that the major subheadings represent a mixed type of classification, including etiologic (nos. 1, 17), anatomic (4, 6, 7–9, etc.), physiologic (3, 11), ill-defined (16), etc. Because these three- to five-digit codes are poorly organized hierarchically they cannot be retrieved by any feasible algorithm. For example, pneumococcal pneumonia is found under code 482, respiratory disease (460–519.9), not under 001–129.8, infectious and parasitic diseases. Tuberculosis, however, is found between 010 and 020.9 and is excluded under respiratory diseases. Numerous other contradictions and inconsistencies can be shown.

Marsden Blois in his classic book on medical descriptions (22) points out that by far most of our knowledge of the world is acquired by direct experience, which he calls "knowledge by acquaintance." Yet it is knowledge by *description*, the use of language, that makes possible the miracle of books and organized knowledge, the means by which we can know things we have never experienced. The process of articulating our experience, that is, converting the first form of knowledge into the second, is fundamental to its verification.

But in this process of translation we range from the almost ideal abstractions of mathematics and physics to the fuzziness and ambiguities of medicine and the human sciences. This gives rise to a knowledge hierarchy reflecting the progressive inexactitude of language as we descend (or ascend) from the world of fundamental particles to cells, medicine, and human beings. This fuzziness and uncertainty is reflected in the richness of our medical vocabulary. There are no synonyms for the words *atom* or *neutron*, but consider how many words we have for cancer: malignancy, carcinoma, tumor, neoplasm, and such closely related terms as papilloma, adenoma, sarcoma, and lymphoma.

The abstractions of mathematics work in physics, therefore, because purely physical processes can be idealized. If words fail us in describing cancer, how often are they largely unsuitable as descriptions of clinical phenomena? This has been captured by Jaki:

> When it comes to biological phenomena, one finds that they are too complex to be represented by ideal cases without destroying their true nature. If, however, their complexity is kept intact, sufficiently powerful mathematical techniques will be lacking for their satisfactory handling (23)

Diagnosis, is, of course, inextricably entwined with these problems of definitions, classifications, and naming. Any nonspecific type of pain, i.e. pain without cause, or any other purely nonspecific symptomatic presentation is a prototypical clinical example of the difficulties and uncertainties of medical classifications and ICD codes. Although these presentations and their numerous clinical relatives just referred to are sometimes called conditions or syndromes, they are not, strictly speaking, diagnoses in the sense that we ordinarily encounter them among ICD codes, let alone in medical textbooks. (Though to be fair, there are symptom codes listed in ICD-9M which, not surprisingly, are rarely used.) Any constellation of symptoms defined in terms of the "we-see-this" syndrome would qualify as a problem of definition or naming. If, as Engel (7) emphasizes, we lack a unitary model for illness, what in fact do we mean by the designation *disease*? Our attempt to identify everything with a name is nothing more than a delusional certitude that everything is indeed nameable, and therefore has an existential reality, "knowledge as description" in Blois' words (22). To name is to know; to know is to control. Without a designation, how can we describe it—without a description—in which case disease becomes "knowledge by acquaintance." Surely, this would not suffice when we come to sign out a chart or fill out an insurance form. The entire medical infrastructure, built around the concept of neatly classified disease names and codes, conspires against the universal clinical logic, which tells us not every patient has a diagnosis; not every condition has a name. But to paraphrase a popular saying, no name, no gain, i.e., no CPT code, no check. The unwitting patient continues to defy our pitiful attempt to put him into some tidy little category. Thus, it is the very richness of medical terminology that tends to become our clinical undoing.

Despite their failings and shortcomings, the ICD codes are a standard in hospital record rooms throughout the United States where they are used to generate diagnosis-related group (DRG) codes for prepayment under Medicare. Since the ICD system is also widely used throughout this country for data collection by, among others, the National Center for Health Statistics (NCHS), we have used it in this text whenever quoting statistics on hospital discharge and procedures data. Not to do so would deprive us of any meaningful data on *nameable*, i.e. disease, conditions.

But although we set considerable store in this data, at heart we continue to be skeptical of any universal applicability of specific naming or coding schemes for the classification of disease, no matter how necessary such schemes would appear for purposes of billing or statistics. Blois (22) expresses this in a parallel set of terms when he discusses the abstraction of disease in the context of the dualistic paradox of disease-as-attribute vs. disease-as-name. As an example, this attribute/nominalist dualism can be expressed on one level as a patient with the attributes of fever, lassitude, anorexia, and adenopathy, and on the other, as a patient who might have, say, lymphoma. In the one case we can visualize the attributes as merely a collection of symptoms, whereas the name lymphoma, if it can be confirmed, is seen as a unifying concept, a powerful abstraction. Seen on one level, we might observe that the motivation to give this collection of symptoms a name is a superior and thus preferable form of conceptualization. But is this really so? The perceived need to diagnose is at the heart of much medical mischief.

In the above example, it is obvious that the lymphomas are decidedly uncommon in clinical practice, whereas the combination of fever, anorexia, lassitude, and mild adenopathy are exceedingly common. Sometimes such symptoms are associated with a viral etiology, but often this cannot be confirmed. Almost always, such collections of symptoms are self-limiting. How frequently do we rush to do gallium scintigraphy, CT, or a bone marrow because such complaints are present and we think it might be nameable, computable, i.e. something serious or at least definable? One is reminded of that most irritating of clinical clichés, a disease to be "ruled out." Today, the nominalist attitude remains more dangerous than the attribute view as a concept of diagnosis. The need to name is the modern reductionist paradigm, the attempt to resolve all uncertainty by means of rendering a diagnosis, reducing collections of symptoms to names. This is not to deny that the attribute theory of disease is without its problems. If by naming something we take the risk that we assume we know what it is, then by describing merely the patient's case history we run the risk of giving every patient a different disease. This perilous state of affairs has been neatly described by Temkin," . . . there is no science of the individual, and medicine suffers from a fundamental contradiction: its practice deals with the individual while its theory grasps universals only" (24).

The nominalist-attribute dichotomy of disease will persist, but this is unavoidable. No view alone will ever provide a completely satisfactory way of dealing with the day-to-day clinical problems of medicine. On the extreme nominalist side we have the epidemiologist, the medical economist, or the coder in the record room, none of whom deal with diseased patients, only disease names. At the other extreme are the analytic psychiatrists to whom no two patients are the same.

Our teaching, our texts, and our literature, which form the foundation of our training as physicians, function primarily in orienting us to the 400-year nominalist concept of disease as a name. This tradition, from the examination room to the record room to the insurance form, underlies a large part of our daily professional lives. If our texts seem to subscribe to this virtually universal medical dogma, our orientation by symptoms and signs, nevertheless, is an acknowledgment that "we see this" is just as common, if not more common, a diagnosis than an ICD code. Not all aspects of medical or any other reality necessarily have a name.

Finally, we come full circle and return to Isaiah Berlin. In a well-known essay he quotes a line from the Greek poet Archilochus: "The fox knows many things, but the hedgehog knows one big thing" (25). He takes this to mean there is one great difference dividing writers, and by extension, thinkers and all human beings in general. There exists a chasm between those on one side who relate everything to a coherent, organizing single central vision, and those on the other who pursue many ends, perceive life on many levels, experience existence in multiple, at time self-contradictory, and incomplete realities. Physicians cannot afford to be either hedgehog or fox; they must, of all people, strive to be both.

REFERENCES

1. Berlin I. The pursuit of the ideal. The Crooked Timber of Humanity. New York: Alfred A. Knopf, 1991.
2. Quoted in Bernstein J. Quantum Profiles. Princeton: Princeton University Press, 1991:37.
3. Casti JL. Searching for Certainty. New York: William Morrow and Company, 1990.
4. Anonymous. Fractals and medicine [Editorial]. Lancet 1991;338:1425–1426.
5. Pool R. Chaos theory: how big an advance? Science 1989;245:26–28.
6. Engel GL. The need for a new medical model: a challenge for biomedicine. Science 1977;196(4286): 129–136.
7. Kellner R. Hypochondriasis and somatization. JAMA 1987;258(19):2718–2722.
8. Kroenke K, Wood DR, Mangelsdorff AD, Meier NJ, Powell JB. Chronic fatigue in primary care. Prevalence, patient characteristics, and outcome. JAMA, 1988;260(7):929–934.
9. Smith Jr GR, Monson RA, Ray DC. Patients with multiple unexplained symptoms. Their characteristics, functional health, and health care utilization. Arch Intern Med 1986;146(1):69–72.
10. Slavney PR, Teitelbaum ML. Patients with medically unexplained symptoms: DSM-III diagnoses and demographic characteristics. Gen Hosp Psychiatry 1985;7:21–25.
11. Kaplan C, Lipkin M, Gordon GH. Somatization in primary care: patients with unexplained and vexing medical complaints. J Gen Intern Med 1988;2:177–190.
12. Stoeckle JD, Zola IK, Davidson GE. The quantity and significance of psychological distress in medical patients. Some preliminary observations about the decision to seek medical aid. J Chronic Dis 1964;17:959–970.
13. Reidenberg MM, Lowenthal DT. Adverse nondrug reactions. N Engl J Med 1968;279(13):678–679.
14. Barsky III AJ. Patients who amplify bodily sensations. Ann Intern Med 1979;91(1):63–70.
15. Rosch PJ. Growth and development of the stress concept and its significance in clinical medicine. In: Gardiner-Hill H, ed. Modern Trends in Endocrinology. New York: Paul J. Hoeber, 1958:278–297.
16. Kroenke K, Mangelsdorff AD. Common symptoms in ambulatory care: incidence, evaluation, therapy, and outcome. Am J Med, 1989;86(3):262–266.
17. Bishop CW. A name is not enough. MD Comput 1989;6(4):200–206.
18. Standard Nomenclature of Diseases and Operations. Chicago: American Medical Association, 1961.
19. Standardized Nomenclature of Pathology. Skokie, III: College of American Pathologists, 1979.
20. Cote RA. Systematized Nomenclature of Medicine. Skokie, Ill: College of American Pathologists, 1979.
21. International classification of diseases (9th revision, clinical modification). Bethesda, Md: Department of Health and Human Services, 1980. (DHHS publication no. (PHS) 80-126).
22. Blois MS. Information and Medicine. The Nature of Medical Descriptions. Berkeley and Los Angeles: University of California Press, 1984.
23. Jaki, SL. Brain, mind, and computers. South Bend, Ind: Gateway Editions Ltd., 1969.
24. Temkin O. The Scientific Approach to Disease: Specific Entity and Individual Sickness. Crombe CC, Ed. New York: Basic Books, 1963.
25. Berlin I. The hedgehog and the fox. In: Hardy H, Kelly A, eds. Russian Thinkers. p 22. Harmondsworth: Pelican Books.

2

General Principles of Diagnosis and Diagnostic Imaging

Medicine is the science of uncertainty and the art of probability.
Quoted by William Bennet Bean
in Sir William Osler Aphorisms, *Ch. 5.*

Misusing Differential Diagnosis. Reliability and Predictability of Tests

We are all familiar with the litany of alternative possibilities often invoked for a given clinical presentation, the so-called differential diagnoses. These are derived from analyzing various combinations of signs and symptoms. Even lengthier lists can be constructed for each individual symptom or sign in terms of its association with specific disorders. Some physicians find such itemizations useful in identifying unsuspected diagnostic possibilities or in reducing the number of options. Nonetheless, this classic approach is usually employed in a careless fashion, because the various choices tend to be viewed as equally likely.

Differential diagnoses must be seen as a *limited order of probabilities*, from common to rare, rather than an endless list of conditions having equal merit. Thus, coronary disease is a possible diagnosis in anyone with chest pain, but less than one such patient in 1000 under 30 years of age turns out to have this condition. The rational diagnostic approach to chest pain must begin by taking the pertinent medical history into account. There must be a significantly high probability of coronary disease before subjecting a patient to expensive or invasive procedures such as stress testing or coronary arteriography.

Balla (1), Sox et al. (2), and others (3) have summarized various intellectual, philosophical, and mathematical ideas bearing on clinical diagnosis. These include complicated concepts such as cognitive heuristics, retrospective memory, interpretation and reliability of data, falsification, information processing, decision analysis, and others that automatically come into play when we attempt to arrive at the correct diagnosis. Because this text is based on the straightforward presentation of the patient rather than considerations of the diagnostic process per se we have simplified this discussion for the sake of brevity and consistency. We will also include opinions based on personal observations of common diagnostic errors.

Before embarking on the specific details of diagnostic imaging, details applicable to any type of clinical studies, we must first acquire some basic understanding of the testing process itself. We cannot do this without reviewing some basic mathematical principles. These fundamental concepts are the so-called new mathematics of medicine which borrow from Bayes' Theorem and classic probability theory and are not really new at all. We ignore these basic principles at our peril, because failure to appreciate them is by far the greatest cause of inappropriate and excessive clinical testing. A more extensive and rigorous mathematical treatment comprises the first appendix of this book and is also thoroughly discussed elsewhere (1, 4–7).

It is amazing how often procedures, special and otherwise, are regarded as so highly reliable by both physicians and patients. On the one hand, patients eagerly await their test results, while physicians plan their next battery of investigations or "workup" with equal expectations that *the* answer will be provided. Most tests are invested with all the confidence we usually reserve for the Almighty without our really understanding the mathematical subtleties affecting the reliability of all clinical testing procedures.

It should be revealing to test our intuitive skills with an example adapted from the mathematician Solomon W. Golomb (8). Let us suppose an imaginary infectious agent, the X poultry virus, affects one out of a thousand chickens in a flock. Now, suppose we have a superb test for this virus, the Whiz test, which is 99% reliable, i.e. it misses only 1% of the infected chickens and incorrectly diagnoses 1% of the uninfected chickens. A chicken is selected at random and proves to have a positive Whiz test. What is the probability that the chicken has the X virus? Many people would answer 99%, and they would, of course, be wrong because they would reason that the reliability of the test is the same as its predictability.[a]

Nothing could be further from the truth. In actual fact there is only a 9% chance that the chicken is infected. How does this come to pass? Let us first assume for purposes of calculation we have a huge flock of 1 million chickens. In this case, we would have 1,000 infected chickens. If the Whiz test is 99% reliable, then we can expect to identify 990 infected birds (99% of 1,000). So far, so good. But what about the other positive Whiz tests that will occur in 1% of the well chickens? One percent of 999,000 (1 million − 1,000) or 9,990 chickens will test incorrectly positive for the X virus! (We stress in this example that the reliability of the test is identical in both sick and well chickens. In practice, this is rarely the case.) Thus, more than 10 times the number of virus-free chickens will test positive compared with those that are virus-infected. In other words, 990 chickens with the virus plus 9,990 without the virus, or 10,980 chickens, will have a positive Whiz test; 990 divided by 10,980 is 9%. The chance of a chicken picked at random having the X poultry virus is about 1 in 11, given that it has a positive Whiz test.

A real life situation is the screening test for the AIDS antibody where the routine enzyme-linked immunosorbent assay (ELISA) test for the human immunodeficiency virus (HIV) is in actuality 84–99% "reliable" in patients positive by the Western blot test, that is, it detects 84–99% of those with the antibody (assuming the Western blot is 100% reliable—which obviously it is not) (9, 10). Furthermore, the ELISA test incorrectly identifies 1–7% of those without the antibody (9). Comparable figures are reported for the immunobinding and agglutination assays (11). From these figures, let us assume a very high performance of the ELISA test of 97% reliability in individuals with the antibody, and of incorrect diagnoses in only 1% of those without the antibody. In the present U.S. population of approximately 250 million individuals, accepting the current prevalence estimate that approximately 1.5 out of 1,000 Ameri-

---

[a]Ordinary speech is imprecise in the world of probability. Thus, not only the word *reliability* but also the term *accuracy* are frequently confused with the concept of *predictability*. This semantic confusion is a constant source of difficulty. The term reliability is used here only for purposes of illustration and in the probabilistic senses of both *sensitivity* and *nonspecificity*, which will be defined with other terms below.

cans are HIV positive (12), what is the likelihood that a person picked at random and testing HIV positive will in fact be correctly identified? We can derive our new calculations from the same arithmetic used above. The number of correct positive tests would be 97% of 0.15% × 250 million. (Recall, incidentally, that 3% of the HIV-positive individuals would be missed.) The total number testing positive would be this number plus those who are actually HIV negative but who will incorrectly test positive. As in the chicken example, the probability of a person with a positive test having AIDS can be easily calculated because it is the fraction of all individuals in the total population tested who test HIV positive correctly, compared to the total who test HIV positive both correctly and correctly. (Recall that 1% of the noninfected individuals will also test falsely positive.)

Let A = HIV-positive individuals testing positive correctly. Let B = HIV-negative individuals testing positive incorrectly. Then the predictability for AIDS of a positive test is A ÷ (A + B), where A = 250 million × 0.97 (test reliability) × 0.15% (fraction of individuals HIV positive). Thus, A = 250 million × 0.97 × 0.0015 = 0.36375 million.[b] B = 250 million × 0.9985 (fraction of people HIV negative) × 1% (those who are actually HIV negative who test positive incorrectly). Thus, B = 250 million × 0.9985 × 0.01 = 2.4962 million: so 0.36375 million ÷ (0.36375 million + 2.4962 million) = 0.364 ÷ 2.86 = 0.127 or 12.7%.

The result indicates that given a random person with a positive test for HIV antibody in the *unselected* U.S. population, there is less than one chance in eight he or she is in fact HIV positive.

What is our chance of correctly identifying an HIV-positive individual in a high-risk group? Suppose, instead of testing a population with a 0.15% prevalence of HIV positivity, we tested a population of inner city drug addicts with a known positive HIV prevalence of 30%, some 200 times that of the U.S. population? If the reader can verify the answer, he will have concluded there is 97.6% probability that a positive test in this population identifies a truly HIV-positive individual. Further examples of the dependence of test predictability on prevalence of disease abound in the literature. One such study reproduced in Table 2.1 shows the predictive value of prostatic acid phosphatase (PAS) in three different populations. Even though the PAS has been supplanted by what has been claimed to be the superior prostate-specific antigen (PSA) test, predictive values do not change significantly without increased prevalence of disease, and the number of false-positive results may increase, a phenomenon we are now seeing with rising frequency. In the case of the PSA test, it turns out that 21% of men with benign prostatic hypertrophy (BPH) had elevated levels (greater than 4 ng/ml), and in another quoted British study 33% of men with BPH had PSA concentrations of more than 10 ng/ml (13). Once again, the latest enhancement is not necessarily better.

We are now prepared to draw a fundamental conclusion: The ability of a test to predict the presence of a condition is dependent on the prevalence of the suspected condition and on the reliability of the test. However, because test reliability seldom varies more than ± 12%, (80 ± 10%), and prevalences may vary several orders of magnitude (0.001% to more than 99%), *prevalence is almost always more important in determining predictability than is test performance.* Even if a test is extremely reliable, the

---

[b]The actual population figures, of course, have no bearing on the calculations because they cancel each other out; the result would be the same regardless of the total population tested if we accept the accuracy of the HIV antibody prevalence data and the pair of test reliability numbers.

Table 2.1. Effect of Prevalence on Predictive Value: Positive Predictive Value of Prostatic Acid Phosphatase for Prostatic Cancer (Sensitivity = 70%, Specificity = 90%) In Various Clinical Settings[a]

Setting	Prevalence (cases/100,000)	Positive Predictive Value (%)
General population	35	0.4
Men, age 75 or greater	500	5.6
Clinically suspicious prostatic nodule	50,000	93.0

[a]From Watson RA, Tang DB. The predictive value of prostatic acid phosphatase as a screening test for prostatic cancer. N Engl J Med 1980;303:497–499.

probability of disease after a positive test result is poor if the prior prevalence of disease is low, (less than 20–25%).

Measuring and Defining Test Performance: Sensitivity, Specificity, Prevalence, and Predictive Indices of Disease

> *Appearances to the mind are of four kinds.*
> *Things either are what they appear to be;*
> *or they neither are, nor appear to be;*
> *or they are, and do not appear to be;*
> *or they are not, yet appear to be.*
> *Rightly to aim in all these cases*
> *is the wise man's task.*
>
> *Epictetus (Second Century A.D.)*

In order to obtain a deeper understanding of the testing process, we must formalize the concepts upon which the above examples are based and define the mathematical terms we will later incorporate in many of this book's illustrative tables. We ask the reader's indulgence because some repetition is unavoidable.

Let us assume that a given patient may have a disease (or, more strictly, a "condition") we are trying to diagnose. This, of course, also implies he or she may not have the condition. The principal reason for ordering a test is to reduce the degree of diagnostic uncertainty. *This should always assume the necessary corollary that making a diagnosis will indeed benefit the patient.* Furthermore, let us assume we have a test to help establish the presence of this condition. We must assume there will always be instances in which such a test gives positive results in patients without the condition and negative results in patients in whom the condition has been unequivocally established. This is illustrated in Table 2.2, which shows the standard 2 × 2 table listing the various combinations of disease presence or absence with a positive or a negative test result. In order to simplify the presentation, the table is reproduced (Table 2.3) with only the abbreviations for true- and false-positive results in the presence (D +) or absence (D −) of disease. As we indicated previously, the word *true* indicates, respectively, the concordance of a positive or negative test result with the presence or absence of disease, that is the correctness of a test result, whereas *false* refers to the incorrectness of a test result. Unfortunately for some, the use of the words true and false in this context can be semantically confusing, but it is consistent. These important definitions follow.

A *true-positive* test (TP) is a positive test result in the *presence* of disease, i.e. a correct positive test.

Table 2.2. Possible Test Results in Patients With and Without Disease

Disease Present	Disease Absent	
No. of TP	No. of FP	Total positives
No. of TN	No. of FN	Total negatives
Total with disease	Total without disease	Total tested

Table 2.3. Abbreviated Form of Table 2.2

Disease present	Disease absent	
Test positive TP	FP	(TP + FP) = total positive tests
Test negative FN	TN	(FN + TN) = total negative tests
Total disease	Total without disease	Total tested
(D + = TP + FN)	(D − = FP + TN)	(= TP + FN + FP + TN)

A *false-positive* test (FP) is a positive test result in the *absence* of disease, an incorrect positive test.

A *true-negative* test (TN) is a negative test result in the *absence* of disease, a correct negative test.

A *false-negative* (FN) test is a negative test result in the *presence* of disease, an incorrect negative test.

Sensitivity is the ratio of patients with disease who test positive compared to the total number of patients with disease; i.e. it is the percentage of patients with disease testing positive. This is expressed either as a decimal between 0 and 1 or, in percentage, as an integer between 0 and 100. (The reader will now note the ambiguity of the term *reliability* used in the chicken and AIDS examples above.) Sensitivity = TP ÷ (TP + FN).

Specificity is defined as the ratio of patients without disease who test negative compared to the total number of patients without disease, i.e. the percentage of patients without disease testing negative. (Again note the ambiguous and incorrect use of the previous term, reliability, which was used above in the dual context of both sensitivity and specificity.) Specificity = TN ÷ (TN + FP).

Thus, measures of sensitivity and specificity describe, respectively, the intrinsic ability of a test to distinguish those patients with and without disease.

If we eliminate all indeterminate or equivocal results, i.e. we exclude all but positive or negative test results, this is in effect a binary situation. However, in real life, this is far from true, as we hope to show later when we consider the problem of analyzing multiple outcomes from a given test or the predictive values of multiple sequential tests. We emphasize that the terms sensitivity and specificity are properties inherent in the tests themselves. As the above examples should have made entirely clear, these indices must not be confused in any way with *predictive* abilities of any given test. They do not tell us the *likelihood* of disease given a positive or negative test. Stated differently, the question, "given this condition is (or is not) present, what are the odds the test is positive or negative?" is an entirely different question from, "given this test result, what are the odds this condition is (or is not) present?"

This ability of a test to predict the presence or absence of disease depends principally on the one crucial factor we have already emphasized, the prevalence of the condition for which we are testing, which, obviously, is completely unrelated to test

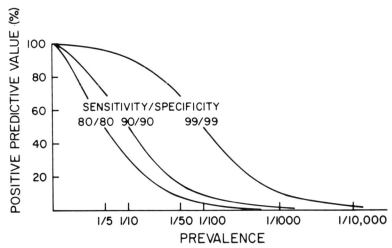

Figure 2.1. Positive predictive value according to sensitivity, specificity, and prevalence of disease. Reprinted from Fletcher RH, Fletcher SW, Wagner EG. *Clinical Epidemiology: the Essentials,* 2nd ed. Baltimore: Williams & Wilkins, 1987:57.

performance. At times we may substitute the terms *prior* or *pretest* probability of disease for prevalence, which is defined as the fraction of individuals with a particular disease or condition in a specified population.[c] The term pretest or prior probability of a disease emphasizes that the probability is defined *before* some event, such as a test taking place. *Posttest* probability is the new likelihood of disease after a test result is *known.* For clinical purposes the most meaningful index of any test is indeed this so-called *predictive* value. It is expressed simply as the new probability of the presence or absence of a disease after the test results are known. This knowledge is fundamental in choosing any test and, as we shall learn, absolutely essential in deciding whether a specific study is indicated or contraindicated in a given clinical setting. The definitions follow:

Positive predictive value of a test (PPV) is the new prevalence or likelihood of disease, given a positive test result.

Negative predictive value of a test (NPV) is the converse, the new prevalence or likelihood of no disease after a negative test result.

One minus the NPV of a test (1 − NPV) is perhaps a less confusing concept than the NPV and is the new prevalence or likelihood of disease after a negative test result.

Both the PPV and 1 − NPV will be used as predictive indices throughout the book and will be expressed as percentages. The fundamental importance of prevalence is clearly demonstrated in Fig. 2.1, which shows the relationship between various matched test performances, prevalence, and positive predictive value (14). Note that even with test sensitivities/specificities approaching 90–95% how predictive values depend so exquisitely on prevalence. With prevalences less than 15–20%, as noted above, the predictive values of even the best tests hover in the 50–70% range. Further explanations along with tables and diagrams are given in the important mathematical section of "Appendixes A and B." These can be used to predict more

---

[c]Prevalence should not be confused with *incidence*, the number of new cases occurring during a specified interval of time. Incidence is often expressed as the number of new cases per 100,000 population occurring during the index year.

precisely the PPV and 1 − NPV, given a condition and its prevalence (prior probability) and an imaging procedure and its known sensitivities and sensitivities.[d]

The ROC Curve and Other Considerations

> *He that would know correctly beforehand those that will recover, and those that will die . . . must be able to form a judgment from having made himself acquainted with all the symptoms, and estimating their powers in comparison with one another. . . .*
>
> *Hippocrates*

An important testing principle, a corollary derived from the above analysis concerns the so-called ROC curve. This somewhat curious acronym stands for "receiver operating characteristics." Its history begins in World War II just after the fall of France during the Battle of Britain, when radar, which had just been invented by the British, was first used to detect German aircraft approaching the British Isles. The job of radar operators was to determine whether small blips that appeared on the radar scopes actually indicated the presence of hostile aircraft. In order to achieve this, amplification on the radar scope frequently had to be increased so much that artifacts such as flocks of birds, storm clouds, or other weather disturbances were detected. It was not long before the military realized there was a trade-off between detecting the signal of enemy planes and the "noise" of other phenomena. In other words, the more sensitive the radar detection, the less specific the blips on the screen became. On many occasions defensive aircraft were scrambled only to discover nothing but a flock of wild geese, hence the term "wild goose chase" (15).

This ROC curve is an inescapable reality in all testing situations and equally familiar to scientists as well as statisticians and economists assessing test procedures and performance for business and government. By plotting the true positive rate against the false positive rate, i.e. the sensitivity against 1 − specificity, one can plot an ROC curve which can be used to describe the accuracy of a test over a range of values or cutoff points. Such a curve is shown in Fig. 2.2, which describes the relationship of various 2-hour postprandial blood sugar levels to the diagnosis of diabetes. If we accept one of the WHO criteria of 140–200 mg/dl as "impaired glucose tolerance," (200 mg/dl being definite diabetes), there remains the very difficult problem of deciding which patients are indeed diabetic. If we require that a blood sugar taken 2 hours after a meal be more than 200 mg/dl, we will miss a large number of diabetics (low sensitivity, high specificity); if we make the cutoff point 110 mg/dl we will overdiagnose diabetes in a significant number (high sensitivity, low specificity). (Before 1979, the University of Michigan, the American Diabetes Association, the U.S. Public Health Service, and other official and semi-official bodies had differing criteria for the diagnosis of diabetes.) In all cases, however, there is no way, using a single blood sugar determination under standard conditions, that one can simultaneously improve both the sensitivity and the specificity of the test. At 110 mg/dl, the false-positive rate for the diagnosis of diabetes will approximate 20%. That is, with a high sensitivity, there will be more wild goose chases. Using 140 mg/dl as the cutoff the false-positive

---

[d]The formula relating sensitivity (sens), specificity (spec) and prevalence (prev) to PPV is derived from Bayes' Theorem of Conditional Probabilities: PPV = (sens × prev) ÷ {(sens × prev) + (1 − spec) × (1 × prev)}.

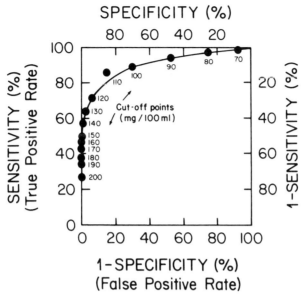

Figure 2.2. A receiver operator characteristic (ROC) curve. The accuracy of 2-hour postprandial blood sugar as a diagnostic test for diabetes mellitus. (Data from *Diabetes Program Guide*, Public Health Service Publication No. 506, 1960.)

rate approaches 0, but this is at the expense of sensitivity, i.e., more cases will be missed.

Thus, in a clinical testing situation where one radiologist "overreads" films, more patients will be reported with an abnormal study and will be subjected to needless anxiety, expense, unnecessary testing, or worse, but fewer diagnoses will be missed. A radiologist who is an underreader will report fewer false-positive studies, but will miss some diagnoses. There is no way to avoid this problem either in the command room or the reading room. Whom is to be preferred in imaging diagnosis, the under- or the overreader? For many reasons, answers to this and other questions dealing with these important "type I" and "type II" errors will be postponed until the last chapter.

In practical terms there is a limit to the sensitivity of any test system. The lower the disease stands in the differential diagnostic lists (the lower the prevalence) and the higher the test sensitivity, the greater the loss of specificity, i.e. the higher the fraction of false-positive results (16).

Indeterminate Tests

> *If a man's wit be wandering, let him study the mathematics.*
> Francis Bacon, "Of Studies"
> Essays *(1625)*

We have already alluded to another thorny problem in interpreting the meaning and reliability of any test finding. This resides in the fact that diagnostic tests do not necessarily yield strictly positive or negative results. Sometimes results are intermediate, indeterminate, uninterpretable, or even meaningless. Because there is no practical way to incorporate such results in the assessment of data, there is no consensus as to the best method for dealing with it. Nonpositive, nonnegative, or indeterminate results are an unfortunate fact of life not only in imaging studies, but in tissue biopsies, in the clinical laboratory and, of course, in clinical histories and examinations obtained from patients. Much of the problem is directly related to the skill and experience of the test interpreter or the clinician. With a blood chemistry test, results may very well depend on the reagents or equipment used as well as the mood of the technologist at the time of performing the test. In radiologic and imaging studies we have similar problems of technical performance: quality of equipment and film, adequacy of views, limitations caused by the condition of the patient, etc. Furthermore, the better the interpreter the fewer nondiagnostic results will be obtained. Here, as in all of medicine, there is no way of escaping this basic fact of life (17).

For our purposes, we have attempted in some examples to take into account the effect of more than two test outcomes when it seems feasible to do so for the calculation of predictive values. Thus, it is not always necessary to ignore these uncertainties; i.e. we will not require in certain examples either a negative or a positive imaging test result. The test deficiencies and limitations, no matter what their cause, will be reflected in any available values for sensitivities and specificities.

Summary of Mathematical Discussion

> *Choosing whether to test the patient is at least as important as choosing the test.*
>
> *Sturman's Law*

The thrust of the foregoing discussion is that the less probable the condition, the less likely one is to find it with any test or combination of tests, no matter how specific or sensitive the test. We emphasize the words *any test*. For many years we have heard claims about some studies such as endoscopy, magnetic resonance imaging (MRI), and angiography being "gold standards" among available testing procedures. But in fact gold, though once a monetary standard (all gold redemption ended in 1971), never represented any ideal, and it is hard to find its relevance for clinical testing. In fact, tests can only be compared with each other in a specific context; it is ingenuous to describe tests in terms of a universal standard. Endoscopy is a terrible test for peptic ulcer but a good test for gastric cancer, just as coronary angiography is an abysmal test for chest pain but useful in some patients with coronary artery disease. It has been amply confirmed that MRI is a miserable test for subdeltoid bursitis but a superb study for cartilaginous injury to the knee joint. Whether, in fact, *any* imaging procedure is intrinsically better for a given condition can only be decided on the basis of multiple factors, including risk, availability, and cost, but in particular the probability of disease, a fact to which we shall continually return throughout this text. The concept of any testing standard, gold or otherwise, is pernicious and misleading, because it tends to trivialize the testing process by false generalization.

One of the best examples of our fundamental testing principle is prefigured, if not immortalized, in Sutton's famous law. Willie "The Actor" Sutton, you will recall, was the notorious bank robber who never used a weapon when he worked. He was once asked why he robbed banks. His reply, frequently quoted at medical rounds was, "because that's where the money is." In other words, banks are more likely to have money, just as patients are more likely to have common conditions. In a wistful commentary on the expectation of the exotic, the actress Rita Hayworth is said to have once remarked, "When men go to bed with Rita Hayworth they wake up and find it's only me."

Thus, rather than looking for the common, students, house staff, and other inexperienced clinicians often search for bizarre or rare conditions. They also tend to be unduly influenced by a recent case. This results in unnecessary testing for the least likely condition, as if the discovery of a rare entity is proof of diagnostic excellence. Predictably, the frequent finding of a false-positive test in a population with a low prevalence of a condition, often leads to more inappropriate testing and a plethora of confusing data. This is a common result of misguided investigation often leading to the well-known "cascade effect," to be discussed later.

The most unambiguous sign of the clinician's weak diagnostic skills is the repeated need to "rule out" a list of diagnoses. This tendency, characteristic of the lazy intellect, is more often the result of faulty clinical instruction. A young physician told us the perfect story illustrating this trend. One of his instructors reminded the class that, "if it looks like a duck, walks like a duck, and quacks like a duck, be very careful; it could be a strange-looking chicken." To paraphrase a medical sage, "in order to explain the obvious, they invoke the obscure." Another problem may be a need to placate the patient or his family or to convince ourselves that everything possible is being done. But is the desire of the physician or family to perform a test a valid reason to do so? If unnecessary studies are ordered for reassurance or to please or impress, who should be responsible for the bill?

The format of this book, therefore, will stress diagnostic strategy in terms of prevalence of disease with emphasis on common conditions. We are not here to discuss ruling out the unexpected or the unlikely by suggesting a plethora of studies, though it will become clear that effective testing frequently does help rule out the *expected*. On the contrary, we hope to show how a thoughtful approach to diagnosis begins with *ruling in* the most likely diagnoses, given the presentation of the patient. This is where cost effectiveness becomes the economic equivalent of common sense.

Cost Considerations in Imaging Procedures

With the tremendous explosion of medical technology in recent years the question of cost of medical diagnosis and treatment has become an increasingly volatile public issue. Terms such as cost effectiveness and cost-benefit ratio are increasingly being applied to problems dealing with health care. Doubilet and his associates (18) have summarized four ways of interpreting "cost effectiveness" in clinical practice as it achieves: (*a*) cost savings; (*b*) effectiveness in improving health care; (*c*) cost savings with an equal (or better) health *outcome*; and (*d*) having an additional benefit worth the additional cost.

We are not convinced that analyses of cost, cost effectiveness, or cost-benefit ratios of medical testing can be neatly isolated from the larger more fundamental issues of rational diagnostic strategies and good medical care (19). Rather, our stress will be on the predictive value of specific procedures in a given clinical setting, and let the costs speak for themselves. We are convinced that clinical common sense and appropriately conceived testing strategy will automatically tend toward cost effectiveness because the two factors are not opposed. The decoupling of medical costs from common sense medical diagnostic strategy never needed to occur, but it would take several social historians, 100 lawyers, and scores of legislators to explain it.

Having stated this, there still remains the metaproblem of what happens to the patient, i.e. the outcome resulting from our intervention. The prior determination of outcome is indeed the central problem in choosing imaging and therapeutic strategies for every patient. Rather than being concerned merely with test sensitivities and other indices of performance or with cost-benefit ratios, we should be asking the question, what are the comparative merits of various methods of imaging for medical management, specifically in terms of patient outcome? This is the so-called "outcomes analysis" approach, an important but heretofore neglected technique for telling us what we are actually accomplishing as physicians and as a society. Precious little work has been done in this vital area, and because of this, the subject cannot command the attention it deserves. In certain important areas of diagnosis, considerations of test performance are not always sufficiently pertinent by themselves. Although the thrust of this book rests firmly on our conviction that prevalence of disease should be the engine driving the diagnostic process, it is also true that the choice of management, both diagnostic and therapeutic, rests finally on considerations of the patient's ultimate welfare. Cost and benefit are rarely discordant, but benefit is theoretical until it has been translated into a specific outcome. This, then, is another "missing data" problem characteristic of much in modern-day medicine. With the advent of ever more expensive, unpleasant, and risky testing procedures, we must unceasingly ask ourselves whether the ends justify the means. If we are to save X lives with a diagnostic or therapeutic procedure at the cost of X + N deaths + Y dollars + Z pain and suffering, should we not consider the numbers before leaping on the bandwagon?

True Clinical Examples of Faulty Diagnostic Reasoning

Case 1.   An 84-year-old woman with a history of angina and coronary disease, including coronary bypass surgery 15 years before, suddenly developed urticaria and angioedema associated with transient vascular collapse about 4 hours after eating a lobster dinner. Immediately hospitalized, she responded promptly to antihistamines and intramuscular steroids. At no time did she complain of chest pain, nor were there any EKG or neurologic changes. Cardiac enzymes were normal. She was normotensive throughout her hospital stay. The following morning, anxious to go home, she was told by her doctor he was "99 44/100% sure" her physician son-in-law was right, that it was an allergic reaction to lobster, but that she should have "some more tests to be absolutely sure there is nothing else going on that we might have missed." In the meantime an arterial blood gas was drawn by mistake, a medication error occurred, and the patient was prepared for brain computed tomography (CT) (contrast material so soon after an anaphylactoid reaction?). Serial cardiograms and enzymes were to be done every 8 hours for the next 24 hours along with other tests.

Her family signed her out immediately against medical advice. (P.S. She did much better after returning home.)

COMMENT

This is a prototypical example of the "ruling out" syndrome, whereby invoking remote and unrelated clinical possibilities results in needless, and in this case, potentially dangerous testing and unnecessary hospitalization. The clinician, trained in defensive medicine or badly lacking confidence in his clinical skills, simply could not accept the obvious. Unfortunately, he could not test for anaphylaxis, but he could test for myriad other possibilities. The ordering of diagnostic tests, according to Wilson's Law (named for Dr. McClure Wilson), often serves no purpose other than confirming the obvious: "The more times you run over a dead cat, the flatter it gets" (7).

Another illustrative feature of this case was the interesting remark by the physician that he was "99 44/100% sure." (Though *sure* does rhyme with *pure* in the Ivory soap commercial, this was clearly a misquote.) The search for certainty in diagnosis—as in life, as we have previously stressed—is among the most dangerous, disappointing, and ultimately foolish clinical pastimes. We expect perfection and omniscience from ourselves, as do our patients. In medicine we must constantly remind ourselves of Edgar Watson Howe's remark, "a reasonable probability is the only certainty."

Case 2.   A 14-year-old girl was referred for gallium scintigraphy because of the presence of fever, generalized lymphadenopathy, and mild weight loss for 4 weeks. The physicians wanted to rule out the diagnosis of Hodgkin lymphoma.

COMMENT

The prevalence or pretest probability of Hodgkin lymphoma in this particular 14-year-old girl is certainly less than 3%. Moreover, though the sensitivity of gallium scintigraphy is about 80% for Hodgkin lymphoma, the specificity is extremely low, certainly less than 50%. This means that in the case of a positive gallium study, the positive predictive value of an abnormal test for Hodgkin lymphoma is well below 1%, lower than the likelihood of disease before testing. Such a rule-out approach is worse than useless. Our knowledge tells us that many more common types of adenopathy, including cat scratch fever, an underlying infectious process, etc., are apt to be gallium-positive. This leaves us with a variation of Cochrane's aphorism: "If the management is the same whether the test is positive or a negative, don't perform the test." Clearly the only helpful test is a lymph node biopsy, but does adenopathy for a month justify this?

Case 3.   A man appears in the nuclear medicine department for a gated cardiac study including left ventricular ejection fraction (EF) 7 days after coronary bypass surgery. He is in congestive failure and doing poorly. No preoperative cardiac imaging studies other than arteriography were performed, despite complaints of mild dyspnea. The radionuclide study demonstrates four-chamber enlargement and severe biventricular dysfunction with a left ventricular EF of 27%.

COMMENT

This is a tragic example of a diagnostic sin of omission. Although the systolic EF is normal in about 30–40% of patients with congestive failure, a low EF is a reliable indicator of left ventricular dysfunction. Though the patient could have developed severe left ventricular dysfunction as a result of a perioperative infarction, the clinical story of dyspnea before coronary bypass surgery was troubling. We can only suspect he had left ventricular dysfunction before surgery, the severity of which was not appreciated by his physicians. (Neither coronary arteriography nor echocardiography are consistently reliable for determining left ventricular dysfunction, particularly diastolic dysfunction.) Vide infra. Many internists and cardiologists, though admitting that a normal EF does not exclude left ventricular dysfunction, would hesitate to submit a patient for bypass surgery with a resting systolic EF below the range of 20–30%.

Case 4.   A request was received for emergency portable ultrasound study of the kidneys to rule out hydronephrosis. The patient, a 44-year-old woman, respirator dependent with renal failure, was in the preterminal stages of AIDS. She had previously undergone multiple imaging studies, including brain CT, bone, perfusion, and ventilation scintigraphy, none of which resulted in the discovery of any treatable complication.

COMMENT

None.

Disclaimers and Cautionary Notes

> *To be perfectly intelligible one must be inaccurate, and to be perfectly accurate one must be unintelligible.*
>
> *Bertrand Russell*

Although sensitivities and specificities of most imaging procedures have been published and are available in the literature (5, 6, 20), the data vary over a wide range and are usually derived from small patient series. Statistically, the data are often suspect, especially since interobservor variability is usually ignored. When we come to the endoscopic or direct imaging modalities such "quantitative," information that does exist is of even more dubious reliability, because the information is almost always subjective from a single observer, and unverifiable, because photographic or videotape records are not usually obtained. Thus, it is not surprising that sensitivity and specificity numbers for these procedures are sparse indeed. Even when endoscopic biopsy is obtained, control biopsy data from large populations are limited. Thus, most quantitative data relating to the accuracy of medical imaging or other testing can only be categorized as an approximation of statistical reality, because factors such as selection bias of the investigators or in population sampling, e.g., healthy vs. sick, geography, age, race, socioeconomic factors, etc., can seldom be taken into account. Epidemiologically speaking, this is not always "hard data." The problem of test performance data has been nicely summarized by Metz (21) and Fleiss (22), who stress the limited usefulness of sensitivity and specificity estimates derived from small patient samples. We therefore remind the reader that whether the numbers are derived from the literature, expert opinion, or a combination of the two—and we will so indicate this—*all* statistical data relating to test performance must be considered a rough approximation only. In our tables we will supply citations when we have been able to obtain numerical data from the published medical literature. With our own estimates we will sometimes give a range. Objections will no doubt be raised, particularly because there continues to be serious dispute among students of probability theory about the very concept of subjective probability with the "Bayesians" against the "Formalists." Our answer to the latter is: far better to have subjective probability than no probability at all.

It should be understood, moreover, that we neither guarantee nor claim any absolute reliability for these numbers, whether the published or our subjective estimates are employed in any clinical or other context. They are to be taken only as a rough guide, with the knowledge that disease prevalence always determines predictive values of a test more than measures of test performance.

An even stickier problem occurs with disease prevalence or prior probability, given various categories of signs and symptoms. After more than 100 years of scientific medicine, the medical literature is still sadly deficient in quantitative information regarding the relative frequencies of diseases or conditions, given certain findings or complaints. An exemplary work by Blacklow et al. (23) deals with signs and symptoms, but disease prevalence is all but ignored.

Outstanding works by Blacklow (23) and the standard classic of Harrison (24) deal with signs and symptoms, but disease prevalence is all but ignored. Barker's fine text (25) emphasizes common conditions, but is not based on clinical presentation. The majority of medical textbooks and most clinical literature deal with specific conditions and thus are almost invariably disease-oriented.

We are attempting the converse here; namely, given the sign or symptom, what is the most likely disease or diseases? Anyone can come up with a list of differential diagnoses simply by consulting French's classic reference (26) or other medical texts (27, 28). But clearly, when faced with a *patient*, the logical move is look up the *finding* or the *complaint*. This text is not organized as a reference for looking up a procedure.

The problem for us is to determine priority. For example, given right lower quadrant pain or anemia or a lump in the axilla, what are the relative probabilities of likely causes? This information is extremely difficult to sort out, let alone find in the medical literature, because, sadly, medicine remains more descriptive or anecdotal than quantitative. Thus, case reports abound, and most clinical literature is devoted to diseases rather than findings. We learn that nonanginal chest pain may be seen in mitral valve prolapse, esophageal reflux, duodenal ulcer, chest wall syndromes, pericarditis, and even primary pulmonary hypertension, but it can be very difficult to discover that, given a patient with nonanginal chest pain, 25% of cases are due to chest wall syndromes, 15% to esophagitis, etc. When we see a patient, we really want to know not what he *might* have among a plethora of choices, but rather what he is *most likely* to have. This is the classic form of question addressed by Bayes' Theorem.

Fortunately, useful information is available for certain categories of clinical presentations, notably abdominal pain, headache, anginal chest pain, jaundice, fever of unknown origin, arterial hypertension, and others. But where these figures are not accessible or available from the general medical literature we will again attempt to derive estimates of these probabilities from hospital discharge data obtained from the NCHS (29), ambulatory care data from the National Ambulatory Medical Care Survey (NAMCS) (30), other epidemiologic surveys, or from experts in the given fields consulted by the author.

Expert clinical opinion based on experience and knowledge has always been respected and is what really counts in the clinical confrontation. Our experience suggests that the best clinicians are often able to summon up these probability estimates without too much hesitation. With the major entities, there is often good agreement between consultants in the same clinical area. Again, however, we can claim no responsibility for the clinical reliability of prevalence estimates either from published or physician sources.

Some General Principles of Diagnostic Imaging

After considering the implication of any clinical findings and results from previous investigations, we must always ask ourselves if further testing is indeed necessary. Is the disease, in fact, *imageable?* Are anxiety, depression, chronic recurrent headache, dyspepsia, constipation, and nonanginal chest pain sufficient reason for ordering extensive neurologic, gastrointestinal, or cardiac work-ups? If we are reasonably certain of the diagnosis from the clinical assessment, why do we need further confirmation? This sounds like a platitude, but in reviews of clinical records it is clear that many unnecessary studies are performed in a setting where there was already ample clinical evidence of a diagnosis.

The other principal cause of unnecessary imaging or laboratory testing occurs when there is no clear diagnostic hypothesis. Electing to do a test *without any disease in mind* is, to repeat, mindless medicine. Equally bad or worse is the habit of attempting to exclude entities that logically should not even be considered. This habit is the last refuge of the diagnostically destitute. Once diagnosis becomes an unjustified search for the bizarre, all rationality is abandoned. The desire to perform a test is never an indication to do so. To summarize:

One should always have a *clinical* reason for suspecting a specific diagnosis before ordering any test or imaging procedure. Corollary: Never use any imaging procedure as a fishing expedition or to rule out the unlikely.

Whenever possible, order the least hazardous and inexpensive studies first, such as plain x-rays or ultrasound, before doing any other imaging (except in specified emergency situations).

Corollary: Except for certain types of trauma and central nervous system disorders, always consider doing routine studies before CT or MRI.

Indications for all procedures with attendant risks of injury or mortality must obviously be carefully weighed against any conceivable benefits.

How Reliable Is Medical Testing?

Let us examine the above question more closely by citing some important real-life examples. Later on we will learn that a very good test indeed is one that has a sensitivity of 85–90% and a specificity greater than 95%. In practice, few imaging studies, whether plain radiographs, endoscopy, CT, or MRI, enjoy this level of sensitivity or specificity, most of them hovering in the 75–85% range. In general, imaging studies rarely have the sensitivities or specificities claimed for them. Further facts should be of interest. According to the American College of Obstetricians and Gynecologists, the Pap test fails to detect cervical cancer or other serious abnormalities up to 40% of the time. In a 1988 study by the Conference of Radiation Control Program Directors and the FDA's Center for Devices and Radiological Health, mammograms of "unacceptable quality" were found in 13% of 286 x-ray laboratories. In another 1988 report by the National Cholesterol Education Program, nearly half of all laboratory cholesterol test results vary by 5% or more from the correct value, and some readings were described as "highly inaccurate." In an oft-quoted paper, one well-known pathologist disagreed with the diagnosis of Hodgkin disease made by colleagues in almost half the cases (31).

It may be that we are interpreting out of context. How many of these reports disclosed poor test performance because of substandard laboratories or poor medical interpretation, and how many because of low prevalence of disease? In the area of medical screening, claims for effectiveness of *all* test procedures must be regarded with considerable skepticism because of low disease prevalence. An important study reported from the Mayo Clinic dealt with preoperative laboratory screening (aspartate aminotransferase, glucose, potassium, platelet count, and hemoglobin) of almost 3800 asymptomatic healthy patients. The investigators found only 4% with an abnormality, but no surgical procedure was delayed and no adverse outcome could be associated with any of these patients. Because of these findings, the Mayo Clinic no longer requires preoperative laboratory screening for healthy patients (32).

It may surprise the reader that, despite our disclaimers, warnings, and general expressions of doubt, we will remain committed to the value of diagnostic testing. But we are convinced that in order to practice sensible medicine in an age of expensive new toys, it is essential to proceed largely on the basis of the clinical encounter. Only after a reasonable probability of disease is suspected based on signs and symptoms can a reasonable diagnostic course be initiated.

REFERENCES

1. Balla JI. The Diagnostic Process. Cambridge: Cambridge University Press, 1985.
2. Sox HC, Blatt MA, Higgins MC, Marton KI. Medical Decision Making. Stoneham: Butterworth Publishers, 1988.
3. Holtzman S. Intelligent Decision Systems. Reading, Pa: Addison-Wesley Publishing Co. Inc., 1989.
4. Gorry GA, Barnett GO. Sequential diagnosis by computer. JAMA 1968;205(12):849–854.
5. Goris GL. Sensitivity and Specificity of Common Scintigraphic Procedures. Chicago: Year Book Medical Publishers, 1985.
6. Griner PF, Panzer RJ, Greenland P. Clinical Diagnosis and the Laboratory: Logical Strategies for Common Medical Problems. Chicago: Yearbook Medical Publishers, 1986.
7. Schreiber MH, Wilson's law of diminishing returns [Editorial]. AJR 1982;138(4):786–788.
8. The Los Angeles Times, 1988, quoted by Root-Berstein RS. Misreading reliability. The Sciences, 1990;Feb:6–8 (N.Y. Academy of Sciences).
9. Spielberg F, Kabeya CM, Ryder RW, Kifuani NK, et al. Field testing and comparative evaluation of rapid, visually read screening assays for antibody to human immunodeficiency virus. Lancet 1989; 1(8638):1325–1326.
10. Francis HL, Mann J, Colebunders RL, Ndongala L, et al. Serodiagnsosis of the acquired immune deficiency syndrome by enzyme-linked immunosorbent assay compared to cellular immunologic parameters in African AIDS patients and controls. Am J Trop Med Hyg 1988;38(3):641–646.
11. Mitchell SW, Souleymane M, Mingle J, Sambe D, et al. Field evaluation of alternative HIV testing strategy with rapid immuno-binding assay and agglutination assay. Lancet 1991;337:1328–1331.
12. Anonymous. HIV prevalence estimates and AIDS case projections for the United States: report based upon a workshop. MMWR 1990;39(RR-16):7.
13. Glenski WJ, Malek RS, Myrtle JF, Oesterling JE. Sustained substantially increased concentration of prostate-specific antigen in the absence of prostatic malignant disease: an unusual clinical scenario. May Clin Proc 1992;67:249–252.
14. Fletcher RH, Fletcher SW, Wagner EG. Clinical Epidemiology. The Essentials. 2nd ed. Baltimore: Williams & Wilkins, 1987;57.
15. Soloway HB. No name, no fame for an important testing principle. Medical Laboratory Observer 1983;Nov:21–23.
16. Robertson EA, Zweig MH, Van Steirteghen AC. Evaluating the clinical efficacy of laboratory testing. Am J Clin Pathol 1983;79(1):78–86.
17. Simel DL, Feussner JR, Delong ER, Matchar DB. Intermediate, indeterminate, and uninterpretable diagnostic test results. Med Decis Making 1987;7(2):107–114.
18. Doubilet P, Weinstein MC, McNeil BJ. Use and misuse of the term cost-effectiveness in medicine. N Engl J Med 1986;314(4):253–625.
19. Eiseman B, Stahlgren L. Cost-Effective Surgical Management. Serving Two Masters. Philadelphia: W. B. Saunders, 1987.
20. McNeil BJ, Abrams HL, eds. Brigham and Women's Hospital Handbook of Diagnostic Imaging. Boston/Toronto: Little Brown, 1985.
21. Metz CE. Constraints on the sensitivity and specificity of "logically" merged test results [Editorial]. J Nucl Med 1991;32(8):1646–1647.
22. Fleiss JL. Statistical Methods for Rates and Proportions. New York: Wiley, 1981·14
23. Blacklow RS, et al. MacBryde's Signs and Symptoms. Applied Pathologic, Pathologic Physiology and Clinical Interpretation. 6th ed. Philadelphia: J. B. Lippincott Company, 1983.
24. Barker LR, Burton JR, Zieve PD, eds. Principles of ambulatory medicine, 2nd ed. Baltimore: Williams & Wilkins, 1986.

25. Petersdorf RG, Adams RD, Braunwald E, Isselbacher KJ, Martin JB, Wilson JD, eds. Harrison's Principles of Internal Medicine 10th ed. New York: McGraw-Hill Book Company, 1983.
26. Hart FD. French's Index of Differential Diagnosis. 11th ed. Bristol: John Wright & Sons, Ltd., 1979.
27. Margulies DM, Thaler MS. The Physician's Book of Lists. New York: Churchill Livingston, 1983.
28. Krupp MA, Schroeder SA, Tierney LM, eds. Current Medical Diagnosis and Treatment. 26th ed. Norwalk: Appleton & Lange, 1987.
29. U.S. Department of Health and Human Services, U.S. Public Health Service, Centers for Disease Control, and the National Center for Health Statistics. National Hospital Discharge Survey (NHDS). Detailed diagnoses, procedures, days of care, diagnoses-related groups for patients discharged from short-stay hospitals. Public Use Data Diskettes, 1985–1990.
30. National Center for Health Statistics, McLemore T, DeLozier J. 1985 Summary: National Ambulatory Medical Care Survey. Advance Data from Vital and Health Statistics, No. 128 DHHS pub. no. (PHS) 87-1250. Hyattsville, Md.: Public Health Service, Jan. 23, 1987.
31. Symmers Sr. WS. Survey of the eventual diagnosis in 600 cases referred for a second histological opinion after an initial biopsy diagnosis of Hodgkin's disease. J Clin Pathol 1968;21(5):650–653.
32. Narr BJ, Hansen TR, Warner MA. Preoperative laboratory screening in healthy Mayo patients: cost-effective elimination of tests and unchanged outcomes. Mayo Clin Proc 1991;66(2):155–159.

3

Concise Descriptions and Comparisons of the Modalities

X-Rays—Their moral is this: that a better way of looking at things will see through almost anything.
Samuel Butler
Note-Books, *Vol. V*
(Further extracts, ed. by A. T. Bartholomew)

What's in a Name?

A word on procedure terminology is indispensable. Specifically, the use of the word *scan* is endlessly confusing to both laymen and physicians. This includes radiologists and other specialists engaged in performing the gamut of imaging procedures. Physicians frequently order studies using the generic term *scan* without specifying sonography, computed tomography (CT), magnetic resonance imaging (MRI), or nuclear medicine studies. Upon receiving request slips, the imaging specialist often does not know which study to perform when a patient arrives in the department. Most patients are equally bewildered and usually have little idea what procedure is required.

Thus, the term *scan* is used loosely to indicate ultrasonographic studies, as in "gall bladder scan," and to describe CT or MR as in "CT head scan" or "MR scan." To complicate matters further, the terms *nuclear, isotope, radionuclide,* or specific organ scan (i.e., liver-spleen scan) have become almost standard. Kidney scan requests, for instance, could refer to ultrasound, nuclear medicine, CT, or MR studies. Thyroid, pancreas, testicular, and pelvic scan requests are also ambiguous.

The word *scan* suggests an imaging study performed by passing some type of movable detector over or around the body. However, semantic difficulty arises when we attempt to determine whether this or some analogous process actually occurs during CT, MRI, or even positron imaging. The words *study* or *imaging* could be appended to any procedure, but this seems redundant. For traditional radiographic procedures, the current nomenclature seems adequate, and for computed tomography and magnetic resonance, the simple acronyms CT and MR (or MRI) should suffice. Why add another descriptor?

We also concur in using the standard descriptive word *sonography, ultrasound,* or even *sono* or *U/S* for all ultrasound procedures, as in gall bladder sonography, ultrasonography of the aorta, pelvic sono, etc. For all radionuclide studies we prefer the use of the terms *scintigraphy* or *scintiscan* (derived from *scintillante,* or sparkling, the flashes of light emitted from a suitable material, usually a sodium iodide crystal, after absorption of gamma or X-rays). *Radionuclide* or *nuclear study* are also clear, although they are somewhat more cumbersome. Thus, one would order renal scintigraphy, resting thallium cardiac scintigraphy (or scintiscan), etc. Although these terms have the disadvantage of extra syllables, they are precise. There is no possibility of confusion with ultrasound studies, CT, or MRI that follow the word scan. It is impossible to be a purist, however, and we will continue to use scan in place of the more awkward scintiscan or scintigraphy so long as the context is unambiguous. Sometimes we will use the modifier nuclear, radionuclear, or radionuclide. The term *isotope* or *isotopic scan* is imprecise. Whenever possible, however, the use of the "S" word without qualification should be avoided. We will follow this system of nomenclature throughout the book.

General Radiography

> *The radiologists' national plant is the hedge.*
>
> *Bernstein's Precept*

INDICATIONS

Conventional radiographic studies or routine X-rays are still the mainstay of diagnostic imaging, accounting for 60–70% of all imaging procedures. When dealing with skeletal trauma, articular, osseous, or back pain, or whenever a bone lesion is suspected, plain films should always be obtained *before* any other imaging procedure is requested.

Plain radiographs should also be the first imaging study in examinations of the chest (heart, lungs, pleura, diaphragm, and ribs), abdomen, gastrointestinal (GI), and genitourinary (GU) tract. For further study of any portion of the GI tract, barium or in some cases water-soluble contrast studies are indicated, except in the case of GI bleeding, in which appropriate procedures will be discussed later. After plain radiographs, barium contrast should *always* be used as the next imaging procedure of the GI tract and, except in GI bleeding, should *precede* any invasive upper or lower endoscopic procedures. We stress that no diagnostic procedure with known mortality and morbidity should ever be performed in preference to a safer procedure providing equivalent information (vide infra).

Contraindications to Radiography

There are no absolute contraindications to general radiographic procedures, and none for those conducted with barium, with the following exceptions: Barium should generally be avoided in suspected viscus perforation where aqueous contrast may be preferable and safer. Oral administration of barium is contraindicated in known or suspected large bowel obstruction. *Pregnancy, regardless of its stage, is not a contraindication to a medically indicated radiologic procedure involving ionizing radiation (X-ray, CT, and nuclear), if to delay the study would subject the patient to any potential risk.* The American College of Radiology and the National Council on Radiation Protection concur that even inadvertent exposure of a fetus to ionizing radiation arising from diagnostic procedures would rarely, if ever, be a cause by itself for terminating a pregnancy (1, 2).

Ultrasonography: General Indications

Like general radiographic procedures, ultrasound is quick, comfortable, and without hazard. No study has ever convincingly demonstrated that sound energies normally used in diagnostic ultrasound are harmful to human beings, with the possible exception of prolonged umbilical Doppler scanning in early pregnancy. Ultrasonography presently is the procedure of first choice for imaging the following structures: (a) the biliary tract (gall bladder, pancreas, and common bile duct); (b) abdominal aorta; (c) kidneys; and (d) the female pelvis and the pregnant uterus.

Ultrasound is also indicated as the first procedure in distinguishing: (a) obstructive from medical jaundice, specifically in differentiating hepatocellular or intrahepatic cholestasis from extrahepatic obstruction due to stone or tumor; and (b) obstructive from medical renal disease, i.e. excluding hydronephrosis as a cause of chronic or acute renal dysfunction, including renal failure.

Furthermore, sonography is unequaled in determining the cystic or solid nature of masses, palpable or otherwise. If a mass, adenopathy, or collection is discovered or suspected in the abdomen and pelvis, CT or MRI may provide additional information, but in almost all cases ultrasonography should be done first in this setting, not only for localization but because, if a cyst or other benign structure is identified, the other modalities may not be required.

Ultrasound is the most sensitive procedure for confirming the presence of ascites and, when upright or decubitus chest films are equivocal, for diagnosing pleural effusion. Generally, organ biopsy, cyst puncture, and drainage of collections are also more easily and safely performed under ultrasonic guidance. CT, however, is usualy indicated for deep-seated masses and osseous lesions.

The unique application of conventional and Doppler ultrasound in studying the heart (echocardiography), the peripheral vascular tree, and other regions will not be dealt with here. We emphasize, however, that these are important areas of diagnosis where this modality has proven indispensable.

Hints on Ordering Sonographic Studies

One must bear in mind that sonographic imaging of the abdomen or pelvis is usually not as informative in obese patients when compared to the images obtained in thin individuals. Fat tissue has strong acoustic impedance, which tends to inhibit full penetration of the sound waves, often resulting in the propagation of spurious echoes. Moreover, because of the physics of high frequency ultrasound in the 3- to 7-MHz range with its very short wavelength, gas or air in the bowel and lung is, for all intents, impenetrable. In addition, bone tissue, barium, and feces are strong sound reflectors and do not transmit the high frequency acoustic beam. A good rule to follow is: watch out for the two G's, girth and gas, and the three B's, bowel, bone, and barium, when considering the potential value of an ultrasound study. Air and gas are the reasons ultrasound is generally of little value in assessing the digestive tract, except in hypertrophic pyloric stenosis of infants. Sonography is virtually worthless in the lungs, except in the detection of pleural effusion, and rarely useful in unsuspected atelectasis. Dilated bowel loops may be noted serendipitously in the adult with an obstructing bowel carcinoma, and some report the ability to detect appendicitis, but these are exceptions. For most patients, sonography of the stomach and small and large bowel is largely useless and should not be ordered

Because barium interferes so strongly with acoustic waves, gamma rays, and possibly MRI, barium studies should be deferred when any other imaging studies of the abdomen and pelvis are anticipated. It may be necessary to wait a day or two after a

GI series or barium enema to get a good gall bladder, pancreas, aortic, or pelvic sonogram.

A good rule of thumb in the abdomen is, in the absence of suspected renal or aortic disease: if you suspect nonintestinal disease *above* the umbilicus, order an *upper abdominal* sonogram. In our laboratory this includes primarily the biliary tract, gall bladder, common duct, and pancreas, with survey of the abdominal aorta, liver, both kidneys, and the left upper quadrant. We also survey both hemidiaphragms, because unsuspected small pleural effusions are a frequent cause of unexplained upper abdominal pain, which, in fact, is pleuritic in origin. (Note that liver ultrasonography is generally a poor imaging technique for that organ.)

If the disease is thought to be *below* the umbilicus, particularly in a female (and again, not of intestinal origin), order a *pelvic* sonogram.

Preparation for Sonography and What to Tell the Patient

Proper preparation is essential for most abdominal sonographic studies. For example, the gall bladder should be examined only in the fasting state, because even fat-free food may occasionally cause the organ to contract. We prefer all our patients to have fasted overnight and schedule them for abdominal (gall bladder/pancreas) sonograms in the morning. Although it is often possible to study patients within 3 or 4 hours after eating, adequate visualization often is not achieved, and the study may have to be rescheduled. We have observed that sometimes even a piece of fruit or a teaspoon of artificial coffee creamer can cause sufficient contraction of the organ to prevent optimal visualization. A good guide is: if the patient has not had a cholecystectomy, failure to visualize the gall bladder is almost always due to surreptitious ingestion of food, because agenesis of the organ occurs in less than one in 3300 cases (3). Other problems occur with a "high," intrahepatic, or the extremely rare left-sided gall bladder, but with careful scanning technique, visualization is usually satisfactory. In the event of failure to visualize the gall bladder or pancreas, we routinely reschedule the examination at no charge. Interfering bowel gas is a frequent cause of failed pancreatic imaging, but with repeat examinations it should be possible, except in obese individuals, to visualize this organ more than 90–95% of the time. Otherwise, abdominal CT is indicated.

For pelvic sonography the patient need not fast. This study does require a full bladder, because the fluid-filled bladder is used as an acoustic window (sound penetrates fluid easily) and as a method of pushing interfering bowel loops away from the pelvic organs. Although this may be uncomfortable at times, inability to fill the urinary bladder adequately may result in a suboptimal study and failure to establish a diagnosis. Sudden hydration has been reported to result in the appearance of a small amount of fluid in the cul-de-sac of some females. This finding by itself, therefore, does not necessarily indicate abnormality. In some cases of suspected early or ectopic pregnancy and adnexal disease an endovaginal probe is often indicated, and transabdominal pelvic sonography may not be required. This obviates the requirement for a full bladder. It is not uncommon to suspect masses in the pelvis because of retained feces or loops of bowel, and we frequently have poorly prepared patients return at no charge for a repeat examination. More often than not, the suspected but spurious mass is found to have disappeared. To prevent such difficulties, it is frequently advisable for patients to take a laxative the night before or a Fleet's enema a few hours before having a pelvic sonogram.

Some patients, particularly older women with poor pelvic supports, cannot be studied adequately because of inability to maintain a full bladder. Other patients, including infants and children, those in renal failure, or others who are unable to drink, must have a catheter inserted to permit filling of the urinary bladder. One must therefore weigh the risk of urinary tract infection when deciding whether to order a pelvic sonography in such instances. Catheterizing a 6-month-old infant is not a routine procedure, and there should be a strong indication for pelvic sonography before it is ordered in infants and uncooperative young children.

Renal sonography, in our experience, requires no preparation. Although some physicians advise hydration before the study, we have occasionally found subtle dilation of the collecting systems in such hydrated patients, which unnecessarily raises the question of minimal hydronephrosis.

Sonography of the aorta, again because of interfering bowel gas, should be done in the fasting state. When using ultrasound for the detection and study of intraabdominal masses, ascites, or pleural effusions, no preparation is usually required.

The most important thing to tell patients undergoing ultrasound examination is that it is easy, quick, completely painless, and without risk or discomfort. In the case of pelvic ultrasound, arriving for the examination with a nearly full bladder will save time.

Scintigraphic Studies: General Indications

Radionuclides are unexcelled for simultaneously studying both anatomy and organ function. Neither plain radiography, CT, MRI, or sonography offers functional information about the thyroid, heart, brain, bone, lung, liver, spleen, and kidneys. It is in this realm of assessing physiology of various organs that scintigraphic examination is unsurpassed. There is no better test for gall bladder function and patency of the cystic and common bile ducts than hepatobiliary scintigraphy. Moreover, despite superior anatomic delineation of the genitourinary tract with the intravenous pyelogram, there is no safer and more sensitive method for measuring kidney function and emptying than the radionuclide renal study. In detecting hepatocellular dysfunction, liver scintigraphy may be more sensitive than liver chemistries in 15–20% of chronic cases (4). Hepatic dysfunction is usually not well demonstrated with scintigraphy in the usual mild case of acute hepatitis, however, and the use of liver/spleen scintigraphy in patients with chemical evidence of primary hepatocellular disease is redundant.

Radionuclide studies of lung ventilation and perfusion retain their preeminence for the diagnosis of pulmonary embolism, the visualization of airways disease, and the study of regional lung function. In addition, there are no other techniques that approach the ability of bone scintigraphy to study metabolic activity of bone, and its sensitivity is unequaled in detecting osseous infections, primary tumors, metastases, and unsuspected and occult fractures. One possible exception may be quantitative CT for assessing osteoporosis.

Scintigraphy has revolutionized cardiac imaging, in particular the study of chamber size, detection of wall motion abnormalities, the quantitative measurement of left and right ventricular function, and the detection and quantification of intracardiac shunts. Moreover, there is no simpler, safer, and more sensitive method to detect and evaluate coronary disease than stress myocardial perfusion scintigraphy. A very few patients with unstable angina, a recent MI, and other emergent cardiac problems may be candidates for early invasive studies, but in *all* other cases of suspected coronary disease, neither coronary angiography, angioplasty, nor, especially, coronary bypass surgery should be performed *without first obtaining myocardial perfusion scintigraphy*.

Safety of Scintigraphic Studies

Radionuclide studies are virtually as harmless as plain radiography and ultrasound. (More will be said later about the so-called "risks" of radiation.) Radiopharmaceutical agents are among the safest compounds a patient is likely to receive in the hospital. In 1984, despite 7 million procedures involving the administration of radiopharmaceuticals, only 21 adverse reactions were reported (5). This represents a consistent decline over the previous decade and is attributable to improvement in quality control and radiopharmaceutical manufacture. Even allowing for noncompliance in reporting by a factor of 2–10, the minimum rate for adverse reactions would be 100 times less than those reported for contrast media (6). Moreover, the rate of less than 1 reaction per 100,000 administrations is far lower than that of most therapeutic drugs and probably even placebos. That this is true, despite the fact that most radioactive drugs must be given intravenously, is quite amazing. The incidence of anaphylaxis is minuscule, with the range of severe reactions over a 4-year period being 2–9 per 10 million cases (only 3% of all reactions), none of which were fatal (6–9).

These statistics demonstrate the overwhelmingly innocuous nature of radiolabeled diagnostic agents. In the case of ionic compounds the actual molar amounts of the ion used are generally in the microgram range or lower, because these materials are virtually free of "carrier." These compounds include indium-111 chloride, gallium-67 citrate (infection and tumor imaging), thallium-201 chloride (myocardial perfusion imaging), iodine-123 and -131 as sodium iodide for thyroid studies, technetium-99m used as pertechnetate or as a radioactive label (liver, kidney, bone, and gated blood pool studies), etc. As every mystery fan knows from Agatha Christie's novel, *The Pale Horse*, thallium in huge (nonpharmacologic) doses is a severe cardiac toxin. But it is impossible to suffer metal poisoning from thallium or any other microgram trace of elemental ionic material received in a radionuclide study.

A word about "iodine allergies" is appropriate here. We occasionally see anxious patients who, on arriving at the laboratory, give a history of reactions to iodine-containing radiographic contrast material. The point to keep in mind, however, is that only large amounts of exogenous iodine can produce delayed allergy by forming iodinated blood proteins; it is incapable of causing allergies or anaphylactic reactions in the microgram amounts used as radioiodine in nuclear medicine, even in patients with known iodine hypersensitivity. Furthermore, the allergic reaction to contrast material is not due to ionic iodine, but rather to the iodinated organic molecule. In clinical practice, it is more often the osmolar effect of the hypertonic contrast preparation itself that causes cardiovascular or circulatory collapse after injection. In fact, a history of such reactions is a prime indication for using scintigraphy rather than contrast pyelography (IVP) in studying renal function.

With respect to those patients with a history of allergy to iodine in seafood or shellfish, their sensitivity is to fish protein rather than to iodine. Such people must be firmly reassured. Thus, there is probably no such thing as a true allergy to radioactive isotopes of iodine or for that matter to any other ionic materials used in nuclear medicine. The safety of iodine- and technetium-labeled renal imaging agents has been attested to by millions of such studies (4, 5).

Hints on Ordering Scintigraphic Studies
THYROID

Thyroid uptake blockade because of prior exposure to significant amounts of stable iodine is a common problem. Yet it is surprising how often physicians ordering thyroid studies forget how long this effect may last in their patients who have had prior intravenous contrast for an intravenous pyelogram, angiogram, or a CT study. Moreover, the ubiquity of iodides in various medications such as expectorants, health foods such as kelp, vitamin preparations, skin creams, antiseptics and douches (in particular Betadine), at the dining table where white bread may contain iodates as a preservative, and in the environment in the form of liquid cleaners, makes it imperative to obtain a careful history before thyroid uptakes or scintigraphy are undertaken. The most common offender is prior injection of contrast material given for pyelography, angiography, and, in particular, CT. Thyroid blockade after intravenous contrast may last anywhere from 4–12 weeks or longer, and oral administration of stable iodides can produce effects that last 4–6 weeks. Though it is possible to perform pertechnetate thyroid scintigraphy within a few days of an iodine contrast study, the examination is frequently suboptimal and may in fact be worthless. Moreover, in a hyperthyroid patient who is blocked with iodides, radioactive iodine treatment will have to be delayed for weeks, often causing serious medical risks, because antithyroid drugs are also frequently ineffective for equally long periods of time after pretreatment with iodides due to slow release of preformed iodinated thyroglobulin.

In the past, and occasionally today, one still sees patients who have received iodized oil rather than aqueous contrast for myelography, salpingography, and even bronchography. In these patients, retention of contrast with slow release of iodine may result in iodine blockage for years—and occasionally for life.

A frequent problem occurs in the patient with an upper mediastinal mass suspected to be thyroid who has already had CT with contrast. In this setting the diagnosis of substernal goiter is almost always more effectively, safely, and economically made with scintigraphy rather than CT. If CT ends up being indeterminate for goiter, a not infrequent result, reliable radionuclide thyroid studies could be delayed for weeks. Here is another example of the wisdom of delaying CT (or MRI) until all information from other studies has been obtained. For thyroid imaging, radionuclide studies should always be performed first.

Thyroid hormone also inhibits thyroid uptake of radioiodine by inhibition of pituitary thyrotropin secretion. If the patient has been on thyroid hormone (T_4 or thyroxine) treatment for any length of time, the suppressive effect generally takes 4–6 weeks to dissipate, for T_3 or triiodothyronine preparations, 3–4 weeks.

HEPATOBILIARY

Another scintigraphic study interfered with by extraneous factors is the hepatobiliary study, notoriously sensitive to fasting or food intake. Because the gall bladder contracts after food, if the test is done in the postprandial state the organ rarely visualizes until 2–4 hours have elapsed. Moreover, in moderate to prolonged fasting, which can be anything beyond 18–24 hours, a distended gall bladder frequently will not fill. This effect is variable and therefore, like food ingestion, results in uncertainty of interpretation. By injecting a small dose of cholecystokinin (CCK), the imaging specialist can partially empty the gall bladder, and within 20 minutes the imaging radiopharmaceutical can be injected. The normal gall bladder should fill within 45–60 minutes. Contrary to expectation, the injection of this amount of CCK even in a patient with acute or chronic cholecystitis is essentially without hazard. Failure to inject CCK before hepatobiliary scanning in a patient who has not eaten in 24 hours can give a false positive test for acute cholecystitis, i.e. nonvisualization. Thus, failure to note such a seemingly trivial event as the time of the last meal may lead to misleading test results.

GALLIUM

Because of its relatively long 78-hour half-life, its radiation characteristics, and its body distribution, radiogallium scintigraphy will seriously interfere with other radionuclide studies for 1 week or more after injection. When indicated, gallium scinti-scanning should always be the *last* of any radionuclide studies to be performed.

Another problem with gallium is its use for tumor staging after lymphangiography, where false-positive results are occasionally seen due to retention of contrast material in nodes and in the lungs. When lymphangiography and gallium scintigraphy are both planned, the gallium study should always be done first.

Preparation for Radionuclide Studies and What To Tell the Patient

In addition to the preparations and precautions noted above for thyroid and hepatobiliary studies, patients should be fasting for all resting or stress myocardial perfusion studies. It is also desirable for patients to omit a meal before gated wall motion studies, because the postprandial state has been shown to falsely elevate the ejection fraction in some patients. We prefer to hydrate our bone scan patients. Otherwise, no preparation, fasting or otherwise, is required for any other scintigraphic studies, except pretreatment with stable iodine before adrenal scintigraphy.

As to time of imaging, bone scintigraphy requires a 2- to 3-hour wait after injection; thyroid uptakes are occasionally done at 4–6 hours, but usually at 24 hours; and gallium scanning is performed 24–72 hours or longer after injection. Adrenal medullary scintigraphy is performed at 24 and 48 hours and adrenocortical scintigraphy anywhere from 2–5 days after injection. For most other imaging studies including lung ventilation/perfusion, cardiac, hepatobiliary, renal, and GI bleeding scans, patients should be told they will receive an injection followed by immediate imaging. Patients can be assured they will experience no sensation aside from venipuncture and no adverse reaction from radiopharmaceutical injection. Anxious patients, particularly those concerned about allergic reactions or idiosyncrasies, should be reassured that such problems are almost never seen and are virtually unknown with radiodiagnostic agents currently in use.

CT and MRI
GENERAL INDICATIONS

Ever since NMR for *nuclear magnetic resonance*, lost the "N" because of public confusion over radiation hazards and became MRI or MR, its growth has exploded. Because CT and MRI are both relatively new modalities, each new generation of scanners demonstrates marked improvements over previous instrumentation. Therefore, studies of the comparative efficacy of MRI and CT will require considerable time and assessment in large numbers of patients with various disorders before the final judgments can be made with respect to superiority for any given clinical situation.

Both of these imaging techniques have reasonably parallel indications at this time, but it is not at all clear to what extent MRI will surpass or replace CT in the future. Economic as well as medical factors are involved. Authorities now agree that MRI is superior to CT for studying most conditions of the central nervous system, especially demyelinating diseases, in articular disease, especially the knee and shoulder joints, in soft tissue (muscle and ligamentous) imaging, and in the intervertebral disk spaces, especially postoperatively. Cardiac applications of MRI are now being actively explored. CT as of this writing appears generally superior in bone, lung, liver, and kidney, though in some instances, the two modalities give complementary information. The relative merits of CT and MRI in the pelvis are still being debated. CT remains superior to MRI in the identification of fresh bleeding in head trauma. The relative effectiveness of the present generation of MRI and CT scanners in other anatomic structures, e.g. lymph nodes, is yet to be established and will no doubt change with improvement in MRI instrumentation.

There remain some intractable problems with MRI which do not appear to have easy solutions. It is frequently impossible to study certain types of patients in an MRI machine. First, there are trauma and other critically ill patients requiring intensive care, those on respirators or cardiac monitors, who cannot be isolated completely for any length of time in an MRI capsule. Second, claustrophobia is noted in a significant proportion of patients who simply cannot tolerate the extreme confinement in an MRI capsule for up to 1 hour or more.

The principal conditions appropriately studied by both CT and MRI are deep masses of any type: intracerebral, intrathoracic, intraabdominal, and organ masses including adenopathy, and as mentioned above, the central nervous system (CNS), major joints, intervertebral disk spaces, and soft tissue. CT (but not MRI) is extremely helpful in localizing early osseous abnormalities, though it should almost never precede bone scintigraphy.

MRI has quickly become a popular imaging procedure and is now available in probably more than 2000 in- and outpatient facilities throughout the United States. At present there are more than 1500 free-standing private imaging centers throughout the country, one-third or more of which offer MRI, a fact that suggests entrepreneurial excesses. Even more so than CT, MRI has been widely abused, because it is far too often employed inappropriately. At present the modality is enormously overused in medical diagnosis by physicians poorly trained in its indications and its use. This explosion in the use of MRI is much more impressive than that of CT, which began 20 years ago. Clearly, the growth of MRI does not appear to have been adversely affected by the wider availability of the less expensive CT, nor by the expense and maintenance costs of MRI facilities. It is of interest that in all of Great Britain at the time of this writing there are only a handful of MRI machines, probably less than 20.

The critical question remains, why replace CT scanners, which can be purchased for about $500,000–800,000, with MRI units that may cost as much as $2–3 million and require their own buildings? Anderson, in an excellent review (10), suggests the principal reason may be that MRI is superior for imaging soft tissue (though this would hardly explain its widespread use for other reasons). He then poses the second question: Why not get rid of the CT scanners altogether and replace them with MRI machines?

Table 3.1. Contraindications to MRI

Strict
Intracranial aneurysm clip
Metallic foreign body in the eye
Staples prosthesis
Cochlear implant
Acute multiple trauma or other condition requiring close monitoring

Relative
Involuntary movement disorder
Claustrophobia
Ferromagnetic material in area of interest
Gross obesity
Condition requiring mechanical ventilation
Risk of apneic spell
Dyspnea at rest, with resulting exaggerated respiratory motion

Reprinted with permission by *Postgraduate Medicine* (1989;85(3):80).

Table 3.1 shows contraindications to MRI scanning, some of which were mentioned above. Under relative contraindications, again note that claustrophobia is listed. Almost 1 out of 20 patients sent for MRI scanning cannot tolerate being enclosed and isolated in the confined space of the machine. The closest person to the patient is usually 40 to 50 feet away in another room behind a console, where there is little opportunity for reassuring close physical contact. This is made even worse by the loud pounding noise caused by huge electrical power surges through the magnetic coils. As one articulate patient described it to us, "It is terrifying when you're lying there entombed in a crypt where you can hardly move and you suddenly begin to hear a jackhammer. If it were not for the occasional voice of the invisible technologist through the intercom I would have gone stark raving mad."

Table 3.2 summarizes Anderson's opinion (10) about the relative advantages of both modalities. Excellent reviews of the applications of MRI in the abdomen and pelvis have been published elsewhere (11–14).

Implications of CT and MRI for Contrast Procedures

Since the introduction of CT and MRI, we have seen a significant decline in the use of arteriography and at least three other invasive procedures employing contrast material: myelography, arthrography, and lymphangiography. A few authorities bemoan this, but on balance one is hard-pressed to make a convincing case for resurrecting these largely outdated procedures. If MRI is available, it is almost impossible, for example, to justify the use of arthrography for joint imaging, especially of the shoulder and knee. Myelography may retain some advantages over CT or MRI for the orthopedist or neurosurgeon in the rare spinal case—i.e. certain patients with herniated cervical disk, postsurgical patients, those with spinal stenosis or in clinically silent thoracolumbar tumors, and in defining the level of subarachnoid blockage usually from metastatic disease—but even these indications are becoming increasingly controversial. Myelography is invasive, entails a finite risk of allergic reactions, aseptic meningitis, or even transverse myelitis, and its overall sensitivity and specificity are no better and may sometimes be inferior to CT or MRI (15). Furthermore, as

Table 3.2. MRI versus CT

Imaging site	Relative advantages of MRI	Relative advantages of CT
Head	More sensitive	Better for trauma
Cervical spine	Images spinal cord and most disk herniations	Better for fractures and small disk herniations[a]
Lumbar spine	Shows disk disease well in sagittal and axial planes	Better for bone detail
Knee	Demonstrates intracapsular and extracapsular diseases	Better for bone detail
Extremities	Shows soft tissues well	Better for bone detail
Chest	Shows heart chambers and great vessels noninvasively	Better for screening lungs and mediastinum
Abdomen	May be useful in diagnosing liver disease	Better for screening
Pelvis	Coronal and sagittal views often helpful	Better for screening

Reprinted with permission by *Postgraduate Medicine* (1989;85(3):80).
[a]Small disk herniations visible only after myelography using water-soluble contrast agent.

with CT, a significant number of normal patients will have an abnormal myelogram (16).

Lymphangiography continues to be preferred over CT or MRI in some settings, but again, the technique is continuing to fall into disfavor for several reasons. It is technically difficult, lasting 2-4 hours and tying up equipment and physician time. It is unpleasant for the patient, may cause serious pulmonary complications, and gives false-positive gallium uptake in the lungs, sometimes for months. The main problem with all modalities used in visualizing lymph nodes is the number of false-negative results that occur in microscopic disease, though lymphangiography, unlike CT or MRI, can sometimes disclose abnormalities in normal sized nodes. The principal advantages of CT, and probably MRI, are the ability to detect the exact location and extent of *enlarged* nodes in all lymph node groups, as opposed to lymphangiography, which only can assess the para-aortic, common, and external iliac chains.

In all three invasive procedures, to whatever degree they may be preferred in the individual patient, the *overall* advantages of CT and MRI are clearly making the other procedures obsolete. We face another significant problem with all diagnostic studies, whether they suffer justified or unjustified obsolescence: as the older procedures begin to be replaced, those skilled in their technologies disappear, and no new physicians are trained in their uses. We call this the "disappearing effect." Whatever arguments can be invoked for retaining these procedures, within a few years' time they will have all but disappeared from the imaging armamentarium. There is a dark side to this phenomenon when newer, more risky technologies threaten older and much superior methods, a fact that we shall discuss when we come to upper GI barium studies vs. endoscopy.

We emphasize that CT and MRI are still to some degree complementary, with MRI clearly showing an advantage over CT in the imaging of soft tissue, CNS, spine, and major joints, and CT still superior in the thorax, as a screening study in the abdomen and pelvis, and in identification of bone lesions. MRI remains significantly more expensive than CT, but as noted it may take several more years before specific advantages of one over the other will be established in different disorders.

Hints on Ordering CT and MRI Studies

When ordering CT and MRI studies, because of the nature of these two imaging techniques, particularly MRI, it is not feasible to scan or survey large areas of the patient. The suspected anatomic location of the abnormality, abscess, or mass must be identified for the imaging physician before ordering these tests. For example, ordering MRI of the lumbar spine is obviously to be preferred to MRI of the spine, whereas, except in lymphomas, CT of the abdomen and pelvis should, when possible, be avoided. Such requests often suggest weak diagnostic indications for the test in the first place. Because of their cost and specific indications, CT and MRI, even more so than other modalities, should never be used as fishing expeditions.

CT of the mediastinum or CT of the lungs should include information about the suspected or known location of the disease. Similarly, when ordering CT or MRI of the abdomen, the suspected organ or site of pathology should be identified. For example, is the suspected problem in the liver, the kidneys, or the pelvis? Indicating an anatomic region is helpful in MRI of the spine, where imaging in different planes and with different pulse sequences is time consuming. Localization of the suspected area of disease to a limited number of vertebral segments permits a more thorough study. This principle also should be observed in CT imaging of the spine.

Preparations for CT and MRI studies and What to Tell the Patient

It is always prudent to prepare the patient for the experience of undergoing CT and MRI as for any other imaging studies. Except for the injection of contrast material in certain CT and MRI studies, the patient will experience no discomfort or inconvenience except for the requirement of lying absolutely still on the imaging table. The physical conditions of the imaging area, however, should be explained carefully to allay any apprehension and to prepare the patient mentally. For example, in both imaging procedures, a very narrow table is used. Patients should be told they will be restricted in motion during the imaging procedure, which may last anywhere from 15 minutes to 1 hour for CT and 45 minutes to 1 hour or more for MRI. Moreover, during MRI the patient is isolated in a room. During CT the patient is closer to the console, but in both CT and MRI he or she is often attended to after contrast material is administered and when there is a need for repositioning.

For the reasons mentioned above MRI is much more stressful for many patients because their isolation is more complete and prolonged, and their only contact with the outside world is by means of an intercom. It is therefore imperative that the patient understand the nature of the test beforehand. A tranquilizer sometimes may be of help before the procedure. Claustrophobia, an unexpected consequence of medical progress, is an unusual contraindication for a medical procedure. Although it is worse with MRI, it is still occasionally seen with CT, and rarely even under the gamma camera detector in a nuclear medicine study.

Safety of CT and MRI

Although doses of ionizing radiation to target organs are significantly higher for CT than for conventional radiography or nuclear medicine procedures, the only real hazard from CT occurs with the almost routine use of intravenous contrast material as part of the study. This risk is small but finite, even with the newer nonionic contrast compounds, and will be discussed in the next chapter. Whenever possible, nonionic contrast should be used. MRI, in our opinion, is without demonstrable risk, because it involves exposure only to magnetic field strengths which have never convincingly been shown to cause detectable harm to humans. The only contrast material now used in MRI, a gadolinium compound, has low toxicity and an exceedingly low rate of adverse reactions, though at least two deaths have already been reported.

Summary of CT and MRI

Both CT and MRI unquestionably have revolutionized medical imaging with respect to the visualization of internal body structure and the delineation of masses. Yet it remains astounding that these modalities are so frequently used in diagnosis. The reason for this is simply that more than 99% of medical conditions affecting human beings are neither imageable masses nor other anatomic abnormalities specifically requiring CT or MRI. Anderson (10) has remarked: "The goal in any new and expensive new technology should be to use it when it is indicated and not because it is interesting or exotic" (10). That is why this book is as much about the frequency of irritable bowel syndrome and tension headache as it is about the occurrence of intraabdominal lymphoma and brain tumors. "When you hear hoofbeats, they are more likely to be horses than zebras."

Postscript: Positron Emission Tomography

Among the problems of assessing "new" imaging technologies is their sudden emergence from obscurity and the rapidity of their clinical development. That these new modalities have great potential application is not disputed, but to know their appropriate place in the diagnostic armamentarium requires time and considerable clinical experience. The hottest new area of interest is positron emission tomography (PET) scanning, which, in fact, was first developed by David Kuhl and coworkers more than 25 years ago at the University of Pennsylvania.

Positron emitters are radionuclides emitting positive electrons from the nucleus which interact with free negatively charged electrons to produce annihilation radiation (high energy, 0.51 million electron volt gamma rays) detectable by special nuclear cameras. The light elements of biological interest, in particular oxygen, nitrogen, carbon, and fluorine, have no usable gamma-emitting radioactive isotopes other than these positron emitters. It is unfortunate indeed that all these radionuclides turn out to have extremely short half-lives. For example, the half-life of oxygen-15 is 2 minutes; nitrogen-13, 10 minutes; carbon-11, 20 minutes; and fluorine-18, 110 minutes. Moreover, these low atomic mass radionuclides can only be made in a particle accelerator, i.e. a cyclotron. Though small cyclotrons can be purchased for as little as $1.5 million today, they require expensive installation and shielding, ample space, high operating costs, and highly qualified personnel, specifically nuclear physicists and radiochemists or radiopharmacists with master's or Ph.D. degrees, to supervise their operation.

The extremely short half-lives of the radioisotopes produced impose severe, inescapable conditions on any PET facility. Because in 10 half-lives, less than $\frac{1}{1000}$ of the original isotope is left (1/2 E + 10 = 1 ÷ 2^{10}), in order to make enough tracer for a study, one would have to produce, say, for nitrogen-13 ammonia (half-time 10 minutes), 1000 mCi or 1 Ci of radioactivity for every millicurie delivered to the patient at 100 minutes! Thus the time of removal of target material from the cyclotron, including incorporation into a chemical compound to the time of injection into the patient, has to be measured in minutes, not hours. Effectively, this means virtually every PET facility has to have its own cyclotron on site or nearby.

Admittedly, the situation could change for some radionuclides. Not all positron emitters, for example, require a cyclotron. New generator "cows," which produce heavier radioelements useful for PET scanning, nuclides such as rubidium-82 for heart scanning, might in the future permit positron emission scanning in community hospitals, and in fact this already has been reported (17, 18). But the logistical problems and cost are real and have only begun to be appreciated by community hospitals eager to enter the foray. A single positron camera, for example, costs about $2–3 million. Medicare and most health insurance carriers have yet to reimburse any but a few select PET studies.

The other and more obvious consideration in PET scanning is the question of clinical usefulness in general medical practice. Since the 1970s principal PET applications have been largely in metabolic research. The power of positron emission scanning lies in the noninvasive in vivo chemical examination of the brain, heart, and other organs. Well-established applications include the study of myocardial and cerebral metabolism with ^{18}F fluorodeoxyglucose, ^{11}C-labeled amino acids, ^{13}N ammonia (NH_3), ^{15}O water, and a variety of other positron-labeled compounds, including therapeutic drugs. Emerging clinical applications of PET scanning include distinguishing treatable dementias, including stroke and depression, from Alzheimer's disease, in imaging victims of Parkinson's disease and anoxic brain damage, to look at opiate receptors in the brain, and in the documentation of psychiatric disorders. By measuring neurotransmitter function in the brain it is may be possible to understand chemically, diagnose, and treat a variety of conditions of heretofore obscure etiology. Thus, it appears PET may permit imaging of distinctive "metabolic fingerprints" in various mental diseases, including schizophrenia, depression, and motor disorders. For the first time it is possible to study a variety of diseases in which no previous pathophysiologic abnormality has been detected by other means (19, 20).

In the heart, the study of metabolic function with PET has begun to shed light on myocardial metabolism as a phenomenon often independent of perfusion as determined by angiographic or even radionuclide study. Thus, there may be improved patient selection for angioplasty or coronary bypass surgery when it becomes possible to distinguish healthy or jeopardized from nonfunctional myocardium. An excellent and less technical review of PET applications may be of interest (20).

Despite these advances, other more practical methods for studying brain and myocardial metabolism are now becoming available. With single photon emission computed tomography (SPECT), using a rotating gamma camera computer system with newly developed radiopharmaceuticals, it is now possible to study conditions once thought to fall only within the purview of PET. For example, cerebral perfusion in strokes, local cerebral blood flow in Parkinson's disease, evaluation of dementias such as Alzheimer's disease, localization of seizure foci, and the effects of cocaine on brain metabolism have been studied with ^{123}I-labeled N-isopropyl-p iodoamphetamine and 99m Tc-labeled hexamethyl-propyleneamine oxime (22). The latter compound also has been used to study sexual aggression and pediatric psychiatric patients (23). Most well-equipped nuclear medicine departments in this country are already doing SPECT imaging, and it is only a matter of time before studies such as those referred to above will be done in most large community hospitals.

It should be apparent, then, that PET imaging, though a leading clinical research tool in the study of cardiac and cerebral metabolism, has significant competition from SPECT, which is growing rapidly with the development of new radiopharmaceuticals. Furthermore, the cost issue remains a significant problem. At the present time a PET scanner costs about seven times as much as a SPECT camera including computer ($3 million vs. $450,000). The total cost of a new PET facility in 1990 dollars is $7–12 million, including cyclotron, camera, site construction, etc., not including significantly increased operating costs in personnel, space, and maintenance. This would seem to be well beyond the budget of most community hospitals, especially since reimbursement criteria have not been established.

Most important in the economic equation are issues of resources allocated and potential reimbursement for patients in clinical categories apt to benefit from PET imaging. Although the metabolic study of Parkinson's disease, Alzheimer's disease, stroke, and mental illness are important medical research areas for these conditions, therapy is likely to be limited for years if not decades to come. Moreover, because many of these patients will ultimately be studied with SPECT (the poor man's PET?), it is likely that for the foreseeable future PET imaging will remain in large academic research centers, funded and supported by grants.

As a practical matter, the total percentage of patients who will benefit clinically from PET imaging will probably remain extremely small. This is not meant in any way to minimize the potential impact of PET imaging on our understanding of disease. Even if the techniques provide significant information which cannot be gleaned from other studies, unless this leads to effective therapy, its practical value will remain elusive.

REFERENCES

1. American College of Radiology, Digest of Official Council Actions 1979–1988 and Bylaws. Sec. G. Public Health and Radiation Protection. 1989:22–23.
2. National Council on Radiation Protection and Measurements: Medical Radiation Exposure of Pregnant and Potentially Pregnant Women. NCRP Report No. 54. Washington, DC: National Council on Radiation Protection and Measurements, 1977.
3. Taylor KJW, Rosenfield AT, DeGraff CS. Anatomy and pathology of the biliary tree. In: Taylor KJW, ed. Clinics in Diagnostic Ultrasound in Gastrointestinal Disease. New York: Churchill Livingstone, 1979:203.
4. Mangum JF, Powell MR. Liver scintiphotography: an index of liver abnormality. J Nucl Med 1973; 14(7):484–489.
5. Atkins HL. Reported adverse reactions to radiopharmaceuticals remain low in 1984. J Nucl Med 1986;3(27):327.
6. Rhodes BA, Cordova, MA. Letter to the editor. Adverse reactions to radiopharmaceuticals: incidence in 1978 and associated symptoms. Report of the adverse reactions subcommittee of the Society of Nuclear Medicine. J Nucl Med 1980;21(11):1107–1110.
7. Shani J, Atkins HL, Wolf W. Adverse Reactions to radiopharmaceuticals. Semin Nucl Med 1976;6(3): 305–328.
8. Atkins HL, Hauser W, Richards P, Klopper J. Adverse reactions to radiopharmaceuticals. J Nucl Med 1972;13(3):232–233.
9. Atkins HL. Adverse reactions. J Nucl Med 1974;5(1):6.
10. Anderson RE. Magnetic resonance imaging versus computed tomography—which one? Postgrad Med 1989;85(3):79–86.
11. Fritzsch PJ, Wilbur MJ. The male pelvis, Semin Ultra CT & MR 1989;10(1):11–28.
12. Chang, YC, Arrive L, Hricak H. Gynecologic tumor imaging, Semin Ultra CT MR 1989;10(1):29–42.
13. Baumgartner BR, Chezmar JL. Magnetic resonance imaging of the kidneys and adrenal glands. Semin Ultra CT MR 1989;10(1):43–62.

14. Weissleder R, Stark DD. Magnetic resonance imaging of liver tumors. Semin Ultra CT MR 1989; 10(1):63–77.
15. Panzer RJ, Black ER, Griner PF. eds. Diagnostic strategies for common medical problems. p329. American College of Physicians. Philadelphia 1991.
16. Hitselberger WE, Witten RM. Abnormal myelograms in asymptomatic patients. J Neurosurg 1968; 28(3):204–206.
17. Goldstein RA, Mullani NA, Wong WH, et al. Positron imaging of myocardial infarction with Rubidium-82. J Nucl Med 1986;27(12):1824–1829.
18. Williams BR, Jansen DE, Wong LF, et al. Positron emission tomography for the diagnosis of coronary artery disease: a non-university experience and correlation with coronary angiography. The Society of Nuclear Medicine 36th Annual Meeting, St. Louis, 1989 (Abstract).
19. Weinberger DR. Structural and functional brain imaging in psychiatry. J Clin Brain Imaging 1990; 1(1):3–9.
20. Baxter LR, Schwartz JM, Buze BH, Bergman BS, Szuba MP. Neuroimaging in obsessive-compulsive disorder. J Brain Imaging 1990;1(1):10–21.
21. Finlayson G. PET: an overview. Appl Radiol 1989;Oct:10–14.
22. Susskind H, Weber DA, Volkow ND, Harold WH. Effect of cocaine on brain uptake of iodoamphetamine in the dog. J Nucl Med 1989;30(suppl 5):830.
23. McEwan AJ, Blackman M, Paterson W, Hooper HR. Quantification of hexamethylpropyleneamine oxime (HMPAO) distribution in pediatric psychiatric patients. J Nucl Med 1989;30(suppl 5):812.

4

The Radiation Question

May you live in interesting times.

Chinese malediction

The patient was in the intensive care unit, a pale, unkempt, jaundiced young woman in her 20s and 6 months pregnant. An IV drug abuser/alcoholic with alcoholic hepatitis and renal failure, she also had, among other problems, a bleeding diathesis. She was surprisingly alert and quite suspicious. When we approached the bed with the portable ultrasound unit, and following a brief explanation, she protested, "Just a minute, Doc, you ain't giving me no radiation, are you?"

In this latter portion of the 20th century, a time that Walter Lippmann once dubbed "the minor Dark Ages," we live in a period dominated by phobias. Unlike Joe in Jerome Kern's famous *Ol' Man River* who was ". . . tired of livin' and skeered of dyin'," our feelings are often inexpressible. We are obsessed more with the risks, not the actuality, of death. Such fears dominate us to a degree unknown in less sophisticated times and quite probably are attributable more to the increasing influence of the media than any sudden changes in the likelihood of health perils and other hazards. These perils, ranging from the "four *C's*" (cancer, cholesterol, crime, and cocaine) to AIDS, radiation, destruction of the environment, and the eradication of minor species, are just a few of the many problems we read about in the newspapers or see on the evening news. It is the uneven perception of these issues as risks that creates confusion in public policy. As Ross Adey remarks, "We dwell in a self-indulgent society without historical parallel. Our anxiety is reflected in an endless pursuit of physical perfection; our insecurities boggle the minds of our colleagues from Third World countries."

This perception of risk is so confused with its reality that many purely scientific issues become distorted by emotional controversy. Although many dangers such as saturated fats, radiation, and contamination of the biosphere by petrochemicals are real, their relative importance in the scale of things is seldom appreciated. Various issues are often linked with conflicting and unverifiable data. Opinion is often based on fact and pseudofact in a confusing melange of information that is incomprehensible to the public—and frequently to so-called experts.

Risks that increase the chance of death and disease by one per million are listed in Table 4.1, where it can be seen that the perils of many well-accepted activities are often much larger than highly feared circumstances. Table 4.2 shows the relationship between occupation and job-related fatal injury. Table 4.3 shows the relationships between lifespan shortening and various conditions. The confused public perception

Table 4.1.   One-in-a-Million Risks

	Risk	Nature
Existence		
Male, age 60	20 min	CVD,[a] cancer
in New York	2 days	Air pollution
in Denver	2 months	Cosmic radiation
in stone building	2 months	Natural radioactivity
Miami water	1 year	Carcinogens
Near PVC plant	10 years	Carcinogens
Travel		
Canoe	6 min	Accident
Bicycle	10 miles	Accident
Car	300 miles	Accident
Airline	1000 miles	Accident
Airline	6000 miles	Cosmic radiation
Work		
Coal mine	1 hr	Black lung
Coal mine	3 hr	Accident
Typical factory	10 days	Accident
Miscellaneous		
Cigarettes	1.4	CVD,[a] cancer
Wine	500 cc	Cirrhosis
Diet soda	30 cans	Carcinogens

Reprinted by permission of *Technical Review* (1979-81:45).
[a]Cardiovascular disease.

Table 4.2.   Average Reduction in Lifespan (in Days)

	For 1 year of working life (Person Aged 40)	For 35 years of working life
Deep-sea fishing	31.9	923
Coal mining	3.6	103
Oil refinery	2.6	74
Railways	2.2	63
Construction	2.1	62
Industry (average value)	0.5	13.5
Occupational exposure to radiation at 5 rem/year	1.3	32
Occupational exposure to radiation at 0.5 rem/year	0.1	3

Source: *IAEA Bulletin* (1980);22:117.

of risk is vividly illustrated in Table 4.4 in which the true mortality of an activity or product is compared with the estimated mortality by three groups, and in the amusing cartoons which are reproduced (Figs. 4.1 and 4.2). Table 4.5 shows the relative risks of fatal injury by occupation and demonstrates the extremely low risk in the nuclear industry, where radiation risk was included.

At the turn of the century, the hazards of ionizing radiation[a] were poorly understood, and the worst offenses occurred during that period, especially before

---

[a]Radiation is any type of energy propagated at a distance through space or matter. This can be purely in the form of waves as in acoustical (mechanical) energy, used in ultrasonography, or electromagnetic energy which exists as waves/particles (see Chapter 1). At the low frequency end of the electromagnetic spectrum are infrared, radiofrequency, visible and

Table 4.3.   Lifespan Shortening Associated with Various Conditions

Condition	Days
Unmarried (male)	3500
Cigarette smoking (male)	2250
Heart disease	2100
30% Overweight	1300
Cancer	980
Stroke	700
Motor vehicle accidents	207
Alcohol (U.S. average)	130
Accidents in home	95
Average job (accidents)	74
Drowning	41
Job with radiation exposure	40
Illicit drugs (U.S. average)	18
Natural radiation (BEIR, 1972)	8
Medical x-rays	6
Diet drinks	2
Reactor accidents (UCS,[b] 1977)	2[a]
Reactor accidents (Wash-1400, 1975)	0.02[a]
Smoke alarm in home	− 10
Air bags in car	− 50

Reprinted by permission from *Health Physics* (Cohen BL, Lee IS. A catalog of risks, 1979;36:707–722). Copyright 1979, Pergamon Press plc.
[a]These items assume that all U.S. power is nuclear.
[b]UCS is Union of Concerned Scientists, the most prominent group of nuclear critics.

and after World War I. At one time radium was considered a cure-all, and radium patent medicines could be purchased at the corner drugstore until well into the 1930s. An amateur golf champion, Eben Byers, faithfully drank 2-ounce bottles of it every day. He died in 1932 of aplastic anemia and a brain abscess, his jaw in decay, from severe radiation toxicity (1). Evidence of the deadly effects of radium accumulated over the years, as Marie Curie fell victim to leukemia and as the tragedy of the watch dial painters at the U.S. Radium Corporation in Newark unfolded. Marie Curie's daughter Irene, also a Nobel Laureate and the co-discoverer of artificial radioactivity, died of leukemia in the 1930s. Early radiologists lost fingers and, like many researchers and patients exposed to large doses of radiation, succumbed to various cancers. Studies of radiologists appeared to document the fact that even in the late 1940s, their life expectancy was shortened. After the explosion of the atomic bomb over Hiroshima in 1945, the dangers of high-level ionizing radiation became well known and the principal task of experts was to determine the safe level of radiation exposure.

Much of the last four decades has witnessed a continuing battle over whether there is indeed a "threshold" level below which no harm is done. Clearly, there must be a safe level of radiation exposure, because everyone is bombarded by background radiation from natural and man-made sources, including cosmic rays, ground radioactivity, electromagnetic fields, even potassium-40 in our bodies. The amount of this radiation varies widely in different geographical areas, but a *significant* relationship

---

ultraviolet light, etc., forms of *nonionizing radiation* associated with MRI and electromagnetic fields, and discussed in the following section. At the higher energies are *ionizing radiation* in the form of X-rays, gamma rays, cosmic rays, and other emissions from radioactivity. *Radiation* in this section, refers to the ionizing form used in plain radiography, CT, and radionuclide procedures.

Table 4.4.   Risk: How People See It[a]

Activity and deaths per year (Est.)	League of Women Voters	College students	Business and professional club members
1. Smoking (150,000)	4	3	4
2. Alcoholic beverages (100,000)	6	7	5
3. Motor vehicles (50,000)	2	5	3
4. Handguns (17,000)	3	2	1
5. Electric power (14,000)	18	19	19
6. Motorcycles (3,000)	5	6	2
7. Swimming (3,000)	19	30	17
8. Surgery (2,800)	10	11	9
9. X-rays (2,300)	22	17	24
10. Railroads (1,950)	24	23	20
11. General (private) aviation (1,300)	7	15	11
12. Large construction (1,000)	12	14	13
13. Bicycles (1,000)	16	24	14
14. Hunting (800)	13	18	10
15. Home appliances (200)	29	27	27
16. Firefighting (195)	11	10	6
17. Police work (160)	8	8	7
18. Contraceptives (150)	20	9	22
19. Commercial avaition (130)	17	16	18
20. Nuclear power (100)	1	1	8
21. Mountain climbing (30)	15	22	12
22. Power mowers (24)	27	28	25
23. High school and college football (23)	23	26	21
24. Skiing (18)	21	25	16
25. Vaccinations (10)	30	29	29
26. Food coloring[b]	26	20	30
27. Food preservatives[b]	25	12	28
28. Pesticides[b]	9	4	15
29. Prescription antibiotics[b]	28	21	26
30. Spray cans[b]	14	13	23

Source: *Sinclair*. Reprinted by permission of *Radiology* (1981;138:8).
[a]The public's idea of what is most risky usually differs widely from the estimated mortality for each activity. When three groups were asked to rank 30 products or activities from most to least risky, they came up with the ordering above.
[b]Data on mortality from these sources are too uncertain to estimate.

between background and low-level radiation and cancer rates has yet to be demonstrated conclusively.

To put the problem in perspective, everyone agrees there is ample evidence of carcinogenicity and mutagenicity of radiation at very high dose levels. But at lower levels of exposure the evidence of this effect is extremely obscure and virtually impossible to document. For example, the natural incidence of cancer varies even in carefully selected control populations, and this variation complicates the identification of increased cancer rates in an irradiated population compared with controls. Two approaches may be used to increase the accuracy of epidemiologic studies of radiation carcinogenesis and mutagenesis. One method is to select populations, such as the subgroups of Japanese who were exposed to relatively large amounts of radiation, and then attempt to infer the effects of low levels by extrapolation. Unfortunately, there is no general agreement on any method of performing this extrapolation. It is difficult if not impossible to prove statistically, for example, that the effects of low-level radiation exposure are reduced in frequency

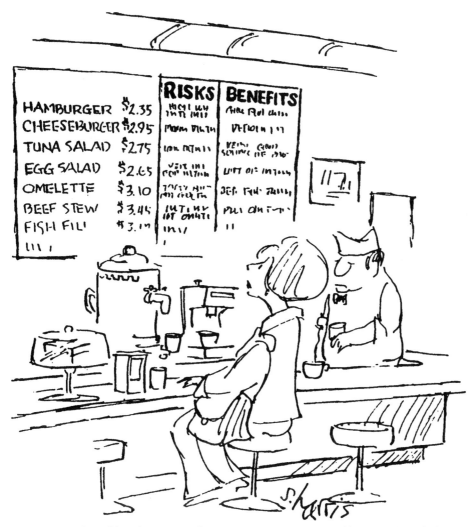

Figure 4.1. Risks and benefits. Drawing by S. Harris; © 1979. Reprinted by permission of The New Yorker Magazine, Inc.

from those of a higher exposure level. This is simply because the population size required for definitive studies would number in the tens of millions of people (2, 3).

There is no accurate way of compiling the data for both irradiated and control groups in such populations, because there are no sources of radiation other than background that affect human populations in such large numbers. The experimenter attempting to do studies with animal populations at various dose levels under controlled conditions must also make a choice between exposure level and population size. Furthermore, a number of factors may make it impossible to transfer animal results to human experience, factors such as difference in species, tumor strains, life span of animals and man, etc. (4).

Several interesting developments from epidemiologic studies cast grave doubts on the assumptions of the danger of low-level ionizing radiation. For example, comparison of cancer rates and infant mortality in three regions of the United States with

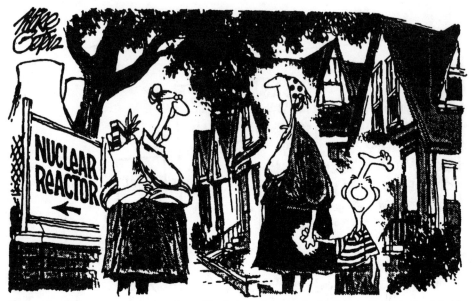

Figure 4.2. He's grown a foot since I saw him last. . . . Drawing by M. Peters; © 1981. Reprinted by permission of United Features Syndicate, Inc.

Table 4.5. Career Chance of Job-Related Fatal Injury

Occupation	Individual probability of accidental fatality (per 10,000)
Mining, quarrying	295
Construction	265
Agriculture	255
Transportation and public utilities	140
All occupations (average)	65
Government	50
Manufacturing	40
Services	35
Nuclear (radiation, calculated)	32
Wholesale and retail trade	30

Source: Lapp and Russ, *Atomic Industrial Forum* (1979; Nov: 6-4B). Reprinted with permission from the Society of Nuclear Medicine.

different background levels varying from 118–210 millirems/year[b] has failed to show any correlation with dose and adverse health effects (5). A similar study was performed in China, examining families living in the same region for many generations. More than 75,000 people who received 196 millirems/year from background radiation were compared with a control group who received 72 mrems/year. Again, no significant difference in morbidity or mortality was found (6). Similar studies have been undertaken in Brazil and India and once more showed negative results (7, 8). The extremely wide variation of background radiation received by various populations is startlingly demonstrated in Table 4.6, which shows differences of more than one order of magnitude for various parts of the world. If indeed there is a relation-

---

[b]A *rem* is a special unit of radiation dosage, equivalent to the rad for X- and gamma rays in man. (The absorption of 100 ergs/g tissue). The average American receives 180–200 millirems (mrems)/year from various sources, of which about half is from natural sources and 30–40% is from diagnostic imaging studies. The more current terminology (in SI units) uses the *Gray* (Gy), equal to 100 rads (1 Joule/kg; J/kg^{-1}), and the *Sievert* (Sv, equal to 100 rems also 1 Joule/kg).

Table 4.6. Natural Background Levels: Cosmic, Terrestrial, plus Internal

Area	Population included	Background level (mrems/year)
U.S. (Atlantic and Gulf Coast)	6,760,000	65–70
U.S. (Noncoastal plains)	46,780,000	80–95
U.S. (Colorado plateau)	1,070,000	125–160
U.S. (Leadville, Colorado)	10,000	235
U.S. (Central Florida and New England areas)		200
Brazil (coastal strips)	30,000	500
France (granite rock areas)	7,000,000	180–350
India (Kerala and Madras states)	100,000	1,300
Niue Island (Pacific)	3,000	1,000
Egypt (northern Nile Delta)	Densely populated	300–400
World (calculated average)	2 billion	80–90

Source: NIH Publication 80-2087 (1980:111).

ship between low-level radiation and cancer or other disease incidence, one would expect further epidemiologic studies to be revealing. Instead, we have virtually nothing but unsupported speculation. Persons living at very high altitudes (>10,000 feet) have whole body exposures from cosmic rays more than four times higher than that of the average person living at sea level. Further, astronauts, pilots, and passengers of jet aircraft experience temporary exposure to very high levels of cosmic rays. Such population exposures have not been shown to be associated with increased disease incidence.

One of the most interesting groups studied has been the Japanese survivors of the atomic bomb, the population number in excess of 100,000 who received 0–600 rems with an average of an almost 200-rem radiation dose to the whole body (9). The epidemiologic findings today show increase in leukemia incidence for those receiving 50 rems (50,000 mrems) or more with an increased incidence beginning 2 years after radiation, which peaked at 7–10 years but with a value of only 5% *above* control incidence and returning almost to control levels by 20 years (10). This level should be compared with the amount of radiation received during an average nuclear medicine or radiological procedure, 50–100 mrems. The interesting fact is that, "for the population receiving lower doses, in the range of 0–9 rem, no significant correlation between radiation exposure and carcinogenesis has been found to date" (3).

Studies of radiation therapy patients are confused by the fact that most of these patients have received doses in excess of 100 rems, in the range of the huge doses received by the Japanese atomic bomb survivors and several orders of magnitude above the amount of radiation received in diagnostic studies, but these doses were not to the whole body and were fractionated over several weeks. Yet a study of over 10,000 patients in Sweden receiving 50–100 rems to the thyroid from ^{131}I in one dose for diagnostic nuclear medicine studies in the late 1950s, when doses used were 50–100 times in excess of those used today, showed no subsequent increase in thyroid cancer incidence as compared to the normal Swedish population (11).

Most radiologists 50–90 years ago were almost completely unaware of the hazards of radiation. As a result, before 1940 there was indeed an increased incidence of malignancies among physicians performing radiological procedures when compared with physicians who did not work with radiation. However, malignancy rates for radiologists in practice since 1960 show no variance from those of other physicians

(12). It is not possible to estimate the amount of radiation a pre-World War II radiologist might have received, but it could have been hundreds or even thousands of rems over a lifetime, whereas today's average radiologists seldom receive more than 1 rem/year (12–14).

It is estimated at present that 16% of Americans can be expected to die of cancer. For each additional rem of radiation an increase in death rate of less than 0.01% has been *assumed* (3), a figure, like all such estimates, based on backward extrapolation from high dose data. All such estimates must be regarded as scientifically suspect, because the available data does not support a value of this magnitude for dose equivalences below 10 rems. This means that the carcinogenicity of small amounts of radiation, amounts routinely encountered by the population, is vastly exceeded by the carcinogenicity of many of the chemical compounds found in our own environment. This was convincingly shown by a study of the incidence of several different cancers and of heart disease in 43 urban areas. There was found to be a *negative* correlation between background radiation levels and disease incidence. This does not mean that higher background radiation levels are associated with less disease, because the study could not rule out the influence of other carcinogens in these urban areas. But the conclusion of the authors is inescapable: the carcinogenic effects of environmental chemicals *vastly overshadow* the effects of low level radiation in urban areas (14).

Early effects of radiation and the causation of mutagenesis have been noted since the 1920s with the classic studies of H. J. Mueller (15) with the short-lived fruit fly, *Drosophila melanogaster*. However, mutagenesis leading to phenotypically expressed abnormalities has never been convincingly detected in human beings exposed to radiation. Ritenour (4) states: "So far, *no correlation* has been shown between radiation and the incidence of genetic disorders in *any* human population at *any* dose level" (emphasis added) (16–18).

For example, no statistically significant increase in the frequency of genetically related abnormalities has been found among the 78,000 children of Japanese survivors of the atomic bomb whose parents received an average gonadal dose equivalent of 50 rems or more (19). According to Ritenour (4), because radiation leaves no unique signature on irradiated chromosomes it is difficult if not impossible to distinguish chromosomal damage caused by radiation from that of other environmental mutagens.

Other barriers include the population size and number of generations required for adequate studies and the fact that there is a significant natural occurrence of genetic diversity in human populations. Some even speculate that an increase in the radiomutations in the population may be beneficial because mutation is one of the mechanisms of evolution.

Related to this speculation are new lines of inquiry well-summarized in an article by Sagan (20), referring to research that paradoxically suggests that very low doses of ionizing radiation, rather than being harmful, may indeed have benefits. In the 19th century a stimulatory effect of low doses of chemical agents on the growth of organisms was noted by two German biologists who assumed this effect to be universal. More recently these observations have been extended to show increased longevity of animals exposed to low doses of agents toxic at higher levels (21). Studies have shown that laboratory animals exposed to low doses of radiation outlive unexposed animals, and human leukocytes exposed to low-dose radiation are protected against high doses (22, 23). In 1940 the term *hormesis* was coined to describe this stimulatory effect, about which there is still considerable controversy. In the absence of any observable effects it has always been assumed that low-level radiation produces the same harmful effects as those seen at high levels, and this assumption has become the accepted radiation paradigm. Yet some 1200 references were collected by Luckey (24) in 1979 supporting the existence of hormesis resulting from exposure to low-level radiation. As a result of uncritical and confused thinking over the unproven dangers of low-level radiation, inappropriate and hysterical efforts have been made over the past 40 years to reduce or avoid even minuscule exposures to workers and members of the public.

Thus, there remains the unsettled question of public policy toward imagined and unproven dangers of low-level radiation. Sagan (20) reminds us that "literally tens of billions of dollars are being sought by one federal program alone for the purpose of reducing exposure to low levels of radiation and chemical wastes on the basis of largely hypothetical health risks."

Roslyn Yalow, nuclear medicine pioneer and Nobel Laureate, has done a remarkable job in refocusing the attention of the scientific community on the fallacious reasoning affecting government policy over the past 30 years (25). She reminds us that a Government report to the Congress in 1981 concluded, after 80,000 papers and $2 billion spent, "there is as yet no way to determine precisely the cancer risks of low-level ionizing radiation, and that it is unlikely that this question will be resolved soon" (26, 27).

Yalow questions whether continued federal or other support of research on the effects of low-level radiation is either cost-effective or desirable, and adds: "To date, no proven body of evidence has established an increase in either human malignancy or other harmful effects as a consequence of radiation dose rates and cumulative exposure comparable to those of natural background or even at doses 10-fold higher. *We simply do not know whether there is a threshold level below which deleterious effects of radiation do not occur. If there are any such effects, they are hidden in the noise of the system,* that is, the natural statistical variation in the occurrence of health effects. Furthermore, from what we have learned during recent years from studies in molecular biology about hitherto unsuspected repair mechanisms, *a threshold might exist, but there is no known way to either prove or disprove it*" (27) (our italics).

Unfortunately, the question of low-level radiation has been politicized for too many years and, like so many issues of public policy, has become involved with vested interests. Federal agencies such as the National Research Council, the Environmental Protection Agency, the Nuclear Regulatory Commission, and especially the Department of Energy, support research and issue pronouncements periodically on low-level radiation. These reports tend to feed our anxieties and distract us from the very real risks posed by nuclear plants, high-level radioactive waste sites, and disposal policies. When one reads BEIR V (28), the latest official report intended to raise our consciousness over the dangers of low-level radiation, and which received considerable press, the knowledgeable expert remains unconvinced. A large number of respected authorities have leveled serious and compelling criticism against the methodology and conclusions, which were in disagreement with many recognized classical epidemiological studies (29). Strangely, even the Nuclear Regulatory Commission, formerly so phobic about radiation, in a surprising reversal, has recently issued a very sensible pamphlet, *Below Regulatory Concern* (30), which finds "radiation so low they do not warrant further regulatory control [sic]" (30).

Summary of the So-Called "Risks" of Low-Level Radiation

Our profound conviction based on the evidence to date is that there is *no scientifically verifiable evidence* demonstrating a danger from low-level radiation up to 20 times the so-called "threshold level." This is the reason for reiterating our position that exposure to ionizing radiation should never be invoked as a reason for omitting or postponing any appropriate medical indication for diagnostic imaging with CT, radiography, or nuclear procedures in any patient. Medical indications for imaging should be the only consideration in the performance of diagnostic imaging. This applies equally to adults, pregnant women, children, and infants. The so-called risks of low-level radiation, being unproven and probably unprovable, do not belong in any risk/benefit equation.

Postulated Risks of Electromagnetic Fields and Other Forms of Nonionizing Radiation

As if ionizing radiation were not fearful enough, we are now in the throes of another radiation controversy, that involving postulated risks of nonionizing radiation. This includes electromagnetic fields (EMF), radiofrequency, gradient, and other fields propagated by everything from long-distance power transmission lines, radio waves, television, long-distance telephone transmission lines, satellites, and microwaves, to hair dryers, microwave ovens, cellular telephones, and MRI machines. Aside from the apparently real risk of close exposure to extremely high power-transmitting sources, i.e. cataracts in workers exposed directly to radar transmitters, evidence of biological risk from the usual range of EMF levels in the environment is at best questionable (31), a controversy that could go on indefinitely and that involves the same difficulties as the low-level ionizing radiation debate. Like other ubiquitous factors in the environment, EMF presents the epidemiologist with almost impossible problems in attempting to sort out real from confounding influences and thus in identifying causal relationships to human disease. We can only wonder at the 35–50 million electromagnetic devices used in industry in this country, the 15–20 million microwave ovens, the 20–30 million radar sources, and the 30 million citizen's band radios, not to mention the television receivers, video display terminals, tens of millions of hair dryers, thousands of radio and television broadcasting stations, etc.

Whether indeed there is a cancer or lymphoma risk from living near high-tension power lines has never been satisfactorily proven, although it is true that men working in electrical jobs are at higher risk of brain tumors and other cancers. (They are also exposed to higher levels of benzene and other carcinogens.) The issue is confused by the fact that electric, electromagnetic, and magnetic fields differ qualitatively and quantitatively in terms of their source, energy emitted, and time variance. Furthermore, the range, type, and dose-response curves of their biological effects, if any, are almost completely unknown. According to Jauchem (32), "At this time, the variability and complicated nature of EMF characteristics do not allow researchers to even *design* definitive studies of EMF health effect." Cartwright (33) has stated, "The criticisms of surrogate measures (of EMF) mean that no proposed study will ever directly address the issue."

In terms of possible medical risks to patients from the electromagnetic fields and radiofrequency energies absorbed from present day MRI machines, the issues are complex and changing. The recent development of ultrafast MRI imagers with spatially encoded gradient field techniques can reduce imaging time and improve resolution by virtually eliminating movement artifacts. Gradient fields, however, may trigger unwanted events such as cardiac arrhythmias or muscle twitching in susceptible patients. In light of the uncertainty, the Food and Drug Administration may impose guidelines that could restrict the development of this new technology (34, 35).

Still, there appears to be no contraindication or documented medical risk associated with the use of conventional MRI, and we take the present view of the FDA and other regulatory bodies that no harm has been proven, and the technique is safe. Almost certainly, however, this issue will receive significant attention in the years to come and will continue to generate research funding, dramatic press announcements and, of course, a new round of public fears.

REFERENCES

1. Caufield C. Multiple Exposures: Chronicles of the Radiation Age. New York: Harper and Row, 1989.
2. Archer VE. Epidemiological studies of low-level radiation effects [Letter to the editor]. Health Phys 1981;40:129.
3. Advisory Committee On The Biological Effects of Ionizing Radiation. The Effects On Populations Of Exposure To Low Levels Of Ionizing Radiation. Washington, DC: National Research Council, National Academy Of Sciences, National Academy Press, 1980.
4. Ritenour ER. Health effects of low-level radiation: carcinogenesis, teratogenesis, and mutagenesis. Semin Nucl Med 1986;16(2):106–117.
5. Frigerio NA, Stowe RS. Carcinogenic and genetic hazard from background radiation. In Biological and Environmental Effects of Low-Level Radiation. Vienna: International Atomic Energy Agency, 1976:385–393.
6. Anonymous. High background radiation research group, China, health survey in high background radiation areas in China. Science 1980;209(4459):877–880.
7. Friere-Maia A, Friere-Maia DV. Mortality rates in a Brazilian area of high background radiation. Preliminary analysis based on official records [Abstract]. Nucl Sci 1968;22:38453.
8. Mills WA, Youmans HD. Population exposures from natural background radiation in Kerala, India [Abstract]. Health Phys 1968;15:188.
9. Beebe GW, Kato H, Land CE. Lifespan study report 8. Mortality experiences of atomic bomb survivors 1950–74. Technical report RERF TR 1-77. Hiroshima: Radiation Effects Research Foundation.
10. Ishimaru T, Hoshina T, Ichimaru M, Okada H, Tomiyasu T. Leukaemia in atomic bomb survivors. Hiroshima and Nagasaki, 1 October 1950–30 September 1966. Radiat Res 1971;45(1):216–233.
11. Holm LE, Lundell G, Walinder G. Incidence of malignant thyroid tumors in humans after exposure to diagnostic doses of iodine-131. Retrospective cohort study. J Natl Cancer Inst 1980;64(5):1055–1059.
12. Matanoski GM, Seltser R, Sartwell PE, Diamond EL, Elliott EA. The current mortality rates of radiologists and other physician specialists: Specific causes of death. Am J Epidemiol 1975;101(3)199–210.
13. Court Brown W, Doll R. Expectation of life and mortality from cancer among British radiologists. Br Med J 1958;21:181–187.
14. Hickey RJ, Bowers EJ, Spence DE, Zemel BS, Clelland AB, Clelland RC. Low level ionizing radiation and human mortality: multi-regional epidemiological studies. Health Phys 1981;40(5):625–641.
15. Muller HJ. Artificial transmutation of the gene. Science 1927;66:84–87.
16. Advisory Committee on the Biological Effects of Ionizing Radiation. The Effects on Populations of Exposure to Low levels of Ionizing Radiation. Washington, DC: National Research Council, National Academy of Sciences, National Academy Press, 1980.
17. Harvey EB, Boice Jr JD, Honeyman M, Flannery JT. Prenatal X-ray exposure and childhood cancer in twins. N Engl J Med 1985;312(9):541–545.
18. Beebe GW. Ionizing radiation and health. Am Sci 1982;70(1):35–44.
19. Upton AC. The biological effects of low-level ionizing radiation. Sci Am 1982;246(2):41–49.
20. Sagan LS. On radiation, paradigms, and hormesis. Science 1989;245(4918):574–621.
21. Boxenbaum H, Neafsey, PJ, Fournier DJ. Hormesis, gompertz functions, and risk assessment. Drug Metab Rev 1988;19(2):195–229.

22. Congdon, CC. A review of certain low-level ionizing radiation studies in mice and guinea pigs. Health Phys 1987;52(5):593–597.
23. Wolff S, Afzal V, Wiencke JK, Olivieri G, Michaeli A. Human lymphocytes exposed to low doses of ionizing radiations become refractory to high doses of radiation as well as to chemical mutagens that include double-strand breaks in DNA. Int J Radiat Biol 1988;53(1):39–47.
24. Luckey T. Hormesis With Ionizing Radiation. Boca Raton: CRC Press, 1980.
25. Yalow RS. Reappraisal of risks associated with low level radiation. Com Mol Cell Biophys 1981;1: 149–157.
26. GAO. Problems in Assessing the Cancer Risk of Low Level Ionizing Radiation Exposure. Report to the U.S. Congress by the Comptroller General. Gaithersburg, Md: U.S. General Accounting Office, 1981;2:XVIII-43.
27. Yalow RS. Low level radiation effects [Foreword]. In: Brill BA, ed. A Fact Book. 2nd ed. New York: Society of Nuclear Medicine, 1982: vii–viii.
28. Health Effects of Exposure to Low Levels of Ionizing Radiation. Committee on the Biological Effects of Ionizing Radiations, Board on Radiation Effects, BEIR V. Washington, DC: National Academy Press, 1990.
29. Yalow RS. Commentary. Concerns with low level ionizing radiation: rational or phobic? J Nucl Med 1990;31(7):17a–18a, 26a.
30. Nuclear Regulatory Commission. Below Regulatory concern. Washington, DC: Superintendent of Documents, 1991:NUREG/BR-0157.
31. Pool R. Electromagnetic fields: the biological evidence. Science 1990;249(4975):1378–1381.
32. Jauchem JR. Electromagnetic fields and cancer [Letter to the editor]. Science 1990;250(4982):739.
33. Cartwright RA. Low frequency alternating electromagnetic fields and leukaemia: the saga so far. Br J Cancer 1989;60:649.
34. Biological Effects and Safety Aspects of Nuclear Magnetic Resonance Imaging and Spectroscopy. Sponsored by the New York Academy of Sciences, held in Bethesda, Md., May 15–17, 1991.
35. Bain L. MRI-Safety issues stimulate concern. Science 1991;252(5010):1244.

5

Risks in Diagnostic Imaging

The feasibility of an operation is not the best indication for its performance.

Lord Cohen of Birkenhead

A fundamental principle underlying any rational diagnostic philosophy must be intelligent avoidance of risky diagnostic procedures. Because the benefit of detecting a treatable disorder must be weighed against any possible risk of making a diagnosis, hazardous studies associated with *any* potential for misadventure or death must be kept to an irreducible minimum. Unnecessary clinical testing is rampant and should be discouraged, but potentially dangerous procedures are often included in a thoughtless approach to diagnosis and are coming under increasing scrutiny and criticism. It may be legally, even morally defensible, for a patient to undergo surgery, even die, as a result of a bowel perforation from *unequivocally indicated* colonoscopy; it is certainly malpractice and therefore actionable for injury or death to result from a hazardous procedure when a much safer study might have provided the necessary information. The most indefensible example is resorting to a risky procedure in a futile attempt to exclude some unlikely conditions, e.g. using endoscopy or arteriography to rule out gastric cancer or coronary disease.

As more sophisticated and dangerous technologies emerge, complications and fatalities from diagnostic procedures will inevitably increase along with adverse publicity. In the past, many such unfortunate consequences were reluctantly accepted as an unavoidable fact of life. But with increasing public education, patient advocacy groups, and skyrocketing malpractice claims, this issue should become more prominent. The predictable result will be increasing litigation. So far, we have been spared some of the lawsuits and adverse publicity. This is because of the conspiracy of silence surrounding diagnostic catastrophes, resulting in low reporting rates and, most important, public ignorance of the problem. Mishaps and deaths from diagnostic procedures are rarely reported in this country. An excellent discussion that comprehensively reviews complications and mortality of diagnostic imaging is the landmark text by Ansell and Wilkins (1). Significantly, two entire chapters are devoted to medico-legal problems. The following discussion omits the important endoscopic procedures, cystoscopy and bronchoscopy.

Intravascular Contrast Agents

Any discussion about the safety of imaging studies should address the largest risk of medical imaging, the widespread use of contrast material in CT, angiography,

Table 5.1. IV Urography Ionic Media Incidence of Reactions

	Minor reactions	Intermediate reactions	Severe reactions	Death
Fischer & Doust (1972) U.S.A.			1/1900	1/52000
Witten et al. (1973) Mayo Clinic	1/18	1/57	1/1000	1/31000
Shehadi, U.S.A. (1980)	1/29	1/60	1/2800	1/15000
Toniolo, Italy (1980)	1/31	1/130	1/1200	1/34000
Ansell et al., U.K. (1980)	1/15	1/77	1/4200	1/45000
Hobbs, Ontario (1981)			1/2000	1/93000
Pinet et al., (1982), France	1/17		1/2800	1/91000
Hartman et al. (1982), Mayo Clinic				1/75000

Reprinted by permission from *Diagnostic Imaging Supplement* (1987;9(4)part 2:12).

pyelography and other procedures. Preinjection allergy testing using classic skin or conjunctival responses to detect potential fatal reactors or using smaller intravenous test doses has failed to offer any protection from adverse reactions and deaths in several large studies. At special risk are those patients with a strong history of asthma and allergies who are more likely to develop bronchospasm or anaphylaxis. The risk of an asthmatic having a fatal reaction to intravenous contrast is conservatively estimated as 1 in 14,000 injections but is probably closer to 1 in 5,000. Some workers have claimed that pretreatment with steroids may lower total adverse reactions by about one-third, but the number of severe life-threatening reactions were the same in both treated and placebo groups (2). The protective effect of steroid treatment on mortality could not be ascertained because of the small size of population studied.

Epidemiologic studies of adverse reactions and deaths from conventional ionic or high osmolality contrast material (HOCM) reveal a significant variation in incidence reported from different centers. In intravenous urography, the rates ranged from 1 severe reaction in 1,000 at the Mayo Clinic (3) to 1 in 4,200 in the United Kingdom (4) and 1 death per 14,000 injections in Shehadi's series (5) to 1 death in 93,000 in the Ontario survey (6). In Ansell's series (7) the mortality rate was midway between these figures, 1 in 45,000. These figures are shown in Table 5.1. It is widely acknowledged that many serious reactions and fatalities are never reported and that the true incidence may be 10 or more times higher. Table 5.2 gives the yearly number of fatal reactions to contrast reported to the Food and Drug Administration between 1985 and 1989 (8) and the author's estimate of the possible true total death rate. In a personal review of a radiologic department by the author, 5 deaths were found after contrast for CT scanning in approximately 10,000 cases, an astounding rate of 1 in 2,000. It is the rare radiologist indeed who has not seen or heard of a death from contrast, yet reports of such deaths are more often suppressed in both the private office and the hospital because of malpractice fears. It seems clear that as imaging procedures such as CT and angiography increase, the numbers of severe reactions and deaths, reported or not, will continue to rise.

Most statistics do not include additional patients who suffer long-term complications which may be delayed in onset. Impaired renal function due to intravenous contrast material has an incidence of almost 0.6% in hospitalized patients without preexisting renal disease, whereas up to 75% of patients with moderate renal insufficiency can have renal function further impaired by contrast. Though much of this is reversible, in juvenile onset diabetic patients up to 90% of patients without normal

Table 5.2. Fatal Reactions to Intravenous Contrast Material Reported to the FDA, 1985–1989 (8)

Year	Number of fatalities	Est. Deaths per 100,000 Injections[a] (Hypothetical)
1985	29	1:8,620–1:17,240
1986	40	1:6,250–1:12,500
1987	19	1:13,160–1:26,314
1988	39	1:6,410–1:12,820
1989 (incomplete)	25	1:10,000–1:20,000

[a]Assuming a conservative reporting rate of 20% and a conservatively inflated total of 1.25–2.5 million injections.

Table 5.3. Clinical Features and Risk Factors of Acute Renal Failure Associated with Contrast Agents

Clinical features:
Rapid onset with oliguria
Fractional excretion of sodium less than 1%
Persistent nephrogram
Risk factors:
High risk
  Preexisting renal insufficiency
  Diabetes mellitus
Moderate Risk
  Dehydration
  Multiple myeloma
  Previous contrast nephrotoxicity
Mild Risk
  Large contrast load
  Advanced age

Reprinted with permission from *Diagnostic Imaging Supplement* (1987;9(4)part 2:12).

renal function develop more severe renal insufficiency after contrast, and up to 50% of these patients never return to their baseline renal function (9). Table 5.3 enumerates the clinical features and risk factors associated with this complication.

One of the most interesting advances in radiology has been the recent development of low osmolar iodine-containing contrast material (LOCM), often referred to as nonionic media. In the past 15 years numerous studies have demonstrated that toxic effects of contrast media can be significantly reduced with the use of these agents (10). High-risk asthmatic and allergic patients, individuals over 50, those with a previous history of adverse reactions, cardiac disease, etc., have a 2- and 5-fold greater incidence of severe reactions with HOCM compared to the newer LOCM agents (11, 12). Serious problems still occur, but the overall incidence of all reactions appears to be at least 50% less than that reported for ionic agents. In a large Japanese study involving almost 340,000 patients (170,000 each in low and high osmolar groups) the authors reported an incidence of all grades of reaction four times higher in the HOCM group, with severe reactions being six times greater (13). The overall risk ratio for severe reactions was approximately 6:1 in favor of LOCM over HOCM in the Australasia and the Japanese series of over 447,000 patients (14). King et al. (10) caution, however, that mortality rates have been difficult to estimate because of lack of large well-controlled studies. They further state that whether LOCM offers any reduction in rates of contrast-associated nephropathy remains to be demonstrated. Others claim that mortality rates for LOCM agents appear to be only 10–20% of those associated with conventional ionic preparations (3, 11, 12).

Although the cost of LOCM agents is high (their average price is 8–15 times that of HOCM media) their added safety, according to Palmer (13) "is such that their ultimate universal acceptance is inevitable." At the present time he and others believe that there are "no patient groups where the continued use of the ionic agents can be justified on scientific grounds" (13). (This may be inaccurate in view of the continuing controversy over the thrombogenic effects of LOCM in arteriography.)

Even if only some of their advantages are acknowledged, the low osmolar compounds will undoubtedly force us to reconsider medical policy. Unfortunately, there will be a long delay before the expense of these new agents comes down sufficiently for routine reimbursement approval by insurers. Until that time the cost will discourage their wider employment. At the present time serious discussions on this issue are taking place between the American College of Radiology, other physician groups, and fiscal intermediaries. One must question whether it is now justifiable to continue using ionic agents in certain high-risk groups, such as the elderly and asthmatics, given our present state of knowledge. The possibility of litigation resulting from reactions to HOCM agents has already been raised, particularly in instances when a patient has *not* been informed of the alternative choice of a *safer* compound. If, as expected, the LOCM agents continue to demonstrate superior safety records, it will be hard to justify the continued use of conventional (HOCM) agents for most patients.

Angiography: General Facts

Systemic reactions to intravascular contrast material are reportedly lower with intraarterial as compared to intravenous administration. This is probably due in part to dilution of the hyperosmolar solution during its passage through the peripheral circulation. Nevertheless, direct organ injury can occur, for example in the brain, or in the heart where stroke, arrhythmias, or cardiac standstill may be induced. Major contributors to risk are patient factors such as age, preexisting disease, bleeding tendencies, hypertension, etc. Catheter problems, postangiographic care, and the skill of the angiographic team all affect complications. Catheter thrombogenicity is a common and troublesome problem with a frequency of thrombus deposition reported to be between 44% and 100% (14–16). Thromboembolic complications caused by red cell clumping have been reported more frequently in *nonionic (LOCM)* contrast material, despite systemic heparinization (16). Major vascular complications from arterial catheterization and injection are relatively infrequent but can include arterial thrombosis, embolism, hematoma, and pseudoaneurysm formation. Moreover, angiographic jets which produce high intravascular pressures always create opportunities for disasters such as perforation and dissection.

Coronary Angiography

Various side effects of direct injection of contrast material into the coronary vasculature include the production of arrhythmias, inhibition of the conducting system, depression of myocardial contractility, and autonomic nervous system disturbances. Several large surveys have revealed a nonfatal complication rate of about 1%. In one series the incidence of ventricular fibrillation was 1.28% (17). Mortality directly related to the action of contrast material occurs with a frequency of 0.05% (18–20), or 1 in 2000 cases. In a cooperative VA study from 13 centers of 1483 patients undergoing cardiac catheterization for valvular heart disease, complications were reported in 6.9% of 1559 preoperative procedures of which 2.6% were major and 0.2% were fatal. Presumably, these results occurred in a highly select group of patients, but no estimated pretest likelihood of operable disease was given (21).

According to a report of the Society for Cardiac Angiography and Interventions (22), of 222,553 patients studied nationally between 1984 and 1987, 218 deaths occurred (0.098%), or almost *1 in 1,000*. This is similar to the Mount Sinai experience in New York (23), with 53,581 patients studied between 1982 and 1984 and reported the same year. Increased risk was related to age over 50, poor functional classification, presence of left main coronary disease, and an ejection fraction less than 30%.

Pulmonary Angiography

Mortality of pulmonary arteriography may be greater than that of coronary arteriography (1). Right heart catheterization with forcible injection of contrast into the pulmonary arteries is most hazardous in patients with significant pulmonary hypertension, the very condition apt to be present in patients undergoing this study because of pulmonary embolism itself. This increases the risk of dangerous arrhythmias, pulmonary edema, and death. *The appropriate use of ventilation and perfusion lung scintigraphy should make pulmonary angiography unnecessary in the overwhelming majority of cases of suspected pulmonary embolism.* The subject has been recently summarized in an excellent review by Juni and Alavi (24). These authors quote studies reporting significant interobserver disagreement in the interpretation of pulmonary angiograms (25) and state that the "V/Q scan and pulmonary angiography have *quite similar reliability* as assessed by agreement between two different interpreters. . . . The patients with greatest disagreement between V/Q scan and pulmonary angiogram, those in the low- and intermediate-probability scan categories, are also those in which there is least certainty in angiography."

Cerebral Angiography

Carotid angiography after cerebral hemorrhage was associated with a complication rate of 1.7% with 1 patient out of 2509 dying of thromboembolism (26). In 242 patients studied for intracranial aneurysms, worsening of the neurological condition occurred in 5.8% of patients, often as late as several days after the procedure (27). In another report, transient complications in cerebral angiography were seen in 4.5% of patients with transient ischemic attacks and 7.7% of patients with evolving strokes. The authors emphasized that a stroke in progress had too high a complication rate to warrant study (28).

A study of 713 patients with 749 catheter arteriographies of aortic arch and cerebral vessels using LOCM showed neurological complications in 6.4% of studies and concluded that nonionic contrast did not drastically lower the rate of these complications (29). Fatal complications of arteriography, although rare, are discussed in an Italian study (30), which describes distal macro- and microembolization with irretrievable loss of tissue perfusion. One of the greatest contributions of CT and MRI to CNS diagnosis has been their significant effect in reducing the number of patients undergoing cerebral angiography.

Direct Imaging. Gastrointestinal Endoscopy: Esophagogastroduodenoscopy (EGD), ERCP, Colonoscopy, and Laparoscopy
UPPER GASTROINTESTINAL ENDOSCOPY AND THE UPPER GI SERIES

> *Every hospital should have a plaque in the physicians' and students'*
> *entrances: "There are some patients whom we cannot help, there are*
> *none whom we cannot harm."*
> *Arthur L. Bloomfield (1888–1962).*
> *Personal communication after iatrogenic tragedy.*

Let us imagine we are living in 1965 and are suddenly transported to the future. The scene is an immaculate, luminous white room containing medical equipment, including a "crash cart" and other resuscitative and monitoring equipment. A physician and a nurse are in attendance. The patient, who is supine and unresponsive, is attached to an electrocardiographic monitor. Extending from his finger is a lead from an oximeter. He is anesthetized. Question: Where are we and what is going on? We are in an operating room, of course, and surgery of some type is being performed. A *diagnostic* procedure you say? Nonsense.

This, of course, is fact, not fiction. A recent survey sponsored by the American Society for Gastrointestinal Endoscopy (ASGE) (31) showed that among more than 200 experienced endoscopists, 99% used electronic monitoring during EGD in the hospital but only 27% in the office. Most patients received "conscious sedation" with Meperidine and intravenous Midazolam, diazepam, or Naloxone. Cardiopulmonary sedation-related complications had a "low annual occurrence rate of 0.5% [sic]." In practice, up to 90% or more of patients undergoing the procedure are given some type of intravenous sedation (usually a benzodiazepam drug) with or without narcotic premedication. This is simply because the procedure is so unpleasant that a struggling patient without proper restraint could easily suffer esophageal or gastric perforation, one of the most common complications even in the anesthetized subject. Because intravenous benzodiazepam with narcotic, despite the euphemism *conscious sedation*, is, in fact, general anesthesia (otherwise, why would patients require monitoring?), there has been the threat of turf battles with the anesthesiologists. The ASGE and the American Society of Anesthesiologists have had discussions after the Joint Commission for Accreditation of Health Care Organizations included "analgesia/sedation that may result in loss of protective reflexes" in its anesthesia and surgical standards. The issue has probably not yet been settled to everyone's satisfaction, and it is probable that the final adjudications will take place in the courts (32). When this will occur depends both on sorely needed and improved legal guidelines for the definitions of malpractice in cases of mishap or death from a diagnostic procedure, and the reporting of these events to families and the authorities. The under-reporting problem is not apt to be resolved without careful epidemiologic surveillance of all patients undergoing various procedures. Because only about 10% of serious drug reactions are reported, one can only guess at the actual number of serious complications and deaths resulting from endoscopic and other diagnostic procedures. We do, however, know certain facts:

1. In one of the largest recently reported series consisting of 252,888 EGDs from a specialty clinic in Switzerland, Miller (33) disclosed 205 serious complications, (cardiovascular, pulmonary, and GI perforations), a rate of 0.081% (1:1,237) and 17 deaths, a mortality rate of 0.007% (1:14,875).

2. For 1987 and 1988, respectively, 27 and 18 endoscopically related deaths were reported per 100,000 examinations in U.S. Vital Statistics (ICD diagnostic code E870.4). This death rate translates to 1 in 3,703 and 1 in 5,555 procedures, respectively (34). The specific endoscopic procedures were not separately coded, so we must assume the figures represent an average that includes both higher-risk (colonoscopy, ERCP, and laparoscopy) and more frequently performed procedures. (EGD is the most commonly performed endoscopic study.) Acknowledging the reporting problem, we can still conclude that 1 death per 3,703–5,555 endoscopic procedures must be taken as an *absolute minimum* figure overall for all endoscopic procedures.

Economic factors by themselves, though important, can never make a convincing argument against the inappropriate use of diagnostic studies. In diagnosis, the more important issue is benefit vs. risk rather than vs. cost. This fundamental principle has been virtually ignored in all the position papers, review articles, and general writings on the subject.

Direct imaging of the upper gastrointestinal tract has increased rapidly and widely throughout Western countries since the introduction of the fiber optic panendoscope by Hershowitz in 1963 (35) and is now the most commonly employed endoscopic procedure. In recent years EGD has become so popular and has replaced upper gastrointestinal barium X-ray studies to such an extent, the astounding suggestion (apparently already heeded) has been made that EGD could be substituted for the upper GI on a routine basis (36). It is understandable that endoscopists are of this opinion, but its indiscriminate acceptance by many physicians and fiscal intermediaries as a routine substitute for prior upper and lower GI barium studies is nothing less than a national disgrace. In a far less captious tone, "Routine diagnostic upper and lower GI endoscopy is enormously costly to the public with little demonstrable benefit" (personal communication, Feb 15, 1993 Dr. David Gelfand, Professor of Radiology, Bowman-Gray School of Medicine). Dr. Gelfand and Dr. David Ott, whose work is later cited, have reviewed published figures on morbidity and mortality rates of EGD and colonoscopy. Gelfand estimates that the total cost to the health care system of failing to perform routine upper and lower GI studies before deciding on the need for endoscopy is between $2–4 billion. Some idea of the problem may be gleaned from the following quote taken from the current classic reference on gastrointestinal endoscopy (37) published in 1987:

> Although EGD is *reasonably* safe, it is not perfectly so. The incidence of untoward events varies somewhat, depending on methods of collecting data ... Three relatively large series representing experience from the United States, Great Britain and Denmark (were) summarized (38–40). ... In more than 250,000 EGD procedures, the incidence of a fatal complication was *3 per 10,000*. The commonest complications (*13 per 10,000*) were aspiration or cardiac problems, or both, that were often related to the effects of sedative drugs. Major morbid events occurred in *20 per*

10,000 cases; in addition, minor complications were associated
with nearly *1*% of procedures (emphasis added).

A national survey in France (41), reporting the results from 150,000 examinations,
indicated similar rates of complications and mortality: 0.1% and 0.03%, respectively.
The complication rate for endoscopy in the upper GI bleeder reported by the ASGE
survey (42) showed a much higher rate of 0.9%, but a rate of 5% with 2% mortality
also has been reported in older patients (43). These are earlier references with astonishingly high complication and fatality rates. Yet the mortality rates of 1972-1979 are
almost *identical* to those reported for total endoscopic deaths by the U.S. Public
Health Service (CDC) in 1987 (34). If one compares Miller's 1987 (33) with Silvis'
1974 ASGE series (44), the complication rate was lower in the latter series (0.08% vs.
0.13%), but the mortality rate was higher (0.007% vs. 0.004%). The two series are
separated in time and place, but they summarize results obtained by skilled endoscopists.

Our literature searches for any large recent American series on complications and
mortality of EGD have been unsuccessful. Since the 1974 series (44) the ASGE surprisingly discontinued collecting statistics on complications and mortality for EGD,
since an inquiry to them elicited this reply: "I am not aware of any recent data reporting complications or mortality rates for upper and lower gastrointestinal endoscopy. Our Standards of Practice Committee has not addressed this issue by survey or
formal literature review" (Keeffe, E. B., Chairman, Standards of Practice Committee,
ASGE, personal communication). Furthermore, the true rates of misadventures and
deaths have always been reported in series by experienced endoscopists, which might
well be falsely low compared to results by the inexperienced, in particular gastroenterologists in training. The reporting problem, however, is unlikely to go away in the
foreseeable future, so we may never know the true risks of EGD. In New York City
alone in 1988, two deaths from upper endoscopy were reported (New York Department of Vital and Health Statistics, personal communication). Assuming a conservative reporting rate of 10% and extrapolating to the U.S. population, this is equivalent
to 250 deaths, almost the same figure one obtains using the U.S. Vital Statistics data
(34).

Thomas Hodgkin, the British physician for whom the disease was named, reportedly once offended a rich patient by charging him too little, a 19th century parable
for our own times. Thus, the quality of medical care is often a blind item, and many
patients equate value with the fee charged. The average EGD costs from $500–1200
and up, compared with $150–275 for an upper GI series. In view of the increased
expense, various complications, including death, and no verifiable diagnostic advantage (45, 46), one must question the logic and motivation for making endoscopy a
routine procedure.

Newer radiographic techniques using air contrast have greatly improved the early
detection of gastric and esophageal malignancies and other lesions so that the overall
sensitivity and specificity of the upper GI series is comparable or superior to that of
EGD. (47) Endoscopy may be required in clarifying equivocal or persistently abnormal upper GI esophageal/barium studies, but it should *never* be used to screen for
conditions with an extremely low prevalence, nor can its use be justified in lieu of the
upper GI study.

There is no epidemiological evidence to suggest that the introduction of upper GI endoscopy has affected the overall survival of gastric cancer patients in Western countries (48). Holdstock and Bruce (49) found that the availability of "open access endoscopy" resulted in a 10-fold increase in endoscopies performed without demonstrable effect on overall prognosis or on the proportion of early gastric cancers diagnosed. As we have emphasized, *all* diagnostic procedures, no matter how sensitive or specific, have *very poor* predictive ability when used in a population with low disease prevalence. In this circumstance, false-positive studies are frequent—and inevitably lead to further expensive and needless investigation. Furthermore, the use of indiscriminate endoscopy in a setting of overwhelmingly common and benign conditions, such as ulcer and nonulcer dyspepsias, motility disorders, nonspecific abdominal pain, and functional GI disease, must be regarded with shock and dismay. This is certainly contrary to the opinion of official, self-appointed committees (again, the *consensus* problem) (50). Ott, Gelfand, and their associates (46, 48, 51) have written extensively on the problem of inappropriate EGD and colonoscopy and the declining use of the upper and lower GI series and have made significant contributions to our appreciation of the problem.

The National Center for Health Statistics (NCHS) procedure data for the years 1985–1989 (52), shown in a later chapter, demonstrate the ratio of EGDs performed in U.S. hospitals to upper GI studies changed from 2:1 in 1985 to more than 5:1 in 1990, associated with more than a 50% decline in the radiographic procedure (52). This steady drop in upper GI series performed demonstrates what is really happening: an expensive, risky, unpleasant *diagnostic* procedure with *known complications and documented mortality* has been permitted to replace an established imaging technique of at least *equal* if not *superior* effectiveness, at a cost to the health care system of $1–2 billion.

If the trend of replacing the upper (and lower) GI barium study with EGD and colonoscopy (vide infra) continues, as it is likely to do without an informed public and profession (this will also require the elimination of self-referral), a familiar disease of medical progress will occur: fewer radiologists in training will become proficient in performing barium contrast studies, as has already been happening, and ultimately the study will disappear by default. If that is permitted to occur, it will be an unprecedented tragedy for medicine and the hapless public, resulting in *billions of dollars* spent and the occurrence of *hundreds of needless deaths* per year.

Endoscopic Retrograde Cholangiopancreatography (ERCP)

To the man with a 'scope, every patient harbors a gastric cancer.
Anonymous

Like its sister modality, upper GI endoscopy, ERCP has enjoyed enormous and uncritical acceptance by the medical community in recent years. (The discussion that follows is not directed toward therapeutic applications.) ERCP is quickly becoming a leading method for studying the pancreas and biliary tract, despite the widespread availability of overwhelmingly easier, safer, cheaper, and generally more consistently reliable sonography, hepatobiliary scintigraphy, and CT. That this has come to pass is again a serious indictment of both the medical profession and third-party payers who have permitted this to take place.

The complication rate of diagnostic ERCP is significantly higher than EGD at 2–7%, with a mortality rate of 0.1–0.8% (53, 54). Hyperamylasemia may occur in up to 60–75% of patients when the pancreatic duct is explored (55), and acute pancreatitis may occur in anywhere from 1.0–17% of patients (56–60). The rate of resultant ascending cholangitis is significant but is difficult to estimate from the literature. The above-quoted important series of Bilbao et al. (54) involving a study of 10,000 cases from 402 owners of duodenoscopes revealed procedure failures occurring in 30%, complications in 3%, and death in 0.2% (55). Although this study was published in 1974, it was based on reports from experienced endoscopists using equipment similar to that used today.

Summary of EGD and ERCP

It is obvious that diagnostic studies carrying significant risk of major complication or mortality should be limited to serious conditions with a high enough pretest probability to justify the risk. Thus, no one would dispute the decision to perform EGD if there is evidence or a high suspicion of esophageal obstruction or gastric cancer based on radiographic findings. However, several major questions arising from the wide-spread use of EGD demand an answer from the endoscopists. Among them are the following:

1. Is EGD, described as a "gold standard" by its devotees, superior to clinical judgment in diagnosing the most commonly encountered gastrointestinal complaints—nonulcer dyspepsia, nonspecific abdominal pain, irritable bowel syndrome, and functional disorders—or is it simply a ruling out strategy?

2. As a corollary, how can endoscopy, which is only an anatomic test, replace radiologic and nuclear studies, which yield both anatomic and physiologic information? Motility disorders are associated with many benign gastrointestinal complaints, both functional and nonfunctional, and therefore are not *imageable* by endoscopy in the first place. What is the justification for using this potentially risky procedure in the largest group of GI patients, those with benign disease?

3. As a rule, only one person looks through the endoscope. Although radiographs are taken during ERCP, who will confirm or contradict EGD findings reported? How often are studies photographed or videotaped? Where indeed is a *permanent record* of the endoscopic study for review, corroboration, or refutation by other experts?

4. With respect to ERCP, why do physicians use a technique with a high potential for complications and death when simpler, more sensitive, safer, and much less expensive procedures are available? On reviewing the index to Sivak's text (61), references to hepatobiliary scintigraphy were absent. Only one passing reference to hepatobiliary scintigraphy was given by the Patient Care Committee of the American Gastroenterological Association in a recent major review on imaging in obstructive jaundice (62).

Colonoscopy

Colonoscopy, endoscopic examination of the entire colon to the ileocecal valve, should be distinguished from flexible sigmoidoscopy ("flex sig"), examination up to the splenic flexure or below. Colonoscopy, unlike flex sig, which is virtually (though not entirely) risk free, is associated with a complication and mortality rate significantly higher than upper GI endoscopy and perhaps even ERCP. Much controversy continues to surround the relative indications for colonoscopy vs. barium enema with or without flex sig in the detection and surveillance of colon cancer.

For example, only 1–2% of polyps 6 mm to 1 cm and only 5% of polyps 1–2 cm are malignant (63–66). Search-and-destroy biopsy/fulguration for polyps smaller than 0.5–1 cm would result in an unacceptable mortality and morbidity, ethically unacceptable in view of any potential benefits. Furthermore, the sensitivity of double-contrast barium enema examination for detection of polyps larger than 1 cm is 82–98%, but the risk of perforation during barium enema examination is less than 1 in 50,000, whereas the risk of perforation during colonoscopy varies from *1 in 50* to *1 in 500* (67, 68). Examination of the distal colon may be incomplete in 16–43% of colonoscopies (69, 70). There is no evidence of any decrease in mortality from the procedure over the past decade, and in point of fact, Gelfand (46, 48) has quoted statistics and estimated that 1 in 5,000 patients can be expected to die as a result of the procedure. There are no unbiased controlled studies comparing double-contrast barium enema examination and colonoscopy in the diagnosis of cancer (68–71). Both methods appear to be equally accurate for well-established cancers with a sensitivity of more than 85%, but barium enema without flexible sigmoidoscopy cannot always be relied upon alone for examination of the lower rectosigmoid. It is highly doubtful that flex sig needs to be extended beyond the sigmoid in the case of a negative barium enema. Of course, those patients with an abnormal barium enema proximal to the splenic flexure will ultimately have to undergo colonoscopy for biopsy or polypectomy.

On balance, we are in favor of barium enema/flex sig as the mainstay in cancer diagnosis, reserving colonoscopy for surveillance (postoperative cancer resection patients), high-risk patients with a familial history or previous polyps, and those with suspicious proximal lesions. This seems to be the most cost-effective and, more important, by far the safer strategy.

Laparoscopy

With diagnostic laparoscopy we again encounter the issues of false expectations, economic influences, and changing practice patterns giving rise to the widespread application of an expensive, risky, and immensely overrated and inappropriately used procedure (72). As with other highly touted endoscopic studies, one is reminded of the humorist Wilson Mizener's remark, "I respect faith, but doubt is what gets you an education."

A wide variety of complications and misadventures may result from diagnostic laparoscopy, including cardiovascular collapse (73, 74), necrotizing fasciitis (75), intraabdominal hemorrhage, peritonitis, hydropneumothorax (76), and even retinal hemorrhage. (77). One 14-year analysis of 1121 diagnostic laparoscopies performed in gastroenterology patients (more than 50% of examinations were for malignant disease) reported 9.8% minor and 1.8% major complications including 1 death. Major complications included abdominal wall hematoma, perforated abdominal viscus, hemoperitoneum, bleeding from liver biopsy, and respiratory depression (78). The authors add in an intriguing understatement (1987), "We observed a trend to decreased use of laparoscopy." This paper underscores the fact that, except for a few centers, diagnostic laparoscopy (for chronic conditions) and outside the pelvis is not currently a popular procedure.

This is changing, however, with the rapid increase in laparoscopic surgery, which has significantly enhanced the value of the procedure as a substitute for open abdominal or pelvic surgery. The use of laparoscopy in diagnosing difficult cases of the acute abdomen is being reassessed, particularly because it may be useful as a combined diagnostic-therapeutic procedure (79). For example, laparascopic appendectomy is increasingly being performed. We enthusiastically endorse the use of diagnostic laparoscopy in the difficult acute abdomen, especially in the aged and in other suitable patients.

Despite the brilliant success in imaging the pelvis with ultrasonography, the use of diagnostic pelvic laparoscopy continues to soar. The mortality rate has been reported as 2.5–10 per 100,000 (1:10,000–1:40,000) (80). Formerly, the major complication rate (any complication necessitating laparotomy) was 4–6 per 1000 (81). An excellent review of this subject can be found in Sivak's text (82).

Medico-legal problems as a consequence of this procedure are not limited to the United States. One French study (83) reported on 200 gynecological cases leading to legal action in the civil or criminal courts. Thirty-two cases stemmed from pelvic laparoscopy, among which more than one-third resulted in death. Although some of these cases were laparoscopic sterilization procedures, the actual percentages are not known. A German legal journal also published a study (84), which included a report of 2 deaths and quoted "international statistics" of 3.5 per 1000 for complications. A 7-year prospective study of the complication rate for diagnostic pelvic laparoscopy in 603 U.S. patients (85) revealed 5.1% minor and 2.3% major complications with 3 (0.49%) deaths. These complication rates are 5- and 7-fold higher than those reported in retrospective studies in the literature. The authors conclude that retrospective studies have underestimated the complication rate of laparoscopy.

It is exceedingly difficult to reconcile the widespread use of *nonacute* diagnostic laparoscopy with the universal availability of ultrasonography, a modality that, combined with the history and pelvic examination, is more than 98% accurate for gynecological diagnosis. We have seen countless patients with obvious pelvic inflammatory disease, endometriosis, ovarian cysts, or nonspecific pelvic pain subjected to laparoscopy. More important, we continue to be alarmed and dismayed about those patients in whom laparoscopy is performed *before* or *instead of* pelvic ultrasound. It is astounding that most health insurers do not even require routine ultrasound before laparoscopy, nor is pelvic laparoscopy in the presence of a normal pelvic sonogram ever questioned, although little or no additional information is likely to be obtained.

Closing Remarks on Upper GI Endoscopy, ERCP, and Laparoscopy

> *The public will choose to believe a simple lie in preference to a complicated truth.*
>
> *Alexis de Tocqueville*

Like the audience who anxiously awaits its diva to appear on stage and perform her famous aria, we have come to expect our invasive specialists to arrive armed with their 'scopes and retinue of assistants and trainees to observe them performing their feats of technical brilliance. Is it any wonder our consultants oblige us by singing their familiar tunes every time the opportunity for their services arises? What can the lowly gastroenterologist or gynecologist offer, a barium meal or a sonogram of the pelvis? Besides, the patient and his family will clamor for the latest test anyway, under the assumption that "newer is better," and the specialist is always right. After all, who worries about cost containment if the insurance will pay? Although all these factors are operating to make us slaves of our technological enhancements, "the fault, dear Brutus, is not in our stars, but in ourselves, that we are underlings." And "lo, men have become the tool of their tools."

In a more modern metaphor we are seeing a phenomenon that the French have long recognized. It is called *deformation professionelle*. The definition given in *Harrap's New Standard French and English Dictionary* is "professional idiosyncrasy: vocational bias." This hints at the term's broader meaning: *a view of reality biased by one's profession*.

If only all specialists could have the valuable experience of a few years in primary care practice before settling into their little niches. Even the rotating internship, which was once a requirement for licensure in most states, remains an educational relic. The world seen through an endoscope is a microcosm, more often reflecting the narrow view of the specialist rather than the clinical reality of the patient's need. Someone has remarked that modern physicians are busier doing things *to* patients than *for* them. This is particularly applicable to the vast majority of endoscopic procedures.

We can think of no more appropriate final quotation for this chapter than that of the great physician and medical educator, Dr. Paul B. Beeson (86), who said:

> There are risks, too, in many of our present invasive diagnostic procedures. In a manner of speaking, the recent scientific and technologic explosion in clinical medicine has created its own kind of pollution. One of the most important qualities needed by today's physician is ability to restrain curiosity. We should adhere to the rule that a potentially injurious diagnostic procedure should be carried out only when its possible benefit to that patient justifies the risk. A test should never be done just for the sake of "thoroughness," that is to say, before someone else suggests that it be done, or because a specialist feels it must be done to protect his or her reputation, "just in case" . . . .

REFERENCES

1. Ansell G, Wilkins RA. Complications in Diagnostic Imaging. 2nd Ed. Oxford: Blackwell Scientific Publications, 1987
2. Lasser EC, Berry CC, Talner LB, et al. Pretreatment with corticosteroids to alleviate reactions to intravenous contrast material. N Engl J Med 1987;317(14):845–849.
3. Witten DM, Hirsch FD, Hartman GW. Acute reactions to urographic contrast medium. Incidence, clinical characteristics and relationship to history of hypersensitivity states. Am J Roentgenol Radium Ther Nucl Med 1973;119(4):832–840.
4. Ansell G, Tweedie MCK, West CR, et al. The current status of reactions to intravenous contrast media. Invest Radiol 1980;15(suppl 6):S32–S39.
5. Shehadi WH, Toniolo G. Adverse reactions to contrast media. A report from the Committee on Safety of Contrast Media of the International Society of Radiology. Radiology 1980;137(2):299–302.
6. Hobbs BB. Adverse reactions to intravenous contrast agents in Ontario, 1973–1979. J Can Assoc Radiol 1981;32(1):8–10.
7. Ansell G. An epidemiologic report on adverse reactions in urography: ionic and nonionic media. Diagn Imaging 1987;9(suppl 4)part 2:6–10.

8. Information obtained from the Food and Drug Administration pursuant to the Freedom of Information Act. Inquiry 1989;F89-32044.
9. Humes HD, Cieslinski DA, Messana, JM. Pathogenesis of radio-contrast-induced acute renal failure: comparative nephrotoxicity of diatrizoate and iopamidol. Diagn Imaging 1987;9(suppl 4)part 2:12–18.
10. King BF, Hartman GW, Williamson Jr B, et al. Low-osmolality contrast media: a current perspective. Mayo Clin Proc 1989;64(8):976–985.
11. Schrott KM, Behrends B, Clauss W, Kaufmann J, Hehnert J. Iohexol in excretory urography: results of the drug-monitoring program. Fortschr Med 1986;104(7):153–156.
12. Katayama H. Report of the Japanese Committee on the Safety of Contrast Media. Scientific Poster Session presented at the Radiological Society of North America Meeting, Chicago, Ill., 1988.
13. Palmer FJ. The RACR survey of intravenous contrast media reactions: final report. Australas Radiol 1988;32(4):426–428.
14. Siegelmann SS, Caplan LH, Annes GP. Complications of catheter angiography: study with oscillometry and "pullout" angiograms. Radiology 1968;91(2):251–253.
15. Jacobsson B, Bergentz SE, Ljungqvist U. Platelet adhesion and thrombus formation on vascular catheters in dogs. Acta Radiol 1969;8(3):221–227.
16. Bjork L, Enghof E, Grenvik A, et al. Local circulatory changes following brachial artery catheterization. Vasc Dis 1965;2(5):283–292.
17. Bettmann M. Ionic vs. nonionic contrast agents and their effects on blood components: clinical summary and conclusions. Invest Radiol 1988;23(Suppl 2):S378–S380.
18. Adams DF, Fraser DB, Abrams HL. The complications of coronary arteriography. Circulation 1973;48(3):609–618.
19. Bourassa MG, Noble J. Complication rate of coronary arteriography. A review of 5250 cases studied by percutaneous femoral technique. Circulation 1976;53(1):106–114.
20. Lebowitz WB, Lucia W. Complications of selective percutaneous transfemoral coronary arteriography. Radiology 1975;116(3):545–547.
21. Folland ED, Oprian C, Giacomini J, et al. Complications of cardiac catheterization and angiography in patients with valvular heart disease. VA Cooperative Study on Valvular Heart Disease. Cath Cardiovasc Diag 1989;17(1):15–21.
22. Lozner EC, Johnson LW, Johnson S, et al. Coronary arteriography 1984–1987: a report of the Registry of the Society for Cardiac Angiography and Interventions. II. An analysis of 218 deaths related to coronary arteriography. Cathet Cardiovasc Diagn 1989;17(1):11–14.
23. Kennedy JW, Baxley WA, Bunnel IL, et al. Mortality related to cardiac catheterization and angiography. Cathet Cardiovasc Diagn 1982;8(4):323–340.
24. Juni JE, Alavi A. Lung scanning in the diagnosis of pulmonary embolism: the emperor redressed. Semin Nucl Med 1991;XXI(4):281–296.
25. Quinn ME, Lundell CJ, Klotz TA, et al. Reliability of selective pulmonary arteriography in the diagnosis of pulmonary embolism. AJR 1987;149(3):469–471.
26. Skalpe IO. Complications in cerebral angiography with iohexol (omnipaque) and meglumine metrizoate (isopaque cerebral). Neuroradiology 1988;30(1):69–72.
27. Zareba A, Sadowski Z, Dowzenko A. The risk of complications of cerebral angiography in patients with cerebral aneurysms in relation to the time of its use. Neurol Neurochir Pol 1988;22(1):55–60
28. Theodotou BC, Whaley R, Mahaley MS. Complications following trans-femoral cerebral angiography for cerebral ischemia. Report of 159 angiograms and correlation with surgical risk. Surg Neurol 1987;28(2):90–92.
29. Gross-Fengels W, Mödder U, Beyer D, Neufang KF, Godehardt E. Complications of brachiocephalic catheter angiography using a non-ionic contrast medium. Radiologe 1987;27(2):83–88.
30. Gasparini M, Arosi OM, Galbiati N, et al. Neurological complications of cerebral angiography. Ital J Neurol Sci 1986;7(3):353–357.
31. Keefe EB, O'Connor. 1989 A.S.G.E. survey of endoscopic sedation and monitoring practices. Gastrointest Endosc 1990;36(Suppl 3):S13–S18.
32. Pollner P. Endoscopy generates a skirmish. Med World News 1989;July 10:10–11.
33. Miller G. Complications of endoscopy of the upper gastrointestinal tract. Leber Magen Darm 1987;17(5):299–304.
34. Vital Statistics of the United States, 1987, 1988. Mortality. U.S. Department of Health and Human Services (Public Health Service, Centers for Disease Control, National Center for Health Statistics). Hyattsville, Md: DHHS Publication (PHS) 90-1102. Section 1-General Mortality, 1988;II:208.
35. Hershowitz BI. A fiber optic flexible oesophagoscope. Lancet 1963;2:388.
36. Dooley CP, Weiner JM, Larsen AW. Endoscopy or radiography? The patient's choice. Am J Med 1986;80(2):203–207.

37. Carey WD. Indications contraindications and complications of upper gastrointestinal endoscopy. In: Sivak MV, ed. Gastroenterologic Endoscopy. Philadelphia: WB Saunders Co., 1987:296–306.
38. Mandelstam P, Sugawa C, Silvas SE, Nebel OT, Rogers BH. Complications associated with esophagogastroduodenoscopy and with esophageal dilation. Gastrointest Endosc 1976;23(1):16–19.
39. Andersen KE, Clausen N. Outpatient gastroscopy risks. Endoscopy 1978;10(3):180–183.
40. Schiller KF, Cotton PB, Salmon PR. The hazards of digestive fiber-endoscopy: a survey of British experience [Abstract]. Gut 1972;13(12):1027.
41. Hancy A, Condat M, Cougard A, et al. Les accidents de la fibroscopic oeso-gastro-duodenale. Enquete nationale portant sur 150,000 fibroscopies oeso-gastro-duodenales. Ann Gastroenterol Hepatol 1977;13:101–110.
42. Gilbert DA, Silverstein FE, Tedesco FJ, and 277 members of the American Society for Gastrointestinal Endoscopy. National A.S.G.E. Survey on upper gastrointestinal bleeding: complications of endoscopy 1981;26(suppl 7):55s–59s.
43. Noel D, Delage Y, Liguory C, et al. Haemorragies digestives d'origine haute chez les sujets de plus de 65 ans. Apport de l'endoscopie. Nouv Presse Med 1979;8(8):589–591.
44. Silvis SE, Nebel O, Rogers G, Sugawa C, Mandelstam P. Endoscopic complications: results of the 1974 American Society for Gastrointestinal Endoscopy Survey. JAMA 1976;235(9):928–930.
45. Shaw PC, van Romunde LK, Griffioen G, Janssens AR, Kreuning J, Eilers GA. Peptic ulcer and gastric carcinoma: diagnosis with biphasic radiography compared with fiberoptic endoscopy. Radiology 1987;163(1):39–42.
46. Gelfand DW, Ott DJ, Munitz HA, Chen YM. Radiology and endoscopy: a radiologic viewpoint. Ann Intern Med 1984;101(4):550–552.
47. Fraser GM, Earnshaw PM. The double-contrast barium meal: a correlation with endoscopy. Clin Radiol 1983;34(2):121–131.
48. Gelfand DW. Radiology and endoscopy. In: Taveras JM, Ferrucci JT, eds. Radiology-Diagnosis-Imaging-Intervention. Philadelphia: J. B. Lippincott Co., 1988:1–10.
49. Holdstock G, Bruce S. Endoscopy and gastric cancer. Gut 1981;22:673–676.
50. Health and Public Policy Committee, American College of Physicians. Position paper. Endoscopy in the evaluation of dyspepsia. Ann Intern Med 1985;102(2):266–269.
51. Ott DJ, Wu WC, Gelfand DW. Reflux esophagitis revisited: prospective analysis of radiologic accuracy. Gastrointest Radiol 1981;6(1):1–7.
52. U.S. Department of Health and Human Services, U.S. Public Health Service, Centers for Disease Control and the National Center for Health Statistics. National Hospital Discharge Survey (NHDS). Detailed diagnoses, procedures, days of care, diagnoses-related groups for patients discharged from short-stay hospitals. Public Use Data Diskettes, 1985–1990.
53. Cotton PB. E.R.C.P. Gut 1977;18(4):316–341.
54. Bilbao MK, Dotter CT, Lee TG, Katon RM. Complications of endoscopic retrograde cholangiopancreatography (E.R.C.P.). A study of 10,000 cases. Gastroenterology 1976;70(3):314–320.
55. Blackwood W, Venes J, Silvas S. Post-endoscopy pancreatitis and hyperamylasemia. Gastrointest Endosc 1978;20:56–58.
56. Cotton PB. Cannulation of the papilla of Vater by endoscopy and retrograde cholangiopancreatography (ERCP). Gut 1972;13(12):1014–1025.
57. Kasugai T, Kuno N, Aoki I, Kizu M, Kobayashi S. Fiberduodenoscopy analysis of 353 examinations. Gastrointest Endosc 1971;18(1):9–16.
58. Kasugai T, Kuno N, Kobayashi S, Hattori K. Endoscopic pancreatocholoangiography. I. The normal endoscopic pancreatocholangiogram. Gastroenterology 1972;63(2):217–226.
59. Ruppin H, Amon R, Ett W, et al. Acute pancreatitis after endoscopic/radiological pancreaticography (ERCP). Endoscopy 1974;6:94–98.
60. La Ferla G, Gordon S, Archibald M, Murray WR. Hyperamylasaemia and acute pancreatitis following endoscopic retrograde cholangiopancreatography. Pancreas 1986;1(2):160–163.
61. Sivak MV. Gastroenterologic Endoscopy. Philadelphia: W. B. Saunders Co., 1987.
62. Frank BB, and members of the Patient Care Committee of the American Gastroenterological Association. Clinical evaluation of jaundice. JAMA 1989;262(21):3031–3034.
63. Fleischer DE, Goldberg SB, Browning TH, et al. Detection and surveillance of colorectal cancer. JAMA 1989;261(4):580–585.
64. Ragozzino MW. Detection and surveillance of colorectal cancer [Letter, comment]. JAMA 1990;263(3):374.
65. Fleischer DE, Goldberg SB, Bond JH. Response. JAMA 1990;263(3):374–375.
66. Kelvin FM, Maglinte DD. Colorectal carcinoma: a radiologic and clinical review. Radiology. 1987;164(1):1–8.

67. Meyers PH [Quoted in]. Encouraging barium screenings can cut colon cancer mortality. Radiol Today 1990;7(2):21.
68. Obrecht Jr WF, Wu WC, Gelfand DW, Ott DJ. The extent of successful colonoscopy: a second assessment using modern equipment. Gastrointest Radiol 1984;9(2):161–162.
69. Gelfand DW, Wu WC, Ott DJ. The extent of successful colonoscopy: its implication for the radiologist. Gastrointest Radiol 1979;4(1):75–78.
70. Gilbert DA, Shaneyfelt SL, Silverstein FE. The national ASGE colonoscopy survey: analysis of colonoscopic practices and yield [Abstract]. Gastrointest Endosc 1984;30:143.
71. Sakai Y. Technique of colonoscopy. In: Sivak MV, ed. Gastroenterologic Endoscopy. Philadelphia: W. B. Saunders Co., 1987:840–867.
72. Sturman MF. Pelvic examination versus fiberoptic laparoscopy: a fictional study of patient preference in 1534 women [Editorial]. J Clin Gastroenterol 1988;10(6):612–613.
73. Brantley JC, Riley PM. Cardiovascular collapse during laparoscopy: a report of 2 cases. Am J Obstet Gynecol 1988;159(3):735–737.
74. Morison DH, Riggs JR. Cardiovascular collapse in laparoscopy. Can Med Assoc J 1974;111(5)a:433–437.
75. Sotrel G, Hirsch E, Edelin KC. Necrotizing fasciitis following diagnostic laparoscopy. Obstet Gynecol 1983;62(suppl 3):67S–69S.
76. Henning H, Look D. Laparoskopie Atlas und Lehrbuch. Stuttgart: Thieme, 1985.
77. Stow PJ. Retinal haemorrhage following laparoscopy [Letter]. Anaesthesia 1986;4(9):965–966.
78. De Groen PC, Rakela J, Moore SC, et al. Diagnostic laparoscopy in gastroenterology. A 14-year experience. Dig Dis Sci 1987;32(7):677–681.
79. Paterson-Brown S, Vipond MN, Simms K, Gatzen C, Thompson JN, Dudley HA. Clinical decision making and laparoscopy versus computer prediction in the management of the acute abdomen. Br J Surg 1989;76(10):1011–1013.
80. Chamberlain FVP, Carron Brown JA, eds. Gynaecological Laparoscopy: Report of the Working Party of the Confidential Enquiry into Gynaecological Laparoscopy. London: Royal College of Obstetricians and Gynaecologists, 1978:151.
81. Phillips JM, Hulka JF, Keith D, Hulka B, Keith L. Laparoscopic procedures: a national survey for 1975. J Reprod Med 1977;18(5):219–226.
82. Lightdale CJ. Indications, contraindications, and complications of laparoscopy. In: Sivak MV, ed. Gastroenterologic Endoscopy. Philadelphia: W. B. Saunders Co., 1987:1030–1044.
83. Soutoul JH, Pierre F. Les risques medico-legaux de la coelioscopie. Analyse de 32 dossiers de complications. J Gynecol Obstet Biol Reprod (Paris) 1988;17(4):439–451.
84. Lignitz E, Puschel K, Saukko P, Koops E, Mattig W. Blutungsk-komplikationen bei gynakoligischen laparoskopien-berichta uber zwei falle mit todlichem Verlauf. Z Rechtsmed 1985;95(4):297–306.
85. Kane MG, Krejs GJ. Complications of diagnostic laparoscopy in Dallas: a 7-year prospective study. Gastrointest Endosc 1984;30(4):237–240.
86. Beeson PB. On becoming a clinician. In: Reynolds R, Stone J, eds. On Doctoring. New York: Simon & Shuster, 1991:176.

6

Imaging by Chief Complaint, Signs, Symptoms, or Conditions

1/ The Dyspepsias: Chronic Upper and Lower Gastrointestinal Complaints and Irritable Bowel Syndrome

---

Confirmed dyspepsia is the apparatus of illusions.

George Meredith

The patient was an anxious spinster, a 55-year-old secretary who had always lived with her parents. A hypochondriacal lady with a variety of somatic complaints during most of her adult life, she had consulted physicians frequently for dyspeptic and other abdominal complaints for over 25 years. In the 4 years after the death of both parents she had experienced an exacerbation of symptoms. During that period she underwent three negative upper gastroduodenal endoscopies, four colonoscopies, two negative and two with removal of "5-mm polyps," plus two negative barium enemas and one negative upper GI series. She finally appeared in our department for her first ultrasonography of the gall bladder and pancreas. Another upper GI endoscopy was planned if the sonography was normal—which it was.

A 20-year-old college student suffering from severe generalized and crippling rheumatoid arthritis had been treated at the National Institutes of Health for 5 years. She had not responded to any medications except steroids in large doses and was bedridden on doses of less than 40–80 mg prednisone daily. As a result of steroid therapy she suffered a series of disastrous complications including sepsis and a peptic ulcer, which bled on several occasions and perforated twice. The unfortunate patient had undergone upper gastroesophageal duodenoscopy (EGD) on several occasions, despite the known presence of ulcers for more than 2 years, and was finally placed under the care of an academic gastroenterologist in Virginia who proceeded to schedule her for monthly upper EGDs in order to "make sure we keep an eye on the ulcers so they don't perforate again." At the time she was seen, she had undergone four successive EGDs in as many months.

(Moral: If you make your living passing 'scopes, make sure you find the right patient. There's nothing like practicing preventive medicine.)

On the Epidemiology of Gastrointestinal Imaging

These true clinical tales are terrifying examples of outrageously risky, costly, and needless investigations. They are a paradigm of our $840 billion health care expenditures for 1992 estimated by the Commerce Department. Even in these times of diagnostic overkill, the number of actual studies done on these unfortunate patients was

EGD vs UGI SERIES
PROCEDURES IN THOUSANDS
NCHS Data (1)

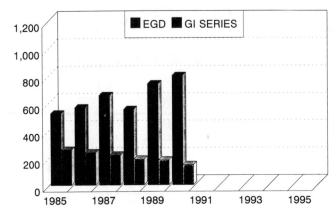

Figure 6.1.1.   EGD vs. UGI Series. Procedures in thousands. NCHS data (1).

EGD vs UGI SERIES
PROCEDURES IN THOUSANDS
NCHS Data (1)

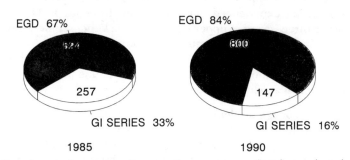

Figure 6.1.2.   Procedures in thousands and comparative percentages of total procedures for the years 1985 and 1990.

(probably) unusual, though the preferred choice of procedures was certainly not atypical. Total cost of investigation for the first patient is estimated at $6700, almost all of which was for endoscopic studies.

Data on diagnostic procedures performed in U.S. hospitals was obtained from NCHS statistics (1). Represented in Figs. 6.1.1–6.1.4 in bar and pie charts are the comparative totals for two sets of procedures performed during 1985–1990, in Figs. 6.1.1 and 6.1.2 upper gastrointestinal endoscopy (EGD) vs. upper GI radiographic studies, and in Figs. 6.1.3 and 6.1.4 colonoscopy vs. barium enema and colonoscopy; 755,000 upper esophagogastroduodenoscopies (EGD), including EGD with closed biopsy (ICD 45.13 and 45.16 (2), were performed in 1990 compared with 147,000 upper GI series, a ratio of more than 5 to 1. In 1985 the numbers were 524,000 and 257,000, respectively, or a ratio of 2 to 1. The stunning increase in rate of EGD and colonoscopic procedures with respect to upper GI series, barium enemas, and flexible

COLONOSCOPY VS FLEX SIG VS BARIUM ENEMA
ALL LISTED DIAGNOSES
(IN THOUSANDS)

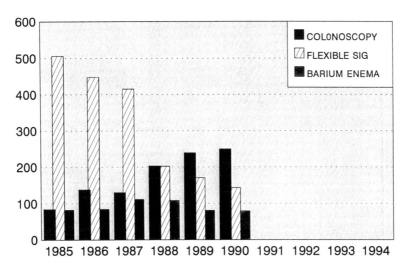

NCHS DATA

Figure 6.1.3. Colonoscopy vs flex sig vs barium enema. All listed diagnoses (in thousands).

Colonoscopy vs Flex Sig vs Barium Enema
Procedures In Thousands
NCHS Data (1)

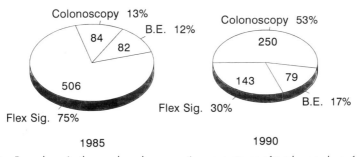

1985   1990

Figure 6.1.4. Procedures in thousands and comparative percentages of total procedures for the years 1985 and 1990.

sigmoidoscopies can be appreciated in Figs. 6.1.1 and 6.1.3 by following the trends into the near future years plotted on the x-axis, which indicate hypothetical extrapolations made forward to 1995. (Unfortunately, NCHS data on some of these procedures are not available before 1985.) The apparent drop in EGD only (ICD 45.13) is really due to the astounding rate of increase in performance of EGD with biopsy (ICD 45.16), showing more than a 5-fold increase in this all-listed procedure in the three years 1988–1990. NCHS data disks list "no data found" when one attempts to access this latter code for any year before 1988 (1).

Table 6.1.1. Comparative Discharge rates per 100,000 U.S. Population and Percentage Group Diagnoses, Major Upper GI Malignancies and Benign Upper GI Conditions 1985 vs. 1990 U.S. Hospital NHDS (NCHS) Data

ICD-9-M Code	Diagnoses	Rates		Total diagnoses	
		1985	1990	1985	1990
150	Malignant neo, esophagus				
151	Malignant neo, stomach	57	45	7%	6%
157	Malignant neo, pancreas				
530	Diseases of esophagus	215	229	26%	30%
531	Gastric ulcer				
532	Duodenal ulcer	232	200	28%	27%
533	Peptic ulcer, site NOS[a]				
535	Gastritis and duodenitis	247	215	30%	28%
536	Stomach function disorder				
537	Other gastroduodenal disease	73	70	9%	9%
Total				100%	100%

[a]Not Otherwise Specified.

There are no available figures on the numbers of respective outpatient procedures performed, although the NCHS is now attempting to address this problem. The contemplated studies, however, will involve only hospital outpatient and allied diagnostic and surgicenters and will not include private offices and other facilities (NCHS, personal communication). Nevertheless, it is clear that upper and lower GI endoscopy are rapidly replacing the respective barium studies in the investigation of GI complaints. One result of this, as previously noted, will be the permanent loss of adequately trained radiologists capable of performing GI barium studies. Figures 6.1.1 and 6.1.3 strongly suggest that by the turn of the century virtually everyone investigated for abdominal symptoms (at the present rate of increase, probably the majority of patients who present themselves) will be subjected to either EGD or colonoscopy rather than barium studies or flexible sigmoidoscopy. The estimated increased annual cost would be in the $2–4 billion range as mentioned previously, perhaps even more.

Epidemiology of GI Disease

The above figures tell us very little about the prevalence of those conditions likely to be invoked as reasons for performing direct or indirect GI imaging. Gastric cancer has continued to show a steady decline since the early 1960s, further dropping from 24,700 to 20,000 cases between 1985–1989 (3–5). The annual incidence of gastric cancer has now fallen to less than 10 per 100,000 population (6), about the same as esophageal malignancy, which has remained essentially stable. Cancer of the pancreas has shown a slow but steady increase in the past few decades, whereas colon cancer has changed little during this period (7).

Discharge rates for the spectrum of benign as well as malignant upper GI conditions have dropped 21% for malignancies, 16% for ulcer disease, and 13% for gastritis, and have increased 13% for esophageal disease for the 6-year period, 1985–1990, as shown in Table 6.1.1. Yet the relative percentages of these major categories among the total diagnoses have changed hardly at all during this interval despite the precipitous drop in upper GI radiography and the almost 50% increase in upper GI endoscopy, including endoscopic biopsy. If invasive studies were detecting a different proportion of disease conditions than radiography, we would have expected far different results. Moreover, the significant *drop* in hospital discharge rates for GI malignancies between 1985 and 1990 is at variance with reported cancer rates and suggests, if anything, that EGD is not as sensitive as assumed.

When we examine the nonhospitalized population we learn that "abdominal pain, cramps, spasms" (RVC code S545) was the 10th most common cause for physician visits in 1989, accounting for 12.3 million visits, based on analysis of physician office records (8). Comparing the outpatient data with discharge totals for the 15 most frequently diagnosed GI diseases suggests that only about 2–4% of patients seen for such upper abdominal complaints are admitted to hospitals.

The Dyspepsias and Functional GI Conditions

> **Indigestion,** *n.* A disease which the patient and his friends frequently mistake for deep religious conviction and concern for the salvation of mankind. As the simple Red Man of the western wild put it, with, it must be confessed, a certain force: "Plenty well, no pray; big bellyache, heap God."
>
> Ambrose Bierce,
> *The Devil's Dictionary*

Shakespeare and Moliere described dyspeptic symptoms long before Bierce, but they were, of course, not the first. We know from archaeological and historical studies of Babylon and even earlier epochs that abdominal ailments have plagued the human race from the time of the earliest civilizations. The word *dyspepsia* (Greek for "bad digestion") from which the name of a world-famous cola drink is derived, has had a multiplicity of definitions. Whether we attempt to define dyspepsia as either "functional" or "organic," the word is such a broad term it defies definition. It has been defined as "episodic, recurrent or persistent abdominal pain or discomfort, or *any other symptoms* referable to the alimentary tract excluding jaundice or bleeding;; (Emphasis added). Included among symptoms in the definition would be one or more of the following: pyrosis or heartburn, regurgitation, dysphagia, globus, anorexia, nausea, vomiting, abdominal pain or discomfort, flatulence (burping, belching, bloating, farting), cramps, diarrhea, symptoms attributed to "wind," early satiety with eating, and all combinations thereof, plus a host of other GI symptoms (9).

Disagreement about taxonomy continues, but we will accept Crean's comprehensive description of dyspepsia, which includes disorders of the GI tract having their source anywhere from the esophagus to the lower colon or rectum (9). Thus, we include irritable bowel syndrome in the dyspepsias. The modifier *functional* is a slippery adjective in medicine. Undoubtedly, the word encourages convenient distinctions, but at the same time we tend far too often to think in terms of the mind-body dualism. Organic symptoms and disease conditions may indeed be provoked by psychiatric causes, but the most profound understanding of the problem has been expressed by Spiro in his writings, in particular a short classic published over 17 years ago (10), which should be required reading for every physician. In this essay he points out the philosophic and semantic problem of even defining and conveying the idea of "pain" and the difficulty faced by the physician who must decide which pain is real or imaginary, "which gets antacids, and which an operation, and which puts the patient to bed and which sends him off to a psychiatrist." To Spiro, the abdomen is "a temple of mystery," yet so many patients complain of pain who may merely suffer from "too delicate an awareness of ordinary sensations." Such pain patients are well-known to virtually every specialty: to the orthopedist, the "low back pain" syndrome; to the urologist, the "urethral syndrome." There is the "headache" patient, the "rheumatic" patient, a whole litany of pain complaints, too many to be discussed. The problem of naming is involved here—the very concept of disease. This has been discussed in Chapter 2 and extensively in the literature.

Whether or not we oversimplify the conceptualization with the descriptor *psychosomatic*, many of these dyspeptic conditions may be indistinguishable from their organic counterparts. For example, the distinction between ulcer and nonulcer dyspepsia has in the past caused a great deal of confusion, simply because in many patients these conditions are identical both clinically and in their response to therapy. Ulcer disease was traditionally distinguished from nonulcer dyspepsia by whether it was *imageable* either by endoscopy or GI series. This gave rise to confusion because some ulcer patients do not have radiographic or endoscopic evidence of disease at the time of symptoms, and conversely, some patients with evidence of ulcer on imaging do not have symptoms.

The distinctions have become even less clear, however, since the discovery of the organism *Helicobacter pylori*, which has been shown to infect the gastric mucous layer of almost all patients with duodenal ulcer, most patients with gastric ulcer disease, and almost all patients with histologic antral gastritis (11). Because the prevalence of antral gastritis and *H. pylori* infection is not increased in patients with nonulcer dyspepsia compared with control groups, it has been implied that this may separate nonulcer from ulcer dyspepsia. However, further studies have shown an extremely high rate of infection in the general population, 20% in whites to more than 60% in some subgroups (12). To complicate the issue even further, among dyspeptic patients, no significant difference has been found in symptom severity between those infected or not infected with *H. pylori* (13). The issue is a thorny one, particularly because the questions which symptomatic patients with *H. pylori* should be treated with antibiotics, for how long, and which antibiotics should be used, have not yet been resolved. (11) Whether *H. pylori* should indeed be sought in dyspeptic patients is certainly a nonissue so far as imaging studies are concerned. The infection can be diagnosed by noninvasive tests such as a sensitive and specific enzyme-linked immunosorbent assay (ELISA) test or by means of 13-C or 14-C urea breath tests. Neither endoscopy nor biopsy is necessary.

As a group, these upper and lower intestinal disorders are a heterogeneous collection of clinical syndromes that include not only irritable bowel and nonulcer dyspepsia, but also chronic recurrent (nonspecific) abdominal pain, irritable esophagus, and a host of other conditions that elude neat classification. These clinical "symptom syndromes" are among the most commonly encountered in practice, affecting some 30% of the population at one time or another (14). Witness the nightly television advertisements and the multibillion-dollar markets for antacids, laxatives, and antidiarrheal and other over-the-counter medications.

The dyspepsias comprise almost half of all office visits for GI complaints (15), resulted in 472,000 hospitalizations totaling almost 2 million hospital days in 1986 alone (16), and account for 40% or more of gastroenterologists' practice (17). Irritable bowel is probably the most common condition seen by gastroenterologists, and

GI complaints are among the major causes of medical illness and lost work time in the United States (18, 19). The symptoms are protean, variable, and often poorly described. Eliciting complaints such as nausea, flatulence, bloating, indigestion, and even cramping and recurrent pain may be so difficult as to tax the skill and patience of the most experienced clinician. In an important study in which 40 experienced gastroenterologists and surgeons were asked to write down their own definitions of "nausea," "flatulence," "bloating," and even "diarrhea," the disagreement in definitions was striking (20). Some patients suffer from gastric emptying disorders and other types of poorly understood autonomic dysfunction such as intestinal or gastric dysrhythmias, abdominal epilepsy, and the like. Many of these syndromes may be related to abnormal responses or overproduction of endogenously produced epinephrine, prostaglandins, or other unknown mediators (21). Whether emotions or stress are a cause or result of these abnormalities remains to be elucidated.

When to Investigate the Patient with GI Complaints

> *Medicine is for the patient. Medicine is the people. It is not for the profits.*
>
> *George Merck*

From the foregoing we can conclude that in the patient with dyspepsia, particularly in those under 50 years old, the probability of medically significant disease is vanishingly small. To investigate or not to investigate is the question. "Whether to desist is nobler of the mind" only the competent physician can answer. Without the courage of our clinical convictions to put a stop to unnecessary "workups," surely many of our patients will end up like the subjects of our introductory anecdotes. Perhaps it even means deferring consultations, for it is well-documented that many specialists are prone to overinvestigate. The problem of self-referral for various lucrative procedures vastly complicates the issue.

With an extremely low pretest probability of GI malignancy, particularly in the patient under 45 years old, the desire to rule out cancer never justifies risky invasive studies, despite "community standards" for endoscopy established and endorsed by over-zealous specialists and prestigious professional bodies (22). Gastritis and esophagitis, like peptic ulcer, are associated with extremely low morbidity and almost no mortality and rarely call for invasive study. It has been shown that the high quality double-contrast upper GI study is highly sensitive and specific and should always be the initial screening test (23), eliminating the need for more than 99% of endoscopies for these conditions. The *unfounded* suspicion of cancer and a host of other rare conditions likewise does not call for mindless testing when most of these patients have self-limiting, benign, treatable diseases. A period of watchful waiting along with symptomatic therapy with antacids or H2-receptor antagonists has repeatedly been advised as the obvious and most cost-effective approach in the low-risk patient likely to have ulcer or nonulcer dyspepsia (24–27). A nationally respected gastroenterologist has stated that: "Since many patients with gastro-duodenitis and dyspepsia will improve on anti ulcer therapy, treatment of dyspeptic patients with classic ulcer symptoms without ascertaining whether an ulcer is present could result in a 70 to 80 percent 'cure' rate" (28).

Although no one denies the possibility of serious disease in the exceptional patient, it is obvious that only symptoms and signs dictate the need for investigation. Certain clinical guidelines have proven extremely helpful in distinguishing functional (including unclassifiable conditions or those without identifiable etiology) from organic causes of GI complaints. Many groups have developed questionnaires and effective computer programs to separate nonulcer dyspepsia from peptic ulcer (29, 30) and dyspepsia from irritable bowel and other organic upper and lower intestinal conditions (31, 32). These authors identified 20 symptoms that helped discriminate functional from organic GI disease.

One of the best examples of an easy method to identify low-risk abdominal symptoms is from Orient et al. (33), who reported that 10 simple features, including age, history of specific diseases, location, constancy and time of pain, vomiting, weight loss, and the presence of occult blood and various physical findings were powerful predictors of serious disease.

Acute gastroenteritis is a frequent cause of dyspepsia. Typical is the presentation of acute or subacute onset of new GI symptoms, often with fever and changes in bowel function. Some of these patients may have symptoms for up to 1 month or even longer. We have noted a surprising and disturbing tendency among some physicians in recent years to substitute early investigation for symptomatic therapy and watchful waiting. In particular, increasing numbers of patients are sent for upper abdominal sonography, hospitalization, even endoscopy before a reasonable time has been allowed for symptoms to subside, sometimes even within 1–2 weeks. This waiting period should be at the very least 4–8 weeks before embarking on any investigation. If we can wait out a postviral syndrome involving the respiratory tract for this long, why not give the GI tract the same respect?

What Imaging Modalities Should be Used in the Dyspepsias?

Three basic studies, time-tested, safe, accurate, inexpensive, and risk-free are the foundation for diagnostic imaging of the GI tract: (a) the esophagram/upper GI series with or without air contrast and small bowel follow-through; (b) the lower GI series or barium enema with or without air contrast; and (c) ultrasonography of the gall bladder, pancreas, and common bile duct. When the barium enema is nondiagnostic or reveals a lesion, or in the presence of occult blood or possible colitis, flexible sigmoidoscopy is also indicated.

We again emphasize that chronic or recurrent dyspepsia, by itself, is never a reason for subjecting a patient to EGD. Furthermore, endoscopic studies should *never* precede or replace upper or lower barium studies of the GI tract. The attempt to sell endoscopy as a routine substitute for radiographic study of the GI tract should be resisted, if not by the profession, then by the public and the health insurers who are paying for it.

If the physician has decided imaging is necessary for a diagnosis, it is always worth attempting to identify the problem as one of either the upper or lower GI tract. Occasionally this strategy works, but often it does not. Most chronic dyspeptics will give a history suggesting *one or more* of five major clinical categories:

1. Esophageal, dysphagic, or globus-type symptoms. Often, these may suggest gastroesophageal reflux.
2. Typical symptoms of ulcer or nonulcer dyspepsia. These two categories are clinically indistinguishable.

3. Irritable bowel or one of its variants: chronic recurrent episodes of dyspeptic symptoms, flatulence, bloating, mid or lower abdominal pain with episodes of bowel dysfunction, in particular constipation, diarrhea, mucoid stools, fecal pellets, etc. Symptoms tend to be more pronounced earlier in the day and are said rarely to waken the patient from sleep.

4. Localizing or nonlocalizing recurrent abdominal pain without significant bowel or other accompanying complaints (acute or chronic nonspecific pain, NSAP). Pain occurs almost anywhere in the abdomen, particularly in the pelvis in women, less often in the groin, flanks, subxiphoid, or upper quadrants.

5. A mixed syndrome of various complaints, including flatulence, nonspecific pain as above, early satiety, nausea, vomiting, or diarrhea.

As a practical matter, for patients in groups 1 and 2 if investigation is indeed warranted on the basis of chronicity or recurrence, an esophagogram and upper GI series with tilt studies should be done first. If upper GI barium studies are normal, gastroesophageal reflux (GER) and radionuclide esophageal scintigraphy (RES) studies should be done to determine the presence of gastroesophageal reflux or an esophageal motility disorder. (These studies are described in Section 3 of this chapter). Gall bladder sonography, but rarely, may be indicated.

In groups 3, 4, and 5 requiring investigation, ultimately all three studies will usually be required i.e. esophagogram with upper and lower GI series, sometimes with small bowel follow-through, gall bladder/pancreas sonography, barium enema and occasionally flex-sig. In the case of patients over 40 years old, it is worthwhile to perform both the upper and lower GI barium studies with air contrast.

The decision to study such patients, however, must be based on sound clinical criteria. New GI symptoms not responding to a month or so of therapy in a previously well patient, particularly in patients over 45 years old with or without accompanying weight loss and other obvious findings, *always* call for appropriate imaging studies. But recurrent, long-standing symptoms with a consistent pattern, especially in the typical patient who has already been investigated, rarely, if ever, justify repeat studies.

If imaging studies are negative, as they are in the over-whelming majority of such patients, further investigation can be terminated. In those patients who demonstrate gall stones, be aware of the high number of asymptomatic individuals with cholelithiasis. In other words, think twice about performing sonography in patients without a history that indicates cholecystitis. One should remain skeptical about attributing symptoms to the presence of gall stones.

A serious problem with the dyspepsias and other chronic complaints is the tendency of patients to consult different physicians over the years and to have negative studies constantly repeated, sometimes with the result that false-positive findings are ultimately reported. Most insurance carriers have been unsuccessful or remiss in keeping records of repeat claims for identical procedures. Moreover, there have been few proposals for secure computer tracking systems for diagnostic procedures accessible to patients and physicians which would at the same time preserve confidentiality. The issue remains a thorny one and cannot be answered by any easy formula.

In general, one can conclude that patients with dyspepsia responding to antacids or H2-receptor antagonists, whether or not an ulcer is demonstrated, do not require repeat barium studies. Patients with negative gall bladder/pancreas ultrasonography rarely should have repeat studies at least for several years (2–5) because of the long, if uncertain, period required for development of cholelithiasis. Patients with obvious, long-standing irritable bowel syndrome should not have to be reinvestigated.

Upper GI Endoscopy (EGD)

When the finger points at the moon, the idiot looks at the finger.
Chinese saying

The most obvious indications for EGD are in patients with ominous findings on the esophageal/upper GI radiographic study. These include constricting and other esophageal lesions, mass lesions, greater curvature gastric ulcers, and other types of gastric ulcers failing to heal within a reasonable time. EGD, usually with biopsy, is essential to establish a diagnosis and to determine the need for surgical treatment. Proponents of the procedure have listed, in addition to these conditions, a bewildering variety of indications such as "iron-deficient anemia with negative results on colon evaluation," "suspected malabsorption," and, of course, dyspepsia. At the same time, the appropriate *prior* use of the upper GI series in determining the need for endoscopy is usually ignored (34).

We readily confess to a strong bias, oft-repeated in this text, against needless invasive studies. To put it succinctly, the present trend in medicine is to employ more and more complicated, expensive, and often dangerous technologies in the investigation of more and more common medical complaints. We are seeing medical costs in this country spiraling ever upward with no end in sight. Yet compared to other Western countries, all of which spend far less on medical care, we do not appear to have increased our longevity or reaped any measurable health benefits from our investment.

Although we have strong feelings about the uncritical acceptance of needless invasive studies, we are also opposed to the widespread overuse of CT and MRI, invaluable but expensive and immensely overrated procedures for the diagnosis of most medical conditions. Slavishly addicted to fashion, many of us have developed a mentality that equates good medicine with extensive investigation, when in fact the opposite is the case: overinvestigation almost always implies poor quality medicine.

REFERENCES

1. U.S. Department of Health and Human Services, U.S. Public Health Service, Centers for Disease Control, and the National Center for Health Statistics. National Hospital Discharge Survey (NHDS). Detailed Diagnoses, Procedures, Days of Care, Diagnoses-Related Groups for Patients Discharged from Short-Stay Hospitals. Public Use Data Diskettes, 1985–1990.
2. ICD-9-CM. International Classification of Diseases, 9th revision, 3rd ed. Clinical Modification, vol 1–3. Los Angeles: Practice Management Information Corporation (PMI), 1989 (U.S. Department of Health and Human Services Publication No. PHS 89-1260).
3. The Surveillance Program, Division of Cancer Prevention and Control, National Cancer Institute. Bethesda: U.S. Department of Health and Human Services. Public Health Service. National Institutes of Health. Cancer Statistics Review 1973–1987. NIH publication 90-2789, 1987.
4. Ca-A cancer journal for clinicians. The American Cancer Society 1985;35(1):26.
5. Ca-A journal for clinicians. The American Cancer Society 1989;39(1):12.
6. Silverberg E, Boring MS, Squires TS. Cancer statistics, 1990. CA 1990;40:9–26.
7. Bourke GJ. The Epidemiology of Cancer. Philadelphia: The Charles Press, 1983.

8. Schappert SM. National Ambulatory Medical Care Survey: 1989 Summary. Hyattsville, Md: National Center for Health Statistics. Vital Health Statistics, 1992:131(110).

9. Crean GP. Towards a positive diagnosis of irritable bowel syndrome. In: Irritable Bowel Syndrome. London: Grune and Stratton, Ltd., 1985:29–42.

10. Spiro HM. Visceral viewpoints: pain and perfectionism: the physician and the "pain patient." N Engl J Med 1976;294(15):829–830.

11. Walsh JH. Helicobacter pylori: selection of patients for treatment [Editorial]. Ann Intern Med 1992; 116(9):770–771.

12. Graham DY, Malaty HM, Evans DG, Evans Jr DJ, et al. Epidemiology of *Helicobacter pylori* in an asymptomatic population in the United States. Gastroenterology 1991;100:1495–1501.

13. Veldhuyzen van Zanten SJ, Tytgat KM, deGara CJ, et al. A prospective comparison of symptoms and five diagnostic tests in patients with *Helicobacter pylori* positive and negative dyspepsia. Eur J Gastroenterol Hepatol 1991;3:463–468.

14. Thompson WG, Heaton KW. Functional bowel disorders in apparently healthy people. Gastroenterology 1980;79(2):283–288.

15. Collins JG. National Center for Health Statistics. Prevalence of Selected Chronic Conditions, United States, 1979–1981 period. Hyattsville, MD: U.S. Department of Health and Human Services, Public Health Service, National Center for Health Statistics. Vital and Health Statistics. 1986: series 10, no. 155. DHHS Publication No. (PHS)86-1583.

16. Lawrence L, National Center for Health Statistics. Detailed Diagnoses and Procedures for Patients Discharged from Short-Stay Hospitals, United States, 1984. Hyattsville, MD: U.S. Department of Health and Human Services, National Center for Health Statistics. Vital and Health Statistics. 1986: series 13, No. 86. DHHS Publication No. (PHS) 86–1747.

17. Mitchell CM, Drossman DA. Survey of the AGA membership relating to patients with functional gastrointestimal disorders [Letter]. Gastroenterology 1987;92:1282–1284.

18. Switz DM. What the gastroenterologist does all day. A survey of a state society's practice. Gastroenterology 1976;70(6):1048–1050.

19. Kirsner JB. The irritable bowel syndrome. A clinical review and ethical considerations. Arch Intern Med 1981;141(5):635–639.

20. Knill-Jones RP. A formal approach to symptoms in dyspepsia. Clin Gastroenterol 1985;14(3):517–529.

21. Dubois A. Gastric dysrhythmias: pathophysiologic and etiologic factors [Editorial]. Mayo Clin Proc 1989;64(2):246–250.

22. Kahn K, Greenfield S (for Health and Policy Committee, American College of Physicians). Endoscopy in the evaluation of dyspepsia. Ann Intern Med 1985;102:266–269.

23. Halpert ARD, Shier C, Waslowski S, Feczko PJ. The radiologic diagnosis of nonspecific gastritis with endoscopic correlation. Appl Radiol 1989;18(2):24–28.

24. Read L, Pass TM, Komaroff AL. Diagnosis and treatment of dyspepsia. A cost-effectiveness analysis. Med Decis Making 1982;2(4):415–438.

25. Clark ML. Investigating young patients with dyspepsia [Letter to the Editor]. Lancet 1988;1(8631): 212.

26. Williams B, Luckas M, Ellingham JHM, Dain A, Wicks ACB. Do young patients with dyspepsia need investigation? Lancet 1988;2(8624):1349–1351.

27. Goodson JD, Richter JM, Lane RS, Beckett TF, Pingree RG. Empiric antacids and reassurance for acute dyspepsia. J Gen Intern Med 1986;1(2):90–93.

28. Lagarde SP, Spiro HM. Non-ulcer dyspepsia. Clin Gastroenterol 1984;13(2):437–446.

29. Horrocks JC, de Dombal FT. Clinical presentation of patients with "dyspepsia." Detailed symptomatic study of 360 patients. Gut 1978;19(1):19–26.

30. Talley NJ, Phillips SF. Non-ulcer dyspepsia: potential causes and pathophysiology. Ann Intern Med 1988;108(6):865–879.

31. Horrocks JC, de Dombal FT. Computer-aided diagnosis of "dyspepsia." Am J Dig Dis 1975;20(5): 397–406.

32. Talley NJ, Phillips SF, Melton III JL, Wiltgen C, Zinsmeister AR. A patient questionnaire to identify bowel disease. Ann Intern Med 1989;11(8):671–674.

33. Orient JM, Kettel LJ, Lim J. A test of a linear discriminant for identifying low-risk abdominal pain. Med Decis Making 1985;5(1):77–87.

34. Morrissey JF, Reichelderfer M. Gastrointestinal endoscopy (medical progress). N Engl J Med 1991; 325(16):1142–1149.

2 Acute Abdominal Pain

> *Beauty cannot disguise nor music melt*
> *A pain undiagnosable but felt.*
>
> Anne Morrow Lindbergh
> "The Stone"

Acute Abdominal Pain: General Remarks

Acute abdominal pain is defined here as abdominal pain of less than 7 days duration. If we include the dyspepsias, it is one of the most important medical symptoms. The complaint is among the three most common in patients presenting to emergency rooms or admitted to hospitals and constitutes a major medical problem. In a British series more than 30% of random adults who were *not* seeking medical care had some type of GI problem or pain (1). No doubt these figures relate primarily to the dyspepsias, a problem we have already discussed. For example, irritable bowel syndrome causing acute or chronic recurrent abdominal pain is the most common condition seen by gastroenterologists and is one of the major causes of absenteeism in this country (2, 3). If one also adds nonspecific abdominal pain, the economic and social consequences of benign abdominal complaints are staggering, because of lost work days, needless hospitalizations, and expensive but unnecessary medical investigation.

On the other side of the coin are diagnostic failures in more serious causes of abdominal pain, resulting in needless morbidity and mortality. For example, between 20–30% of patients operated on for appendicitis do not have this disease confirmed at surgery (4). Although this was acceptable in the past, this false-positive figure is no longer justifiable (vide infra). Moreover, the death rate for intestinal obstruction in this country still ranges from 10% in the small bowel to 20% in colonic obstruction (5). The mortality rate for uncomplicated pancreatitis remains around 5% but can rise to over 85% in complicated cases in which the diagnosis is delayed or missed (6, 7). Diagnostic errors in the early diagnosis of cholecystitis, diverticulitis, and other dangerous conditions also have been amply documented (8, 9).

It is instructive to review the causes of acute abdominal pain seen in an emergency clinic in Leeds, England (Table 6.2.1) (10). Almost half the cases were "nonspecific abdominal pain," an important condition about which we will have more to say. In another large series of 1000 consecutive patients presenting to an emergency room at the University of Virginia, the authors reported similar findings (11). Of note is the number of conditions involving the urinary and female genital tract, which accounted for 10–15% of abdominal pain complaints. Diagnoses may vary with demographics. For example, in an urban U.S. population one would anticipate much higher numbers of patients with pelvic inflammatory disease, ectopic pregnancy, and pancreatitis than those encountered in the Leeds experience. In certain series abdominal trauma may be the principal cause of surgical abdominal disease (12). Although numerous intra- and extra-abdominal conditions may cause acute abdominal pain (Table 6.2.2), virtually all patients with this complaint will fall into one of the categories listed in Table 6.2.1.

Table 6.2.1. Causes of Abdominal Lesions Seen in an Emergency Clinic in England

Diagnosis	No. of cases	% of total
Nonspecific abdominal pain	545	45.6
Appendicitis	187	15.6
Dyspepsia	91	7.6
Cholecystitis	69	5.8
Mesenteric adenitis	43	3.6
Urinary tract infection	38	3.2
Small bowel obstruction	31	2.6
Constipation	29	2.4
Perforated peptic ulcer	27	2.3
Salpingitis	25	2.1
Gastritis	25	2.1
Renal colic	18	1.5
Pancreatitis	16	1.3
Diverticular disease	13	1.1
Dysmenorrhea	13	1.1
Ovarian cyst	6	0.5
Ectopic pregnancy	2	0.2
Incomplete abortion	1	0.1
Other, miscellaneous	17	1.4
Total	1196	100.0

Reprinted by permission from *British Journal of Surgery* (1977;250:252), Butterworth & Co. (Publishers) Ltd.

Table 6.2.2. Less Common Causes of Nontraumatic Acute Abdominal Pain (Partial List)

Intraabdominal conditions	Extraabdominal conditions
Ruptured hepatic abscess	Pneumonia
Fistula	Pleural effusion
Ruptured omphalocoele	Pulmonary embolism
Hemorrhage into omentum	Coronary disease
Ruptured corpus luteum cyst	Lead poisoning
Ovarian cyst	Diabetic acidosis
Twisted or ruptured ovarian cyst	Uremia
Meckel's Diverticulum	Collagen vascular disease
Penetrating gastric or duodenal ulcer	Porphyria
Hepatitis	Neurologic lesions
Intraabdominal malignancy	Herpes Zoster
Perinephric abscess	Hyperlipemia
Pseudomembranous colitis	Arachnidism
Hemorrhage into rectus muscle	etc.

DeDombal and colleagues (13–16) have written extensively about the clinical and epidemiologic aspects of abdominal pain, particularly with respect to surgical disease, and have developed computer-assisted diagnostic programs. We also have developed and tested a diagnostic microcomputer program which, like deDombal's, has the approximate accuracy of the average clinician's initial diagnostic assessment, given the presence or absence of specific signs and symptoms (17). Thus, whether carrying out the diagnostic process in the examination room or emulating it on a computer, the clinical history and physical examination remain central to the process, and they remain the *best tests* for acute abdominal pain (18). A routine complete blood count (CBC), urinalysis, and occasionally serum amylase and pregnancy tests are obviously useful, but the optimal approach to diagnosis will continue to be based on the pretest

Table 6.2.3. What Physicians See in Their Offices: Major GI, Genitourinary, and Female Pelvic Disorders Based on the National Ambulatory Medical Care Survey, United States, 1985 (19)

Diagnostic category[a]	Percentage of all cases	Running total (%)
1. Functional GI disorders	16	
2. Other symptoms involving abdomen and pelvis	15	31.
3. Gastric, duodenal, peptic ulcer	10.5	41.5
4. Pain and other symptoms associated with female genital system	8.7	50.2
5. Gall bladder disease	8.2	58.4
6. Diverticular disease	6.7	65.1
7. Noninflammatory disease of the ovary and adnexae	5.4	70.5
8. Salpingitis, including inflammatory disease of ovary and adnexae	5	75.5
9. Calculus of the kidney and ureter	4.8	80.3
10. Disorders of function of stomach and other disorders of stomach and duodenum	4.7	85
11. Symptoms involving digestive tract, including, nausea, vomiting, dysphagia, heartburn, flatulence, etc.	4.1	89.1
12. Endometriosis	3.2	92.3
13. Appendicitis	3.2	95.5
14. Infections of the kidney	2.3	97.8
15. Intestinal obstruction	1.2	99
16. Pancreatitis	1	100

Totals from statistical sample extrapolated to 17,991,065 out of 636,000,000 visits.
[a]ICD-9 codes: 1, 564; 2, 789; 3, 531–534; 4, 625; 5, 574–575; 6, 562; 7, 620; 8, 614; 9, 592; 10, 536, 37; 11, 787; 12, 617; 13, 540–543; 14, 590; 15, 560; 16, 577.

probability of the most common disorders. This dictum applies equally to all presentations, signs, and symptoms.

In acute abdominal pain diagnosis invasive studies are almost never indicated. The only exception is laparoscopy, which has a limited place in older patients or those with complicating intercurrent disease suspected of having surgical problems. The investigation of abdominal trauma is quite another matter, often requiring CT, MRI, or laparoscopy, but will not be discussed here. In almost all cases of suspected appendicitis, intestinal obstruction, perforation, diverticular disease, cholecystitis, pancreatitis, acute pelvic disease, or ectopic pregnancy, four classes of studies form the cornerstone of diagnostic imaging:

1. Supine and upright films of the abdomen (left lateral decubitus if the patient is unable to stand);
2. Upper GI contrast series, preferably with aqueous media, if perforation is suspected, and the barium enema;
3. Ultrasonography of the upper abdomen and pelvis;
4. Hepatobiliary scintigraphy.

At the same time, we cannot overemphasize the surgical dictum that *signs of peritoneal irritation unexplainable in terms of extraabdominal disease, by and large, make it incumbent to explore.* In contemporary medical practice the misuse of technology threatens to replace clinical acumen and surgical bedside diagnosis. To paraphrase Pasteur, symptoms and signs "favor the prepared mind." It is unfortunately true that far too many patients with an obvious surgical abdomen are going for CT examination before a surgeon is even called in attendance.

During our study of acute abdominal pain we often found essential parts of the physical examination neglected to the patient's detriment. For example, many did not have a rectal examination, and in the case of females with lower abdominal pain, pelvic examination was frequently omitted. The old adage, "put your finger in it before you put your foot in it," was amply confirmed in several of our patients with salpingitis, appendiceal disease, and especially fecal impaction and distended bladder (17).

Acute abdominal pain may be classified into "innocuous" (benign) and "serious" (life-threatening) conditions. In the serious group we include "pure" surgical disease such as appendicitis and ectopic pregnancy, other conditions which might not require immediate surgery, i.e., some cases of cholecystitis and obstruction, and finally, conditions rarely requiring surgical intervention, such as diverticular disease, salpingitis, and pancreatitis. An anatomic classification might divide presentations according to location of pain and tenderness. The purpose of these schemata, both of which we will explore, is merely to help organize and orient what Zachary Cope refers to as the "tables of the mind."

Common Causes of Acute Abdominal Pain Seen in the Physician's Office

The abdomen is the reason why man does not easily take himself for a god.

Nietzsche

The Leeds and University of Virginia series indicate the generally innocuous nature of most acute abdominal pain presentations. Almost half of all acute abdominal diagnoses seen in the emergency room are accounted for by "nonspecific" pain and another quarter by "dyspepsia," "gastritis," constipation, urinary tract infection, ovarian cyst, dysmenorrhea, and the like. Table 6.2.3 shows the major abdominal disorders for which patients seek attention in physician's offices in the United States (19). A high percentage of these conditions may present as acute abdominal pain, but in contrast to the emergency room data, no true prevalence of this symptom may be inferred from these statistics. Still, it is obvious that patients seen in office practice likely to present with acute abdominal pain are similar to those seen in the emergency room in usually having benign conditions. Note that the first 10 conditions of the GI/GU tract account for 85% of such visits. The data represent those obtained from a cross-sectional survey of all physician specialties. Approximately three out of five office visits in 1985 were to doctors, such as family practitioners, internists, pediatricians, and obstetricians/gynecologists, the physicians most likely to encounter these conditions. The importance of these 16 entities cannot be overestimated because they represent almost 5% or an estimated 20 million visits to these physicians (20).

These conditions or diagnoses lend convincing statistical support of our concepts on medical nosology put forward in Chapter 1. Five of the major categories, including the two most frequent diagnostic codes, "functional GI disorders" (ICD-9, 564), and "other symptoms involving abdomen and pelvis" (ICD-9, 789), are descriptive categories rather than disease names and account for almost one-third of all cases (21). The ICD classification scheme attempts to deal with this important distinction, but in fact, compared with outpatient data, the overwhelming preponderance of hospital discharge diagnoses are coded as diseases and not conditions-as-descriptions. We emphasize again that most abdominal pain seen by physicians is the "we-see-this" syndrome and can *more accurately be described by symptom* than classified as disease.

It is appropriate here to discuss the single most important benign cause of acute abdominal pain, followed by a discussion of the most important serious causes of this complaint.

Nonspecific Abdominal Pain (NSAP)

This category of acute pain, often called "no sweat abdominal pain" for the above acronym, undoubtedly includes a heterogeneous group of conditions, both functional and organic, and goes by a variety of names. There are disagreements as to terminology and usage between the European and the American literature. These may be among several reasons the subject has been so grievously neglected in our medical textbooks and literature. Ask a physician to define nonspecific abdominal pain and you are apt to draw a puzzled look. Under the ICD-9M codes 780–799, "symptoms, signs, and ill-defined conditions," two of which are included in Table 6.2.3, one indeed finds 789.0, "abdominal tenderness, colic, cramps, epigastric and umbilical pain" (21). But the descriptor *nonspecific* does not appear. Thus, epidemiological study of the condition based on hospital discharge data becomes virtually impossible in this country. Yet a retrospective British study using the old ICD rubric 785.5 showed that "abdominal pain without definite explanation"—the most accurate definition of nonspecific abdominal pain—ranked 6th among all causes of hospital admission for women and 10th for men (22).

Thus, nonspecific abdominal pain is disease-as-description masquerading as disease. This is one of many conditions or "syndromes" in search of a diagnostic code. Most patients with NSAP experience subsidence and disappearance of their complaints with or without treatment within a few days to 1 week. The vast majority of these patients never prove to have any significant disease despite numerous presentations and frequently exhaustive workups. In a prospective study of 230 patients followed up for 5 years after hospital admission for acute NSAP, 77% were free of any symptoms during the observation period. Of the remaining 53, 5 out of 7 patients rehospitalized had appendicitis. Only 15% had diagnosed recurrences of nonspecific pain, usually of benign colonic or gynecologic origin, though malignant disease did develop in 4% of patients over age 50 (23). In an important series of 5675 patients presenting with acute undiagnosed abdominal pain, again, only a small number, just less than 2%, later proved to have intraabdominal cancer, more than half of these being of the large bowel and almost all in patients over age 50. By including those patients with NSAP subsequently developing malignancy, the rate of cancer in this older age group was 10.7% (24). There was no control series, so it is unknown what number of patients without a history of an attack of NSAP would have developed malignancy anyway. This is important because increased cancer rates in this group may have largely reflected age-related factors.

The exclusion of gastroenteritis as a separate diagnosis may be questioned, though most of these patients do not present with the chief complaint of abdominal pain. Moreover, in that small subset where pain is the presenting feature, the patients are usually clinically indistinguishable from those with NSAP. That they should be thus classified is further supported by studies linking viruses with acute abdominal pain,

Table 6.2.4. Principal Nontraumatic Surgical Causes of Acute Abdominal Pain Seen in the Emergency Room[a]

	Av % surgical cases	% Total cases
Appendicitis	58	10–15
Cholecystitis	21	3–7
Small and large bowel obstruction	14	2–4
Perforation including predominantly perforated peptic ulcer and diverticulitis	6	1–2
Ectopic pregnancy	<1	<1
	100	16–29

[a]Abstracted from combined data (7, 8)

especially in children (25). Perhaps the most important etiological factor is psychological or emotional stress in a susceptible patient (26). The diagnosis of nonspecific pain often resolves itself into a problem of semantics, because other presentations of acute abdominal pain described as acute gastritis, dyspepsia, or GI upset might well be included under the rubric of NSAP.

A Strategy for Studying the Epidemiology of Serious Acute Abdominal Pain in Hospitalized Patients

Table 6.2.4 summarizes the percentage of principal surgical conditions reported among patients with acute abdominal pain in the emergency room, numbers that are discordant with the hospital data (vide infra). Important surgical emergencies, in particular abdominal catastrophes such as ruptured aortic aneurysm, intraabdominal abscesses, perforations, twisted or ruptured ovarian cyst, etc., do not appear because the combined percentage of such causes of acute abdominal pain is usually less than 0.5%. It is in this small but important subset of abdominal pain presentations that the alert clinician may save his stricken patients the perils of unnecessary diagnostic delay.

Missing from this list are three additional conditions which, curiously, do not account for significant numbers in the above emergency room surveys but comprise an important percentage of hospital discharge diagnoses: salpingitis or pelvic inflammatory disease (PID), pancreatitis, and diverticular disease.

There is no inclusive inpatient hospital data dealing with the occurrence of acute abdominal pain per se. In attempting to establish relative occurrence or period prevalences of various intraabdominal conditions as a basis for diagnostic imaging *by symptom*, one must therefore infer a relationship based on data *by disease*. This method, despite its limitations, has been used throughout this text. There are some problems with this approach, because it can by no means be assumed that all cases of these conditions indeed present with, *or only with*, acute abdominal pain. Furthermore, it may be argued that hospital discharge diagnoses do not consistently reflect true prevalence among the nonhospitalized population. There is also the problem of readmission for the same diagnosis; i.e. it might be argued that the total diagnoses for a given condition may be falsely raised because of the tendency for recurrences. Thus, patients with cholecystitis, pancreatitis, and diverticulitis might well be discharged more than once the same year; patients with acute appendicitis would almost never be discharged more than once with that diagnosis. Patients also may suffer an attack of cholecystitis, salpingitis, or other serious conditions without being hospitalized. Nonetheless, our focus is deliberately restricted to inpatient data, because our purpose is to estimate the relative importance of those conditions in the spectrum of acute abdominal pain *severe enough to require hospitalization*. This method is epidemiologically consistent and useful if it can lead to some approximation of statistical reality. Certainly, from clinical experience one may infer that the great majority of patients presenting to hospitals with these seven conditions, appendicitis, cholecystitis, pancreatitis, intestinal obstruction, salpingitis, diverticular disease, and ectopic pregnancy, do in fact present initially with acute abdominal pain.[a] Any questions as to the completeness of our list can be answered by a careful review of discharge data for all relevant ICD codes, i.e. Diseases of the Digestive System (520–579) and Genitourinary System and Female Genital Tract (580–629) (27). Tabulation of government data derived from the National Hospital Discharge Survey (NHDS) indicates that at the very least, the above seven major conditions comprise more than 95% of all likely hospital diagnoses for acute abdominal pain.

In order to accomplish our analysis, we were exceedingly fortunate in having available the expert assistance and advice of statisticians and epidemiologists at the NCHS, a branch of the Centers for Disease Control (CDC). Its hospital discharge and other data are probably the most exhaustive and reliable epidemiological data in the world on disease occurrence in hospitalized patients.[b]

Occurrence of Leading Surgical and Medical Conditions

In the All-Listed NHDS data for the above seven pertinent diagnoses by sex in Tables 6.2.5 and 6.2.6, the relative occurrences of serious acute abdominal disease diagnoses in the hospitalized population are listed. The first two columns should be read vertically in order to compare relative frequencies of the listed diagnoses combined for all ages. To determine the percentage of patients by age for each condition, read the numbers by row. Note the subset "Other," which was explained above. This category will be necessary for all subsequent tables in order to complete the list of all possibilities. Thus, there will always be innumerable uncommon conditions causing a given symptom or sign, but which in toto rarely account for more than a few percentage points of the total cases. To emphasize the thrust of this text, given a specific sign or symptom, *only a few common conditions, rarely more than five or six, comprise more than 95% of cases likely to be encountered.* Long differential diagnostic lists tend to falsify this statistically verifiable fact by constantly invoking the unusual. A truism, often forgotten, is that rare conditions occur rarely. Common sense dictates that the only rational diagnostic strategy is to search first for the most likely.

The tables show that in females, cholecystitis is the most common serious intraabdominal condition causing acute pain, followed by salpingitis, intestinal obstruction, and appendicitis. PID is almost as common as cholecystitis and occurs more than three times

---

[a] The objection that possible coexisting symptoms will affect conditional probabilities is dealt with in Appendix A. In order to base this text on clinical findings and simultaneously avoid the mathematical problem of "dependency," we have had to assume throughout the presence of a *solitary sign or symptom*. Thus, in discussing the likelihood of a disease given acute abdominal pain, we are making the assumption—not always justified on probabilistic grounds—that *only* acute abdominal pain is the presenting complaint.

[b] The NHDS data are based on random sampling of more than 6,000 U.S. acute-care hospitals, using unimpeachable statistical methods and design, and are employed throughout this book (27). The disease frequencies (totals) and the rates per 100,000 U.S. population represent total diagnoses, procedures, and other data derived from an analysis of 31–34 million hospital discharges. The figures were normalized by inflating reciprocals of the probabilities of sample selection. The rates are based on the entire U.S. population as supplied by the Bureau of the Census for the indicated years. NHDS diagnostic data are available in two forms, either "first-listed," meaning that only the initial ICD-9 code is tallied, or "all-listed," indicating the ICD code is counted if it occurs in any of the first seven listed discharge diagnoses. In general, we will use the all-listed data but will indicate which database is used.

Table 6.2.5. Percentage (Rounded Off) of Total All-Listed (First Seven Diagnoses): Major Intraabdominal Conditions Causing Serious Acute Abdominal Pain, by Age, Females, U.S. Acute Care Hospitals, 1988 (Adapted from NHDS) (27)

Diagnostic category[a]	% Total diagnoses	% Age group				
		<15[b]	15–44	45–64	65 +	Total
1. Cholecystitis	28	b	36	29	35	100
2. Salpingitis	26	b	89	11	—	100
3. Intest. obstruction	15	5	16	22	57	100
4. Appendicitis	8	21	59	10	10	100
5. Diverticulitis	7	b	9	28	63	100
6. Pancreatitis	6	b	33	33	34	100
7. Ectopic pregnancy	5	b	100	—	—	100
8. Other[c]	5					
Total % of cases	100					

[a]ICD-9 code: 1, 574 (omitting 574.2 and 574.5), 575.0, 575.1; 2, 614; 3, 550.1, 560; 4, 540–543; 5, 562.11; 6, 577.0, 577.1; 8, 633.
[b]Estimates below 5000 patients statistically unreliable.
[c]Clinical estimate based on expert opinion.

Table 6.2.6. Percentage (Rounded Off) of Total All-Listed (First Seven Diagnoses): Major Intraabdominal Conditions Causing Serious Acute Abdominal Pain, by Age, Males, U.S. Acute Care Hospitals, 1988 (Adapted from NHDS) (27)

Diagnostic category[a]	% Total diagnoses	% Age group				
		<15[b]	15–44	45–64	65 +	Total
1. Intest. obstruction	28	6	16	21	57	100
2. Cholecystitis	24	b	36	29	35	100
3. Appendicitis	21	21	60	10	9	100
4. Pancreatitis	15	b	33	33	34	100
5. Diverticulitis	7	b	10	27	63	100
6. Other	5					
Total % of cases	100					

[a]ICD-9 codes: 1, 550.1, 560; 2, 574 (omitting 574.2 and 574.5), 575.0, 575.1; 3, 540–543; 4, 577.0, 577.1; 5, 562.11.
[b]Estimates below 5000 patients statistically unreliable.

as frequently as appendicitis. It is not at all surprising that the greatest number of patients operated on mistakenly for appendicitis are females who prove to have PID at surgery (vide infra). The row totals show that cholecystitis is almost evenly distributed in both sexes in age groups over 15 years (though the age range 15–44 is too broad to show the increasing incidence of the disease over age 30). Intestinal obstruction rises rapidly with age. Over half of all patients of both sexes with obstruction and almost two-thirds of those with diverticular disease are over age 65. In children, 75–80% of surgical abdominal disease is accounted for by appendicitis and most of the remaining by obstruction due to various causes. However, in children, nonsurgical causes of acute abdominal pain still predominate over surgical causes.

The pie charts, Figures 6.2.1 and 6.2.2, show graphically the percent distribution of serious abdominal disease by sex and illustrate the similar occurrence of cholecystitis in both sexes and the similar frequency of salpingitis in females and intestinal obstruction in males. These two pairs of conditions, cholecystitis with either salpingitis or obstruction, account respectively for more than half of all serious abdominal disease in both sexes. Intestinal obstruction followed closely by cholecystitis and appendicitis are the most frequent serious abdominal diseases in males, accounting for

Serious Causes of Acute Abdominal Pain in U.S. Males
Percentage of All-Listed Hospital Discharges
1988 NHDS Data (27)

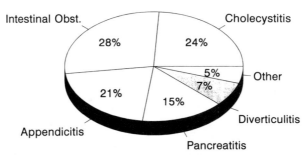

Figure 6.2.1. Serious causes of acute abdominal pain in U.S. males. Percentage of all-listed hospital discharges, 1988 NHDS data (27).

Serious Causes of Acute Abdominal Pain in U.S. Females
Percentage of All-Listed Hospital Discharges
1988 NHDS Data (27)

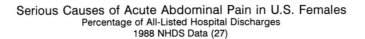
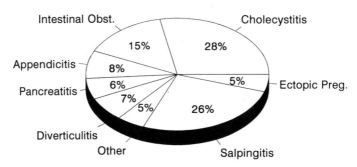

Figure 6.2.2. Serious causes of acute abdominal pain in U.S. females. Percentage of all-listed hospital discharges, 1988 NHDS data (27).

three-quarters of all cases.[c] Pancreatitis, ectopic pregnancy, and diverticular disease occur with about equal frequency in women, 5–7% each, but pancreatitis is seen in almost 15% of men with serious abdominal pain. Other useful information can be derived from the NHDS data, for example, the overall frequencies of the various conditions seen in both sexes, which for 1988 are listed in Table 6.2.7 and illustrated graphically in Figure 6.2.3, which shows the comparative frequency of these major conditions in males and females. They must be regarded as close approximations of the totals (estimated NHDS accuracy is ±3%), because it was not always desirable to

[c] The absence of perforated ulcer from the list, clear testimony to the effectiveness of histamine antagonists, may still be surprising for those of us in practice more than 20 years. Yet of the more than 507,000 All-Listed discharge diagnoses for gastric, duodenal, peptic, and gastrojejunal ulcer disease in 1990 — diagnoses we have deliberately omitted from our tabulations for "serious" disease — only 11,000 diagnoses of perforation were recorded by the NHDS. This is an insignificant number (0.5%) out of the more than 2 million total discharge diagnoses for the above seven major serious conditions (23).

Table 6.2.7. Total Sex Distribution of Discharged Patients with Serious Abdominal Disease: All Age Groups; 1988 (Adapted from NHDS) (27)

	Females (%)	Males (%)
Cholecystitis:	70	30
Diverticular disease	64	36
Intestinal obstruction	59	41
Pancreatitis	45	55
Appendicitis	42	58

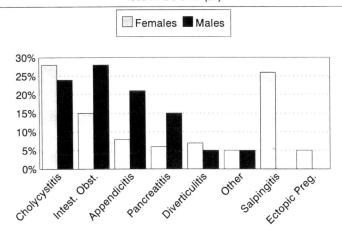

Serious Causes of Acute Abdominal Pain in U.S.
Percentage of All Listed Hospital Discharges
1988 NHDS Data (27)

Figure 6.2.3. Serious causes of acute abdominal pain in U.S. Percentage of all-listed hospital discharges, 1988 NHDS data (27).

split up etiological categories and therefore diagnostic codes.[d] The following sections describe our approach to imaging in these serious acute abdominal conditions. We stress once again that only when the physician has ascertained the significant likelihood of one of the following conditions *on clinical grounds* is imaging either desirable or necessary.

Medical Imaging in Specific Acute Abdominal Conditions
SUSPECTED CHOLECYSTITIS

Because cholecystitis is the most common cause of acute surgical abdominal disease in women and the second in men, it is not surprising that cholecystectomy is the third most frequently performed abdominal operation, more than 522,000 in the United States during 1990. (What *is* surprising: cesarean section is now the number-one abdominal operation performed in this country, more than 944,000, followed by hysterectomy, 552,000; vide infra.)

Real-time ultrasonography is the procedure of first choice in the diagnosis of cholecystitis, because 90–95% of patients with acute inflammatory disease of the gall

[d] For example, ICD-9M diagnostic and procedure codes have been designed to be exhaustive and exquisitely precise, so that ICD-540, "acute appendicitis," also includes 540.0, "with generalized peritonitis," 540.1, "with peritoneal abscess," etc. A similar situation holds for the other conditions. ICD-9 codes are indicated when appropriate, though compromises had to be made in order to select the pertinent data.

bladder have cholelithiasis, and the overall sensitivity of sonography in detection of gall stones is more than 92% with a specificity of 95%. This is to be compared with CT, which is only 79% sensitive (28). Two difficulties must constantly be kept in mind, however. First, a significant percentage of the population, estimated to be 2–6% for men and 2–12% for women, have cholelithiasis (29–31). Second, *only about one-third of patients with acute right upper quadrant pain will have acute cholecystitis* (32, 33). Thus, the presence of gall stones is of little significance without accompanying clinical signs and symptoms pointing to acute inflammatory disease of the gall bladder. Conversely, the *absence* of cholelithiasis on sonography is strong evidence *against* acute cholecystitis, because acalculous cholecystitis accounts for *less than 5–10%* of all cases. In a large series, three criteria were used to establish the diagnosis of acute cholecystitis with virtually 100% certainty. If the following criteria were present, no further imaging tests were felt indicated (34): (a) presence of cholelithiasis; (b) tenderness elicited with pressure of the transducer over the right upper quadrant (a positive "sonographic Murphy" sign); and (c) a thick gall bladder wall, on sonography (32). (The sonographic finding of a thick-walled gall bladder in acute cholecystitis, however, probably occurs in less than half the cases.)

The authors found that even if stones were present, if all three of these criteria were not met, hepatobiliary scintigraphy would have been indicated in one-quarter of their series of almost 500 patients. This group would include not only patients with acalculous cholecystitis, but most of those without clinical findings sufficient to justify surgical exploration. Some of these latter patients are in the younger age group with viral hepatitis, but a variety of other conditions, especially peptic ulcer, pancreatitis, NSAP, or viral enteritis, are associated with acute presentations of right upper quadrant or epigastric pain and tenderness.

Thus, when neither stones nor thickened gall bladder wall can be demonstrated and there is still clinical suspicion of acute cholecystitis, hepatobiliary scintigraphy must be performed. Failure of the gall bladder to visualize within 2–3 hours of injection (and after proper preparation with cholecystokinin in patients who have been fasting more than 18–24 hours) is virtually 100% sensitive and specific for the diagnosis of acute cholecystitis. In order to reduce the time of the study, some physicians use intravenous morphine to cause contraction of the Sphincter of Oddi. In this instance, failure of gall bladder visualization within 1 hour indicates acute cholecystitis. Because normal physiological contraction of the gall bladder after food ingestion prevents visualization of the organ, both sonography and scintigraphy may have to be postponed 3–6 hours if the patient has eaten.

SUSPECTED APPENDICITIS AND SALPINGITIS

Appendicitis is the third most common serious abdominal disease in both sexes, but in men its frequency rivals that of cholecystitis and obstruction, whereas in women it accounts for only 8% of all serious abdominal pain. Not all patients are as helpful as the Newfoundland Eskimos who, it is said, often paint the offending part of their anatomy in an attempt to relieve their pain. Thus, Eskimos with appendicitis often present with a circle drawn around the umbilicus and an arrow pointing to the right lower quadrant (35).

Patients with typical appendicitis present with right lower quadrant pain and tenderness about 75% of the time, but the clinical diagnosis all too often remains elusive. More than 100 years after the description of the disease the false-positive rate for surgery still varies from 8–33% with an average of 20% (36–38). The 20% figure is important and even today is often accepted, because surgeons who remove too few normal appendixes have been regarded as likely to miss the diagnosis. This is a tacit recognition of the trade-off between nonspecificity and sensitivity, our old friend the ROC curve. But times change; false-negative appendectomies, at least in females, in whom the majority of cases occur, should be regarded with far less tolerance than in the past.

Plain abdominal films and barium enema examinations have sometimes proven to be helpful in advanced disease such as abscess formation and perforation, but majority opinion holds that because of their low sensitivity and specificity, in the early and uncomplicated cases, these studies are unreliable and "almost without merit" (39). The barium enema is still regarded as risky in the diagnosis of uncomplicated appendicitis because of the danger of perforation, but plain films disclosing a fecalith occasionally may be diagnostic.

Three additional imaging procedures have been proposed for the direct visualization of acute appendicitis, and in difficult or complicated cases may have a place in diagnosis: CT scanning (39), indium-111-labeled leukocytes (40), and compression ultrasonography (41–43). In the ultrasound technique it has been claimed that with graded compression, using a specially designed high-frequency transducer, overlying bowel gas and fluid will be eliminated, and the incompressible inflamed appendix will be brought into view. Of interest is the observation that in a group of patients in whom clinical signs subsided and ultrasound findings regressed, acute appendicitis may have been reversible.

As of this writing, the use of ultrasound in the direct diagnosis of appendicitis is still undergoing clinical study in some major centers. The procedure has so far failed to incite general interest because it requires meticulous technique, state-of-the-art equipment, and clinical experience for validation of accuracy. This is likely to remain a problem in the average center, because of the limited opportunity to study and verify a significant number of cases of acute appendicitis. Yet, with the rapid spread and improvement of ultrasound imaging skill and technology, there is a distinct possibility this method may well be applied more widely within a few years. Our own experience with the technique so far has not been encouraging.

When confronting the young female patient with lower quadrant pelvic pain and tenderness, it is essential for the clinician to keep in mind that acute adnexal disease, usually salpingitis, is three times as likely as appendicitis and is the second most common cause of serious abdominal pain in women. In the important subset of females from 15–40 years, in whom the clinical differentiation of inflammatory adnexal or ovarian disease from appendicitis may be extremely difficult, it is not surprising that removal of normal appendixes occurs with the highest frequency, in 35–59% of cases (37, 38, 44). Thus, ultrasonography is at present more reliable in excluding, rather than confirming, the diagnosis of appendicitis.

The most important use of pelvic ultrasonography in the differential diagnosis of lower abdominal or pelvic pain is therefore in this group of young women. *The high sensitivity and specificity of sonographic diagnosis of acute pelvic conditions should make this procedure virtually mandatory in women with suspected appendicitis.* We stress that transvaginal pelvic sonography is generally to be preferred to the transabdominal study in visualization of the adnexae.

HOW OFTEN DO OVARIAN CYSTS CAUSE ABDOMINAL PAIN?

An enormous number of discharge diagnoses were recorded for ovarian cysts in the United States, more than 188,000 in 1989, putting it well ahead of pancreatitis and diverticular disease. In the same year there were astounding numbers of ovarian operations and combined salpingectomies, excluding those performed with hysterectomies. It is impossible to estimate from the ICD codes how many operations were performed solely for ovarian cysts, but the number must have been significant. The total number of tuboovarian operations, 288,000, should be compared with 127,000 appendectomies performed in women in 1990 and an additional 112,000 "incidental" appendectomies performed during pelvic surgery (27).

Our decision not to include ovarian cyst as a significant cause of serious abdominal pain may raise a few eyebrows but is no oversight. First, most so-called ovarian cysts are in fact Graafian follicles. Normal size for these physiological structures may reach 2.0–2.5 cm. After observing more than 15,000 pelvic ultrasonographies (we routinely witness almost all ultrasonographic examinations in our department), we have concluded that perhaps 90% or more of recurrent chronic or acute pelvic pain in women referred to us is of undetermined or unverifiable origin. Most of these cases would be classified as some type of chronic or recurrent nonspecific type pain or, in the opinion of many, "nondisease". It is hard to escape the clinical impression from the histories of these patients that they have either some underlying emotional source of their pain, some variant of irritable bowel syndrome, or else some chronic equivalent of NSAP. This has been amply documented in the literature, particularly in young women with right-sided pelvic pain (45). Many of these unfortunate patients, some of whom already have had unnecessary appendectomies, often consult numerous physicians and may undergo needless and multiple laparoscopies and failed pelvic operations, usually ovarian cystectomies or total hysterectomies.

Because physicians, like other mortals, are cause-seeking animals, there is a temptation among the ingenuous to ascribe unexplained pelvic pain to the presence of an incidental ovarian cyst. However, because small physiological ovarian cysts smaller than 2.5 cm are found almost routinely in pelvic sonography of patients in their menstrual years, and most patients with such cysts are asymptomatic, a cause-and-effect relationship remains doubtful. Moreover, a significant number of women with larger cysts up to 4–6 cm or more discovered incidentally are completely asymptomatic. We continue to see numerous patients operated, sometimes repeatedly, for "symptomatic" ovarian cysts, only to return with continued pain.

A well-known gynecological dictum is that, in addition to small physiological cysts, larger cysts, often up to 6 cm or more, frequently disappear spontaneously, within a few weeks. This is the basis for responsible gynecological opinion, which holds that asymptomatic ovarian cysts in this size range generally should not be operated upon unless they fail to show regression in a period of no less than 6–8 or even 12 weeks.

We do not minimize the potential for trouble with larger cysts or deny that ovarian cysts may indeed cause pelvic pain, even abdominal catastrophe. A fair number may bleed causing transient symptoms, but the majority of these cysts resolve without difficulty and can be followed with sonography. There is always the rare case of significant hemorrhage, rupture, or twisting on a pedicle, all verifiable ovarian causes of lower abdominal pain, *sometimes* requiring immediate surgical intervention. We stress, however, that most physiological and larger cysts that have bled, leaked, or ruptured days or even weeks before sonographic discovery do well without any intervention. The clinical history in these cases is typical. Recall, too, that the most common cause of painful ruptured ovarian cyst is ovulation causing Mittelschmerz, a frequently overlooked diagnosis in young women.

When the sonographic criteria of a "pure" ovarian cyst are satisfied, i.e. one without any internal echoes, etc., we hold that the *diagnosis of symptomatic ovarian cyst should be made with caution and is an uncommon cause of pelvic pain.*

IMAGING IN PANCREATITIS

Pancreatitis ranks next to last in frequency as a cause of serious abdominal conditions, accounting for 15% and 6% of all such cases in men and women, respectively. Yet, because of its mortality and morbidity, and its frequent confusion with surgical emergencies, it remains an important condition. Acute pancreatitis has many causes, and in fact its association with gall stones deserves separate mention in terms of diagnostic imaging. In uncomplicated pancreatitis, imaging is usually not required, especially when a typical history and physical findings are accompanied by an elevated serum or urinary amylase or lipase. In pancreatitis complicated by gall stones, hemorrhagic disease, pseudocyst formation, infection, or when the patient is seen late and chemical findings are normal, imaging is essential.

Real-time ultrasonography is the study of first choice because of its ease, safety, and effectiveness. With newer equipment and techniques, the organ can now be visualized more than 95% of the time in the nonobese patient. In a retrospective series of 278 patients studied over a 3-year period, CT was proclaimed superior to ultrasound, whereas 300 patients were studied *prospectively* for 2 more years with CT and ERCP—but not with sonography (46). In fact, ERCP should *never* be used in patients with acute pancreatitis, because it is not only of doubtful effectiveness but exceedingly dangerous, with the ability to cause or exacerbate the very disease it is meant to diagnose (47–49). Angiography is indicated only in differentiating chronic pancreatitis with a mass effect from tumor, or when assessing vascular complications of pancreatitis preoperatively in the rare case when surgical management is called for. Studies dealing with the sensitivities of CT and ultrasound report a morphologically normal pancreas in approximately 10–28% of patients with acute uncomplicated pancreatitis (50). The failure rate, sensitivity, and specificity of both modalities in *complicated* cases varies with the series, but overall, CT is indicated only if ultrasound imaging fails to provide a diagnosis.

Table 6.2.8 should be studied carefully, because it is the prototype for many of those to follow. The purpose of these tables is to indicate the predictive values of a specific imaging study based on the assumed prevalence of the condition and the known or estimated sensitivity of the procedure. The mathematical bases for the various calculations, in particular the derivation of nonspecificity, PPV, and 1-NPV are derived from Bayes' Theorem, which is discussed at length in Appendix A. In the first column we have indicated the hypothetical prior probability (prevalence) of acute pancreatitis as 67%. In this example we are assuming the clinician feels, based on his findings, there are two chances out of three the patient has pancreatitis and one chance out of three he has some other condition causing

Table 6.2.8.   Comparison of Ultrasonography and CT in Diagnosing Pancreatitis

| Test | Prevalence | Name of disease: pancreatitis | | PPV | 1-NPV |
		Sensitivity	Nonspecificity		
Ultrasonography	67	78	5	97	32
CT	67	92	5	97	15

Prevalence is the probability of disease. Sensitivity is the probability of positive test result given the disease. Nonspecificity is the probability of positive test result given not the disease. PPV is the probability of disease given a positive test result. 1-NPV is the probability of disease given a negative test result.

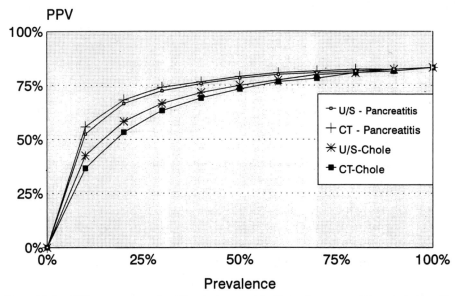

Figure 6.2.4.   PPV vs. prevalence for CT and ultrasound in diagnosing pancreatitis and cholecystitis.

acute abdominal pain. Nonspecificity represents the estimated percentage of false-positive tests and is assumed to be low for an imaging procedure. Both ultrasound and CT, with reported sensitivities of 0.78 and 0.92, respectively (51), have the same high PPV of pancreatitis, 97%, despite what appears to be the significantly better sensitivity of CT. In Figure 6.2.4 PPVs for CT and ultrasound for both pancreatitis and cholecystitis are plotted graphically against disease prevalence. Sensitivities for cholecystitis are estimated as 0.72 for CT vs. 0.92 for sonography, and nonspecificities 0.10. Note the typical shape of all four curves and the minimal spread between CT and ultrasonography for each pair of diseases. The curves demonstrate a recurring theme of this text, namely that disease prevalence much below 20% results in very poor predictive value of even a good test with high sensitivity and low nonspecificity.

Overall, however, if ultrasound is *negative* and the diagnosis of pancreatitis is still suspected, CT should be performed next. The effectiveness of MRI compared with CT in pancreatic diagnosis has yet to be established.

IMAGING IN SUSPECTED LARGE AND SMALL BOWEL OBSTRUCTION

The supine and upright, or if the patient is unable to stand, the lateral decubitus radiographs of the abdomen, are the mainstay of imaging in intestinal obstruction, but in the small bowel plain films alone may be misleading. Pathognomonic findings in small bowel obstruction may be present in only one-third to half of cases early in the disease, and the differentiation of partial or early mechanical small bowel obstruction from adynamic ileus may be impossible. In the majority of cases of suspected intestinal obstruction, a barium enema should be done *first* to exclude colonic obstruction. Once confirmed that the problem is not in the large bowel, aqueous contrast may be given orally. This may be useful in the rare case in which the patient is not vomiting, but contrast is generally more helpful if given through a Cantor or Miller-Abbott tube. Most radiologists prefer barium in the patient with suspected mechanical small bowel obstruction in whom plain films are not sufficient for diagnosis. Surgeons, however, are apprehensive if operation is contemplated on the barium-filled small bowel. Oral barium should *never* be used in suspected large bowel obstruction.

Large bowel obstruction with a competent ileocecal valve is easily recognized because distension with gas is mainly confined to the colon, otherwise the films in proximal colonic obstruction may resemble distal small bowel obstruction. Here, as in most cases of bowel obstruction, a careful barium enema is invaluable in determining the site or nature of the lesion, even in the presence of suspected perforation. (In toxic megacolon the barium enema should be avoided.) Again, however, the surgeon approaches the barium-filled bowel with trepidation and often prefers aqueous contrast. This poses a problem, because the radiologist prefers barium due to poor visualization with aqueous media. In general, careful clinical examination combined with plain abdominal radiographs and, if necessary, barium or aqueous contrast enema should establish the diagnosis and location of large bowel obstruction in the vast majority of patients.

Two large recent studies dealt with the radiologic diagnosis of intestinal obstruction. In one retrospective series of 229 patients with a final diagnosis of small-bowel obstruction (52), in 84 patients or 37%, the clinical history and plain abdominal films were sufficient for diagnosis and subsequent management. The remaining 145 patients were studied with an upper GI series, barium enema, or both, and accurate diagnostic information was obtained in 125 or 86%. Only three false-negative and two false-positive studies were obtained. In the second study (53), either upper GI contrast or barium enema examinations were performed in only 96 or 27% of 342 patients with small bowel obstruction, suggesting that plain films had a much higher accuracy in their series. The results with upper GI studies predicted complete small bowel obstruction in 34 of 34 operated cases, whereas barium enema demonstrated obstruction in only 13 or 33% of 39 cases. Yet in 19 of 23 patients with large-bowel obstruction, barium enema showed the level of obstruction in all cases. Three recovered with barium enema reduction of intussusception or volvulus. The choice of aqueous contrast over barium, however, remains an unsettled issue. In small bowel and even large bowel obstruction aqueous contrast is diagnostically so inferior to barium that radiologists whenever possible prefer the latter, whereas surgeons dislike and sometimes abhor the use of barium if they anticipate an operation.

Perhaps in no other serious intraabdominal condition are frequent clinical observation and clinical judgment more important for a successful outcome than in the patient with intestinal obstruction. Although we would prefer to have some perfect test for obstruction, we must acknowledge that even the basic studies outlined above may complement but never substitute for bedside clinical skill and experience.

IMAGING IN SUSPECTED PERFORATION AND DIVERTICULITIS

In suspected acute perforated peptic ulcer, plain and upright abdominal films remain the premier imaging procedure. Air will be seen under the diaphragm in more than 90–95% of cases (though the sign may be absent in the first few hours). As noted above, however, this is no longer an important cause of acute abdominal pain presentations. With lower intestinal perforations, most of which occur as a result of diverticulitis, the presence of air under the diaphragm is much less reliable because it occurs rarely. However, the plain film is still important in assessing the presence of coexistent problems such as large bowel obstruction.

The majority of patients admitted to hospitals with left lower quadrant and left-sided peritonitis and suspected diverticulitis will tolerate a careful early barium enema, a study that will immediately confirm the diagnosis and help eliminate complications and lengthy hospital stays. Some authors advocate that this be done with aqueous material such as Gastrografin (54). Though Shinya (55) suggests the examination be delayed until the attack subsides or when it is felt safe to perform the procedure, we prefer early barium studies in most cases.

The use of flexible sigmoidoscopy or even colonoscopy in the diagnosis of acute diverticulitis is a dangerous exercise and should be condemned. We will merely quote from Shinya's classic text on colonoscopy (55): "With acute diverticulitis, treatment of the bowel disease precedes elective colonoscopic evaluation. After the attack subsides, a barium enema is obtained to exclude carcinoma, obstruction or a sealed perforation, which may require early surgery. *If there is no clinical or radiologic evidence of diverticulitis or other complications* . . ., endoscopic evaluation *may be done*." (our emphasis). Other diagnostic studies, in particular CT, ultrasound, or gallium/indium white blood cell (WBC) scintigraphy, may be required in the presence of an intraabdominal collection resulting from diverticular perforation. This subject will be discussed in a later chapter.

We have omitted other important but unusual causes of acute abdominal pain here because we continue to emphasize the most common conditions likely to be encountered. Other diagnostic methods, however, may become necessary in an important, if small, subset of patients with acute abdominal pain who are acutely ill. These are predominantly older patients, usually those with significant complicating conditions, in whom the risk of needless laparotomy makes it unacceptable. In some of these patients there is a place for CT and, in particular, diagnostic laparoscopy. In one series of more than 200 patients, emergent laparoscopy helped avoid useless laparotomy in 21% of cases (56). An important surgical text devoted entirely to laparoscopic diagnosis of abdominal disease deals with the application of this technique in abdominal pain (57). At present we are witnessing an explosion in the use of laparoscopic abdominal surgery. In patients with indications for diagnostic laparoscopy, treatment, either open or laparoscopic surgery, if indicated, may be carried out at the same sitting. A good example would be the use of pelvic laparoscopy for the diagnosis (and treatment?) of appendicitis and ectopic pregnancy. We must, however, add that laparoscopy is undoubtedly overused and overrated in the diagnosis of chronic conditions of the female pelvis.

Aside from these difficult or unusual cases, and in the elderly or those with complicating medical conditions, *in competent clinical hands, successful imaging, with plain abdominal radiographs, contrast studies, ultrasonography, and hepatobiliary scanning, suffices for abdominal diagnosis in 85–95% of cases of serious acute abdominal pain.*

A Reasonable Clinical Diagnostic Approach to Acute Abdominal Pain

Having said that most patients presenting with acute abdominal pain will have benign conditions not requiring further testing, we conclude by outlining a basic imaging approach for the significant serious diseases listed above. We stress again the list is not meant to be exhaustive, but that overall it covers the great majority of serious conditions.

At the risk of repeating ourselves, we continue to emphasize that rational imaging strategy depends on *pretest probability* of disease. Only the physician can estimate this in light of his knowledge of the prevalence, symptoms, and signs of various conditions combined with his clinical skills. For the initial approach to the patient with abdominal pain, it is obviously critical to establish, first and foremost, two facts:

1. Is one dealing with a serious or a benign condition, and if the former, is it an urgent (operative) or a nonurgent problem?

2. Are the pain and tenderness concordant, and if not, what is the relationship between their locations? Is the disease more likely to be localized in the upper abdomen, in the right or left abdomen, in the central or lower abdomen or pelvis, or is it generalized?

It goes without saying that in acute intraabdominal disease, frequent observation and examination of the patient over a period of several hours are sometimes required to answer the above questions. However, almost nowhere else in diagnosis is early treatment so critical to the successful outcome, because unjustifiable delay in diagnosis, perhaps even 8–10 hours, is gambling with a life. Sir Zachary Cope, in his classic work (58), stated a priceless clinical dictum: ". . . the majority of severe abdominal pains which ensue in patients who have been previously fairly well, and which last as long as six hours, are caused by conditions of surgical import."

The Anatomical Geography of Serious Abdominal Pain: The Patient with Localizing Complaints or Findings

If significant localizing abdominal pain and/or tenderness are present, including that on rectal and pelvic exam, it is helpful to attempt to estimate the likely diagnoses and indicated imaging studies by abdominal regions.

Localizing Upper Abdominal Pain, Including the Periumbilical Region, Epigastrium, and Right Upper Quadrant: Both Sexes

Peptic ulcer disease, nonulcer dyspepsia, acute gastritis, and NSAP are, of course, the most common causes of epigastric, right upper quadrant, and periumbilical pain, but we are assuming the clinical indications are of *serious* and *new* disease. Admittedly, these benign conditions may be difficult to exclude, but if in doubt, think of cholecystitis *first*, pancreatitis *second*, with appendicitis, perforation, and intestinal obstruction far down the list, and pelvic conditions, diverticular, and all other causes very far down the list. In this situation, ultrasonography of the biliary tract, including gall bladder, common bile duct, and pancreas, is unsurpassed. In the presence of a negative examination, acute cholecystitis and pancreatitis can be excluded with more than 90% confidence.

In the presence of gall stones and a thick-walled gall bladder on ultrasound, and with a convincing clinical history and physical findings, the diagnosis of cholecystitis can be made without resorting to hepatobiliary scanning. In the presence of convincing right upper quadrant or epigastric tenderness, *without gall stones* by ultrasound, or if all three criteria are not met, the hepatobiliary scan always should be done to exclude or rule in the diagnosis of acute cholecystitis with more than 99% confidence.

Localizing Right-Sided Abdominal (Right Half), and Right Lower Quadrant Pain: Males

The most likely serious causes here are cholecystitis, pancreatitis, and appendicitis, and least likely, intestinal obstruction. Diagnosis is essentially the same as above: sonography of the gall bladder, biliary tract, and pancreas to exclude cholecystitis and pancreatitis. Sonography of the appendix is still of unproven reliability, and the diagnosis of appendicitis remains a clinical one, except in those few difficult patients in whom diagnostic laparoscopy is felt justifiable in order to avoid possible exploratory surgery. If appendiceal and biliary tract disease are unlikely, and particularly in patients with previous abdominal surgery, the method outlined above for intestinal obstruction should be followed.

Right-Sided Abdominal Pain and Right Lower Quadrant: Females

In all female patients in the menstruating years (including young girls likely to be close to menarche) with acute right-sided pain and accompanying findings, always perform pelvic ultrasonography to exclude pelvic disease, in particular salpingitis, and ectopic pregnancy. Ectopic pregnancy is 99% excluded with a negative β-subunit human chorionic gonadotropin (but not with the routine urinary pregnancy test). Whether one chooses pelvic or upper abdominal ultrasound first depends entirely on clinical suspicion of disease location. Suffice it to say that if one study is negative, the other may have to be performed, but again only if indicated on reasonable clinical grounds. For example, in a young woman with strong suspicion of appendicitis, if pelvic sonography is negative, upper abdominal sonography is obviously not indicated.

Note: Except under unusual or emergent circumstances *do not send a woman of menstrual age for appendectomy without first obtaining pelvic sonography.*

Lower Abdominal or Pelvic Pain: Females

Pelvic ultrasound again is the modality of choice. We do not feel acute pelvic pain generally calls for ultrasonography in the male patient.

Left-Sided Abdominal Pain

In the younger age group, most left-sided pain is benign, except for the rare possibility of pancreatitis. Cholecystitis and appendicitis virtually *never* present with exclusively left-sided findings or complaints. Obstruction always remains a possibility. In the older patient, left-sided abdominal pain, particularly in the lower left quadrant with signs of peritoneal irritation, usually indicates diverticular disease, with obstruction the second most likely diagnosis. Imaging procedures, as outlined, include plain abdominal X-rays, sonography in a patient at risk for pancreatitis, and upper or lower GI barium studies in the presence of suspected intestinal obstruction or diverticulitis. In young females, of course, left lower quadrant pain should be regarded as pelvic pain and ultrasonography performed.

Nonlocalizing or Generalized Abdominal Pain and Tenderness

Like abdominal pain with localized findings, a reasonable diagnostic approach to nonlocalizing abdominal pain does not require mindless ordering of tests. The first approach, obviously, is the plain abdominal film, followed by surgical consultation. Depending on likelihood of disease based on age, sex, and history, the diagnoses of ruptured appendix, acute pelvic inflammatory disease, ectopic pregnancy, perforation, diverticulitis, acute cholecystitis, and intestinal obstruction often can be made with a high degree of confidence.

If plain abdominal films are not helpful, sonography always should be performed to help exclude gall bladder, pancreatic, and pelvic disease. If, as is sometimes the case, it is difficult to image the pancreas by ultrasound in the presence of significant tenderness or distension, abdominal CT is recommended when the clinical findings and amylase or lipase studies are nondiagnostic for pancreatitis.

General Summary of Imaging in Acute Abdominal Pain
BENIGN ABDOMINAL PAIN

1. Careful clinical assessment of the patient should obviate the need for diagnostic studies in more than 90% of all patients with abdominal pain under 7 day's duration. Approximately half the patients presenting will have NSAP, and more than 98% of these will recover without specific treatment and without a cause being found.

This, therefore, should elicit no anxiety except in the patient over age 50. About 10% of patients in this age group with unexplained abdominal pain ultimately will turn out to have an intraabdominal malignancy. These patients, when they recover, should have air contrast barium studies of the upper and lower GI tract.

2. In young women with unexplained pelvic pain, a pregnancy test is mandatory. In upper or midabdominal pain in high-risk groups such as alcoholics, the serum or urinary amylase or lipase should be obtained.

A cautionary word about amylase. It is now well-appreciated that serum amylase is elevated significantly not only in pancreatitis but in more than half the cases of appendicitis and in a variable percentage of patients with other serious intraabdominal and even extraabdominal pathology, in particular intestinal obstruction, perforated ulcer, cholecystitis, peritonitis, renal insufficiency, cerebral trauma, burns, postoperative patients, and especially ruptured ectopic pregnancy (59). However, if we keep the nonspecificity of the test in mind, the highly consistent early elevation of amylase in pancreatitis is still an enormous help in diagnosis of that condition. Yet this remains a classic example of the perils of ordering an inappropriate test. A high serum amylase in a clinically suspect case of appendicitis, intestinal obstruction, or ectopic pregnancy is worse than meaningless—it is misleading.

SERIOUS ABDOMINAL PAIN

In the presence of significant clinical findings, particularly localizing or nonlocalizing tenderness *whether or not fever or leukocytosis are present*, and especially with persistent severe pain for more than 6 hours in a patient who has been previously well, consider the following:

1. In the case of an obvious surgical abdomen, the kind that "cries out to be explored," do not waste time; first call the surgeon. While waiting for him, it is perfectly reasonable to order supine and upright films of the abdomen, and appropriate sonography, if gall bladder or pelvic disease is suspected. But time is of the essence. In general, for nontraumatic acute abdominal pain *do not order CT or MRI, both of which are virtually useless in this setting and result only in unnecessary delay. Upper GI endoscopy or sigmoidoscopy have virtually no place in the diagnosis of acute abdominal pain.*

2. Never overlook the possibility, especially in younger patients, of a lower lobe pneumonia causing an acute abdomen. The simple chest radiograph usually can settle the issue. Moreover, in the older patient, myocardial infarction can occasionally masquerade as acute abdominal disease, especially cholecystitis.

3. For all patients under the age of 15, by far the single most common cause of acute surgical abdomen is appendicitis. In the age group under 5, think also of small bowel obstruction, usually secondary to intussusception. However, note again from Table 6.2.6 that less than 5% of all cases of intestinal obstruction occur in patients under 15 years old. Imaging in children with acute abdominal pain always should include plain abdominal and chest films. If obstruction is suspected, the barium enema is virtually mandatory and may, in cases of volvulus and intussusception, be therapeutic.

4. For all other patients, cholecystitis is the most common cause of surgical abdomen in both sexes, and its age distribution is fairly uniform over the age of 30.

5. Intestinal obstruction due to strangulated hernia is common at all ages, *and this may be inguinal or femoral in both sexes.* Other types of intestinal obstruction are increasingly common with age, with more than 80% of cases occurring in patients over age 45. Diverticular disease also is exceedingly rare in younger patients, with more than half the cases occurring over age 65. Free perforations due to peptic ulcer have become increasingly less common in the past few years.

The single most valuable study in upper or lower intestinal obstruction, diverticulitis, and perforation, is the supine and upright plain radiograph of the abdomen, followed by upper or lower barium (occasionally aqueous) contrast studies. Abnormal findings on plain radiographs may not always be present, and, if findings are present, they are often nonspecific. Therefore, in these three conditions, imaging studies cannot replace clinical assessment. This may cause consternation in some quarters but should reassure those who worry about physicians being replaced by machines.

Final Remarks and Possible Omissions

We have not included pyelonephritis and renal calculus in the above discussion. Unquestionably, these entities are responsible for a significant number of acute abdominal pain presentations, perhaps 10–15%, but they will be covered in subsequent chapters dealing with GU pain and urinary findings. Suffice it to say these two important urinary tract diseases may mimic any one of our principal seven significant causes of abdominal symptoms. If a careful history and examination are done, however, *along with a urinalysis,* diagnostic errors should be kept to a minimum. Note that urinary tract pain does not always present typically in the "flank," and that CVA tenderness as well as tenderness over the kidneys anteriorly should largely be distinguishable from true abdominal tenderness. The problem is that one man's midlateral quadrant may be another man's "flank" — and vice versa. *A normal urinalysis virtually excludes a GU cause of abdominal pain.*

Acute duodenal ulcer and nonulcer dyspepsia rarely should cause difficulty in the diagnosis of new, acute upper abdominal pain, but it is always wise to keep these possibilities in mind. The real talent in abdominal diagnosis consists of listening to the patient, skillful examination of the abdomen, and a knowledge of serious medical and surgical disease prevalence by age, sex, and even ethnic origin. For example, Hispanics have a high incidence of cholelithiasis and presumably cholecystitis.

Whether to image, and, if so, what procedure to choose, can only be determined in light of clinical findings and good clinical judgment.

REFERENCES

1. Thompson WG, Heaton KW. Functional bowel disorders in apparently healthy people. Gastroenterology 1980;79(2):283–288.
2. Switz DM. What the gastroenterologist does all day. Gastroenterology 1976;70(6):1048–1050.
3. Kirsner JB. The irritable bowel syndrome. A clinical review and ethical considerations. Arch Intern Med 1981;141(5):635–639.
4. Jess P. Acute appendicitis: epidemiology, diagnostic accuracy, and complications. Scand J Gastroenterol 1983;18(2):161–163.
5. Silen W. Acute intestinal obstruction. In: Petersdorf RG, Adams RD, Braunwald E, Isselbacher KJ, Martin JB, Wilson JD, eds. Harrison's Principles of Internal Medicine. 10th ed. New York: McGraw-Hill, Inc., 1983:1767.
6. Ranson JH, Acute pancreatitis — where are we? Surg Clin North Am 1981;61(1):55–70.
7. Wilson C, Imrie CW. Deaths from acute pancreatitis: why do we miss the diagnosis so frequently? Int J Pancreatol 1988;3(4):273–281.
8. Schofield PF, Hulton NR, Baildam AD. Is it acute cholecystitis? Ann R Coll Surg Engl 1986;68(1):14–16.
9. Wexner SD, Dailey TH. The initial management of left lower quadrant peritonitis. Dis Colon Rectum 1986;29(10):635–638.
10. Wilson DH, Wilson PD, Walmsley RG, Horrock JC, deDombal FT. Diagnosis of acute abdominal pain in the accident and emergency department. Br J Surg 1977;64(4):249–254.
11. Brewer BJ, Golden GT, Hitch DC, Rudolf LE, Wangensteen SL. Abdominal pain. An analysis of 1,000 consecutive cases in a university hospital emergency room. Am J Surg 1976;131(2):219–223.
12. Jordan Jr GL. The acute abdomen. In: Jordan Jr GL ed. Advances in Surgery Chicago: Year Book Medical Publishers, Inc., 1980;14:259–315.
13. Leaper DJ, Horrocks JC, Staniland JR, deDombal FT. Computer-assisted diagnosis of abdominal pain using "estimates" provided by clinicians. Br Med J 1972;4(836):350–354.
14. DeDombal FT. Computer-based assistance for medical decision making. Gastroenterol Clin Biol 1984;8(2):135–137.
15. Staniland JR, Ditchburn J, deDombal FT. Clinical Presentation of Acute Abdomen: Study of 600 Patients. Br Med J 1972;3(823):393–398.
16. Adams ID, Chan M, Clifford PC, et al. Computer-aided diagnosis of acute abdominal pain: a multicentre study. Br Med J 1986;293(6550):800–804.
17. Sturman MF, Perez M. Computer-assisted diagnosis of acute abdominal pain. Compr Ther 1989; 15(2):26–35.
18. deDombal FT. Picking the best tests in acute abdominal pain. J R Coll Physicians Lond 1979;13(4):203–208.
19. Cox K, ed. The National Ambulatory Medical Care Survey. United States, 1975–81 and 1985 Trends. Hyattsville, MD: U.S. Department of Health and Human Services. Public Health Service. Centers for Disease Control. National Center for Health Statistics, June 1988. Data from the National Health Survey. DHHS Publication (PHS) 88–1754.
20. NCHS Advancedata. From Vital and Health Statistics of the National Center for Health Statistics Jan 23, 1987, no. 120.3.
21. ICD-9-CM. International Classification of Diseases. 9th revision, 3rd ed. Clinical Modification, volumes 1, 2, and 3. Los Angeles: Practice Management Information Corporation (PMI), 1989. (U.S. Department of Health and Human Services Publication PHS 89-1260).

22. Rang EH, Fairbairn AS, Acheson ED. An enquiry into the incidence and prognosis of undiagnosed abdominal pain treated in hospital. Br J Prev Soc Med 1970;24(1):47–51.
23. Jess P, Bjerregaard B, Brynitz S, et al. Prognosis of acute nonspecific abdominal pain. A Prospective study. Am J Surg 1982;144(3):338–340.
24. deDombal FT, Matharu SS, Staniland JR, et al. Presentation of cancer to hospital as "acute abdominal pain." Br J Surg 1980;67(6):413–416.
25. Pullan CR, Halse PC, Sims DG, Alexander FW, Gardner PS, Codd AA. Viruses and acute abdominal pain in childhood. Arch Dis Child 1979;54(10):780–782.
26. Jorgensen LS, Bonlokke L, Christensen NJ. Life strain, life events, and autonomic response to a psychological stressor in patients with chronic upper abdominal pain. Scand J Gastroenterol 1986; 21(5):605–613.
27. U.S. Department of Health and Human Services, U.S. Public Health Service, Centers for Disease Control, and the National Center for Health Statistics. National Hospital Discharge Survey (NHDS). Detailed diagnoses, procedures, days of care, diagnoses-related groups for patients discharged from short-stay hospitals. Public Use Data Diskettes, 1985–1990.
28. Barakos JA, Ralls PW, Lapin SA, et al. Cholelithiasis: evaluation with CT. Radiology 1987;162(2): 415–418.
29. Friedman GD, Kannel WB, Dawber TR. The epidemiology of gall bladder disease: observations in the Framingham study. J Chronic Dis 1966;19(3):273–292.
30. Gracie WA, Ransohoff DF. The natural history of silent gall-stones: the innocent gallstone is not a myth. N Engl J Med 1982;307(13):798–800.
31. Wilbur RS, Bolt RJ. Incidence of gallbladder disease in "normal" men. Gastroenterology 1959;36: 251–255.
32. Laing FC, Federle MP, Jeffrey RB, Brown TW. Ultrasonic evaluation of patients with acute right upper quadrant pain. Radiology 1981;140(2):449–455.
33. Shuman WP, Mack LA, Rudd TG, Rogers JV, Gibbs P. Evaluation of acute right upper quadrant pain: sonography and 99mTc-PIPIDA cholescintigraphy. AJR 1982;139(1):61–64.
34. Ralls PW, Colletti PM, Lapin SA, et al. Real-time sonography in suspected acute cholecystitis. Radiology 1985;155(3):767–771.
35. Talbert JL, Zuidema GD. Appendicitis—a reappraisal of an old problem. Surg Clin North Am 1966; 46(5):1101–1112.
36. Berry Jr J, Malt RA. Appendicitis near its centenary. Ann Surg 1984;200(5):567–575.
37. Bongard F, Landers DV, Lewis F. Differential diagnosis of appendicitis and pelvic inflammatory disease. Am J Surg 1985;150(1):90–96.
38. Lau WY, Fan ST, Yiu TF, Chu KW, Wong SH. Negative findings at appendectomy. Am J Surg 1984;148(3):375–378.
39. Balthazar EJ, Gordon RB. CT of appendicitis. Semin Ultrasound, CT, MR 1989;10(4):326–340.
40. Navarro DA, Weber PM. Indium-111 imaging in appendicitis. Semin Ultrasound, CT, MR 1989; 10(4):321–325.
41. Abu-Yousef MM, Franken Jr EA. An overview of graded compression sonography in the diagnosis of acute appendicitis. Semin Ultrasound, CT, MR 1989;10(4):352–363.
42. Jeffrey RB. New imaging tools improve diagnosis of appendicitis. Diagn Imaging 1988;10(5):100–103.
43. Jeffrey Jr RB, Laing FC, Lewis FR. Acute appendicitis: high resolution real-time US findings. Radiology 1987;163(1):11–14.
44. Harding HE. A notable source of error in the diagnosis of appendicitis. Br Med J 1962;2(5311):1028–1029.
45. Ingram PW, Evans G. Right iliac fossa pain in young women. Br Med J 1965;2:149–151.
46. Freeny PC, Marks WM, Ball TJ. Impact of high-resolution computed tomography of the pancreas on utilization of endoscopic retrograde cholangiopancreatography and angiography. Radiology 1982; 142(1):35–39.
47. Ruppin H, Amon R, Ett W, et al. Acute pancreatitis after endoscopic/radiological pancreaticography (ERP). Endoscopy 1974;6:94–98.
48. La Ferla G, Gordon S, Archibald M, Murray WR. Hyperamylasaemia and acute pancreatitis following endoscopic retrograde cholangiopancreatography. Pancreas 1986;1(2):160–163.
49. Kasugai T, Kuno N, Aoki I, Kizy M, Kobayashi S. Fiberduodenoscopy; analysis of 353 examinations. Gastrointest Endosc 1971;18(1):9–16.
50. Van Dyke JA, Stanley RJ, Berland LL. Pancreatic imaging. Ann Intern Med 1985;102(2):212–217.
51. Freeny PC, Lawson TL. Radiology of the Pancreas. New York: Springer-Verlag, 1982:427.
52. Riveron FA, Obeid FN, Horst HM, Sorensen VJ, Bivins BA. The role of contrast radiography in presumed bowel obstruction. Surgery 1989;106(3):496–501.

53. Ericksen AS, Krasna MJ, Mast BA, Nosher JL, Brolin RE. Use of gastrointestinal contrast studies in obstruction of the small and large bowel. Dis Colon Rectum 1990;33(1):56–64.
54. Wexner SD, Dailey TH. The initial management of left lower quadrant peritonitis. Dis Colon Rectum 1986;29(10):635–638.
55. Shinya H. Colonoscopy. Tokyo: Igaku-Shoin, 1982:79.
56. Kononov AG, Makarov VI, Sotnichenko BA. Effectiveness of laparoscopy in the diagnosis of disease simulating "acute abdomen." Vestn Khir 1989;143(7):37–39.
57. Salky BA, Berci G. Laparoscopy for Surgeons. Tokyo: Igaku-Shoin 1990.
58. Cope, Z. Cope's Early Diagnosis of the Acute Abdomen. 16th ed. Revised by William Silen. New York: Oxford University Press, 1983.
59. Salt II WB, Schenker S. Amylase—its clinical significance: a review of the literature. Medicine 1976; 55(4):269–289.

3/ Thoracic Pain

Classification and General Discussion: Coronary vs. Other Thoracic Pain

Much of your pain is self-chosen. It is the bitter potion by which the physician within you heals your sick self.

Kahlil Gibran
"On Pain," The Prophet *(1923)*

Chest pain is one of the three most common causes of emergency room presentations, preceded only by fracture and abdominal pain. In one British study (1) anterior chest pain was the presenting complaint in one out of four medical cases.

The etiologies and epidemiology of thoracic pain are difficult to unravel because there are an almost limitless number of clinical presentations, both classifiable and obscure, representing coronary, "quasi-coronary," and other types of chest pain. The complaint is strongly reminiscent of abdominal pain in the large preponderance of "we-see-this" and other innocuous, nonspecific, and ill-defined examples. As we observed in Chapter 1, *most of these presentations can be described but not named, and therefore cannot receive ICD-9 codes.* Noncoronary or "no sweat" chest pain is overwhelmingly more common in younger patients complaining of chest pain and predominates over coronary or anginal pain even in the elderly. The logical basis of a diagnostic approach to chest pain is similar to our classification of abdominal pain and is based on the concept of serious or potentially life-threatening vs. benign or innocuous disease.

Table 6.3.1 illustrates this approach. Note the large number of entities included even in this partial tabulation and the difficulty in maintaining consistency in a mixed anatomic/etiological classification. For example, chronic obstructive pulmonary disease, asthma, and hypoxia may not always belong under innocuous pain, many cases of chest wall pain classified as "nonspecific" may be "cross-over" syndromes, i.e. mitral valve prolapse, psychogenic pain, panic attacks, etc. (vide infra). Furthermore, pulmonary embolism has to be classed as both "pleuritic" and "serious" pain. Table 6.3.2 is an abridged list of the most common causes of chest pain in probable order of frequency. We again emphasize that this section deals with a specific *given* symptom, thoracic or chest pain, not the listed conditions per se. We recognize that most patients with pulmonary embolism do not present with pain, pleuritic or otherwise, any more than do all patients with esophagitis or heart attacks. In all of Chapter 6, we are

Table 6.3.1.   Principal Causes of Innocuous and Serious Thoracic Pain, in Probable Order of Frequency

---

Generally innocuous chest pain
1. Nonspecific, including:
   Psychogenic, (anxiety, depression, panic attacks,)
   Idiopathic/undecidable
   Mitral valve prolapse
2. Upper GI-induced chest pain, including:
   Reflux or other esophagitis, (hiatus hernia), esophageal motility disorders, esophageal spasm,
      "nutcracker" esophagitis
   Peptic and nonulcer dyspepsia
   Cholecystitis, pancreatitis etc. (rare)
3. Chest wall pain, including:
   Chest wall syndrome, muscle strain, costochondritis (Teitze's),
   Trauma, rib fractures, etc.
   Intercostal or radicular pain
      (neuritis, thoracic disk, zoster, Bornholm's)
4. Pleuritic and pulmonary pain, including:
   The pneumonias, pleurisy, asthma, chronic obstructive pulmonary disease (COPD), pneumothorax,
      hypoxia
   Pulmonary embolism (also see below)

Serious pain
1. A. Common (ischemic) cardiovascular pain:
      Angina pectoris
      Variant angina, unstable angina
      Acute myocardial infarction
      Syndrome X or microvascular angina
   B. Rare causes (ischemic and nonischemic) of cardiovascular pain:
      Aortic valve disease, aortic dissection
      Pericarditis, Dressler's syndrome
      Vasculitis
      Hypoxia
      Cardiomyopathy
      Myocarditis, etc.
2. Pulmonary and medistinal pain, including:
   Pulmonary embolism (pleuritic)
   Pulmonary hypertension, Intrathoracic tumor, mediastinitis, subdiaphragmatic abscess
3. Miscellaneous
   Drug or chemical toxicity (cocaine, etc.)

---

interested only in the *most likely diagnoses* and therefore the *most effective imaging strategy* given a patient with a *single* specific complaint or finding. It would be desirable to list each group of causes of chest pain by overall frequency, but this, obviously, is not possible in the present state of epidemiological knowledge. What we have done is rank the major subdivisions in a subjective order of importance, acknowledging there may be some minor but not substantive disagreements.

Another even simpler approach omits all the subcategories and divides thoracic pain into two main classes: a) innocuous or generally non-life-threatening thoracic pain, nonischemic, nonanginal, or noncardiac pain, including all other presentations of chest pain (Table 6.3.1, no. 1–4); and b) serious or potentially life-threatening thoracic pain, ischemic, anginal, or cardiac, and by implication all other serious causes: cardiovascular, pulmonary, and miscellaneous chest pain (Table 6.3.1, serious pain no. 1–3). Admittedly, there are indeterminate patients who will defy classification, but they will be regarded as potentially classifiable with clinical followup.

Table 6.3.2. Most Common Causes of Thoracic Pain, in Probable Order of Frequency (Abridged List)

Generally innocuous chest pain
1. Nonspecific, including:
   Psychogenic, (anxiety, depression, panic attacks)
   Idiopathic/undecidable
2. Upper GI-induced chest pain, including:
   Reflux or other esophagitis (hiatus hernia)
   Peptic and nonulcer dyspepsia
3. Chest wall pain, including:
   Chest wall syndrome, muscle strain
   Costochondritis (Teitze's)
4. Pleuritic and pulmonary pain, including:
   Pleurisy and pneumonia

Serious pain
Common (ischemic) cardiovascular pain:
1. Angina pectoris and its variants
2. Acute myocardial infarction

Because more than over 90–95% of serious chest pain encountered will be of ischemic cardiovascular origin, and is extremely age and sex dependent, we can summarize our approach by describing the best "test" for this entity—the clinical history.
The diagnosis of ischemic, coronary, or anginal-like pain can generally be made,
based on the answers to three simple questions obtainable from the patient:

1. Is the discomfort substernal or in the anterior chest?
2. Is it precipitated by exertion?
3. Is there prompt relief with rest or nitroglycerin?

When all three questions are answered "yes," the patient's chest pain is considered
typical angina. If only two of the three answers are affirmative, the pain is classified as
atypical angina, and when only one or no answer is "yes" the pain is probably not
anginal. A preferable and more inclusive definition is modified from Detrano et al.
(2) and Diamond et al. (3):

   Typical angina or anginal chest pain is located substernally, in the anterior chest,
neck, shoulders, jaw, or arms. The pain is often described as tightness, squeezing, or
a heaviness. The pain (or sensation) must be precipitated by exertion, emotional ex-
citement, or a heavy meal, and relieved within 1–5 minutes by rest or nitroglycerin.

   Atypical angina is pain in one of the above locations and either precipitated by the
above influences or relieved by rest or nitroglycerin within 5–10 minutes.

   Nonanginal, (noncoronary) or generally innocuous chest pain is *any other type of
chest pain*. Whether or not it is situated in any of the above locations, it is not related
to exertion and lasts less than 10 seconds or longer than 10 minutes.

Recognizing Innocuous or Nonanginal Chest Pain

   We stress that very few patients in the younger age groups with nonanginal or
benign chest pain have coronary disease. This is simply another way of stating that in
patients under age 50 with chest pain, rarely are we dealing with a cardiac or other
serious etiology. Diamond and Forrester's very instructive Table 6.3.3 (4) shows the
prevalence of coronary stenosis in accident victims (presumed not to have had chest
pain), at autopsy by age and sex, based on data from 3000–5000 patients in each

Table 6.3.3. Prevalence of Coronary Stenosis at Autopsy

Age	Men (%)	Women (%)
30–39	1.9 ± 0.3	0.3 ± 0.1
40–49	5.5 ± 0.3	1.0 ± 0.2
50–59	9.7 ± 0.4	3.2 ± 0.4
60–69	12.3 ± 0.5	7.5 ± 0.6

Reprinted by permission of *The New England Journal of Medicine* (1979;300:1350).

Table 6.3.4. Pretest Likelihood of Coronary Artery Disease in Symptomatic Patients According to Age and Sex (Rounded Off)

Age	Nonanginal chest pain (%) Men	Women	Atypical angina (%) Men	Women	Typical angina (%) Men	Women
30–39	5.5	1.0	22	4	70	26
40–49	15	3.0	46	13	87	55
50–59	22	9	60	33	92	80
60–69	28	20	67	55	94	91

Reprinted by permission of *The New England Journal of Medicine* (1979;300:1350).

subset. Their Table 6.3.4 is an invaluable guide for the clinician, because it compares these frequencies of coronary disease in the general population with the pretest likelihood of coronary artery disease in patients with various types of chest pain according to age and sex.

Table 6.3.4 shows that only 5.5% of men under age 40 and only 15% between ages 40 and 50 with *nonanginal* chest pain are found to have coronary artery disease. The respective numbers for women are 1% and 3%. This means that more than 94% of men and 99% of women under age 40 and 85% of men and 97% of women between ages 40 and 50 with nonanginal-type chest pain will not have coronary disease. Even in men over age 60, the pretest likelihood of coronary disease with nonanginal chest pain is still only 28% compared with 94% with typical angina. Although we should be on the alert for an ischemic cause in the older patient with nonanginal chest pain, we must be aware that the presence of coronary disease cannot always be proven in such individuals. The reason for this is that many such patients submitted to coronary angiography disease display minor or subcritical abnormalities in the coronary vasculature. The actual percentage of patients with nonanginal pain and myocardial infarctions cannot be calculated directly from the NCHS data or even from Diamond and Forrester (4), because an unknown number of patients with heart attacks do not present with chest pain at all. However, it is interesting to note from the NCHS statistics of 1990 that 786,000 patients in U.S. hospitals bore the discharge diagnosis of acute myocardial infarction, whereas 1,274,000 had the diagnosis of chest pain (5). The pie chart, Figure 6.3.1, summarizes these figures by age and demonstrates the high percentage of admissions for nonischemic or noncoronary chest pain in younger age groups. In 1989, 8.4 million patients were seen in medical offices with the complaint of chest pain (6). A 1989 study of 1,000 patients seeking help from internists found that the *most common symptom, chest pain, signified a medical problem in only 11% of cases* (7).

Over the past 20 years a subtle but unmistakable shift in public and medical thinking has occurred, which tends to view with alarm any type of chest pain in patients of

MYOCARDIAL INFARCTION vs CHEST PAIN
DISCHARGE DIAGNOSES BY AGE (IN THOUSANDS)

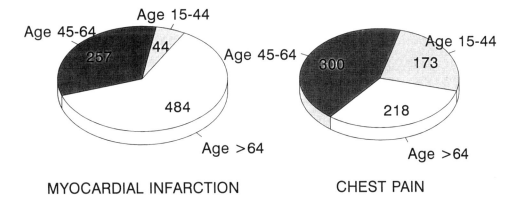

MYOCARDIAL INFARCTION   CHEST PAIN

NHDS, All Listed Discharge Data, U.S. 1990 (5)

Figure 6.3.1. Myocardial infarction vs. chest pain. Discharge diagnoses by age (in thousands).

both sexes and all ages. This is no doubt largely inspired by well-meaning agencies and official bodies, such as the Surgeon General, the American Heart Association, the media, and others who have made us all too aware of the dangers of diabetes, hypertension, cholesterol, and premature deaths from heart attacks, among other perils. The pervasive fear of high cholesterol, coronary disease, and other health risks is demonstrated by the fact that Americans are quite content to spend billions of dollars in health food stores. (A few faddists even prefer to eat like natives of Third World countries in order to forestall heart attacks.) The phobias that drive public behavior and perceptions also inspire physician fears of malpractice actions and lead to cardiac neuroses, not to mention unnecessary stress tests, hospitalizations, and even cardiac catheterizations, in hundreds of thousands of patients with low pretest likelihood of disease. Cardiac stress studies with and without radionuclides are being performed on patients in their 30s and 40s with no other indication than the presence of some type of clearly nonanginal pain.

Pretest probability of coronary disease can, in fact, be estimated with a considerable degree of accuracy from the above tables based solely on the absence or type of chest pain and age and sex of the patient. Furthermore, the presence or absence of coronary risk factors such as smoking, hypertension, family history, diabetes, elevated cholesterol or plasma lipids, type A behavior, etc., can be incorporated in this approach.

We have attempted to embed these findings in a computer program in order to predict the probability of coronary disease in patients by age, sex, different types of chest pain, and four principal risk factor (8). The decision tree is given in Figure 6.3.2 and shows 32 different permutations and combinations of risk factors and their ab-

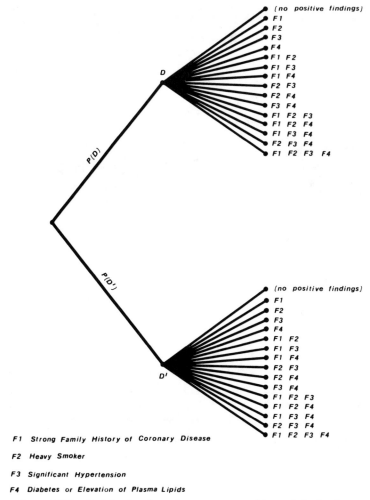

F1 Strong Family History of Coronary Disease

F2 Heavy Smoker

F3 Significant Hypertension

F4 Diabetes or Elevation of Plasma Lipids

Figure 6.3.2.   Decision tree for a given age, sex, and type of chest pain.

sence. These, of course, would have to be multiplied by each age, sex, and pain subset taken from combining Tables 6.3.3 and 6.3.4, giving in our schema 512 possible outcomes. The Framingham data (9), unfortunately, tell us only about risk factors per se and nothing about probability of coronary disease given the presence or absence of chest pain, whereas the figures of Diamond and Forrester (4) deal only with the probability of coronary disease given chest pain. Even though the data sets are disjointed, estimates indeed can be made by experts. Table 6.3.5 shows such estimated probabilities of coronary disease in 16 risk subsets for men and women in the 40–49 age group compiled from several cardiologists. This approach to medical decision making in patients with chest pain has been studied extensively. In one large multicenter clinical trial (10), clinical and laboratory data were used to identify a large subgroup of patients for whom a 12-hour period of observation was usually sufficient to exclude acute myocardial infarction.

The most helpful clue to the presence of serious vs. innocuous chest pain must remain the age and sex prevalence of angina and atypical angina, as demonstrated in the above tables. The clinical gamut of various types of chest pain must be learned

Table 6.3.5. Estimated Probabilities of Coronary Disease in 40–49-Year-Old Patients with Nonanginal Chest Pain by Risk Subset

Risk subset	Logical code	Men	Women
ABCD	YYYY	0.32	0.15
BCD	NYYY	0.30	0.14
ABD	YNNY	0.28	0.12
ABC	YYYN	0.26	0.12
ACD	YNYY	0.26	0.11
AB	YYNN	0.25	0.10
BD	NYNY	0.24	0.10
AD	YNNY	0.24	0.09
BC	NYYN	0.23	0.09
AC	YNYN	0.22	0.08
CD	NNYY	0.21	0.08
A	YNNN	0.20	0.07
B	NYNN	0.18	0.06
D	NNNY	0.17	0.06
C	NNYN	0.16	0.05
None	NNNN	0.14	0.03

A is strong family history; B is heavy smoker; C is significant hypertension; and D is diabetes or elevated serum lipids.

thoroughly in order to be recognized, because they are great masqueraders in clinical medicine and, perhaps, with the possible exception of abdominal pain and dyspepsia, the cause of more diagnostic and therapeutic mischief than any other symptoms. We deceive ourselves as physicians if we fail to appreciate that the *clinical description elicited from the patient remains the first and most reliable test for identifying the cause of chest pain*.

In one interesting report a 6-month survey of 588 patients presenting with chest pain to an emergency room revealed some 85 different diagnoses (11). Psychiatric disorders were extremely common, more so in women. Esophageal spasm was also common and equally prevalent in both sexes. It is well known that chest pain of undetermined origin is the final diagnosis in many patients admitted to coronary care units (12), that psychological chest pain is frequent in children (13), and the digestive tract is an important cause of nonanginal chest pain in adults (14). In addition, there remain important groups about which speculation continues to abound. Among these are patients with ischemic-type chest pain with normal coronary angiograms, the so-called microvascular or small vessel angina, also named "syndrome X," and patients in whom the final common pathway of pain etiology may well be pharmacologically evocable myocardial ischemia or esophageal spasm (15). Innumerable papers have discussed various etiologies and clinical aspects of nonanginal thoracic pain. Among important causes are the so-called chest wall syndrome (16, 17), panic disorder, depression, hyperventilation syndrome, and the controversial mitral valve prolapse (MVP) (11–14, 18–25).

Rosch (26–28) has made valuable contributions to our understanding of the relationship of stress to some of these conditions, in particular, panic disorder and pharmacologically evocable angina. It appears likely that the common denominator is increased secretion of adrenaline and noradrenaline, which produces disturbing symptoms of chest pain or discomfort and/or palpitations. Some patients may even fear they are suffering heart attacks. In one study (29), 99 patients with chest pain and a presumptive diagnosis of coronary disease were assessed blindly within 24 hours of angiography, using standardized psychiatric interviews and personality assessments. More than 40% had normal coronary arteries or insignificant disease. Approximately two-thirds of these patients had predominantly psychiatric rather than cardiac disorders; "the symptoms in these patients are more likely to represent the somatic manifestations of anxiety and overbreathing than the consequences of underlying cardiac disease." Anxiety and panic attacks are most common in young women in the 20- to 40-year age group but may also occur as a result of stressful events in both sexes and all ages, often appearing at the time of divorce, job loss, or death, or in the case of military personnel being ordered into combat (26, 27). It may be difficult or impossible to distinguish panic attacks from hyperventilation syndrome, to which it bears many similarities. The two conditions could, in fact, be variants of the same clinical constellation, which no doubt includes at least some patients with other ill-defined chest pain syndromes.

The GI Tract and Chest Pain

GI, particularly esophageal, causes may be involved in as many as 25% or more of cases with nonanginal chest pain. An excellent summary reviewed controversial issues including mechanisms of esophageal pain and in particular its diagnostic assessment (30). Esophageal dysmotility, a finding frequently seen in patients with noncardiac chest pain, comprises a heterogeneous group of possibly interrelated disorders, including achalasia commonly presenting as dysphagia, so-called diffuse esophageal spasm, "nutcracker esophagus" (prominent, nonpropulsive contractions of the distal esophagus), "hypertensive lower esophageal sphincter," nonspecific esophageal pain, etc.

A variety of studies have been proposed to investigate esophageal dysmotility and acid reflux. These include, among others, prolonged monitoring of intraesophageal pressure and pH and balloon distension of the lower esophagus. These tests, which are invasive, exceedingly unpleasant, expensive, and sometimes even risky, offer little if any assistance in diagnosing chest pain. The use of these approaches is all the more puzzling because of the availability of simpler, safer, and more direct techniques (vide infra). Numerous studies have shown that 20–60% of patients with noncardiac chest pain will have an abnormal baseline manometric finding (31–34). Other studies have reported that even in normal individuals postprandial reflux is common, though symptoms are rare, and that "among patients with esophagitis, intraesophageal pH monitoring frequently shows excessive reflux, but patients do not have chest pain or heartburn during most episodes of reflux" (30). Other invasive procedures include the Bernstein test, which employs acid perfusion of the lower esophagus as a provocative test. One report, in which only 7% of noncardiac chest pain patients had their symptoms reproduced by this technique (31), suggests the test deserved to be completely abandoned. Other provocative tests include the use of ergonovine, which increases esophageal contractions and reproduces chest pain in some patients, but with the risks of cardiovascular side effects. This test is not routinely recommended (30). Tensilon (IV Edrophonium) also has been used to reproduce a postulated esophageal origin of chest pain, but this test, like many of the others, has not predictably distinguished patients with chest pain from healthy subjects (35). Balloon distension of the esophagus has resulted in chest pain, but like manometry, pressures do not distinguish patients with chest pain from controls. Richter et al. (36) suggest there may be a lower pain threshold in these patients similar to the sensitivity to balloon distension of the rectum in patients with irritable bowel syndrome. Last, we emphasize the in-advisability of endoscopy or EGD in the study of pain of suspected esophageal origin. Mucosal disruption with inflammation may be contributory, but 30–60% of symptomatic patients are shown to have a normal esophagus by endoscopy (37, 38). This is not surprising, because function and physiology, and not anatomy, play a predominant role in the etiology of most thoracic GI pain syndromes.

Patients with nutcracker esophagus and irritable bowel had significantly higher scores than other patients on psychological testing, i.e. somatic anxiety and GI susceptibility scales. It was suggested that these patients had excessive concern about somatic functions and tended to have more severe and frequent GI symptoms under stress. Again, there is a definite relationship between emotional distress and esophageal motility, a fact recognized for more than 100 years since Kronecker and Meltzer (39) reported that psychic upset induces esophageal contractions.

In summary, there are a variety of expensive, unpleasant exceedingly unreliable, and occasionally risky procedures available to determine an esophageal origin of chest pain. This category undoubtedly also includes patients with psychosomatic, motility, spastic sphincter, and reflux disorders. It hardly makes sense to study these patients, if at all, with any but the most direct, safe, pleasant, and inexpensive procedures.

Practical Imaging Studies for Chest Pain of Postulated Esophagogastric Origin

A few years ago the following statement would have been regarded as a medical cliché; today, thanks to the misuse of "hi-tech" and invasive procedures, it deserves to be restated: *The single best imaging procedure for a suspected esophagogastric origin of chest pain is the barium swallow combined with the upper GI series.* Unquestionably, this time-tested, effective procedure always should be done first, simply because it is easily the most effective overall screening examination in all patients with the most common GI causes of chest pain: esophageal motility disorders, hiatus hernia, gastroesophageal reflux, and peptic ulcer disease. If gall bladder disease is a consideration, (an unlikely cause of nonanginal pain), abdominal sonography should be done. When these studies are unrevealing and an upper GI cause is still considered a strong possibility, the much-neglected noninvasive radionuclide studies for esophageal motility and gastroesophageal reflux should be performed next (40, 41). These radionuclide tests, to be described below, are available in any adequately equipped nuclear medicine department. In the past, the diagnosis of esophageal motility disorders has rested primarily on the barium swallow, more recently combined with cine esophagography. However, though conventional barium studies or "bread barium" (42) are highly sensitive for anatomical causes of dysphagia, these studies are often normal in patients with chest pain or dysphagia secondary to motility disorders.

In radionuclide esophagogram scintigraphy, RES, 15 ml water containing a small amount of technetium-99m-labeled sulfur colloid is administered in a single swallow, followed by swallowing every 15 seconds on command for 10 minutes. Using a gamma camera and dedicated computer, an esophageal area of interest is identified, and the count rate change is used to determine the rate of transit after serial swallows. In normal subjects, almost no visible activity remains in the esophagus within 10 seconds after the first swallow.

RES can demonstrate and distinguish a large variety of esophageal motility disorders causing chest pain, including diffuse spasm, achalasia, and those caused by other conditions, such as polymyositis, scleroderma, and dysautonomias (e.g., diabetes). Surprisingly, in a review by Chaudhuri et al. (40), the radionuclide examination was abnormal in 64% of a group of dysphagic patients who had normal manometry!

In addition, the radionuclide gastroesophageal reflux test (GER) is extremely useful in studying suspected esophageal causes of nonanginal chest pain in the large group of patients with heartburn and reflux problems with negative radiographic studies. In this procedure, the patient lies supine under a gamma camera after drinking orange juice containing the same type and amount of radioactive material used for RES (esophageal scintigraphy). Pressure over the upper abdomen is provided by a large sphygmomanometer cuff which is inflated at 20-mm Hg increments from 0 to 100 mm Hg, with 30-second timed images obtained at each level of pressure. The percent of GE reflux is calculated from the net esophageal activity (counts) divided by initial gastric activity. Normal patients show less than 4% of the radioactivity refluxed into the esophagus even at the highest abdominal pressures applied. In one report (41) the GER study was positive in 90% of subjects with heartburn and a positive acid reflux test. In comparison, only 50% of patients with GE reflux shown by GER were detected by fluoroscopic reflux, and only 40% showed endoscopic esophagitis. The entire study takes about 15 minutes.

If there is any question as to the appropriate study for investigating these principal GI causes of chest pain, we strongly recommend consultation with the radiologist/nuclear medicine specialist who will tailor the imaging study to answer the clinician's question. For example, some patients, particularly those over age 40, should have an air contrast upper GI, whereas others in whom hiatus hernia is suspected should have special views of the GE region in the tilt position during a Valsalva maneuver. Almost all patients whose symptoms are due to GE reflux and in whom the radiographic study is negative will show a positive GER study.

Does Mitral Valve Prolapse (MVP) Cause Chest Pain?

A 42-year-old woman diagnosed as having long-standing MVP at age 14 was referred for a stress thallium myocardial scintiscan for intermittent nonanginal-type chest pain. She had experienced recurrent symptoms of bizarre left upper chest and shoulder pain, breathlessness, and attacks of palpitations over the years, which she denied being related to extraneous stress. Yet these episodes were capricious, sometimes coming on frequently over a period of weeks or months, only to disappear for years at a time. Specifically, the pain had frequently been disabling during a failed first marriage between the ages of 21 to 28, but did not recur again until 7 years later. After a hysterectomy 6 months before referral, she developed an arrhythmia postoperatively, but without pain, and had no further trouble until 2 months later, when she lost her closest friend, who died of lung cancer. Shortly after this, she developed a severe recurrence of her symptoms, particularly bizarre attacks of chest pain, dyspnea, and palpitations. On auscultation she had a questionable diastolic click at the mitral area. The stress study was normal.

This fairly typical clinical example suggests either that a patient with MVP can develop typical anxiety attacks, or people with anxiety attacks may have true MVP or "clicks." Proof of a cause-and-effect relationship, in other words, would appear to be indeterminate or undecidable. Whether MVP is in fact a cause of chest pain remains controversial, but a superb review of the subject including the results of a prospective study of 800 patients from Cornell Medical Center (25) appears to resolve many of the uncertainties surrounding this condition. Devereaux and his colleagues deserve to be quoted:

> Although mitral valve prolapse has been associated with many clinical features in studies of highly selected patients, controlled studies have not supported this association ... (but have) substantiated the high prevalence of cardiac and psychiatric symptoms in patients with (the condition) in tertiary care hospitals. ... However, chest pain, dyspnea, psychological symptoms and prolongation of the electrocardiographic Q-T interval occurred equally often among patients with mitral valve prolapse and cardiovascularly normal individuals who were evaluated in the same clinical setting. Furthermore, mitral valve prolapse appears to be no commoner in patients with panic and anxiety disorders than in control subjects when similar precautions are taken (25).

The authors in their conclusion state that, "Mitral valve prolapse is associated with thoracic bony abnormalities, low body weight, low blood pressure ... syncope, palpitations, and atrial arrhythmias, *but not with nonspecific symptoms (such as) atypical chest pain*, dyspnea, anxiety or panic attacks" (25) (emphasis added). Still, many cardiologists continue to hold that atypical chest pain *is* associated with MVP.

Estimating the Prevalence of Possible Causes of Nonanginal Chest Pain

Estimating the frequency and therefore the relative importance of various causes of nonanginal chest pain remains an important task for the individual clinician, though a glance at Table 6.3.1 shows that, aside from the rare case of pulmonary embolism presenting with pleuritic pain, very few serious conditions are encountered. The prevalence of clinically significant causes of anginal or coronary disease can be inferred primarily by the age and sex data of Diamond et al. (3) and to a some extent by NCHS hospital discharge statistics, but almost nothing is known about the epidemiology of various causes of nonanginal or benign chest pain. A selection process is always operating whereby patients are referred either by themselves or their physicians to various destinations, i.e. emergency rooms, cardiologists, and gastroenterologists. This often, unfortunately, determines the choice of a diagnostic work-up. The medical specialist may not always be the ideal first person to consult in the presence of such a protean symptom as chest pain. Despite these problems, however, it is possible to construct simplified hypothetical tables based on likely causes of nonanginal chest pain postulated by the physician. A few examples will demonstrate this point.

Let us assume the patient has pleuritic pain, and the immediate concern is the possibility of PE. What is the relative place of chest radiography and lung scintigraphy in studying this individual? We have some helpful data, because pleuritic pain, according to McNeil et al. (43, 44), represents only about 10% of all nonanginal pain in patients under age 40 and is caused by pulmonary embolism in such patients only about 10–15% of the time. Thus, given a young patient with pleu-

Probability of disease given a positive test   (PPV)
SENSITIVITY=1

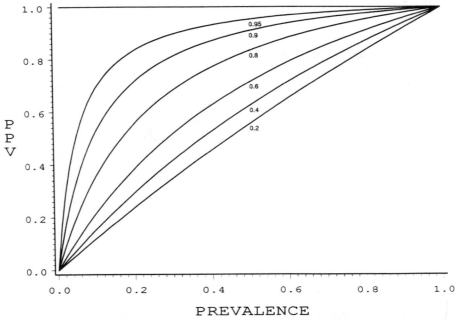

Figure 6.3.3.   Probability of disease given a positive test (PPV) (sensitivity = 1).

ritic pain, the prior probability of PE is only in the 1–2% range. Even this may be excessive, because McNeil's figures are derived from patients with accompanying pleural effusion or predisposing factors. What imaging studies should be used in this type of patient?

Figure 6.3.3 indicates the positive predictive values for various prevalences of PE and other likely conditions depending on a range of sensitivities for a variety of possible tests, given a patient only with pleuritic chest pain. An acceptable sensitivity of perfusion/ventilation scintigraphy is between 80–90% (0.8–0.9). At a likely prevalence of less than 5% in the unselected young patient with pleuritic chest pain, note the PPV or predictive value of a positive scan is in the 20–35% range, hardly worth the trouble. However, pneumonia or pneumonitis is a much more likely diagnosis in this setting, and with the sensitivity of the radiograph at 70–90%, this is obviously the test to be performed. Again, we stress that the likelihood of disease, not test performance, determines the study to be done. This should be intuitively obvious when confronting the usual patient with pleuritic or nonanginal chest pain. Of course, neither chest radiography nor lung scintigraphy are of much help in diagnosing other causes of nontraumatic pleuritic chest pain.

As an important corollary, except for GI and traumatic causes, *virtually all other causes of nonanginal chest pain*, namely nonspecific, chest wall pain, anxiety, costochondritis, intercostal pain, Tietze's syndrome, MVP, etc., are essentially *nonimageable*.

Then how often is the chest radiograph indeed indicated in the patient presenting with nonanginal chest pain? The answer is most of the time. Despite the rarity of pneumonia and other treatable thoracic conditions presenting primarily as chest pain, the consequences of missing such a condition must be weighed against the nominal cost, ease, and universal availability of the plain radiograph. In one series of 120 consecutive patients with anterior chest pain presenting to the emergency room, a total of 14% had clinically significant radiological abnormalities (1). Obviously, missing a serious disease such as PE or pneumonia can have deadly consequences. When the prior probability for PE rises to 50% the probability of disease with positive lung scintigraphy (high probability study) rises to more than 90%.

The reader must remain aware of the obvious fact that PE, GI, and many cardiopulmonary conditions in our initial chart do not necessarily present with nonanginal chest pain. The reasons for this have already been emphasized. Because this text is not about diseases per se, we must accept a tradeoff in our formalized presentation. Instead of each patient being regarded as an example of a *disease*, complete with complaints and findings, we continue to regard the patient as a presenter of complaints and findings, *all of which can share diseases*. Thus, a patient with pulmonary embolism can present with pleuritic chest pain, but more often with weakness, dyspnea, cough, cardiovascular collapse, etc., or various combinations thereof. Likewise, GI conditions may appear with symptoms referable to the thorax, but more often present with abdominal symptoms, which are discussed separately. We acknowledge that no classification schemata based on disease, symptomatology, or physical findings will be wholly satisfactory. This is another example, discussed previously, of the dualistic paradox of disease-as-name (diagnosis) vs. disease-as-attribute (as description, i.e. signs and symptoms). Our conviction reflected throughout this text, is that as physicians we never escape the problems of reconciling these conflicts. Most of the time, chest pain is just we-see-this chest pain; sometimes it is indigestion, occasionally it is PE or a heart attack.

Summary of Imaging Approach to Cases of Nonanginal Chest Pain

1. For unexplained, recurrent, or persistent nonanginal thoracic pain, i.e. chest wall, costochondritis, pleuritic, and nonspecific type pain, a routine chest radiograph with or without rib X-rays is sufficient. In the event other less common entities are suspected, the following is a quick guide for the clinician:

2. For suspected GI causes of nonanginal chest pain, (esophageal disorders, GE reflux, hiatus hernia, and peptic ulcer), the barium swallow and upper GI series with or without air contrast are the most efficacious and easiest imaging procedures. Occasionally, but rarely, gall bladder sonography is indicated. If esophageal dysmotility is suspected and not diagnosed with the barium swallow or cine esophagogram, the RES is indicated. If GE reflux is suspected but not diagnosed by esophagogram and the upper GI, including special tilt studies, an appropriate radionuclide GER should be performed.

3. Even though less than 1% of pleuritic pain in patients under age 40 is caused by PE, and probably less than 10% of patients with PE present with this symptom, certain clinical settings should alert the clinician to PE. Without convincing clinical or radiographic signs of pneumonia, PE becomes a significant possibility in any high-risk patient with pleuritic pain, i.e. those with effusion, postoperative patients, cardiacs, those with phlebitis or venous disorders, lower extremity, and other trauma, etc. In these patients, perfusion and ventilation lung scanning should *always* be performed to establish the diagnosis of PE, which would otherwise be unrecognized.

4. In cases of possible intercostal or thoracic root pain origin, one should always anticipate the possibility of herpes zoster with a typical rash to come in a week or so.

For otherwise unexplained intercostal-type thoracic pain, especially in the older patient, one must not overlook the rare possibility of a herniated thoracic disk or an arthritic spur. It would seem prudent to obtain plain films of the thoracic spine in such patients, and if symptoms such as radicular pain persist, CT or MRI should be considered.

5. Even though less than 2–3% of nonanginal pain can result from conditions such as pericarditis, vasculitis, pulmonary and systemic hypertension, aortic valve disease, cardiomyopathy, etc., many of these conditions cause anginal- rather than nonanginal-type pain (see below). The resting and stress ECG studies are obviously useful screening procedures. For cases of suspected MVP, not diagnosable clinically, or other valvular disease and pericardial effusion, echocardiography is the diagnostic procedure of first choice.

6. Rarer causes of chest pain have not been addressed, but relevant clinical information and abnormal ECG or radiographic findings would obviously alert the physician to their presence. Furthermore, chest pain due to industrial toxins or cocaine would be more likely in an inner city emergency room than in a suburban office.

7. CT and MRI are an enormous waste of time and money and are generally *not indicated* in the diagnosis of chest pain. These studies are indicated only in the rare case of chest pain in which there is radiographic evidence of a mass, aortic aneurysm or dissection, history of significant trauma, or clinical suspicion of discogenic or spinal disease. This latter cause of chest pain, however, is extremely rare, probably accounting for less than 0.3% of cases.

CORONARY AND CORONARY-TYPE PAIN

The frequency of coronary disease and of anginal and nonanginal chest pain by age and sex in Tables 6.3.3 and 6.3.4 continue to dominate our approach to diagnosis in this second major category of chest pain. Two distinct issues are involved in the diagnosis of chest pain of ischemic origin. First, is the pain in fact due to vascular occlusive disease of the major coronary arteries, and, if so, is the patient, acutely or nonacutely, a candidate for thrombolytic therapy, surgical intervention (coronary bypass or angioplasty), or medical therapy?

STRESS TESTING

Screening diagnosis of coronary artery disease (CAD) rests *primarily* on the results of cardiac stress testing with or without myocardial perfusion imaging using thallium-201 or one of the newer compounds (technetium-99m-labeled sestamibi, an isonitrile). (We will use the term *thallium* synonymously with *sestamibi* when referring to myocardial perfusion scintigraphy.) Coronary arteriography is indicated in only a small percentage of patients before or instead of stress testing. In the large majority of patients the diagnosis of coronary disease can be made on the basis of the history and stress testing alone.

How the radionuclide portion of the stress test should be performed is coming under increasing scrutiny at present. Two methods are available, first, the standard *planar* method, in which images are taken in three two-dimensional views with a standard gamma camera. The other more exacting but precise technique employs SPECT, mentioned in Chapter 2. With this method, a much more sophisticated gamma camera rotates around the patient and with the use of dedicated computer

Table 6.3.6. Estimated Posttest Probabilities of Coronary Disease vs. No Coronary Disease Given a Positive or Negative Stress Test Performed with and without 201-Thallium in Patients with Various Pretest Probabilities of Disease

Prevalence (%)	Stress testing alone (Sens. 50%, spec. 85%)		Stress testing + 201-thallium (sens. 80%, spec. 90%)	
	PPV[a] (%)	1-NPV[a] (%)	PPV[a] (%)	1-NPV[a] (%)
5	13	97	30	99
10	27	94	47	97
20	45	87	67	94
30	59	80	77	91
40	69	72	84	87
50	77	63	89	82
60	83	53	92	75
70	89	42	95	66
80	93	30	97	53

Sensitivities and specificities from Detrano et al., Tables 2 and 3 (2).
[a]PPV is likelihood of disease given a positive test; 1-NPV is the likelihood of disease given a negative test.

software reconstructs images of the heart, which can then be displayed in the form of successive slices in three major axes. SPECT myocardial imaging has significantly improved the sensitivity and specificity of stress myocardial scintigraphy and is definitely preferred to conventional planar imaging.

Table 6.3.6 shows the posttest probability (PPV) of disease and of no disease (1-NPV) given a positive stress test result. Two choices are given, the cardiac stress test with and without thallium (sestamibi) perfusion scintigraphy in patients with various pretest probabilities of coronary disease. Sensitivity and specificity of stress testing alone are approximately 50% and 85%, respectively, if positivity is defined as greater than 1.5 mm ST-segment-depression, whereas the respective values of combined thallium scintigraphy (reversible defect) are approximately 80% and 90%, respectively (2, 45, 46). Many cardiologists, however, now consider abnormal any ST depression greater than 1 mm. This results in greater sensitivity of the ECG but reduced specificity, i.e. more false positives for ischemia.

Table 6.3.6 suggests numerically the best choice of imaging procedure, as outlined above, for various pretest probabilities of coronary disease, but unfortunately it does not indicate other essential information necessary to help us make the decision as to whether or when stress testing with the ECG should be performed alone or combined with perfusion scintigraphy. Specifically, we do not learn which choice is preferable in terms of convenience, cost, and efficacy. Moreover, this chart does not identify the most critical element in our decision to perform laboratory studies: What is the cutoff point or pretest probability for pursuing an imaging, or for that matter, any further diagnostic strategy? Again and again we confront the facts of probability and the impossibility of certainty in medical testing. In the case of ruling out coronary disease, we must keep in mind the prior probability of disease before resorting to any type of testing, invasive or noninvasive.

Because one does not want to miss a potentially life-threatening problem, obviously the testing threshold for coronary disease, like that for PE, will be lower than that for duodenal ulcer. Yet, as always, there has to be a minimum threshold probability of disease before testing can predict its presence. This usually can be ascertained by clinical judgment combined with data from some of the tables presented.

A case in point would be a young woman with atypical angina and a pretest probability of 4–5% in whom a positive stress test and would increase probability of disease only to 13%, and a positive thallium stress test would only give a posttest probability of 23%. The striking fact to be noted is the strong negative predictive value of a normal or negative study, and this is one of the important diagnostic areas where the "rule out" strategy might occasionally be justifiable. By glancing at the numbers listed under "1-NPV" it is easy to understand why the coronary arteriogram is rarely justified in a patient with a negative stress test and almost never justified when a negative stress myocardial perfusion scintigraphy has been obtained. In Detrano et al.'s series (2), only 1 in 154 patients would have been diagnosed as having treatable coronary disease, and 32 normal arteriograms would have resulted if a cutoff point of 0.20 had been selected. As a result he proposes that, *"all subjects with a pretest disease probability of less than 0.2 (should) undergo neither noninvasive testing nor coronary angiography"* (2) (emphasis added).

We encounter difficulties in some subjects with anginal-like pain without significant disease of the major coronary arteries. Many of these patients have small vessel disease (microvascular angina), systemic or pulmonary hypertension, cardiomyopathies (especially idiopathic hypertrophic subaortic stenosis), and other rare conditions and may or may not have positive stress tests. These patients along with a subset of younger females comprise the principal group of patients with false-positive stress tests.

When stress testing is indeed indicated, the question of combined myocardial perfusion imaging remains largely an issue of cost and convenience. This issue has been addressed by Berman (47), who suggests that in patients with a likelihood of less than 10% after stress testing alone, CAD is essentially ruled out for practical purposes. If the likelihood of disease after testing is more than 90%, CAD can be considered present and again perfusion scintigraphy is not required. The numbers in Table 6.3.6, however, suggest this may not be the optimal strategy. Obviously, thallium/ sestamibi should be used whenever the resting cardiogram is altered such that ST-T changes cannot be assessed, for example, in patients with hypertension, electrolyte disturbance, complete left bundle branch block and Wolff Parkinson White syndrome.

The problem remains with those patients in whom stress testing without perfusion imaging does not confidently diagnose or exclude CAD. Here, the stress test has to be repeated with radionuclides to increase the predictive index. There are no data as yet to demonstrate that the detection rate of patients with subsequent cardiac events is increased by using thallium in the low probability subsets, (<20–30%), and this again becomes a question of cost effectiveness. Particularly if there is overconcern on the part of the physician or patient, and an intermediate probability of coronary disease (20–60%), it is preferable to perform the stress test with thallium/sestamibi perfusion imaging if only to avoid having to repeat the test with radionuclides in the case of an intermediate PPV.

What to Do When Conventional Stress Testing Cannot Be Performed

The sensitivity of exercise stress testing in revealing stress-induced ischemia is directly dependent upon the level of stress the subject achieves. Certain patients cannot reach an adequate level of stress on a treadmill or bicycle. Others, particularly the aged and those with complicating diseases such as pulmonary problems, arthritis, amputations, and debility, cannot perform any significant exertion. For many of these patients the use of dipyridamole (Persantine) or adenosine with thallium-201 or 99m-Tc sestamibi is an adequate substitute for treadmill exercise. It has been shown that if thallium is injected during the peak effect of intravenously administered Dipyridamole that the results of the myocardial perfusion scan are equivalent to those of a maximal exercise study (45). It is indefensible for patients who cannot undergo standard stress testing to be referred directly for coronary arteriography without benefit of Persantine or adenosine testing, which often obviates invasive studies.

Coronary Arteriography in the Diagnosis of CAD

In general, coronary arteriography is indicated primarily in those patients with CAD in whom coronary bypass surgery or angioplasty is seriously contemplated as an alternative to medical therapy. A subset of patients with unstable angina or non-Q-wave infarction may require invasive studies before or instead of stress testing. The principal purpose of arteriography is to determine the extent and location of coronary disease in order to make critical management decisions with respect to thrombolytic therapy, transluminal angioplasty, or coronary bypass grafting vs. medical therapy.

Although coronary arteriography continues to be viewed as the gold standard for detection of coronary occlusive disease, we hold this opinion to be ingenuous. There is little confirmatory data on the accuracy of determining the degree of vascular narrowing and the relationship of such narrowing to actual myocardial perfusion. Little and his colleagues (46) have found there is no correlation between severity of initial stenosis and the time from the first catheterization until infarction. They have concluded that *coronary angiography does not have the ability to predict the site or timing of a subsequent myocardial infarction.* The use of arteriography should be viewed with the same amount of skepticism as any other procedure. It is unlikely the coronary arteriogram is more than 70–80% sensitive or specific in determining the presence of physiologically significant or life-threatening disease. Show a series of coronary arteriograms to any group of invasive cardiologists or angiographers and see how often they agree. Furthermore, because its predictive value for subsequent myocardial infarction is so poor, one wonders to what degree the need for surgery or percutaneous transluminal angioplasty (PTCA) can be assessed without combining arteriography with physiological (stress) testing. We are shocked at the number of patients in some institutions undergoing PTCA or coronary bypass surgery without prior stress testing. Pitfalls of coronary arteriography have been mentioned in Chapter 5 and include technical problems visualizing the left coronary artery, osteal stenosis, early bifurcation of the left coronary artery, catheter-induced spasm, flow artifacts, eccentric stenoses, unrecognized occlusions at branch points, superimposition of branches, recanalization, etc. (48).

Coronary-Type Pain and the Negative Arteriogram

An increasingly recognized clinical entity is the syndrome of angina or angina-like chest pain with a normal coronary arteriogram, a finding that occurs in up to 10 20% of all patients undergoing arteriography (49–52). One of the most revealing discussions is Cannon's paper (53), in which he examines chest pain in these patients. Referring to "the eye of the beholder," he addresses the problem of patients initially referred for anginal-type pain who subsequently demonstrate angiographically normal coronary arteries.

Cannon admits that most physicians and patients are reassured because of the implication of no cardiac involvement, but the continued complaint of pain and disability in many patients "confuses and frustrates" (53). Of particular interest is his observation that over the years a multitude of etiologies have been suggested with respect to this clinical subset. He notes that investigators frequently report a high incidence of abnormalities referable to the organ system germane to their particular specialty.

In contrast, Cannon et al. (54) found that more than 75% of such patients referred to the Cardiology Branch of the National Heart, Lung and Blood Institute (admittedly a highly select group) had a dynamic abnormality of coronary flow reserve, which can be unmasked by certain stimuli such as ergonovine. This disorder may be due to an abnormal function of the coronary microcirculation, a condition characterized as "microvascular angina." There is evidence of abnormal esophageal motility in these patients along with impaired forearm flow responses to blood pressure cuff ischemia, suggesting a generalized abnormality of smooth muscle (55). Yet questions of etiology remain a thorny problem, because chest pain of this nature appears to evoke alterations in mood and behavior (23) and may even be induced by them.

As William Harvey noted over 350 years ago (56): "Every affection of the mind that is attended with either pain or pleasure, hope or fear, is the cause of an agitation whose influence extends to the heart." A large body of anecdotal evidence recently supported by scientific research confirms that emotions and psychological distress such as stress, anxiety, fright, panic, etc., can cause coronary vasospasm, direct myocardial damage, and serious as well as lethal disturbances in heart rhythm (24, 28, 29). The famous 18th century surgeon and anatomist, John Hunter, who once remarked, "I am at the mercy of any fool who wishes to annoy me," and who dropped dead in the heat of an argument in the committee room of St. George's Hospital, was only one of the more famous to succumb to an acute emotional experience.

The Study of Patients with Known Coronary Disease and Coronary-Prone Patients Before Surgery

Noninvasive testing should be the standard method for studying the large group of patients with presumptive or suspected coronary heart disease whose future management must be determined, as well as those high-risk patients about to undergo elective vascular surgery. The first group includes patients with highly diagnostic histories (angina and atypical angina) and/or evidence of a prior myocardial infarction. In this setting certain questions and concerns can be answered using perfusion stress myocardial scintiscanning.

When should cardiac catheterization be performed? According to one report (57), thallium defects on stress testing were even more valuable than arteriographic anatomic abnormalities in predicting future coronary events. Moreover, Kaul et al. (58, 59) have shown that there is complementary information derived from catheterization and scintigraphic data in determining subsequent prognosis of patients with coronary disease, and that all such data have been concordant. Based on clinical history and the information derived from stress testing, it should be possible in the majority of patients to determine those likely to benefit from PTCA or bypass surgery. Coronary angiography is clearly indicated in this group. Its appropriateness in the majority of other nonacute cardiac patients should be regarded with great skepticism.

After coronary arteriography has been performed, what is the functional significance of "borderline" arterial stenosis (70–80%)? There appears to be strong evidence that the normal thallium scan is an excellent predictor of a favorable prognosis (only 3% of patients had subsequent cardiac events over a 1-year period) and that abnormal thallium studies are highly predictive of future events (45, 46). Evidence is accumulating with PET and SPECT scanning that when there are significant disparities between anatomical and functional abnormalities the physiological data are often the more important predictor.

Should coronary bypass surgery or PTCA be performed on the basis of catheterization alone? No. Radionuclide studies can supply additional relevant physiological information that might alter an option based solely on anatomical considerations. This is true both in patients who show limited extent of ischemia with thallium and those with scintigraphic evidence of extensive loss of viable myocardium. Either of these findings may favor medical over surgical management of coronary disease.

STRESS TESTING AFTER A RECENT MYOCARDIAL INFARCTION

This is a special case, with recommendations varying from stress testing in most patients to almost routine angiography, generally without stress testing. We cannot recommend the latter approach, which would subject the majority of patients to the unjustifiable and unnecessary expense and risk of coronary arteriography. We offer the following as the most reasonable approach to such patients:

For the majority, (perhaps 70–80%) of patients with an uncomplicated myocardial infarction who do not experience pain beyond 24 hours, perform thallium stress testing just before discharge, usually by the 7th to 10th day. Do not perform arteriography unless stress testing indicates significant reversible ischemia, especially involving more than one coronary vascular territory. In the older patient, over 75–80 years, who is asymptomatic after an MI without evidence of failure, stress testing is not generally indicated.

If chest pain persists beyond 24 hours or *recurs at any time prior to that*, go to catheterization directly. *Do not stress. Never stress an unstable patient.*

If a patient has significant systolic dysfunction as shown by gated blood pool studies, i.e. left ventricular ejection fraction less than 20–30%, he or she may not require catheterization unless it is felt the benefit of coronary artery bypass grafting is worth the considerably higher surgical mortality of the procedure in patients with such poor systolic function, approaching 15–20%. However, there is evidence of potentially salvageable myocardium as shown by improved postsurgical systolic ejection fractions in a small number of patients who have been presumed to have "fixed" defects on myocardial perfusion scanning.

Stress Testing After Angioplasty and Preoperatively in Vascular Surgery

Stress testing with thallium after angioplasty is extremely important prognostically and as a method to determine whether restenosis has occurred. This happens in up to 30% of patients within 6 months of PTCA. In fact, stress testing with perfusion scanning has now become a mainstay and to a large extent has replaced repeated catheterization in the majority of patients who have undergone angioplasty as well as bypass surgery.

Table 6.3.7. Pretest Likelihood of Coronary Artery Disease Exceeding 20% (0.2) in Symptomatic Patients According to Age and Sex (Rounded Off)

Age	Nonanginal chest pain (%)		Atypical angina (%)		Typical angina (%)	
	Men	Women	Men	Women	Men	Women
30–39			22		70	26
40–49			46		87	55
50–59	22		60	33	92	80
60–69	28	20	67	55	94	91

Reprinted by permission of *The New England Journal of Medicine* (1979;300:1350).

Paradoxically, angioplasty itself has significantly increased the number of arteriograms being performed, because patients previously considered poor surgical risks can be offered an alternative effective therapy for coronary occlusive disease.

Myocardial infarction accounts for nearly 50% of the mortality and morbidity after peripheral vascular surgery (60). In order to avoid routine coronary angiography, which has been shown to demonstrate severe coronary stenoses in 40–50% of these patients (61, 62), noninvasive evaluation of cardiac risk has been increasingly employed in preoperative assessment. In a study of 100 consecutive patients admitted for elective surgery of peripheral vascular disease, the dipyridamole-thallium imaging study was found to be a powerful predictor of postoperative myocardial infarction and death. Fourteen of 15 patients who had a postoperative myocardial infarction, and all 11 patients who underwent coronary angiography had an abnormal thallium study (stress and redistribution) (63). Moreover, combined dipyridamole thallium scintigraphy is an excellent predictor of future cardiac events after acute myocardial infarction (64).

It is frequently desirable, as implied above, to assess myocardial function noninvasively with the radionuclide gated wall motion study combined with the left ventricular ejection fraction. In some cases unnecessary surgery may be avoided in patients who may not want to accept a high mortality in the face of uncertainty in restoring significant cardiac function.

Summary: Guidelines for Imaging Patients with Angina and Angina-Like Chest Pain

Most patients with a prevalence or prior probability of coronary disease exceeding 0.2 (20%) should have a stress test. It is debatable, however, whether stable angina requires routine stress testing. This would include, but not necessarily be limited to, the following groups (see Table 6.3.7):

1. Any man or woman with new typical angina, regardless of age;
2. Any man with atypical angina, regardless of age;
3. Any woman over age 50 with atypical angina; and
4. Any man over age 50, and any woman over age 60, with any type of unexplained chest pain, anginal or nonanginal.

The combined use of thallium (or sestamibi) myocardial perfusion imaging is generally preferred in women, in certain patients with systemic or pulmonary hypertension, lung problems, and in those with confounding cardiographic abnormalities involving the ST-T wave segments. In patients with a reasonably high or low pretest probability of disease, some physicians would argue that thallium may be omitted. If this is done, however, the cardiologist should be prepared to repeat the test with thallium if there is a significant pretest probability of disease and a negative stress ECG study.

In patients unable to undergo maximal treadmill or bicycle exercise testing, intravenous dipyrimadole/adenosine with thallium or sestamibi is the preferred alternative.

Because of significant pretest probability of coronary disease even with nonanginal chest pain (9% for women over age 50 and 15% for men over age 40), we recommend stress testing with thallium in those patients with strong coronary risk factors, particularly hypertension, heavy smoking history, hypercholesterolemia, diabetes, or strong family history.

Because 30–50% of coronary arteriograms fail to show anatomically significant disease (>70–80% narrowing), except in certain emergency situations, the stress thallium myocardial scintiscan is the safest and most reliable test for making the diagnosis of coronary disease.

Because a negative stress thallium myocardial scintiscan generally is such a strong predictor of the absence of significant coronary disease, arteriography is almost never indicated with a negative stress test. Exceptions occasionally might include patients in certain hazardous occupations (i.e. airline pilots) and patients with a history of frequent bouts of prolonged chest pain (frequent emergency room visits or hospitalizations). Those patients unable to achieve a satisfactory heart rate during stress testing now can be studied with dipyrimadole. Finally, there is the rare patient with persistent unexplained anginal-like pain who cannot be reassured any other way. Most of these patients will turn out to have normal coronary arteries (microvascular angina or "syndrome X"); a few will have variant angina.

Summary of Clinical Approach to Chest Pain

Eliciting the type of pain, whether anginal or nonanginal, is the best single test for diagnosing the cause of chest pain and has profound consequences for patient management. Without some idea whether the patient is suffering from coronary or noncoronary-type thoracic pain, the physician is unable to pursue a rational imaging strategy. One of the most frequent clinical mistakes is to use cardiac stress testing to exclude coronary disease in a patient with a low pretest probability of disease, i.e. a woman under age 60 or a man under age 50 with nonanginal chest pain. It should be obvious that the ability to distinguish anginal from nonanginal pain by a careful clinical history is the key to the etiological diagnosis of thoracic pain.

REFERENCES

1. Russell NJ, Pantin CF, Emerson PA, Crichton NJ. The role of chest radiography in patients presenting with anterior chest pain to the Accident and Emergency Department. J R Soc Med 1988;81(11): 626–628.
2. Detrano R, Yiannikas J, Salcedo EE. Bayesian probability analysis: a prospective demonstration of its clinical utility in diagnosing coronary disease. Circulation 1984;69(3):541–547.
3. Diamond GA, Staniloff HM, Forrester JS, Pollock BH, Swan HJ. Computer-assisted diagnosis in the noninvasive evaluation of patients with suspected coronary artery disease. J Am Coll Cardiol 1983; 1(2)(pt.1):444–455.
4. Diamond GA, Forrester JS. Analysis of probability as an aid in the clinical diagnosis of coronary-artery disease. New Engl J Med 1979;300(24):1350–1358.
5. U.S. Department of Health and Human Services, U.S. Public Health Service, Centers for Disease Control, and the National Center for Health Statistics. National Hospital Discharge Survey (NHDS).

Detailed diagnoses, procedures, days of care, diagnoses-related groups for patients discharged from short-stay hospitals. Public Use Data Diskettes, 1985–1990.

6. Schappert SM. National Ambulatory Medical Care Survey: 1989 summary. National Center for Health Statistics, 1992; Vital Health Stat 131 (110).
7. Goleman, D. Patients refusing to be well: a disease of many symptoms. The New York Times August 21, 1991; section c:10.
8. Sturman MF, Perez M. Probability of cardiac disease: Framingham revisited. Rev Port Cardiol 1990; 9(5):455–461.
9. Kannel WB, Gordon T, eds. The Framingham Study: An Epidemiological Investigation of Cardiovascular Disease. DHEW Publication (NIH) 79-618. May 1973; section 28.
10. Lee TH, Juarez G, Cook EF, et al. Ruling out acute myocardial infarction. N Engl J Med 1991; 324(18):1239–1246.
11. Levene DL. Chest pain–prophet of doom or nagging neurosis. Acta Med Scand [Suppl] 1981;644:11–13.
12. Taylor R, Wright DS, Watson H. Chest pain of uncertain origin in patients admitted to a coronary care unit [Letter]. Lancet 1982;1(8277):911.
13. Asnes RS, Santulli R, Bemporad JR. Psychogenic chest pain in children. Clin Pediatr 1981;12:788–791.
14. Long WB, Cohen S. The digestive tract as a cause of chest pain. Am Heart J 1980;100(4):567–572.
15. Cannon RO, Hirszel R, Cattau EL, Epstein SE. Abnormalities of coronary flow reserve and esophageal motility in syndrome X: a systemic disorder of smooth muscle reactivity? [Abstract]. J Am Coll Cardiol 1987;9(2):249A.
16. Fam AG, Smythe HA. Musculoskeletal chest wall pain. Can Med Assoc J 1985;133(5):379–389.
17. Epstein SE, Gerber LH, Borer JS. Chest wall syndrome. A common cause of unexplained cardiac pain. JAMA 1979;241(26):2793–2797.
18. Hickam DH, Sox Jr HC, Marton KI, Skeff KM, Chin D. A study of the implicit criteria used in diagnosing chest pain. Med Decis Making 1982;2(4):403–414.
19. Rutledge JC, Amsterdam EA. Differential diagnosis and clinical approach to the patient with acute chest pain. Cardiol Clin 1984;2(2):257–268.
20. Selmonosky CA, Byrd R, Blood C, Blanc JS. Useful triad for diagnosing the cause of chest pain. South Med J 1981;74(8):947–949.
21. Beitman BD, Basha I, Flaker G, et al. Atypical or nonanginal chest pain. Panic disorder or coronary artery disease? Arch Intern Med 1987;147(9):1548–1552.
22. Bett JH, Davies P. Non-ischaemic chest pain. Aust Fam Physician 1984;13(5):338–340.
23. Young LD, Barboriak JJ, Anderson AJ. Chest pain and behavior in suspected coronary artery disease. Cardiology 1988;75(1):10–16.
24. Buell JC, Eliot RS. The heart and emotional stress. In: The Heart. 6th ed. New York: McGraw-Hill, 1986:1520.
25. Devereux RB, Kramer-Fox R, Kligfield P. Mitral valve prolapse: causes, clinical manifestations, and management. Ann Intern Med 1989;111:305–317.
26. Rasch PJ. Stress, angina, and syndrome X. The Newsletter of the American Institute of Stress 1988;1:4.
27. Rasch PJ. Stress, panic disorder, and depression. The Newsletter of the American Institute of Stress 1989;2:5.
28. Rosch PJ. Growth and development of the stress concept and its significance in clinical medicine, In: Gardiner-Hill H, ed. Modern Trends in Endocrinology, New York: Paul J. Hoeber, London: Butterworths, 1958:278–297.
29. Bass C, Wade C. Chest pain with normal coronary arteries: a comparative study of psychiatric and social morbidity. Psychol Med 1984;14(1):51–61.
30. Richter JE, Bradley LA, Castell DO. Esophageal chest pain: current controversies and pathogenesis, diagnosis and therapy. Ann Intern Med 1989;110:66–78.
31. Katz PO, Dalton CB, Richter JE, Wu WC, Castell DO. Esophageal testing in patients with noncardiac chest pain or dysphagia: results of three years' experience with 1161 patients. Ann Intern Med 1987;106(4):593–597.
32. Brand DL, Martin D, Pope II CE. Esophageal manometrics in patients with angina-like chest pain. Am J Dig Dis 1977;22(4):300–304.
33. Herrington JP, Burns TW, Balart LA. Chest pain and dysphagia in patients with prolonged peristaltic contractile duration of the esophagus. Dig Dis Sci 1984;29(2):134–140.
34. Orr WC, Robinson MG. Hypertensive peristalsis in the pathogenesis of chest pain: further exploration of the "nutcracker" esophagus. Am J Gastroenterol 1982;77(9):604–607.

35. Richter JE, Hackshaw BT, Wu WC, Castell DO. Edrophonium: a useful provocative test for esophageal chest pain. Ann Intern Med 1985;103(1):14–21.
36. Richter JE, Barish CF, Castell DO. Abnormal sensory perception in patients with esophageal chest pain. Gastroenterology 1986:91(4):845–852.
37. Richter JE, Castell DO. Gastroesophageal reflux: pathogenesis, diagnosis, and therapy. Ann Intern Med 1982;97(1):93–103.
38. Robinson MG, Orr WC, McCallum R, Nardi R. Do endoscopic findings influence response to H2 antagonist therapy for gastroesophageal reflux disease? Am J Gastroenterol 1987;82(6):519–522.
39. Kronecker H, Meltzer S. Der Schluckmechanismus, seine erregung und seine hemmung. Arch Anat Physiol 1883;7(Suppl):328–362.
40. Chaudhuri TK, Fink S, Bird JA. Radionuclide study of esophageal disorders: current clinical status and future directions. Appl Radiol 1988;Nov:70–77.
41. Fisher RS, Malmud LS, Robert GS, Lobis IF. Gastro-esophageal (GE) scintiscanning to detect and quantitate GE reflux. Gastroenterology 1976;70(3):301–308.
42. Davies HA, Evans KT, Butler F, McKirdy H, Williams GT, Rhodes J. Diagnostic value of "bread-barium" swallow in patients with esophageal symptoms. Dig Dis Sci 1983;28(12):1094–1100.
43. McNeil BJ, Hessel SJ, Branch WT, Bjork L, Adelstein S. Measures of clinical efficacy: 3. The value of the lung scan in the evaluation of young patients with pleuritic chest pain. J Nucl Med. 1976;17(3):163–169.
44. McNeil BJ. Ventilation-perfusion studies and the diagnosis of pulmonary embolism: concise communication. J Nucl Med 1980;21(4):319–323.
45. Leppo JA, O'Brien J, Rothendler JA, Getchell JD, Lee VW. Dipyridamole-thallium-201 scintigraphy in the prediction of future cardiac events after acute myocardial infarction. N Engl J Med 1984; 310(16):1014–1018.
46. Little WC, Constantinescu M, Applegate RJ. Can coronary angiography predict the site of a subsequent myocardial infarction in patients with mild-to-moderate coronary artery disease? Circulation 1988;78(5, pt. 1):1157–1166.
47. Berman DS. Clinical application of nuclear cardiology in chronic coronary artery disease. Myocardium (Dupont) 1989;1(3):3–8.
48. Braunwald E. Heart Disease. A Textbook of Cardiovascular Medicine. 3rd ed. Philadelphia: W.B. Saunders Co., 1988:281–286.
49. Ockene IS, Shay MJ, Alpert JS, Weiner BH, Dalen JE. Unexplained chest pain in patients with normal coronary arteriograms. N Engl J Med 1980;303(22):1249–1252.
50. Papanicolaou MN, Califf RM, Hlatky MA, et al. Prognostic implications of angiographically normal and insignificantly narrowed coronary arteries. Am J Cardiol 1986;58(13):1181–1187.
51. Kemp HG, Kronmal RA, Vliestra RE, Frye RL, and participants in the Coronary Artery Surgery Study. Seven-year survival of patients with normal or near normal coronary arteriograms: A CASS Registry study. J Am Coll Cardiol 1986;7(3):479–483.
52. Cannon III RO, Leon MB, Watson RM, Rosing DR, Epstein SE. Chest pain and "normal" coronary arteries—role of small coronary arteries. Am J Cardiol 1985;55(3):50B–60B.
53. Cannon III RO. Causes of chest pain in patients with normal coronary angiograms: the eye of the beholder. Am J Cardiol 1988;62(4):306–308.
54. Cannon III RO, Bonow RO, Bacharach SL, Green MV, Rosing DR. Left ventricular dysfunction in patients with angina pectoris, normal epicardial coronary arteries and abnormal vasodilator reserve. Circulation 1985;71(2):218–226.
55. Sax FL, Cannon III RO, Hanson C, Epstein SE, Impaired forearm vasodilator reserve in patients with microvascular angina. Evidence of a generalized disorder of vascular function? N Engl J Med 1987; 317(22):1366–1370.
56. Harvey W. Exercitatio de motu cordis et sanguis (1628). In: Braunwald E, ed. Heart Disease. A Textbook of Cardiovascular Medicine. 3rd ed. Philadelphia: W.B. Saunders, 1988:1391.
57. Brown KA, Boucher CA, Okada RD, Guiney TE, et al. Prognostic value of exercise thallium-201 imaging in patients presenting for evaluation of chest pain. J Am Coll Cardiol 1983;1(4):994–1001.
58. Kaul S, Lilly DR, Gascho JA, et al. Prognostic utility of the exercise thallium-201 test in ambulatory patients with chest pain: comparison with cardiac catheterization. Circulation 1988;77(4)745–758.
59. Kaul SJ, Finkelstein DM, Homma S, Leavitt M, Okada RD, Boucher CA. Superiority of quantitative exercise thallium-201 variables in determining long-term prognosis in ambulatory patients with chest pain: a comparison with cardiac catheterization. J Am Coll Cardiol 1988;12(1):25–34.
60. Hertzer NR. Fatal myocardial infarction following peripheral vascular operations: a study of 951 patients followed 6 to 11 years postoperatively. Cleve Clin Q 1982;49(1):1–11.

61. Tomatis LA, Fierens EE, Verbrugge GP. Evaluation of surgical risk in peripheral vascular disease by coronary arteriography: a series of 100 cases. Surgery 1972;71(3):429–435.

62. Hertzer NR, Beven EG, Young JR, et al. Coronary artery disease in peripheral vascular patients. A classification of 1,000 coronary angiograms and results of surgical management. Ann Surg 1984; 199(2):223–233.

63. Leppo J, Plaja J, Gionet M, Tumolo J, Paraskos JA, Cutler BS. Noninvasive evaluation of cardiac risk before elective vascular surgery. J Am Coll Cardiol 1987;9(2):269–276.

64. Eagle KA, Singer DE, Brewster DC, Darling RC, Mulley AG, Boucher CA. Dipyridamole-thallium scanning in patients undergoing vascular surgery. Optimizing preoperative evaluation of cardiac risk. JAMA 1987;257(16):2185–2189.

4/ Back and Neck Pain

> *Who, except the gods,*
> *can live time through forever without any pain?*
>
> *Aeschylus*
> Agamemnon

Primary Back and Neck Pain

Back and neck pain may arise in the anatomic structures of the spine from purely mechanical causes such as fractures, musculoskeletal-ligamentous injuries, instability syndromes (spondylosis, spondylolisthesis, and scoliosis), intervertebral disc herniations and annular tears, etc. Far more common causes, however, include the well-known *nonspecific* back and neck pain ("low back pain syndrome") or pain secondary to minor or inapparent trauma, psychological stress, and a host of other causes. Tables 6.4.1 and 6.4.2 show a few of the psycho-social, physical, and occupational factors that are major contributors to low back pain. Nachemson's words (1) ring as true today as when he wrote them two decades ago: "For 98% of patients, . . . knowledge of the psychologic, social, and mechanical stress factors . . . should be utilized for proper counseling, together with *attempts at correction with any type of noninvasive modality* according to the preference of the individual physician" (emphasis added).

Again, we confront the naming ("diagnostic") problem wherein the patient with a cardinal symptom, pain, often defies our attempts to fit him into some neat classification or etiological scheme. We have already encountered this phenomenon in abdominal and chest pain. An entire spectrum of chronic recurrent pain syndromes in otherwise well patients is thus revealed in which the majority of patients fall into the "we-see-this" or "nonspecific" categories. This group includes not only individuals with backache, but also those with a bewildering variety of other musculoskeletal problems, headaches, and other complaints unaccompanied by significant clinical findings. Not surprising, therefore, is the fact that in 1990, 267,000 patients received various nondescript discharge diagnoses such as "cervicalgia," "lumbago," "sciatica," "lumbosacral neuritis," "backache," "disorders of sacrum," and "other back symptoms" (2).

Symptoms involving the back are the ninth most common cause for physician office visits. According to the National Ambulatory Medical Care Survey (NAMCS), in 1985 an estimated 11.3 million Americans consulted physicians for back problems (3). This should be compared with the NCHS (NHDS) statistics for all-listed hospi-

Table 6.4.1. Psycho-Social Factors Associated with Low Back Pain

1. Anxiety and depression
2. Personality disorders
3. Divorce
4. Job dissatisfaction
5. Education
6. Fatigue
7. Alcoholism and addiction
8. Litigation ("compensation neurosis")
9. Malingering

Adapted from Ref. 1 with permission.

Table 6.4.2. Physical and Occupational Factors Contributing to Recurrent or Chronic Low Back Pain

1. Obesity
2. Pregnancy
3. Forward stooping position
4. Repeated lifting of heavy loads
5. Prolonged sitting, standing, or fixed postures
6. Sudden maximal physical stress
7. Vibrational stresses
8. Unaccustomed exercise or physical activity

Adapted from Ref. 1 with permission.

tal discharge diagnoses in the same year for a variety of principal causes of back and neck pain (2). Critics may object that the data sets are disjoint, i.e. that tabulations of symptom presentation in an office population cannot be related to hospital discharge data. However, when we enumerate the diagnoses *most likely to cause acute back and neck pain* represented by the ICD-9 codes 721–724, our approach appears to be validated. These diagnoses are listed in Table 6.4.3 and include totals for both NAMCS and NCHS data. Note that ICD 724, "other and unspecified" back disorders, makes up almost half the listed causes of outpatient back pain and one-third of the hospital discharge diagnoses. Of these latter diagnoses, the majority are benign conditions. As expected, however, intervertebral disc disorders are the largest group, 40% of the hospitalized patients. Although one out of four outpatients with back pain had discogenic disease, total hospitalizations for all the listed codes accounted for less than 15% of all outpatients, and disc discorders made up just less than 6% of all patients hospitalized in the four ICD groups, with "other and unspecified" a close second. If there are further doubts about the tabulations, note that the list of specific diagnostic categories includes 94% of all outpatients listed in the NAMCS totals for back pain (10.6 million out of 11.3 million) (3). We have not included other less common diagnoses, likely to present with chronic, not acute, pain and almost always associated with other complaints.

The 6% of all outpatients with discogenic disease (644,000 hospitalized patients divided by 11.3 million office visits for back complaints) represents roughly that fraction of patients likely to have the most important treatable clinical entity. This number is very close to clinical estimates given by family practitioners, orthopedic surgeons, and others and indicates that CT/MRI studies for discogenic disease in patients complaining of back or neck pain without specific clinical findings is a mindless diagnostic exercise.

Table 6.4.3. Principal Causes of Back Pain Resulting in Physician Visits or Hospitalization and Disc Surgery, 1985 (in Thousands).

Diagnosis	Outpt. visits (3)	Hosp. disch. (2)	% Total patients with back pain hospitalized
Spondylolysis and related disorders (ICD 721)	1842 (17%)	311 (20%)	3
Intervertebral disc disorders (ICD 722)	2680 (25%)	644 (41%)	6
Other disorders, cervical region (ICD 723)	1132 (11%)	86 (6%)	0.8
Other and unspecfied back disorders (ICD 724)	4937 (47%)	513 (33%)	4.8
Totals	10,600 (100%)	1,554 (100%)	14.6%
Total operations on intervertebral discs		246 (ICD 80.5)	
Spinal fusions		102 (ICD 81.0)	

Thus, up to 85% of patients with low back pain will improve rapidly with little or no medical intervention, and a specific diagnosis rarely can be made (1). The symptom of back pain is one of the most ubiquitous of ailments, with 80% of all people afflicted at some time during their lives. Of these only 1–2% become chronically impaired (4, 5), a figure astonishingly close to that percentage of all patients with back pain (1985) undergoing intervertebral disc surgery (Table 6.4.3).

We again stress that clinical findings alone should alert the clinician to the likelihood of a serious condition. Along with severity and poor response to 4–6 weeks of conservative therapy, *physical signs and symptoms of nerve root irritation remain the most reliable indicator of a significant condition*, i.e. exacerbation of pain by coughing, sneezing, or straining, radiation to the extremities, neurological deficits such as motor weakness and sensory changes, plus limited straight leg raising.

The Place of Plain Radiography

Plain films of the spine are, like the chest radiograph, inexpensive and easily available, and one might assume they should be ordered routinely in patients with recurring or persistent complaints of back pain. Yet in a 10-year Swedish study only about 1 patient in 2500 under the age of 50 had unexpected findings on plain radiography (1). Various congenital anomalies and "degenerative changes" of dubious importance are frequently visualized. For example, narrowing of the disc spaces, disc calcifications, osteophytes, changes in the apophyseal joints, transitional vertebrae, Schmorl nodes, mild scoliosis, and other incidental radiographic findings are often invoked as causes of back or neck pain. Yet these are unlikely causes of low back or neck pain and have been found as commonly in patients without back symptoms (1). A tabulation of irrelevant, questionable, and significant radiologic findings on plain X-ray are presented in Table 6.4.4.

The Quebec Task Force on Spinal Disorders (6) concluded that plain radiography was contraindicated during the first week of an acute episode of back pain and was of uncertain value during the first 7 weeks. Despite these studies, at least one set of plain films of the lumbosacral spine will ultimately be taken in most patients with chronic or recurring symptoms. The yield of explanatory findings in all patients will invariably be extremely low and the false-positive rate high because of the frequent disclosure of such unrelated findings as those enumerated above. If plain radiographs

Table 6.4.4.   Radiologic Abnormalities in the Lumbar Spine with Significance for Low-Back Pain

Classification	Abnormality
Irrelevant	Single disc narrowing and spondylosis
	Facet arthrosis, subluxation and tropism
	Disc calcification
	Lumbarization, sacralization
	Intraspongy disc herniation (Schmorl)
	Spina bifida occulta
	Accessory ossicles
	Mild-moderate scoliosis
Questionable	Spondylolysis
	Retrolisthesis
	Severe lumbar scoliosis (>80°)
	Severe lordosis
Definite	Spondylolisthesis
	Lumbar osteochondrosis (Scheuermann)
	Congenital/traumatic kyphosis
	Osteoporosis
	Marked multiple disc narrowing
	Ankylosing spondylitis

Reprinted by permission from *Spine* (1976;1:59–71).

are obtained, anteroposterior and lateral views including a coned-down lateral view of the L5-S1 junction should be done. Oblique views for spondylolysis may be necessary. In the case of chronic cervical pain, in addition to the routine anteroposterior and lateral views, radiographs should routinely include the oblique views to visualize the foramina.

The most appropriate candidates for plain radiography would obviously be those patients likely to have an underlying malignancy, inflammatory (infectious) condition, ankylosing spondylitis, or fracture. Indications for plain radiographs also would include new back pain in older patients and patients with systemic illness, a history of malignancy, neurologic deficits, drug and alcohol abuse, and significant trauma (7, 8).

CT and MRI

Among several reasons CT or MRI should not be performed without specific neurological or other indication is that CT (and myelography) will show herniated discs in approximately 20% of patients who never had back pain (9, 10). Further, MRI imaging shows herniated discs in almost 10% of asymptomatic young women and bulging discs in 45% (11). Figure 6.4.1 shows the estimated yield of CT/MRI in correctly diagnosing discogenic disease at various prevalences or pretest probabilities of the disease and demonstrates the poor predictive value of a positive study unless there is a significant chance of herniated disc (25–35% or better).

There is only one possible conclusion: In the overwhelming majority of patients with back complaints, CT or MRI studies of the spine in the absence of a significant history or clinical findings *are an enormous and unjustifiable waste of time and money.*

Another fact to keep in mind: The nuclear bone scintiscan is almost never indicated in primary back pain in the absence of a history of trauma, except in suspected back pain of secondary origin, discussed below. Several reports discuss relative effectiveness of various imaging procedures for discogenic disease and low back pain (12–15).

POSITIVE PREDICTIVE VALUE (PPV) OF CT / MRI
FOR DIAGNOSIS OF HERNIATED DISC

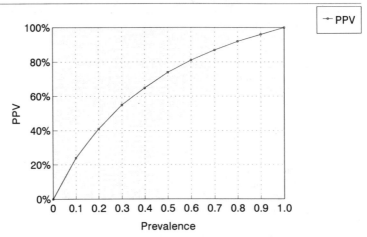

Estimated sensitivity 85%, specificity 70% (11-15)

Figure 6.4.1.   Positive predictive value (PPV) of CT/MRI for diagnosis of herniated disc.

Secondary Back and Neck Pain

A large number of specific conditions other than those arising from purely anatomic derangements may cause back and neck pain. However, these are extremely
uncommon causes. Included here would be rare conditions of unknown cause (inflammatory arthropathies due to ankylosing spondylitis, Crohn's and Paget's diseases, and epiphysitis), cardiac, vascular, and GI conditions such as spinal hemorrhage, dissecting aneurysm, myocardial infarction, peptic ulcer, cholecystitis, pancreatitis, and renal conditions. Parenthetically, gynecological conditions, if they cause
back complaints at all, are usually associated with a nagging or heavy sensation in the
lower back. *The importance of pelvic disease is highly exaggerated as a primary cause of back
pain in women.* Among the more serious secondary causes of back pain are tumors of
the cord and spine, both benign and primary malignant and metastatic tumors, and
infections, in particular, osteomyelitis.

In patients with known malignancy and neck or back pain, total body bone scintigraphy always should be performed. We emphasize the sensitivity and superiority
of bone scintigraphy in this setting, because radiographic abnormalities are rarely
seen except in advanced metastatic cancer.

Conversely, many primary bone tumors, for example osteo- and chon-
drosarcomas, can be diagnosed by their radiographic appearance alone, and bone
scintigraphy is rarely helpful. An exception is osteoid osteoma of the spine, which,
when it is possible to visualize radiographically, may mimic other bone lesions radiographically and require bone scintigraphy. In suspected early osteomyelitis, the radiographs are often normal for up to 2–3 weeks after onset, and bone scintigraphy
should always be the *second* imaging study. In the presence of obvious radiographic
evidence of osteomyelitis, however, we feel as with typical primary tumors, bone and
gallium scintigraphy are superfluous and therefore unnecessary. Spinal cord tumors

suspected because of the presence of neurological complaints or findings always call for CT or MRI.

One of the most common causes of back pain in the older patient, particularly among postmenopausal women is, of course, osteoporosis. Here, plain films of the spine are the mainstay of diagnosis. Bone scintigraphy is useful in the detection and age determination of compression fractures. Dual photon absorptiometry seems to have lost its popularity in diagnosing osteoporosis because of serious questions about its accuracy, but new methods and equipment may revive interest in this technique. Quantitative CT remains useful in diagnosing osteoporosis.

The Imaging Approach to Neck and Back Pain

In covering the subject of neck and back pain, we can only emphasize, as we have in other sections, the most common and important conditions. Like NSAP, most back pain is also "nonspecific" or self-limiting and rarely requires investigation at the outset. More than 90% of patients with back or neck pain will belong to the "primary" group of etiologies, namely the nonspecific category, anatomic musculoskeletal abnormalities and injuries. Only 5–6% of patients will turn out to have discogenic disease, and the rest will have a heterogeneous group of disorders. As a guide, we recommend the following approach to the patient with symptoms referable to the spine.

Summary

If imaging is indeed indicated, plain radiographs of the spine should be performed before any other study. In the aged, patients with serious systemic illness such as cancer and trauma, and in some patients with persistent or recurrent pain, plain radiographs of the appropriate spinal region are indicated as the first imaging study.

Bone scintigraphy and CT/MRI are poor screening studies for nonspecific back and neck pain and should virtually never be performed except with the following clinical indications.

BONE SCINTIGRAPHY

Always perform in the presence of negative radiographs when there is a strong clinical suspicion of secondary causes of bone pain, i.e. infection, fracture, primary or metastatic tumors, etc. In particular, bone scintigraphy is indicated in any patient who may have suffered inapparent trauma (alcoholics, the aged) or those with a history of malignancy, particularly of lung, breast, prostate, or kidney.

If the diagnosis of primary tumor, fracture, or osteomyelitis is made radiographically, further studies, obviously, are *unnecessary*. In the case of vertebral compression, however, the radiograph rarely distinguishes recent from old fractures, and here the bone scintiscan is invaluable.

CT/MRI

Perform on any patient with signs or symptoms of nerve root irritation. These clinical findings are the only reliable predictors of disc disease or other significant neurological condition.

Other indications for CT/MRI include patients in whom the extent of disease is not apparent from X-rays, e.g. spinal cord tumor suspects, spinal stenosis, etc.

If CT/MRI Is Indicated, Which Is Better?

In general, both CT and MRI have comparable sensitivity and specificity not only with respect to each other, but together with myelography in herniated disc, spine, and cord imaging. Because CT of the spine is usually performed without contrast, no risk is involved. Moreover, CT is less expensive and more generally available. MRI, however, seems to be gaining more adherents among surgeons dealing with the gamut of spinal problems including discogenic, osseous, and extraosseous conditions. MRI is particularly useful in studying patients who have undergone previous spinal surgery. In the setting of postoperative scarring and other changes, MRI is clearly superior to CT.

Whatever Happened to Myelography?

There are still adherents of myelography. They advocate the procedure in some symptomatic patients with malignancy, in demonstrating epidural tumors or metastases, and in showing the level of cerebrospinal fluid blockage necessary to guide surgical intervention (16). In addition, many orthopedists and neurosurgeons still use myelography for patients with cervical discogenic disease in whom surgery is contemplated. Despite this, CT and MRI are making the procedure increasingly obsolete. It is indeed arguable whether even in some cases of spinal stenosis or in patients with intradural abnormalities or multiple back operations that myelography can add any useful clinical information. In discogenic disease, because both CT or MRI are noninvasive and have sensitivities and specificities comparable to myelography, they should always be the procedures of first choice (17). In most cases CT/MRI will render myelography unnecessary.

REFERENCES

1. Nachemson AL. The lumbar spine. An orthopaedic challenge. Spine 1976;1(1):59–71.
2. U.S. Department of Health and Human Services, U.S. Public Health Service, Centers for Disease Control, and the National Center for Health Statistics. National Hospital Discharge Survey (NHDS). Detailed diagnoses, procedures, days of care, diagnoses-related groups for patients discharged from short-stay hospitals. Public Use Data Diskettes, 1985–1990.
3. McLemore T, DeLozier J. National Center for Health Statistics, 1985 Summary: National Ambulatory Medical Care Survey. Advance Data from Vital and Health Statistics. Hyattsville, Md: Public Health Service, 1987;no. 128, DHHS pub. (PHS) 87-1250.
4. White III AA, Gordon SL. Synopsis: workshop on idiopathic low-back pain. Spine 1982;7(2):141–149.
5. Shearn MA. Arthritis and musculoskeletal disorders. In: Krupp MA, Schroeder SA, Tierney LA, eds. Current Medical Diagnosis & Treatment. 26th ed. Krupp MA, Schroeder Norwalk: Appleton & Lange, 1987:492–531.
6. Spitzer WO, LeBlanc FE, Dupui M. Scientific approach to the assessment and management of activity-related spinal disorders: a monograph for clinicians. Report of the Quebec Task Force on Spinal Disorders. Spine 1987;12(Suppl 7):S16–S21.
7. Deyo RA. Early diagnostic evaluation of low back pain. J Gen Intern Med 1986;1(5):328–338.
8. Deyo RA, Bigos SJ, Maravilla KR. Diagnostic imaging procedures for the lumbar spine [Editorial]. Ann Intern Med 1989;111(11):865–867.
9. Hitselberger WE, Witten RM. Abnormal myelograms in asymptomatic patients. J Neurosurg 1968; 28(3):204–206.
10. Weisel SW, Tsourmas N, Feffer H, Citrin CM, Patronas N. A study of computer-assisted tomography. I. The incidence of positive CAT scans in an symptomatic group of patients. Spine 1984;9(6):549–551.
11. Weinreb JC, Wolbarsht LB, Cohen JM, Brown CE, Maravilla KR. Prevalence of lumbosacral intervertebral disk abnormalities on MR images in pregnant and symptomatic nonpregnant women. Radiology 1989;170:125–128.

12. Haughton VM, Eldevik OP, Magnaes B, Amundsen P. A prospective comparison of computed tomography and myelography in the diagnosis of herniated lumbar disks. Radiology 1982;142(1):103–110.
13. Hudgins WR. Computer-aided diagnosis of lumbar disc herniation. Spine 1983;8(6):604–615.
14. Kent DL, Larson EB. Magnetic resonance imaging of the brain and spine. Is clinical efficacy established after the first decade? Ann Intern Med 1988;108(3):402–424.
15. Pelz DM, Haddad RG. Radiologic investigation of low back pain. Can Med Assoc J 1989;140(3):289–295.
16. Portenoy RK, Galen BS, Salamon O, et al. Identification of epidural neoplasm: radiography and bone scintigraphy in the symptomatic and asymptomatic spine. Cancer 1989;64(11):2207–2213.
17. Haughton VM, Eldevik OP, Magnaes B, Amundsen P. A prospective comparison of computed tomography and myelography in the diagnosis of herniated lumbar disks. Radiology 1982;142(1):103–110.

5/ Bone and Joint Pain

So much are our minds influenced by the accidents of our bodies, that every man is more the man of the day than a regular and consequential character.

Lord Chesterfield
Letters to his son, Aug. 30, 1748

The patient was understandably upset. On disability and out of work for chronic shoulder pain, but without health insurance, he had just received a $900 bill for an MRI of the shoulder after being told "we find nothing wrong." An examination subsequently demonstrated exquisite tenderness over the biceps tendon and extreme limitation of motion on elevation of the shoulder. Plain radiographs of the shoulder demonstrated calcification within the subdeltoid bursa.

The above story again demonstrates the diagnostic if not financial overkill of unnecessary diagnostic studies. If any imaging study was indeed indicated for this straightforward case of subdeltoid bursitis—and this is arguable—it certainly was not MRI. Yet we are seeing an increasing misuse of high-tech procedures since the explosion of corner CT and MRI centers.

The point will be made repeatedly throughout this book: If medical imaging studies are indeed indicated, *the first choice should almost always be plain X-rays*, followed, where indicated, by ultrasonography. In the musculoskeletal system, thorax, and abdomen, the first study is *always* the plain radiograph. It is never justifiable to perform CT, MRI of the bones or joints, or bone scintigraphy before plain X-rays are taken.

An exhaustive review of the causes of bone and joint pain will not be attempted here, but in order to cover the major conditions likely to result in osseous and articular pain, some general categorization is necessary. We have chosen a mixed classification based on: a) anatomy (monarticular vs. polyarticular disease) and b) etiology (trauma, infection, and tumor). Given a patient with bone or joint pain, what is the best approach to diagnosis? Although the diagnostic strategy is dependent on the conditions most likely to be present, we emphasize that not all instances of these conditions will present with the given symptom. Thus, it should be clear that diagnostic reasoning derives first and foremost from clinical findings, *which are themselves the best tests for disease*. Only when a degree of uncertainty exists after clinical assessment does any testing becomes necessary.

Bone and Joint Trauma

Obviously, the plain radiograph remains the single most important imaging modality to establish the presence of fracture. However, a negative radiograph does not exclude fracture, because in a significant but unknown percentage of such patients the X-ray will either remain normal or become abnormal only after a few days. This is especially true in injuries to cancellous bone, i.e. the small bones of the wrists, hands, ankles, feet, vertebrae, and ribs.

Moreover, in older patients, especially those with osteoporosis, negative X-rays are often seen in the presence of vertebral, subcapital fractures of the femoral head and impacted femoral neck fractures. Athletes and joggers show a high incidence of stress fractures or subperiosteal bone injury (shin splints), which usually do not show up on plain films. Parenthetically, musculoskeletal injuries occur in about 75% of runners (1, 2). It is therefore essential in all patients with a strong suspicion of fracture and negative radiographs that the most sensitive imaging procedure should be performed, namely bone scintigraphy.

In the assessment of joint trauma, plain radiographs again are the mainstay of diagnosis. CT/MRI imaging is important in assessing trauma associated with sports and occupational injuries but, as with virtually all studies, only if the findings will affect management. It is in the major joints, particularly the back, knees, and shoulders, that MRI is especially helpful. Some minor joints can be imaged successfully with CT or MRI, but imaging is advisable only if plain radiographs and clinical findings suggest the need for further anatomic definition. In most cases in which the injury is not serious or likely to result in surgical intervention, or when discontinuation of the activity does not become a serious economic decision, as in professional athletes, CT and MRI are superfluous and not indicated.

ARTHRITIS: MONARTICULAR

Clearly, "medical" arthritis must be distinguished from joint trauma. But if the distinction is confidently made on history, radiographic films are seldom indicated in acute monarticular arthritis. The most common cause of this condition is peritendinitis or bursitis. In a much smaller subset of patients with acute pain in or near a single joint, the diagnosis is usually gout, pseudogout, or some type of inflammatory arthritis. In these conditions plain radiographs again are either not indicated or of little use except in the presence of sepsis.

Even in septic arthritis, however, early destruction of the cartilage, as indicated by narrowing of the joint space, destruction of subchondral bone, and extensive periosteal new bone formation do not show up on X-ray for at least 8–9 days. In the event that deep-seated sepsis of the hip, shoulder, or sacroiliac joints or septic arthritis of other joints is suspected, bone scintigraphy combined with gallium or indium-111-labeled WBCs is indicated. These studies are positive with osteomyelitis and septic arthritis. Because activity crossing the joint space is more characteristic of arthritis than osteomyelitis, scintigraphy is helpful in distinguishing the two conditions.

If nonseptic inflammatory arthritis is present, the gallium or indium-111 WBC scintiscan will show less focal and more generalized uptake, whereas in degenerative and nonseptic joint diseases, the bone scan but not the gallium/indium study may be positive (3). In some cases of acute, and sometimes even chronic arthritis, such as gout or rheumatoid, when both gallium and bone scintigraphy may be positive and therefore strongly suggestive of a septic joint, the plain radiograph often helps settle the issue. Clinical judgment in these cases pays a huge dividend, because sensible clinicians would assiduously avoid scintigraphy if they suspected a nonseptic arthritis such as gout or degenerative disease.

ARTHRITIS: POLYARTICULAR

Acute synovitis may occasionally present as polyarthritis. Its abrupt onset followed by generally spontaneous remission in a few days or weeks can differentiate it from other more serious forms of arthritis. These latter diseases would include a wide variety of conditions such as gonococcal and other infectious arthritides, rheumatoid and other collagen vascular diseases, Reiter's syndrome, viral arthritis (rubella, mumps, and hepatitis B), hypersensitivity states, inflammatory bowel disease, etc. Plain radiographs are often helpful, but in general, other types of medical imaging are not indicated in these conditions.

CHRONIC AND SUBACUTE FORMS OF ARTHRITIS

Plain X-rays are the single most appropriate imaging method in the patient with chronic or subacute arthritis. CT and MRI have essentially no place in the imaging of medical arthritic conditions and should be soundly discouraged. Bone scintigraphy, likewise, is contraindicated except when extent of involvement is questioned and when the radiographic *and clinical* findings are negative or equivocal.

Plain radiographs help distinguish patients in whom the diagnoses of rheumatoid, degenerative joint disease, gout, "atypical" osteoarthritis, and the spondyloarthropathies are entertained (3). Patients with these conditions comprise the majority of those with chronic arthritis. Radiography of the joints of patients with known forms of chronic or subacute arthritis may be helpful when it is clinically difficult to assess the extent and distribution of joint involvement.

Osteomyelitis

If bone films indicate an acute or chronic osteomyelitis, bone scintigraphy is *not necessary* for diagnosis and therefore *should be omitted*. However, in assessing the activity of osteomyelitis, particularly in patients who have completed a course of antibiotic therapy, gallium/indium scintiscanning is extremely helpful.

It is in the patient with suspected *early* osteomyelitis, particularly infants and children, where bone scintigraphy is most useful. In acute osteomyelitis, the plain radiograph may not become abnormal for up to 3 weeks or more. If bone scintigraphy is positive in this setting and the clinical diagnosis thus confirmed, gallium scintigraphy is not indicated.

A great deal of confusion exists over the use of combined bone and gallium scintigraphy in osteomyelitis. Generally, the diagnosis requires *both* imaging modalities in the following patients:

1. Those with chronic deep ulcerations overlying bone, especially in the greater trochanter, tibiae, feet, and hands, where bone scintigraphy may be falsely positive;
2. In the differentiation of osteomyelitis from nonseptic conditions when the radiograph is nondiagnostic or atypical for osteomyelitis and the bone scintigram is positive;
3. In treated osteomyelitis in determining the persistence of active infection after a course of antibiotic treatment; and

4. In postfracture patients, particularly those who have suffered comminuted fractures, open reduction, nonunion, and other complications where radiographs cannot be relied upon to exclude the diagnosis of osteomyelitis.

Once the diagnosis of osteomyelitis has been established either by radiographs, scintiscanning, or both, bone scintigraphy usually need not be repeated, because abnormalities on the bone scan persist long after complete healing. Thus negative bone scintigraphy would signal the end of the healing process. However, this could take as long as 6–18 months or more after normalization of the gallium study, an earlier, more specific indication of healing. (Gallium or indium WBC scans may be falsely negative or indeterminate in patients on long-term antibiotic therapy, which tends falsely to normalize scintigraphy.) If gallium scintiscanning is to be used to determine persistence of bone infection, it is best performed when the patient has been off antibiotic therapy for at least 1–2 weeks.

In order to maintain some perspective about the problem it is important to remind ourselves of some sad but inescapable facts about osteomyelitis. In most cases of extensive disease, particularly of the long bones and that resulting from serious trauma such as compound fractures, and in adequately treated cases persisting for more than 6 months, the outlook for ultimate cure is dim. Repeated scintigraphy in these patients is almost always an exercise in futility and a waste of money when activity can be followed clinically and radiographically. We have had numerous patients referred for scintigraphy when the diagnosis of chronic osteomyelitis was obvious, as for example, the 72-year-old gentleman with a chronic draining sinus of the tibia since an auto accident in childhood.

TUMORS

Most primary benign and malignant tumors of bone can be diagnosed from the plain X-ray alone, which usually establishes or excludes the need for biopsy. Among the exceptions are osteoid osteoma, particularly of the cancellous bone (spine, ribs, and distal extremities). Here, when the radiographic appearance is not always typical, positive bone scintigraphy is helpful. In the rare patient, CT or MRI may help to exclude malignancy in the presence of negative radiographs. These studies are more sensitive than radiography for detecting cortical destruction indicating a malignant lesion.

Metastatic Tumors of Bone

In most patients, the diagnosis of malignancy already should have been made before the search for osseous metastases is launched. It is surprising how frequently malignant metastatic bone involvement is painless, sometimes even in fairly advanced stages. We discourage bone scintigraphy as a screening test for neoplasm. The fear of missing cancer or the obsession with malignancy *in the absence of specific signs or symptoms* almost always results in needless testing of patients with a low pretest probability of disease, most often in the aged, the neglected, and in patients with depressive illness.

If cancer is strongly suspected on clinical grounds, i.e. a breast mass in a postmenopausal woman, or a prostatic nodule, results of bone scintigraphy would have implications for therapy once the biopsy results are known (vide infra). Moreover, in patients with weight loss, bone pain, and other findings that suggest malignancy, bone scintigraphy should be done, but only when accompanied by appropriate organ-specific imaging, e.g. radiographic studies of the GI or GU tract in patients with accompanying GI or GU symptoms. With localized bone pain, plain radiographs should always be performed first.

In the case of bone pain and negative X-rays in a high cancer suspect, bone scintigraphy is indicated, as it is in patients with an established diagnosis of *certain cancers* (see Chapter 9). In the latter case, when scintigraphy is performed, it need not be preceded by the plain radiograph. We stress that many types of malignancy, especially adenocarcinomas with unknown sites of origin or tumors originating in the GI or female reproductive tract, rarely metastasize to bone, or if so, only late in the course of disease.

Summary

The following is meant only as a general guide in the imaging approach to patients with clinically significant bone or joint pain:

TRAUMA

1. If plain radiographs are negative when fractures are suspected, this diagnosis should not be excluded until bone scintigraphy has been performed.

2. In chronic, recurrent, or complicated joint trauma, especially involving the spine, knee, or shoulders, perform CT if MRI is not available. This is especially important in cases where surgical or arthroscopic intervention is contemplated.

3. CT or MRI is also indicated in athletic and occupational injuries when the extent and type of injury cannot be adequately ascertained by radiographic examination, and also when proscribing further physical activity could have serious economic consequences, as in physical laborers or professional athletes.

ARTHRITIS

1. In most cases of acute monarticular arthritis, imaging is not indicated. In suspected septic arthritis, plain films may be helpful (though not usually in the acute patient). If typical findings confirm the diagnosis, no further imaging is required, especially if diagnostic joint aspiration is successful. However, if findings have been present less than 8–9 days, radiographs may be negative, and bone scintigraphy should be performed.

2. If scintigraphy fails to show bone involvement, do not assume septic arthritis has been excluded if strong clinical indications persist. In a few patients with septic arthritis, bone scintigraphy may be falsely negative for a time and only the gallium or indium-111 WBC study will be abnormal. If bone scintigraphy is positive, gallium imaging will be abnormal in septic but not in degenerative disease. However, both bone and gallium scintiscans may be positive in acute forms of nonseptic arthritis such as rheumatoid and gout.

3. In acute polyarticular arthritis, imaging is almost never revealing. In chronic or subacute polyarticular arthritis one should depend primarily on the plain X-ray to distinguish the major causes (rheumatoid, gout, degenerative joint disease, atypical osteoarthritis, and the spondyloarthropathies). Bone scintigraphy and CT or MRI are rarely, if ever, of help in the chronic arthritides.

OSTEOMYELITIS

1. If bone radiographs are typical for acute osteomyelitis, further imaging is unnecessary. If radiographs and the clinical findings indicate chronic osteomyelitis, further imaging is rarely indicated.

2. In patients with suspected *early* osteomyelitis where symptoms or clinical signs have been present for less than 3–4 weeks and radiographs are negative, bone scintigraphy should be performed. Negative bone scintiscans do not always exclude osteomyelitis, because in some patients, early osteomyelitis, like septic arthritis, may not result in a positive bone scintiscan. In these cases gallium or indium-111 WBC studies will almost always be positive. However, tuberculous osteomyelitis of the spine is frequently negative on bone and gallium scintigraphy.

3. Combined three-phase bone and gallium or indium-111 WBC scintigraphy are generally required only in the following settings:

(a) In differentiating septic from nonseptic conditions where radiographs fail to confirm the diagnosis of osteomyelitis and bone scintigraphy is positive.
(b) In patients with chronic deep ulcerations overlying bone when radiographs are nonspecific. We emphasize, however, that particularly in a subset of diabetics with foot ulcers, *the diagnosis of osteomyelitis, short of bone biopsy, is sometimes difficult if not impossible even with radionuclide studies.*

Gallium/indium-WBC scintigraphy alone is indicated in patients with known osteomyelitis *after* a course of antibiotic treatment, to determine persistence of active infection or if healing has occurred.

PRIMARY AND METASTATIC BONE TUMORS

1. Most primary benign and malignant tumors of bone have a fairly typical diagnostic radiographic appearance. Further imaging in these cases is not indicated. If, however, extent of involvement cannot be determined, especially in the spine, CT or MRI should be performed. Bone scintigraphy is helpful in demonstrating osteoid osteoma in cancellous bone, especially where the radiograph may not be diagnostic.

2. Osseous metastatic malignancy should be suspected in all cancer patients with unexplained bone pain. Radionuclide bone scanning is the imaging method *par excellence* for the diagnosis of metastatic bone disease, particularly in tumors of the breast, prostate, lung, and kidneys, which have a frequent predilection for osseous spread. Tumors originating in the GI tract or female pelvis seldom metastasize to bone, and, therefore, bone scintigraphy is not generally recommended in such patients (vide infra).

3. Bone scintigraphy is a poor screening test for the presence of primary malignancy and should not be used for this purpose.

REFERENCES

1. Jones BH. Overuse injuries of the lower extremities associated with marching, jogging, and running: a review. Milit Med 1983;148(10):783–787.
2. Temple C. Sports injuries: hazards of jogging and marathon running. Br J Hosp Med 1983;29(3):237–239.
3. Branch WT. Monoarticular arthritis and acute polyarticular synovitis, and Chronic arthritis, In: Branch WT, ed. Office Practice of Medicine. Philadelphia: W.B. Saunders Company, 1987:829–865.

6/ GU Tract Pain: Urolithiasis and Other Causes

> *Macduff: What three things does drink especially provoke?*
> *Porter: Marry, sir, nose-painting, sleep, and urine.*
> *William Shakespeare*
> Macbeth, *II:3*

Acute flank pain is usually attributed to pyelonephritis or renal calculus. Although this assumption has almost attained the respectability of a medical axiom, it continues to cause diagnostic confusion in the minds of the clinically inexperienced who puzzle over the anatomic location of "flanks" and who disassociate this important complaint from a critical laboratory test, the urinalysis.

The word *flank* is sometimes misinterpreted to mean the lateral abdominal quadrants, even extending into the lumbosacral region. Yet pain of renal origin (pain that is predominantly caused by stone), is classically felt in the posterior subcostal and costovertebral region. As with other visceral pain, urinary tract pain is usually not as well localized as somatic pain involving the same dermatomes, and the accuracy of description increases with body awareness. Children, for example, are poor at localiz-

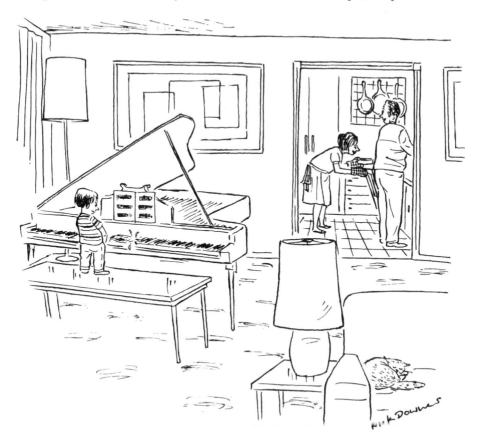

"Could that be our Ritchie tinkling on the piano?"
Reproduced by permission of *Punch*.

ing urinary tract problems (1). Indeed, pain radiation may occur anteriorly around the flank in the lower and upper abdominal quadrants, and even rebound tenderness may occur with spasm of the abdominal muscles. Nausea, vomiting, and occasionally ileus may be seen. Thus, as we have previously noted, pain of GU origin may mimic that of intraabdominal conditions in up to 10–15% of cases presenting as acute abdominal pain. Some cases of acute pyelonephritis or renal stone may be confused with intestinal obstruction, retrocecal appendicitis, pelvic inflammatory disease, and even perforation. Conversely, however, the pain of these and other intraabdominal conditions, even aortic dissection, may be confused with that originating in the GU tract.

Owing to the anatomic extent of the urinary tract, pain arising in the kidney, ureters, and bladder will present with many faces. The classic character, severity, and radiation of ureteral colic is seldom missed, but confusion commonly arises with less severe presentations of urinary tract pain. We have seen occasional patients with recurrent renal or ureteral stones who did not present with classic renal colic, but with more protracted and ill-defined flank pain syndromes. Of notable importance, clinical blunders result from the *failure to distinguish renal and ureteral pain from musculoskeletal pain arising from the back*, particularly the lumbosacral region. One of the most common causes of unnecessary referral for renal imaging is the presence of mid- and lower back pain, *without urinary findings*. The overwhelming majority of these patients have clinical symptoms and signs pointing to musculoskeletal disease, usually a history of recurrent "strain" or back trouble associated with localized tenderness (easily distinguishable from costovertebral angle (CVA) punch tenderness), plus spasm, limitation of motion, and/or pain induced by straight leg-raising tests.

GU pain associated with acute lower tract problems, i.e. the bladder and urethra, is almost always characterized by the presence of the classic symptoms of urgency, frequency, tenesmus, or dysuria. These urinary complaints, of course, frequently accompany acute ureteral colic as well. Women with acute urethral syndromes or vaginitis and men with prostatitis cannot easily be distinguished from patients with cystitis.

One test alone can identify patients with pain of suspected GU tract origin: urinalysis. If there are less than four or five red cells or two or three WBCs (five WBCs in women) per high-power field, the likelihood of any clinically significant urinary tract disease is almost nil (1). The definitions for significant pyuria or hematuria, however, may be more stringent (one or two cells per high-power field, respectively) following the precise method of centrifugation of a midstream specimen quoted by Brenner and Rector (2). The Hemastix test for hematuria is used extensively by nephrologists and is probably at least as useful and is far easier to perform than the microscopic examination for red cells.

The prior probability of disease given abnormal findings on urinalysis, with or without urinary tract pain as a secondary complaint, is obviously different from patients presenting with urinary tract pain as a *primary symptom*. The imaging approach to patients with painless proteinuria, hematuria, pyuria, or bacteriuria is outlined in another section.

Given the patient with acute or subacute flank pain as a principal complaint associated with gross or microscopic hematuria, it is appropriate to review the diagnostic approach to one of the most prevalent and important GU conditions.

Table 6.6.1. Discharge Rates per 100,000 Population, Urinary/Ureteral Calculus. NCHS Data, U.S. Hospitals, 1990.

All-listed ICD-9-CM	Total	Male	Female	Age <15	Age 15–44	Age 45–64	Age 65+
592.0 Calculus of kidney	52	55	49	0	41	83	133
592.1 Calculus of ureter	88	123	55	0	96	151	120
592.9 Urinary calculus NOS	4	5	0	0	0	0	0

Total Discharge in Thousands, Urinary/Ureteral Calculus. NCHS Data, U.S. Hospitals, 1990.

All-listed ICD-9-CM	Total	Male	Female	Age <15	Age 15–44	Age 45–64	Age 65+
592.0 Calculus of kidney	129	66	63	0	47	39	42
592.1 Calculus of ureter	220	149	71	0	111	71	38
592.9 Urinary calculus NOS	9	6	0	0	0	0	0

NOS, Not otherwise specified.

Urolithiasis

> *Rather suffer than die is man's motto.*
>
> *de La Fontaine*

Table 6.6.1 shows the all-listed hospital discharge data giving rates and frequency by age and sex in the United States for renal or ureteral stones in 1990 (3). It is impossible to estimate from the data the number of patients having both ureteral and renal calculi. Note the preponderance of ureteral but not renal calculi in males, the virtual absence of the condition in the young, and the rates preponderance in the age group over 45. According to some writers, 12% of the population will have at least one stone during a lifetime (4), an unexpectedly high figure.

The true prevalence of urolithiasis is more difficult to determine. In a geographically well-defined region of Great Britain a prevalence rate of 3.8% was found in 2000 adults based on the presence of renal calcification on plain abdominal radiograms (5). In point of fact, urinary tract stones have been identified in 5% of carefully studied autopsies (6), further indicating the significant number of asymptomatic people.

We must therefore conclude that renal calculi, like gall stones, are frequently present without causing clinical complaints. The precise numbers of such individuals cannot be estimated from the data available in the literature, but they are considerable. If one assumes the autopsy figure of 5% of the population with urolithiasis out of a U.S. population of approximately 250 million, then approximately 12.5 million Americans would have urolithiasis. The above hospital discharge data of approximately 358,000 discharge diagnoses for renal or ureteral stone must be compared with this figure, giving a hypothetical ratio of nonhospitalized to hospitalized patients with renal or ureteral stone of 35 to 1. This does not prove, of course, that all nonhospitalized patients are asymptomatic, but it is reasonable to conclude from these figures that at the very least more than 95% of patients harboring renal calculi will never be hospitalized. Of these, a significant (though unknown) majority will never develop clinical symptoms. This is consistent with clinical experience. In our large population of unselected renal sonograms, most of which were otherwise nor-

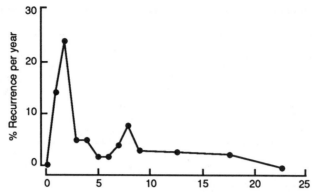

Figure 6.6.1. Rate of stone recurrence in patients who have formed a single calcium stone. (Reprinted by permission from Coe FL. *Nephrolithiasis: Pathogenesis and Treatment.* Chicago: Year Book Publishers, 1978.)

Table 6.6.2. Metabolic and Clinical Disorders in 460 Consecutive Calcium Stone Formers[a]

	No. of Patients	(%)
Idiopathic hypercalciuria	95	(20.7)
Marginal hypercalciuria[b]	53	(11.5)
Hyperuricosuria[c]	67	(14.6)
Hypercalciuria and hyperuricosuria[d]	54	(11.7)
Hyperuricemia	26	(5.7)
Primary hyperparathyroidism	24	(5.2)
Renal tubular acidosis[e]	17	(3.7)
Inflammatory bowel disease[f]	21	(4.6)
Medullary sponge kidney	7	(1.5)
Sarcoidosis	3	(0.7)
No disorder found	93	(20.2)
Total	460	

[a]Reprinted by permission from Coe FL: *Nephrolithiasis: Pathogenesis and Treatment.* Chicago, Year Book Medical Publishers, 1978.
[b]Urine calcium >140 mg/g creatinine but less than 250 mg/24 hours in women and 300 mg/24 hours in men.
[c]Urine uric acid above 800 mg (men) and 750 mg (women), in at least one of two 24-hour urine collections.
[d]Marginal hypercalciuria not included.
[e]Distal, hereditary form.
[f]Regional enteritis, ulcerative colitis, granulomatous ileocolitis.

mal, we have identified calcifications in the renal collecting system in an impressive number of patients without any history or symptoms of renal calculus.

The likelihood of stone recurrence varies with different series, but appears to be generally low after the second year. This is shown in Figure 6.6.1. In patients with calcium-containing stones and one or more recurrences within 1 year there is a 60% probability of having some treatable metabolic disorder (7). Identifiable metabolic and clinical disorders accounted for almost 80% in a large series of stone formers shown in Table 6.6.2. The simple expedient of performing a urinary pH may give an immediate clue to a treatable condition, i.e. the presence of a morning pH less than 6.0 in a fasting patient is typical of uric acid calculi.

Imaging in the Management of Renal and Ureteral Calculi

Most patients with renal colic can be managed outside the hospital with analgesics and forced hydration. In addition to relief of pain, the thrust of managing urolithiasis is observation for secondary infection and to determine if stones have passed or if surgical intervention will be required. The choice and timing of imaging procedures are therefore critical in caring for the small minority of patients with larger stones that do not pass within the first few days or so. In general, stones smaller than 5 mm will pass spontaneously, those between 5 and 10 mm have a 50% chance of passing, and those larger than 10 mm usually require surgical removal (8). The three principal sites of obstruction are the ureteropelvic junction, the pelvic brim, and most frequently the ureterovesical junction. Fifteen percent of ureteral calculi in a selected series measuring 5–8 mm lodged at the ureterovesical junction (9). These stones usually can be located with intravenous urography and removed successfully with endoscopic manipulation with a success rate of 75% on the first attempt (10).

The radiodensity of urinary calculi depends on their size, shape, and composition (11). However, from a practical standpoint, calculi larger than 2 mm in size and containing some calcium are radiopaque. This means that *90–95% of clinically significant stones should be detectable with a good quality plain abdominal film*. If there is any doubt as to location within the urinary tract, oblique films should be taken. Previous abdominal plain films, if available, may be of particular help. The intravenous pyelogram (IVP), however, continues to be preferred by most physicians. This study is certainly crucial in those patients with radiolucent (usually urate) or other obstructing stones, and in determining the need for urological intervention. Such intervention will be required in the presence of persistent complete or partial obstruction, urinary extravasation due to pyelosinus rupture, or with large stones (larger than 10 mm), most of which are unlikely to pass (8).

Whether all patients with renal calculi should routinely have IVP is debatable. In view of the availability and ease of ultrasonography, it would make sense to use it along with plain radiography to decide if pyelography is indeed indicated. There is little question that sonography should be preferable in patients experiencing mild or repeat attacks, pregnant women, those in whom pyelography has been previously performed within a reasonable time period, and, of course, those with contraindications to the IVP, for example, a history of allergy to contrast material, presence of decreased renal function, etc. When the diagnostic accuracy of sonography and excretory urography was compared in a study of acute flank pain in 61 patients, 41 of whom were completely or partially obstructed, a correct diagnosis of obstruction was made by urography in 85% and by sonography in 66% (12). This is surprising in view of the reported sensitivity of sonography in ureteral obstruction of more than 95% (13, 14). Further follow-up studies were not performed, because most patients were not hospitalized and none required subsequent surgery. *In every case the plain radiograph was positive for stone*. The authors concluded that sonography in conjunction with the plain radiograph is "a useful alternative to the excretory urogram." If renal sonography is *normal*, then urography can be omitted unless the stone is not passed, i.e. obstruction develops. This can be determined on the basis of repeat sonography and serial plain abdominal films, if necessary, to note the progression of the stone. In the event of obstruction shown with ultrasound and in those patients in whom pyelography is contraindicated and plain films are not helpful, there is a place for radionuclide scintigraphy in locating the level of obstruction.

Retrograde pyelography may be required when excretory urography fails to visualize the collecting system adequately because of poor renal function, or the suspected stone is radiolucent and cannot be identified. In this instance, however, radionuclide studies may suffice. Invasive retrograde studies should be performed *only* in those patients who have a *reasonable probability of requiring surgical intervention*, i.e. those with obstructing ureteral stones or nonobstructing stones that do not pass within 4–6 weeks. In 1990, 61,000 transurethral procedures for ureteral obstruction (ICD 56.0) and 114,000 retrograde pyelograms (ICD 87.84) were performed in the United States (3). These numbers represent a significant percentage of patients admitted for renal or ureteral calculus.

The place of CT in the management of urolithiasis is limited to a very small group of patients with small, indistinct, or suspected calculi not visualized by other methods. It is usually employed for localization of nonopaque intrarenal calculi before nephrolithotomy (15–17).

Summary of the Imaging Approach to Patients with Acute Flank Pain Thought to be of GU Origin

1. In patients presenting with acute or chronic flank pain, in general, *do not suspect a GU origin of pain, and do not perform imaging studies without abnormal findings on urinalysis.* The overwhelming majority of patients thought to have "flank" pain and with a normal urine will turn out to have lumbosacral pain due to a musculoskeletal condition of the back and spine.

2. In patients with flank or abdominal pain of suspected GU origin, the two most likely diagnoses are pyelonephritis and urolithiasis. Virtually all patients with urinary tract conditions will have an abnormal urinalysis.

3. Acute pyelonephritis usually can be distinguished from renal colic clinically (fever, prostration, pyuria, and positive urine culture) and the absence of significant hematuria. Renal imaging studies are seldom helpful in adults with suspected acute pyelonephritis and should rarely if ever be relied upon to make the diagnosis; pyelography is not usually indicated (vide infra). (Pyelography has been advocated in the diagnosis of chronic pyelonephritis, but we disagree.)

4. Without gross or microscopic hematuria, the diagnosis of ureteral stone is for all intents excluded. (Hematuria, however, may be absent with an intrarenal stone.)

5. In all cases of suspected calculi, a plain or oblique abdominal film should be the first imaging study, because it has a 90–95% sensitivity for stone detection. A negative *good quality* plain abdominal film is strong evidence against urolithiasis. If a stone is seen, its size is a good indication of its prognosis. Stones smaller than 3 mm almost always pass; 5-mm stones have a greater than 50% chance of passing spontaneously; stones larger than 10 mm are likely to require urological intervention.

6. After abdominal films, renal sonography should be performed to exclude obstruction, even if no stone is seen on plain films.

7. In the presence of obstruction demonstrated by sonography (more than 24–48 hours) with failure of a stone to pass, or in the presence of any stone demonstrated to be larger than 5 mm on abdominal radiography or in any patient with continuing symptoms, IVP always should be performed. Most obstructing stones will be found at the ureteropelvic or especially at the ureterovesical junction.

8. Plain abdominal radiography and renal ultrasonography alone or combined with radionuclide scintiscans usually can provide adequate clinical information even in the presence of obstruction in the majority of patients with absolute or relative contraindications to pyelography.

9. Retrograde pyelography should rarely, if ever, be used to determine the need for urological intervention, something which can usually be done using serial plain films, IVP, and sonography. Rather, this invasive procedure should be used principally to visualize urinary tract anatomy *once the need for endoscopic manipulation has been established.*

REFERENCES

1. Perlmutter AD, Blacklow RS. Urinary tract pain, hematuria, and pyuria. In: Blacklow RS, ed. Mac-Bryde's Signs and Symptoms. 6th ed. Philadelphia: J.B. Lippincott Co., 1983:181–193.
2. Brenner BM, Rector FC. The Kidney. 4th ed. Philadelphia: W.B. Saunders Co., 1991:948.
3. U.S. Department of Health and Human Services, U.S. Public Health Service, Centers for Disease Control, and the National Center for Health Statistics. National Hospital Discharge Survey (NHDS). Detailed diagnoses, procedures, days of care, diagnoses-related groups for patients discharged from short-stay hospitals. Public Use Data Diskettes, 1985–1990.
4. Sierakowski R, Finlayson B, Landes RR, et al. The frequency of urothithiasis in hospital discharge diagnoses in the United States. Invest Urol 1978;15:438–441.
5. Scott R, Freeland R, Mowat W, et al. The prevalence of calcified upper urinary tract stone disease in a random population—Cumbernauld Health Survey. Br J Urol 1977;49:589–595.
6. Rosenow EC. Renal calculi: study of papillary calcification. J Urol 1940;44:19–28.
7. Williams G, Chisholm GD. Stone screening and follow-up are necessary? Br J Urol 1975;47:745–750.
8. Burton JR, Smolev JK. Urinary stones. In: Barker LR, Burton JR, Zieve PD, eds. Principles of Ambulatory Medicine. 2nd ed. Baltimore: Williams & Wilkins, 1986:532–542.
9. Anderson EE. The management of ureteral calculi. Urol Clin North Am 1974;1:357–363.
10. Witherspoon JM, Smith MJV. Urolithiasis. In: Branch Jr WT, ed. Office Practice of Medicine. 2nd ed. Philadelphia: W.B. Saunders Co., 1987:580–607.
11. Roth R, Finlayson B. Observations on the radiopacity of stone substances with special reference to cystine. Invest Urol 1973;II(11):186–189.
12. Hill MC, Rich JI, Mardiat JG, Finder CA. Sonography vs. excretory urography in acute flank pain. AJR 1985;144:1235–1238.
13. Maillet PJ, Pell-Francoz D, Laville M, Gay F, Pinet A. Nondilated obstructive acute renal failure. Diagnostic procedures and therapeutic management. Radiology 1986;160:659–626.
14. Naidich JB, Rackson ME, Massey RT, Stein HL. Non-dilated obstructive uropathy: percutaneous nephrostomy performed to reverse renal failure. Radiology 1986;160:653–657.
15. Roth RA. Surgery of renal calculi. Semin Urol 1984;2:45–63.
16. Brennan RE, Curtis JA, Kurtz AB, et al. Use of tomography and ultrasound in diagnosis of nonopaque renal calculi. JAMA 1980;244:594–596.
17. Wickham JE, Fry IK, Wallace DM. Computerized tomography localization of intrarenal calculi prior to nephrolithotomy. Br J Urol 1980;52:422–425.

7/ Headache

The bigger a man's head, the worse his headache.

Persian proverb

When you're lying awake with a dismal headache, and repose is tabooed by anxiety,
I conceive you may use any language you choose to indulge in without impropriety.

W. S. Gilbert
Iolanthe

Headache was the 10th most common reason for visits (S210) to ambulatory care physicians in the United States in 1989, accounting for approximately 9.7

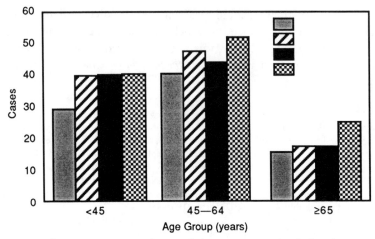

Figure 6.7.1. Prevalence (per 1000 population) of chronic migraine headaches, by patient age and region—United States, 1986–1988. Reprinted from *MMWR* (1991;May 24:338).

million or 1.4% of all visits in that year (1). In 1990, the all-listed NCHS discharge frequency for brain tumors was 18 cases per 100,000 population, or about 1 per 5,500 (2).

These figures have obvious implications for the investigation of patients with headache. Because headache is such a common symptom and brain tumor is such a rare condition, it is obvious why one does not investigate headache in the absence of other findings. Balla (3), using Bayes' Theorem with estimated independent probabilities, calculates the likelihood of brain tumor given a patient who presents with *both headache and papilledema* as approximately 0.33 (3). Calculation shows that the positive predictive value of an abnormal MRI scan in a patient complaining only of headache, assuming a sensitivity of 0.94 and a specificity of 0.98 is 0.01 for brain tumor. That is, given a patient only with headache and an abnormal MRI scan, the chances the patient indeed has a brain tumor is only 1 in 10,000. In the case of a patient with both headache and papilledema, a positive MRI has a predictive value of 0.96 for brain tumor.

In patients with sudden severe headache, by far the most common conditions are migraine, toxic vascular headaches, and the effort-induced headaches (benign exertional, cough, and coital cephalalgia). Almost all such patients give a previous history of similar headaches. Figure 6.7.1 shows the prevalence of chronic migraine headaches through 1989 by patient age and region in the United States, figures that have increased nearly 60% from 1980 (4). Note that approximately 4% of the population is afflicted. It is impossible to estimate the prior probability of other causes of benign headache, but clearly migraine would rank among the most common.

Ominous but much less frequent causes of "the worst headache ever" must, of course, be kept in mind when deciding on the necessity for investigation. In particular, the diagnoses listed in Table 6.7.1 should be considered when clinical signs and symptoms of these ominous conditions summarized by Edmeads in Table 6.7.2 are present (5–7). Confirmation of the diagnosis based on these danger signals obviously

Table 6.7.1. Ominous Causes of ''the Worst Headache Ever''

Subarachnoid hemorrhage
Meningitis
Increased intracranial pressure
High blood presure
Vasculopathies
Acute purulent sinusitis

Reprinted by permission from *Postgraduate Medicine* (1989;86(1):94).

Table 6.7.2. Danger Signals of Ominous Headache

A ''first'' headache
Headache beginning during exertion
Headache accompanied by fever
Headache in a drowsy or confused patient
Headache in a patient whose neck is not perfectly supple
Headache in a patient with abnormal physical signs
Headache in a patient who looks ill

Reprinted by permission from *Postgraduate Medicine* (1989;86(1):103).

rests on the results of examination followed by sinus films, lumbar puncture, and/or CT or MRI.

High blood pressure is often considered a cause of headache, yet this symptom is no more common in patients with mild or moderate hypertension than in age-matched controls (8). Headaches due to chronic hypertension do not occur until diastolic blood pressure exceeds 120 mm Hg, and these patients seldom seek emergency treatment because the headache is usually mild. Severe hypertensive headaches, of course, may result from acute severe idiopathic hypertensive encephalopathy, the secondary form, i.e. pheochromocytoma, or from drugs such as cocaine, amphetamines, certain antidepressants with tyramine release, etc.

Headache Associated with Head Trauma

The question of performing CT or MRI on patients with headache associated with acute head trauma cannot be addressed by any easy set of rules. Minor head *injury* such as a bump on the head is not equivalent to minor head *trauma* and must be distinguished from it. The latter condition has specific diagnostic criteria, including loss of consciousness, confusion, and amnesia. A few specialists still recommend skull roentgenography for these patients, but the vast majority of neurologists and neurosurgeons no longer use plain skull radiographs. Major head trauma, in fact, is one of the few conditions in which CT or MRI *should be performed as first studies*, and where plain X-rays are *largely useless*.

Significant head trauma is defined by the clinical features of the patient and by the results of neurological examination. Even minor head injury can be followed by major neurological dysfunction, whereas onset of serious symptoms can be delayed for 24 hours or more. The Glasgow coma scale (9) may be very helpful in assessment.

Summary

1. The overwhelming majority of patients with recurrent headaches need not be investigated.

2. In the patient with sudden severe headache, clinical distinction should be made between the innocuous causes such as migraine, toxic vascular headache, and the effort-induced headaches and the ominous causes listed in Table 6.7.1. Danger signals of ominous headache are given in Table 6.7.2.

3. Lumbar puncture is clearly indicated first in suspected meningitis and other neurological causes of acute headache if significantly increased intracranial pressure is not present.

4. CT and MRI are the imaging mainstays of neurological diagnosis of headache secondary to severe trauma, increased intracranial pressure, and space-occupying masses.

5. In suspected acute sinusitis, if plain radiographs of the paranasal sinuses are normal or nondiagnostic, proceed to CT and MRI. These studies are superior in delineating the sinuses and in disclosing intracranial complications such as bony destruction secondary to osteomyelitis, expansion or destruction by tumor, mucocele, etc.

REFERENCES

1. Schappert SM. National Ambulatory Medical Care Survey: 1989 Summary. Hyattsville, Md: National Center for Health Statistics. Vital Health Statistics 1992;131(110):16.
2. U.S. Department of Health and Human Services, U.S. Public Health Service, Centers for Disease Control, and the National Center for Health Statistics. National Hospital Discharge Survey (NHDS). Detailed diagnoses, procedures, days of care, diagnoses-related groups for patients discharged from short-stay hospitals. Public Use Data Diskettes, 1985–1990.
3. Balla JI. Decision making. In: Balla JI, ed. The Diagnostic Process. Cambridge: Cambridge University Press, 1985:63–66.
4. Prevalence of chronic migraine headaches—United States, 1980–1989. MMWR 1991;40(20):331, 337–338.
5. Edmeads J. The worst headache ever. 1. Ominous causes. Postgrad Med 1989;86(1):96, 93–104.
6. Edmeads J. The worst headache ever. 2. Innocuous causes. Postgrad Med 1989;86(1):107–110.
7. Mandel S. Minor head injury may not be "minor." Postgrad Med 1989;85(6):217, 220, 225.
8. Badran RH, Weir RJ, McGuiness JB. Hypertension and headache. Scott Med J 1970;15(2):48–51.
9. Miller JD. Minor, moderate and severe head injury. Neurosurg Rev 1986;9(1–2):135–139.

8/ Arterial Hypertension

Medicine makes people ill, mathematics makes them sad and theology makes them sinful.

Martin Luther

Hypertension is the 13th among 60 principal reasons for physician office visits, resulting in more than 10 million visits in the United States in 1989, yet first in principal diagnoses, accounting for 27.7 million or 4% of all visits reported by physicians in the same year (1). Of almost 31 million discharges from acute care hospitals in the United States in 1990 there were more than 10% or 3.3 million total all-listed diagnoses for essential hypertension (2). Table 6.8.1 displays the

Table 6.8.1. Elevated Blood Pressure Among Persons 20–74 Years of Age, According to Race, Sex, and Age: United States, 1960–1962, 1971–1974, and 1976–1980

| | Percent of population with systolic pressure at least 160 mmHg or diastolic pressure at least 95 mmHg | | | | | | | | |
| | All races | | | White | | | Black | | |
Sex and age	1960–62	1971–74	1976–80	1960–62	1971–74	1976–80	1960–62	1971–74	1976–80
Female[a]									
20–74 years, age adjusted	18.6	18.0	15.4	16.9	16.3	14.4	33.2	33.0	23.5
20–74 years, crude	19.3	18.3	15.2	18.0	16.8	14.5	32.3	30.9	21.0
20–24 years	1.9	1.9	2.5	2.1	1.7	2.0	1.3	3.5	4.4
25–34 years	3.4	4.8	3.8	2.5	4.0	3.4	9.7	11.2	6.0
35–44 years	10.8	12.2	11.0	8.3	10.0	9.7	29.8	28.2	17.5
45–54 years	21.5	21.9	22.3	18.7	18.8	20.0	44.3	49.4	43.4
55–64 years	34.1	33.9	25.2	32.5	32.0	24.3	50.5	54.2	34.2
65–74 years	55.4	44.4	35.4	53.8	42.9	34.9	79.0[b]	59.8	40.0

Data are based on physical examinations of a sample of the civilian noninstitutionalized population. Percents are based on a single measurement of blood pressure to provide comparable data across the three time periods. Source: Division of Health Examination Statistics, National Center for Health Statistics, unpublished data.
[a]Excludes pregnant women.
[b]Percents based on fewer than 45 persons are considered unreliable. Percents based on fewer than 25 persons are considered highly unreliable and are not shown.

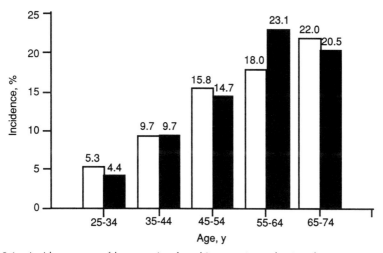

Figure 6.8.1. Incidence rates of hypertension for white men (*open bars*) and women (*cross-hatched bars*) with average follow-up of 9.5 years (follow-up study National Health Epidemiologic Follow-up Study (NHEFS). (From Cornoni-Huntley J, LaCroix AZ, Havlik RJ. *Arch Intern Med* 1989;149:780).

prevalence of various blood pressure levels of different age, sex, and racial groups in the United States from 1960–1980. Figure 6.8.1 shows the estimated *incidence* rates (new cases per 100,000/year) of significant hypertension (either systolic blood pressure 160 and/or diastolic pressure 95 or higher for white males and females) (3). Examining the source data between the years 1960–1980, one finds a drop in prevalence of significant hypertension in the older age groups and a rapidly falling disparity between the races over the 20-year period, with blacks showing a sizable drop in percentages. The statistics also show the enormous number of Americans afflicted, with the prevalence of hypertension increasing from 11%

Table 6.8.2. Frequency (%) of Various Diagnoses in Hypertensive Subjects

	Gifford	Berglund	Budnick	Danielson	Sinclair
Essential hypertension	89	94	94	95.3	92.1
Chronic renal disease	5	4	5	2.4	5.6
Renovascular disease	4	1	0.2	1.0	0.7
Coarctation	1	0.1	0.2		
Primary aldosteronism	0.5	0.1		0.1	0.3
Cushing's syndrome	0.2		0.2	0.1	0.1
Pheochromocytoma	0.2			0.2	0.1
Oral contraceptive-induced		(Men only)	0.2	0.8	1.0
No. of patients	4339	689	665	1000	3783

Compiled from Gifford J RW. *Milbank Mem Fund Q* 1969;17:170, Berglund G, Andersson O, Wilhelmsen L. *Br Med J* 1976;2:554, Rudnick KV, Sackett DL, Hirst S, et al. *Can Med Assoc J* 1977;117–492, Danielson M, Dammstrom BG. *Acta Med Scand* 1981;209:451, Sinclair AM, Isles CG, Brown I, et al. *Arch Intern Med* 1987;147:1289. Reprinted by permission from *Archives of Internal Medicine* (1987;147:(1289–1293).

at 35–44 years to 35% in the 65- to 74-year age group, for an approximate average of 20% of the adult population (4).

These figures have important implications for the investigation of hypertension, for they must be contrasted with the prevalence of secondary forms of the condition. Clearly, with almost all hypertension of the idiopathic or "essential" variety, the overwhelming majority of patients with high blood pressure should not be subjected to needless investigation. Table 6.8.2, also taken from Kaplan's classic text (5), shows the relative frequency of various causes of hypertension summarized from several series. Although more than 50 causes of hypertension can be listed, for all practical purposes chronic renal disease and renovascular and adrenal disease account for more than 99% of secondary hypertension, that is, hypertension with known cause. *Only in this tiny subset of patients with a high pretest probability of secondary hypertension should diagnostic imaging or other testing be considered.*

That the percentages in Table 6.8.2 are indeed biased can be inferred from the fact that they are derived from tertiary referral medical centers where there is a much higher prevalence of secondary hypertension than occurs in the general population. This can be verified from NCHS statistics giving all-listed diagnoses in frequencies and rates for primary and principal causes of secondary hypertension in the United States in 1990 in Table 8.6.3. The only figures for secondary hypertension available are for the four conditions listed: Cushing's syndrome, hyperaldosteronism, "secondary hypertension," and renovascular hypertension. Note that other endocrine causes of hypertension (adrenogenital, Bartter's syndrome, and pheochromocytomoma) are so rare in the discharge data that they are regarded as statistically unreliable and are not listed in 1990. Because one cannot disassociate renal disease caused by long-standing hypertension from hypertension arising as a result of primary renal disease, we have omitted "hypertensive renal disease" (ICD 403) from the tabulations (Ledingham, J.M., personal communication). From the all-listed hospital data the combined totals for secondary, renovascular, and adrenal hypertension are approximately 42,000 cases or slightly more than 1% of all hospital admissions for essential and secondary hypertension. Yet this number in no way reflects the true prevalence of these conditions in the total population of hypertensives. This value can be roughly approximated from the

Table 6.8.3. Primary and Secondary Hypertension All-Listed Diagnoses, 1990

All-listed ICD-9-CM		Total	Male	Female	Age <15	Age 15–44	Age 45–64	Age 65+
255.0	Cushing's syndrome	13	0	9	0	0	8	0
255.1	Hyperaldosteronism	5	0	0	0	0	0	0
401.	Essential hypertension	3296	1388	1908	9	272	1023	1993
402.	Hypertensive heart disease	308	119	189	0	7	71	229
403.0	Mal hypertens renal disease	7	0	0	0	0	0	0
404.	Hypertens heart/renal disease	38	18	20	0	0	9	26
405.	Secondary hypertension	15	6	9	0	0	0	8
405.91	Renovasc hypertension	9	0	6	0	0	0	5

All-Listed Diagnoses in Rates per 100,000, 1990

All-listed ICD-9-CM		Total	Male	Female	Age <15	Age 15–44	Age 45–64	Age 65+
255.0	Cushing's syndrome	5	0	7	0	0	17	0
255.1	Hyperaldosteronism	2	0	0	0	0	0	0
401.	Essential hypertension	1322	1148	1485	16	235	2180	6309
402.	Hypertensive heart disease	124	98	147	0	6	151	725
403.0	Mal hypertens renal disease	3	0	0	0	0	0	0
404.	Hypertens heart/renal disease	15	15	16	0	0	19	82
405.	Secondary hypertension	6	5	7	0	0	0	25
405.91	Renovasc Hypertension	4	0	5	0	0	0	16

Reprinted from Ref. 2.

ratio of hospital discharges for secondary hypertension to the total number of people with hypertension in the U.S. population, approximately 50 million, and gives us a figure of 0.08%. This means that probably only about 1 person with hypertension out of 1,190 is likely to have a *diagnosable* cause of the condition. The discharge rates, however, indicate much lower figures for adrenal disease. For example, discharges for Cushing's syndrome are reported as 1 out of 20,000 population, hyperaldosteronism as 1 in 50,000.

Of further interest are the figures for aortorenal bypass and total abdominal arterial endarterectomies performed in this country in 1987, 3000 each; such low numbers (less than 5000 cases) are considered statistically unreliable by the NCHS, and the total numbers of such procedures are not reported after 1987. No figures are presently available for angioplasty of the renal artery, because this is classified with multiple other vessel repair procedures including vein plications (ICD-9M 39.55), but the procedure has lost favor in the treatment of renal artery stenosis, particularly in the most common types where occlusion is near the site of origin of the renal arteries. It can be assumed that total procedures are well under 5000 per year.

If we are to accept these figures, indicating that probably 99.9% or more of people with hypertension do not require clinical testing, how do we decide which ones belong in the important subsets deserving further investigation? And having decided that a patient deserves study, which tests are indicated for screening? One should keep in mind that by far the more likely secondary cause of hypertension are renal parenchymal and renovascular disease, principally renal artery stenosis, and therefore

Table 6.8.4.   Clinical Features Suggestive of Secondary Hypertension

No family history of hypertension
Abrupt onset of hypertension rather than gradual (over the course of months or years)
Onset of hypertension before the age of 20 or after the age of 50
Sudden acceleration of previously existing hypertension or development of malignant hypertension *de novo*
Rapid deterioration of renal function despite well-controlled hypertension or following treatment with converting enzyme inhibitors
Unresponsiveness to standard antihypertensive therapy
Rapid development of hypokalemia with standard doses of diuretics
History of renal trauma, flank pain, and hematuria, suggesting renal infarction
Sudden onset of hypertension in a patient with systemic emboli or vasculitis
Development of hypertension in association with lower extremity ischemia, calf or buttock claudication, and erectile incompetence, abdominal angina, or aortic aneurysm
Nocturnal polyuria
Periodic paralysis or muscle weakness

Reprinted by permission from Saddler MC, Black HR. *The Yearbook of Nuclear Medicine*. Chicago: Mosby-Year Book, Inc. (1990:xiii–xxxiv).

appropriate imaging procedures for all intents are limited to the kidney. Adrenal imaging procedures should never be performed unless there is clinical followed by chemical evidence of adrenocortical or adrenomedullary hyperfunction. For example, one would never invoke the possible diagnoses of Cushing's syndrome, primary aldosteronism, or pheochromocytoma in the absence of confirmatory biochemical tests, and therefore CT, MRI, or radionuclide studies of the adrenal in this setting would be unjustified (vide infra).

Specific Studies for Renal and Renovascular Hypertension

Renal disease, either primary or secondary to hypertension itself, especially acute glomerulonephritis, pyelonephritis, polycystic disease, diabetic nephropathy, vasculitis, etc., usually can be recognized by the history and the presence of urinary and biochemical abnormalities, but clearly the issue of whether to image these patients has to be addressed. Because renovascular hypertension is a subset of renal disease, sui generis, and may have other surgically correctable causes (for example, obstructive urinary tract disease), one can argue convincingly that all such patients deserve to be studied by one or more imaging techniques.

Returning to the critical question, how do we decide which patients to study, Tables 6.8.4 and 6.8.5 are extremely helpful (6, 7). These important charts list in order of importance strong indicators which should make one suspect the possible presence of secondary (renovascular or adrenal) hypertension (Table 6.8.4) or, more specifically, atherosclerotic renal artery stenosis (Table 6.8.5). Without one or more of these indicators, it is doubtful the low pretest likelihood of any treatable causes would justify investigation of the patient with high blood pressure. This list should serve as a helpful guide, in addition to the presence of known renal disease, in deciding when to image the hypertensive patient.

One should take careful note of some of the most important clinical features suggesting secondary hypertension: (*a*) Abrupt onset of hypertension or (*b*) acceleration of known hypertension, (*c*) development of malignant hypertension; and (*d*) onset of

Table 6.8.5. Clinical Findings Suggestive of Atherosclerotic Renal Artery Stenosis

1. Resistant, severe or accelerated hypertension
2. Hypertension initially presenting in patients aged over 60 years
3. Previously well-controlled hypertension which has become difficult to control
4. Evidence of vascular disease elsewhere:
   a. Coronary artery disease
   b. Cerebral vascular disease
   c. Peripheral vascular disease
5. Presence of abdominal bruits, especially if systolic and diastolic
6. History of heavy cigarette smoking (>25 pack-years)
7. Caucasian race
8. Unexplained renal dysfunction in a patient with recent onset of hypertension

Reprinted by permission from (7).

hypertension before age 20 or after age 50. Other warning signs would include deterioration of renal function despite well-controlled hypertension, occurring especially with the use of angiotensin-converting enzyme (ACE) inhibitors such as Captopril (see below).

Specific Diagnostic Studies for Renal or Renovascular Hypertension
IVP

Having decided there is a significant pretest likelihood of treatable renal or renovascular causes of hypertension, what imaging procedure of procedures are indicated? The rapid-sequence hypertensive intravenous urogram or pyelogram (IVP) enjoys the respectability of long usage in the study of hypertension, but its present use for this purpose can no longer be justified. Aside from the clear-cut danger of contrast media in causing deterioration of renal function in subjects with already compromised kidneys, the IVP has been shown by numerous studies to be a poor predictor of disease. In one study, useful information that changed the course of management was found in only 1% of 952 hypertensive patients studied by IVP (8). Thornbury et al. (9) at the University of Michigan found a false-negative rate of almost 42% in patients undergoing pyelography who had renal artery stenosis subsequently proven by arteriogram. Even as a predictor of surgical outcome, the IVP is notoriously poor. In the Cooperative Study on Renovascular Hypertension (10), 83% of those whose blood pressure fell after renovascular surgery had an abnormal urogram, compared with 81% who failed to respond to surgery.

ULTRASONIC DUPLEX SCANNING OF THE KIDNEYS

This relatively new noninvasive technique which combines high resolution B-mode ultrasound imaging with a pulsed Doppler spectral analysis flow probe to detect flow velocity information from medium and large arteries has been tried for detection of renal artery stenosis. Although this technique ultimately may become a useful screening test for the condition, in its present state of development, its application is questionable. Technical problems concerned with imaging the renal arteries and with the interpretation of the source and form of flow patterns observed strongly suggest that this technique in the abdomen nowhere approaches its proven value in the peripheral vasculature.

RADIONUCLIDE RENAL IMAGING

The radionuclide angiogram and renal imaging study and conventional renogram using either 99m-Tc DTPA, "MAG-3," [131]I- or [123]-I-labeled Hippuran (O-Iodohippurate), or both, have been tried extensively for the detection of renovascular hypertension and for predicting outcome from revascularization procedures (11, 12). Though it is possible with radionuclide methods to determine renal morphology, differential bilateral renal function, individual renal blood flows, effective renal plasma flow, and glomerular filtration rate (GFR), confusing results are often obtained in patients with renal disease, obstruction, or low urinary flow rates. The sensitivity of the radioactive renogram for detecting functional renovascular lesions ranges from 79–85% and the specificity from 74–81% (13). Principally because of the low pretest probability even in the reported studies and the resulting large number of false-positive results, the positive predictive value of this test is lower, though certainly better than the IVP (14).

RADIONUCLIDE RENAL IMAGING WITH CAPTOPRIL

The search for an easy noninvasive test for renal vascular hypertension will continue, but for the present at least, the best single test appears to be standard renal scintigraphy combined with the administration of the drug Captopril.

Captopril, introduced in the late 1970s, belongs to a class of compounds known as ACE inhibitors, which also includes Enalapril and Lisinopril. Initially it was assumed these drugs reduced blood pressure only through inhibition of the renin-angiotensin-aldosterone system because they inhibited production of the powerful vasoconstrictor angiotensin II, which also stimulates the release of aldosterone, the salt- and water-retaining hormone. In actual fact, these drugs will reduce blood pressure in patients with low plasma renin levels, and it is becoming clear they also act through other mechanisms, in particular the bradykinin and prostaglandin systems (15, 16).

In the normal kidney, after the administration of ACE inhibitors, renal blood flow is preserved, or even increased, but in the kidney with fixed reduction of arterial perfusion because of functionally significant renal artery stenosis (FSRAS), the glomerular filtration rate usually decreases markedly because of efferent arteriolar dilatation. This is the reason these drugs should not be given therapeutically to patients with suspected uni- or bilateral RAS. *Renal failure coming on after treatment with these drugs calls for investigation for renovascular hypertension.*

The effect of ACE inhibitors on the kidney with FSRAS forms the basis for testing with Captopril. The effect of one 25–50 mg dose of the drug is to lower GFR and total peak activity and to prolong or even increase renal retention of radioactivity with time in the involved kidney. Different protocols have been tried, and various investigators have used DTPA, iodohippurate, or both, but the effect of Captopril has been consistent, and in a series of 50 patients in whom the prevalence of RAS was 46% by subsequent arteriography the test had a sensitivity of 91% and a specificity of 93% (7). The actual number of patients subsequently operated and the success rate is

PROBABILITY OF RENAL ARTERY STENOSIS
GIVEN A POSITIVE (PPV) OR NEGATIVE (1-NPV) CAPTOPRIL RENOGRAM

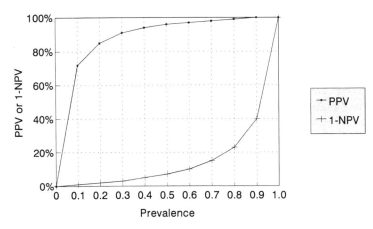

Sensitivity 0.93, Specificity 0.96 (18)

Figure 6.8.2. Probability of renal artery stenosis given a positive (PPV) or negative (1-NPV) captopril renogram.

not mentioned in the paper. Other workers have reported even higher values, a sensitivity of 93% and a specificity of 96% (17).

As we continue to emphasize, Captopril renal scintigraphy, like any other test or imaging procedure, is far from perfect, and its usefulness will depend on how and in what clinical setting it is performed. The principal value of the study is to *save patients with a high pretest probability of FSRAS from undergoing unnecessary renal arteriography.* A shocking statistic is revealed from the NCHS survey (2), which discloses that 28,000 renal arteriographies were performed in the United States in 1987, yet only about 6,000 diagnoses of renovascular hypertension were made, and less than 3,000 aortorenal bypasses performed. This is a devastating criticism of our diagnostic approach to renovascular disease. Clearly, for every patient diagnosed more than 5 patients are being subjected to needless arteriography. Furthermore, only 1 out of 10 patients subjected to the procedure ends up being a candidate for renal bypass surgery. Figure 6.8.2 shows the relationship between prevalence (pretest probability) of renal artery stenosis and the PPV and 1-NPV of a positive Captopril renal scintigraphy study.

RENAL ARTERIOGRAPHY

Renal arteriography, *if indeed indicated*, is optimally performed using the digital subtraction technique, preferably with intraarterial injection. The study, however, continues to be mistakenly regarded as the gold standard for the diagnosis of FSRAS. We profess no admiration for the late Hermann Goering of Hitler's Third Reich, but we are tempted to paraphrase him. When we hear the phrase "gold standard" we feel like reaching for our revolver.

No single test, of course, be it arteriography, endoscopy, CT, MRI, chest radiography, or even tissue biopsy, can be consistently relied upon for diagnosis. Each procedure has its limitations *based primarily on prevalence of disease in the population studied* and only secondarily on innate test sensitivity and specificity. In this sense, the concept of gold standards is falsifiable. This is equally true for the prosaic tests as well as more invasive and dangerous procedures, particularly when they are used in the wrong clinical settings.

Renal arteriography, for example, is indicated when surgery or angioplasty is contemplated for *what has already been determined with a high degree of confidence to be functionally significant renal arterial occlusive disease.* In this event, arteriography is merely used to delineate anatomically and confirm the presence of surgically-repairable vascular narrowing. Arteriography per se can never indicate with any reliability the *functional* significance of RAS, i.e. that a kidney is overproducing renin or is indeed the cause of hypertension. The number of failed endarterectomies, aortorenal bypasses, and renal angioplasties is ample evidence of this fact.

This is probably the principal reason some patients subsequently shown to have RAS do not have a positive Captopril radionuclide studies; the anatomical stenosis is not dynamically significant, i.e. not more than 70–80% in area. In Sadler and Black's series (7) of 50 patients, of 2 patients with false-positive results, 1 had a dysplastic right kidney, and the other patient was thought to have been dehydrated. Of 2 false-negative results, 1 patient had a branch RAS, and the other had only 50% stenoses of both kidneys with poststenotic dilatation.

In this series of patients suspected clinically of having FSRAS, with the final prevalence of disease a respectable 46%, a convincing case can be made for mandatory screening of all high probability RAS patients with Captopril renal scintigraphy before ever subjecting them to renal arteriography. At present, there is no reliable method for avoiding the study of patients with secondary hypertension due to nonvascular-related unilateral renal disease. However, by using Captopril scintigraphy it should be possible to save most patients the expense, discomfort, and danger of arteriography.

Summary of the Imaging Approach to Hypertension

1. Almost all patients presenting with high blood pressure have essential or primary hypertension and do not require diagnostic imaging.

2. Of the less than 0.1% (1 out of 1,000) of people with secondary hypertension, more than 90% of these will have some type of chronic renal disease, and most of the remaining will have renovascular disease. A very tiny number (probably less than 0.01% or 1 out of 10,000 of all people with hypertension) will have treatable RAS. Between 1 in 20,000 to 1 in 50,000 hypertensive patients will prove to have an adrenal cause such as Cushing's syndrome, primary hyperaldosteronism, or pheochromocytoma.

3. Imaging of the adrenals for hyperfunction, in particular for Cushing's syndrome, pheochromocytoma, and aldosteronism, should only be performed in the presence of biochemical evidence of endocrine dysfunction.

4. Patients who should undergo imaging would include those belonging to categories enumerated in Tables 6.8.4 and 6.8.5.

5. IVP and conventional radionuclide renography without Captopril have no place in the investigation of hypertensive patients or in the diagnosis of RAS.

6. Captopril radionuclide scintigraphy is now the best test for the detection of functional RAS.

7. Renal arteriography, or preferably digital subtraction angiography with intraarterial injection, is rarely, if ever, warranted in the patient with a negative Captopril study.

8. Even in patients with a positive renal arteriogram, a significant percentage will not have their hypertension relieved by corrective surgery.

REFERENCES

1. Schappert SM. National Ambulatory Medical Care Survey: 1989 Summary. Hyattsville, Md: National Center for Health Statistics. Vital Health Statistics 1992;131(110).

2. U.S. Department of Health and Human Services, U.S. Public Health Service, Centers for Disease Control, and the National Center for Health Statistics. National Hospital Discharge Survey (NHDS). Detailed diagnoses, procedures, days of care, diagnoses-related groups for patients discharged from short-stay hospitals. Public Use Data Diskettes, 1985–1990.

3. Kaplan NM. Clinical Hypertension. Baltimore: Williams & Wilkins, 1990:15–16.

4. U.S. Department of Health and Human Services. Health United States, 1989:170.

5. Kaplan NM. Clinical Hypertension. Baltimore: Williams & Wilkins, 1990:18.

6. Baxter JD, Perloff D, Hsueh W, Biglieri EG. In: The endocrinology of hypertension. Felig P, Baxter JD, Broadus AE, Frohman LA, eds. Endocrinology and Metabolism. 2nd ed. New York: McGraw-Hill Book Company, 1987:733.

7. Saddler MC, Black HR. Captopril renal scintigraphy: a clinician's perspective. In: The Yearbook of Nuclear Medicine, 1990. Chicago: Year Book Medical Publishers, Inc., 1990:xiii–xxxiv.

8. Atkinson AB, Kellet RJ. Value of intravenous urography in investigating hypertension. J R Coll Physicians Lond 1974;8(2):175–181.

9. Thornbury JR, Stanley JC, Fryback DG. Hypertensive urogram: a non-discriminatory test for renovascular hypertension. AJR 1982;138(1):43–49.

10. Bookstein JJ, Maxwell MH, Abram HL, Buenger RE, Lecky J, Franklin SS, et al. Cooperative study of radiologic aspects of renovascular hypertension-bilateral renovascular disease. JAMA 1977;237(16):1706–1709.

11. Burbank MK, Hunt JC, Tauxe WN, Maher FT. Radioisotopic renography: diagnosis of renal arterial disease in hypertensive patients. Circulation 1963;27:328–338.

12. Chervu LR, Blaufox MD. Renal radiopharmaceuticals—an update. Semin Nucl Med 1982;12(3):224–245.

13. Shovlin M. Radionuclide screening for renovascular hypertension. J Nucl Med 1980;21(1):104–106.

14. DeGrazia JA, Scheibe PO, Jackson PE, et al. Clinical applications of a kinetic model of hippurate distribution and renal clearance. J Nucl Med 1974;15(2):102–141.

15. Millar JA, Johnston CT. Sequential changes in circulating levels of angiotensin I and II, renin and bradykinin after captopril. Med J Aust 1979;2:R15–R17.

16. Zusman RM. Renin- and non-renin-mediated antihypertensive actions of converting enzyme inhibitors. Kidney Int 1984;25(6):969–983.

17. Fommii E, Ghione S, Bertelli P, et al. Renal scintigraphy captopril test: comparison of scintigraphic and angiographic data and preliminary observations in chronic glomerulonephritis [Abstract]. J Nucl Med 1988;29:907.

9/ Cough and Hemoptysis

> *A custome lothesome to the Eye, hatefull to the Nose, harmfull to the Brain, dangerous to the Lungs, and in the black stinking fume thereof, nearest resembling the horrible, stigian smoke of the pit that is bottomlesse.*
>
> *King James I (England)*
> *1604, on the use of tobacco*

Cough

An indication of the importance of the symptom *cough* can be appreciated from the following statistics: Cough, exclusive of head colds and upper respiratory symptoms was the most common *symptom* resulting in office visits to ambulatory care physicians, amounting for about 25 million out of 692.7 million such visits in 1989. (The first 5 nonsymptomatic reasons were general medical, physical, gynecological, prenatal, and well baby examinations). Almost 10% of the first most common diagnoses out of a total of 417.5 million office visits were for symptoms referable to the respiratory system (1, 2).

Although diagnostic data merely allow us to *infer* a relationship to a cardinal symptom, the exercise is most useful in helping us answer the question: Given a patient complaining of cough, what is the likelihood of a serious condition? The

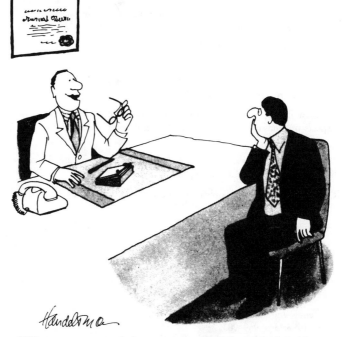

"What we propose to do is remove your head, have a look inside your neck, and then close you up again. It is a brand new technique and it would be less than candid of me to pretend that it does not involve certain dangers. The question is: How badly do you want to get rid of that cough?"

Table 6.9.1. All-Listed, Clinically Significant Respiratory Diseases, Discharges in Thousands, U.S. Hospitals, 1990 (3)

All-listed ICD-9-CM	Total	Male	Female	Age <15	Age 15–44	Age 45–64	Age 65 +
162. Mal neo trachea/lung	442	276	166	0	15	174	253
465. AC URI mult sites/NOS	180	83	97	83	42	22	33
466. AC bronchitis/bronchiol	503	244	259	156	54	82	210
473. Chronic sinusitis	157	75	81	22	55	46	34
474. Chr T & A dis	189	88	102	134	51	0	0
478. Oth uppr respiratory dis	116	63	53	20	48	26	22
482. Oth bacterial pneumonia	287	164	123	14	32	46	194
486. Pneumonia, organism NOS	1022	526	496	188	130	148	555
490. Bronchitis NOS	125	51	74	22	34	18	51
491. Chronic bronchitis	293	146	147	0	22	89	177
492. Emphysema	234	136	98	0	7	64	162
493. Asthma	835	337	498	240	217	172	206
496. Chr airway obstruct nec	1356	781	575	0	28	334	990
507. Solid/liq pneumonitis	136	71	65	7	13	18	99
511. Pleurisy	483	235	249	9	47	101	326
515. Postinflam pulm fibrosis	127	61	67	0	12	22	92
518. Other lung diseases	915	456	460	63	103	215	534

RESPIRATORY TRACT DIAGNOSES
ALL LISTED DATA, NHDS 1990 (3)

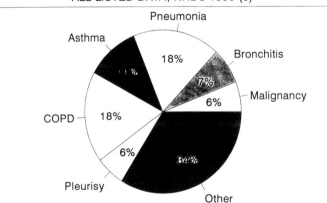

Figure 6.9.1. Respiratory tract diagnoses, all-listed data, NHDS, 1990 (3).

prevalence of clinically significant respiratory tract diseases, that is, serious enough to require hospitalization, can be determined from NCHS statistics. Table 6.9.1 shows the 17 most common respiratory conditions given as all-listed hospital discharge diagnoses in 1990 (3). Figure 6.9.1 shows that more than two-thirds of all these conditions can be accounted for by seven diagnoses, with chronic airway obstructive disease, asthma, and the pneumonias contributing half the total. Figure 6.9.2 normalizes these seven diagnoses for a comparison of their relative frequency to each other. To simplify the presentation we have not tabulated 21 other ICD codes, all accounting for less than 70,000 discharges or 1% of total respiratory disease discharge diagnoses. The pneumonias are grouped together, but Pneumocystis (ICD 136.3) is omitted (4).

Although these figures focus only on primary diseases of the respiratory tract, a multitude of systemic conditions may involve the respiratory system secondarily. An

PRINCIPAL RESPIRATORY TRACT DIAGNOSES
ALL LISTED DATA, NHDS 1990 (3)

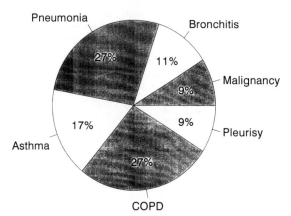

Figure 6.9.2.   Principal respiratory tract diagnoses, all-listed data, NHDS, 1990 (3).

unknown percentage of these conditions may result in cough symptoms. Moreover, other much more common entities such as chest wall, rib, and spinal conditions, especially trauma, along with pulmonary embolism and heart failure, are important causes of cough. For example, in 1990 the number of all-listed discharge diagnoses for congestive heart failure was more than 2.0 million, higher than any category of primary lung conditions. We cannot begin to estimate how many such patients complained primarily of cough. (Pulmonary embolism accounted for only an additional 116,000 cases despite the claim that this condition is reported to have caused 200,000 deaths in the United States in 1974 (5).)

In the case of cough, it is difficult if not impossible to calculate the percentage of office visits resulting in hospitalization, not only because of unknown ratios of revisits to rehospitalizations, but also because of multiple additional etiologies of the symptom not even considered in the above statistics. For example, among important additional causes of acute cough would be aspiration of foreign bodies (primarily in children) and exposure to irritating agents and noxious gases.

Cough that does not clear up in 2–4 weeks or recurs periodically every 6–12 months is considered chronic, the most common cause of which is chronic bronchitis due to cigarette smoking. Smokers, obviously, have the highest risk for most respiratory problems, including neoplasm. In nonsmokers, unquestionably the most common causes of chronic cough are postnasal drip, asthma, obstructive airways disease, bronchitis, heart failure, and psychogenic cough, followed by pneumoconioses and, in children, cystic fibrosis (6).

It is safe to assume that only a small percentage out of all patients presenting with cough will have a condition ultimately requiring hospitalization. For example, even though 6% of the total 7.4 million diagnoses for lung disease are for malignant neoplasms of the trachea and lung (447,00 cases), less than 170,000 of these diagnoses or 2.4% represent new cases. Note the overwhelming number over age 44 in Figure 6.9.3 (7).

The reason for this statistical flight, as usual, is to explore the most probable causes of cough and reach some generalizations about a reasonable diagnostic ap-

Respiratory Tract Malignancies by Age
Hospital Discharges in Thousands
1990 NHDS Data (3)

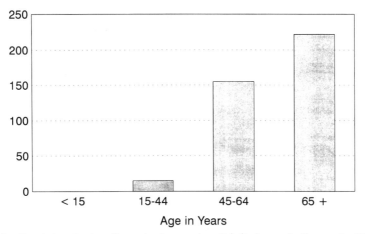

Figure 6.9.3.   Respiratory tract malignancies by age, hospital discharges in thousands, 1990, NHDS Data (3).

proach to this cardinal symptom. Regardless of the pathophysiological explanations of cough, the ineluctable facts of disease prevalence remain the clinician's only reliable guide.

If we accept that the overwhelming number of patients with cough do not require investigation, in those patients who do, what are the best techniques for determining the etiology of the complaint? Beyond the clinical examination of the expectorate, there is, of course, the laboratory study of the sputum for bacterial, viral, mycological, cytological, and chemical offenders. If we were to choose one test, above all others, this would be the most important one. The posteroanterior and left lateral chest radiograph would be the single most important imaging procedure. It is quick, inexpensive, without hazard, and universally available. What is there left after the chest X-ray? MRI, CT, bronchoscopy, bronchography, gallium scintigraphy, lung scintigraphy?

The answer is, further studies rarely need to be done after the chest radiograph except for appropriate follow-up X-rays, because the overwhelming majority of patients with clinically significant new cough will have pneumonia, bronchitis, or some other form of acute infectious disease of the respiratory tract. In those patients with old or chronic cough, particularly smokers, failure to obtain chest X-rays would be difficult to justify under any circumstances.

A note of caution is necessary, however. It is often unappreciated that *a negative chest radiograph does not rule out a pneumonia or cancer any more than a negative bone radiograph excludes fracture*. In a study of 5000 chest radiographs ordered from emergency rooms, only 25% of those suspected of having pneumonia were abnormal (8). Furthermore, *the majority of lung cancers are missed on the plain chest X-ray until their sizes are appreciable, usually larger than 1.0 cm*. The reasons are limitation in resolution of the plain radiograph and the fact that most cancers are in the central lung fields and obscured by hilar markings. Nor does the negative film exclude bronchitis or bronchiolitis. Whether a pneumonitis is visible depends very much on the timing of the radiograph, the extent of disease, and other variables. In plain radiography *as in all imaging and other testing procedures*, we have the problem of the ROC curve. That is, we are stuck with the sensitivity and specificity of the test in a specific clinical setting. Both these measurements of test performance depend, as always, on the skill and temperament of the interpreter—specifically, is he or she an "under-" or an "over-reader"?

The unavoidable consequences of this fact already have been alluded to in Chapter 2. Reading too little into a film will obviously result in an excess of missed or false-negative diagnoses; reading too much, a preponderance of phantom or false-positive diagnoses, the "wild goose chase effect." Although it is arguable, we have observed that because in most clinical settings a benign condition is much more likely than a serious one, more harm is likely to be caused by invoking a diagnosis than in missing one.

To restate: *if pneumonitis or antibiotic-sensitive infection is suspected clinically, obtain the sputum specimen and treat despite the presence of a negative chest radiograph.*

Pneumonia may present with symptoms but without X-ray findings or, conversely, may be seen radiographically in the *absence* of significant symptoms or signs. Anecdotally, we have seen several patients with pulmonary infiltrates discovered incidentally who presented with symptoms of an upper respiratory infection, but without cough, sputum, or other lower tract symptoms. No doubt most of these patients had some type of viral pneumonia. This suggests that the division of respiratory tract viruses into those of either the upper or the lower tract may occasionally be inexact or arbitrary. Moreover, it is known that infectious agents other than those typically afflicting the respiratory tract may at times result in asymptomatic pulmonary infiltrates, for example certain GI or generalized viral infections.

The diagnostic approach to patients with findings other than a pulmonary infiltrate or benign abnormalities such as increased vascular or peribronchiolar markings is discussed in Chapter 8. Specifically addressed are further diagnostic approaches to be taken in the presence of various types of intrathoracic masses.

Hemoptysis

Conventional wisdom once held that hemoptysis, the production of frankly bloody or blood-tinged sputum, justified an immediate call to the bronchoscopist. This reflexive response reflected classic teaching that assumed neoplasms of the respiratory tract were among the most common causes of this symptom. Nothing could be further from the truth, of course. If every patient under age 45 with hemoptysis and without a lung mass were to be bronchoscoped, the yield of cancer diagnoses would be virtually zero and the false-positive rate intolerable. Certainly, the extremely low pretest likelihood of disease would result in a horrendously low positive predictive index for bronchoscopy. We must now ask the same fundamental clinical question as we do for all signs and symptoms: Given hemoptysis, what are the most important causes?

Here again, without the requisite epidemiological data, we are compelled to examine hospital discharges. This is revealing at least in terms of respiratory tract malignancies. Out of 442,000 all-listed diagnoses for malignancies of the trachea and lung in 1990, less than 4% of all cases were in patients under 45 years of age. What are the most common causes of hemoptysis in the general medical population? Unquestionably, new hemoptysis is most often secondary to the acute onset of viral or bacterial infections of the respiratory tract, specifically acute pharyngitis, laryngitis, tracheobronchitis, pleurisy, or pneumonia. Less common but still important causes include, as with cough, inhalation of noxious agents, pulmonary edema, pulmonary embolism, rheumatic heart disease with mitral stenosis, and, especially in children, aspiration of foreign bodies. The importance of the chest X-ray in the investigation of this symptom is underlined by an important study which found that among presenting pulmonary symptoms hemoptysis was one of the complaints associated with the highest number of abnormal radiographs (42–79%), the others being cardiovascular symptoms including failure, dysrhythmia, and hypertension (8).

When is fiberoptic bronchoscopy indicated in the patient with hemoptysis? This question, still an important subject of debate, was addressed by an excellent study of 196 patients with hemoptysis and normal or nonlocalizing chest radiographs referred for bronchoscopy (9). Significantly, three-quarters of the patients were active or previous smokers. The authors examined the relationship of age, sex, smoking, nonspecific roentenographic findings, and amount, duration, and previous bouts of hemoptysis to bronchoscopic findings. They found that 12 patients (6%) had bronchogenic cancer, and in another 33 (17%) a specific cause of bleeding was found. Thus, in only 23% was a cause identified. Not unexpectedly they found that 3 factors, age over 50, male sex, and smoking history of more than 40 pack years, were the best predictors of cancer. Two of these factors together with bleeding of more than 30 ml daily raised the predictability of cancer to 100%. They concluded that use of these criteria could reduce their use of fiberoptic bronchoscopy by 28%. In another study of 48 patients with hemoptysis and a normal chest radiograph, fiberoptic bronchoscopy provided a diagnosis other than endobronchial inflammation in only 4 cases, one a benign polyp, another with tuberculosis, and 2 with carcinoma (10). Again, risk factors were age, significant smoking history, and duration of hemoptysis longer than 1 week. The authors concluded weakly that routine fiberoptic bronchoscopy "may not always be indicated" in patients with hemoptysis and a normal chest X-ray.

Another study examined the use of CT in hemoptysis and concluded that its use other than in selected patients with radiographic abnormalities was generally of very little use (11). This must be strongly questioned, however. In older patients with hemoptysis, particularly smokers, the chest radiograph, as mentioned, is highly unreliable in excluding a small mass lesion. In all such patients with negative chest X-rays, CT scanning should be performed first, *not bronchoscopy*. Further diagnostic approaches to lung masses are discussed in Chapter 8.

Summary of the Diagnostic Approach to Cough and Hemoptysis

1. The PA and left lateral chest radiograph with appropriate follow-up films remains the single most important imaging procedure for diagnosing the principal causes of cough and major hemoptysis.

2. A negative chest X-ray does not exclude pneumonia.

3. CT, MRI, gallium, and pulmonary perfusion and ventilation scintigraphy and other indirect imaging procedures are almost never indicated for a principal complaint of cough or hemoptysis with the following exceptions:

(*a*) Patients with AIDS or HIV-positive individuals with constitutional symptoms who should always have gallium scintigraphy whether or not the chest radiograph is normal; and

(*b*) Patients with specific clinical indications of pulmonary embolism (lung scintigraphy) or those with radiographic findings of a mass lesion (CT).

4. Do not suspect respiratory cancer in a patient under age 45 without a smoking history. The vast majority of patients with minor hemoptysis have acute endobronchial causes, usually an acute infectious condition of the respiratory system, and should not be subjected to further study.

5. Any patient with a negative chest X-ray who is a tumor suspect, i.e. patients with hemoptysis over 45 years of age with or without a significant smoking history, should first have lung CT.

6. Fiberoptic bronchoscopy is indicated after radiography only in patients with significant hemoptysis (more than 15 ml per day, lasting more than 1 week, or unexplained recurrent hemoptysis) with negative or nonlocalizing chest radiographs or if there is suspicion of foreign body aspiration, particularly in infants and children.

7. Bronchoscopy is otherwise indicated only after CT and only if:

a. CT is negative; or
b. CT is positive for a lesion within reach of the bronchoscope, i.e. in a major bronchus (reasonably close to the hilum) (vide infra).

As a general rule, fiberoptic bronchoscopy is not a "routine" procedure and should not be performed for hemoptysis in patients under age 45 without strong clinical suspicion of significant endobronchial disease or foreign body aspiration.

REFERENCES

1. Schappert SM. National Ambulatory Medical Care Survey: 1989 Summary. Hyattsville, Md: National Center for Health Statistics. Vital Health Statistics, 1992:131(110).
2. A reason for visit classification for ambulatory care (RVC). Vital and Health Statistics, Feb. 1979; series 2, No. 78.
3. U.S. Department of Health and Human Services, U.S. Public Health Service, Centers for Disease Control, and the National Center for Health Statistics. National Hospital Discharge Survey (NHDS). Detailed diagnoses, procedures, days of care, diagnoses-related groups for patients discharged from short-stay hospitals. Public Use Data Diskettes, 1985–1990.
4. ICD-9-CM. International Classification of Diseases. 9th revision, 3rd ed. Clinical Modification. Volumes 1, 2, and 3. Los Angeles: Practice Management Information Corporation (PMI), 1989. (U.S. Department of Health and Human Services Publication PHS 89-1260).
5. Dalen JE, Alpert JS. Natural history of pulmonary embolism. Prog Cardiovasc Dis 1975;17(4):257–270.
6. Wartak J, Sproule BJ, King EG. Differentiating causes of cough: an algorithmic approach. J Respir Dis 1989;10(2):77–94.
7. Cancer Facts & Figures. American Cancer Society, 1988.
8. Buenger RE. Five thousand acute care/emergency department chest radiographs: comparison of requisitions with radiographic findings. J Emerg Med 1988;3(6):197–202.
9. Poe RH, Israel RH, Marin MG, et al. Utility of fiberoptic bronchoscopy in patients with hemoptysis and a nonlocalizing chest roentgenogram. Chest 1988;93(1):70–75.
10. Jackson CV, Savage PJ, Quinn DL. Role of fiberoptic bronchoscopy in patients with hemoptysis and a normal chest roentgenogram. Chest 1985;87(2):142–144.
11. Haponik EF, Britt EJ, Smith PL, Bleecker ER. Computed chest tomography in the evaluation of hemoptysis. Impact on diagnosis and treatment. Chest 1987;91(1):80–85.

10/ Dyspnea: Cardiac or Pulmonary?

*Sophie Tucker, the vaudevillian, torch singer, and one of the origi-
nal "red hot mammas," was once asked the secret of her longevity. She
replied without hesitation, "Just keep breathin', honey."*

Dyspnea: General Remarks

Dyspnea remains difficult to define, but like good and evil, everyone knows what it
is. The most serviceable definition is unpleasant, uncomfortable, or difficult breathing. Dyspnea, however, should not be confused with *tachypnea*, rapid breathing, or
hyperpnea increased ventilation in excess of physiological needs. We need not delve
here into the complicated physiological nature of dyspnea, especially the difference
between breathlessness of healthy subjects and that of sick patients, e.g. whether the
sensations of a person after swimming a mile are similar to those of a patient experiencing asthma or heart failure (apparently they are not). Rather, it is sufficient to
acknowledge pathological breathlessness as a cardinal disease symptom but, as with
nausea, vomiting, and fever, one of frequently nonspecific nature.

For example, dyspnea that occurs so frequently in heart conditions as a subsidiary
or secondary symptom can invite comparisons with nausea and vomiting, which are
so regular an accompaniment of intraabdominal disease. Yet, true dyspnea per se is
an extremely reliable symptom of organ-specific dysfunction, in particular of the
lung.

The reader may well ask what purpose is served by these observations. First, our
intent has been to define individual signs and symptoms as precisely as possible in
order to explore their implications for medical diagnosis. Only then is it possible to
conceptualize useful approaches for diagnostic imaging, given a specific presentation.
Unless signs and symptoms are regarded as the engine which drives diagnosis, the
term "clinical medicine" becomes an oxymoron, and the physician assumes the passive role of a mindless test orderer. One must be constantly aware that imaging and
other diagnostic procedures may or may not be indicated in a particular setting. On
balance, our present zeal for ordering testing procedures far exceeds their frequency
of appropriateness.

What pathological conditions are suggested by the patient with dyspnea? First and
foremost, of course, are acute and chronic disorders of the lung, probably the most
common cause of difficult breathing. The second most important category is heart
disease. We emphasize, however, that dyspnea occurs predominantly in cardiac diseases associated with pulmonary congestion. Prime examples would be left ventricular failure due to hypertensive or coronary artery disease, mitral stenosis, and other
conditions causing elevated pressure in the left atrium and therefore throughout the
pulmonary vascular bed. Very often these pressures are not elevated at rest, but appear only during exercise. Other physiological factors are at work in heart failure,
among which are changes in air flow resistance, decreased lung compliance, and secondary changes in the lung parenchyma and pulmonary vasculature. These need not
concern us here except insofar as they have implications for distinguishing between
pulmonary and cardiac causes of dyspnea.

Three other important etiologies of dyspnea deserve mention: Psychogenic, hematological (anemia), and neurological. The most important is dyspnea of psychological origin in which individuals fail to display any objective changes to account for their complaint. These patients usually have a grossly irregular pattern of breathing, often presenting with a history of frequent sighing at rest or after exertion. They often describe tightness or constriction in the chest, a "smothering" sensation, or being unable "to take in a deep breath." Not surprisingly, this is often accompanied by classic hyperventilation syndrome with clear-cut attacks of rapid breathing associated with dizziness, faintness, collapse, and circumoral and distal extremity paresthesias. Many of these patients are reminiscent of those previously discussed with bizarre forms of nonanginal chest pain. Thus, dyspnea and nonspecific thoracic pain may present as a sort of "crossover" syndrome. This broad category is mentioned again, not only because of its frequent occurrence, but because it should be easily recognized from the clinical history. There is never a justification for performing laboratory or imaging studies on such patients.

Dyspnea associated with the anemias, though its mechanism is poorly understood, should likewise be easily suspected on the basis of clinical and hematological finding.

Finally, disordered breathing, changes in respiratory pattern (apnea, Cheyne-Stokes, and Biot's respiration), and dyspnea are commonly found in a wide variety of neurological and neuromuscular conditions. Here, dyspnea becomes a secondary or incidental symptom, and as such it should be clearly recognized. The effects of neurological disease on breathing depend on the anatomical distribution of the abnormality rather than on a specific disease. Thus, various lesions of the cortex and forebrain, midbrain, pons, medulla, spinal cord, peripheral nerves, and respiratory muscles all may produce dyspnea and other breathing disturbances. The diagnostic approach to these patients rests first and foremost on clinically identifying the cause as neurological. If this is done, the investigation becomes appropriately focused. One of the major mistakes in deciding what imaging tests to employ, a problem already alluded to, is the tendency to invoke causes or diagnoses that are inconsistent with the clinical presentation. In a patient with hyperventilation and rapid changes in level of consciousness and neurological status, the alert clinician would be more inclined to look for a brain lesion in the upper pons than search for an associated pulmonary or cardiac problem.

Pulmonary Dyspnea

The most prevalent types of respiratory problems causing dyspnea are *pulmonary restriction* associated with fibrosing conditions, alveolitis, and infiltrations, and *obstructive disorders*, the result of retained secretions, chronic bronchitis, emphysema, or airways obstruction, particularly asthma. In young patients, of course, acute pneumothorax is common. Because lung conditions causing the symptom of dyspnea do so by disturbing pulmonary function, it is obvious that, aside from clinical assessment and the chest radiograph, pulmonary function testing remains the primary diagnostic modality.

There is a place for gallium scintigraphy in searching for a possible etiological category in the subset of patients with pulmonary functional abnormalities in whom clinical and radiographic findings are normal or nonspecific. This group with negative radiographs consists of a significant percentage of patients with unsuspected pulmonary fibrosis and/or interstitial pneumonitis secondary to chemo- or radiotherapy, or a wide variety of organisms, one of the most important of which is *Pneumocystis carinii* in patients with AIDS.

Other important conditions which may or may not be demonstrable on chest X-ray include pneumonia, sarcoidosis, mediastinal adenopathy causing obstructive symptoms, lymphangitic lung metastases, atelectasis, and a variety of other conditions. We stress that gallium uptake in the lung and/or mediastinum is, strictly speaking, nonspecific, but in practical terms this finding is invaluable in narrowing the set of diagnostic possibilities or in excluding certain conditions.

Pulmonary embolism (PE), previously discussed, is another important cause of dyspnea, but in its various clinical presentations it defies easy categorization by signs or symptoms. That is, PE shares too many important clinical features with other major cardiopulmonary disorders, e.g. symptoms such as dyspnea, tachypnea, tachycardia, cough, cyanosis, hemoptysis, collapse, etc. Given *only* dyspnea, one would have to ask when is it appropriate to perform lung perfusion and ventilation scintigraphy. The answer to this question clearly relates to the presence of other clinical elements. Thus, the suspicion of pulmonary embolism rests not so much on complaints or findings as it does on predisposing factors already discussed, namely, factors indicating a high-risk patient, for example, hospitalized and postoperative patients, the elderly, cardiac patients, those with phlebitis, lower extremity fracture, or other trauma, etc. In the postoperative patient with sudden unexplained dyspnea, it is obvious that pulmonary ventilation/perfusion scintigraphy is usually mandatory. In general, however, retained secretions, easily demonstrated on ventilation scintigraphy using the aerosol technique, are found much more often in these patients than PE. This is particularly true in coronary bypass patients who develop sudden dyspnea in the early postoperative period.

Cardiac Dyspnea and Congestive Heart Failure

The patient, a successful musician, morbidly obese all his life but previously well, was 60 years of age and 330 pounds when he had a severe heart attack from which he apparently recovered. Put on a 450-calorie liquid diet, he lost 70 but then regained 30 pounds. In the ensuing year he struggled with his weight sporadically but was convinced he had regained permanent health when his physician repeatedly announced with pride that "we got all the tests back to normal": cardiogram, blood sugar, cholesterol (down to 120), etc. This shared obsession with his tests continued during a period of sudden weight gain, development of edema, dyspnea, and persistent "exhaustion." The patient, with the encouragement of his physician, continued to have bimonthly liver profiles, cholesterol, blood sugars, and resting ECGs, but when his symptoms worsened despite the normal tests he was sent to a psychiatrist for "depression." After 1 week of psychotherapy, he called me, an old high school friend living 1500 miles away, who immediately referred him to a cardiologist for treatment of worsening edema, orthopnea, and weight gain. His congestive heart failure in the presence of "normal" tests responded promptly to treatment.

Moral 1: Normal cholesterol, blood sugar, and ECG do not exclude heart failure any better than a negative MRI rules out meningitis.

Moral 2: Sometimes a normal test is worse than no test at all.

Nowhere in medicine is clinical skill more essential than in assessment of the cardiac patient, particularly in differentiating pulmonary from cardiac causes of dyspnea. It is axiomatic in cardiology that the diagnosis of congestive heart failure is almost

Table 6.10.1. Conditions Involving Increased Resistance to Filling of One or Both Ventricles (Diastolic Heart Failure) (Adapted from Grossman; 93)

1. Mitral or tricuspid stenosis
2. Constrictive pericarditis
3. Cardiomyopathies
4. Ischemic heart disease
5. Hypertrophic heart disease (chronic hypertension, hypertrophic cardiomyopathy, aortic stenosis)
6. Volume overload (mitral or aortic regurgitation, AV-fistula, etc.

always made or suspected on clinical findings. The only exceptions are in those patients who can be diagnosed on chest X-ray before clinical findings have occurred or in patients with early or mild diastolic dysfunction detectable by radionuclide techniques. If the radiologist uses the subtle radiographic signs of left ventricular failure as enumerated by Logue et al. in a long-forgotten paper (1), a large number of patients will be diagnosed on the plain chest X-ray. An important study of 113 patients with proven myocardial infarction showed radiographic evidence of pulmonary edema in one-third. In 38% of these patients *radiographic evidence preceded clinical onset of cardiac failure* (2). Yet perhaps with no other condition have we seen such an unprecedented growth in testing, a grossly misplaced reliance on technology as a substitute for the clinical history and examination.

We refer especially to the misplaced reliance on the left ventricular *systolic* ejection fraction (EF) as determined by radionuclide ventriculography (multigated acquisition, the so-called MUGA) study as an indicator of heart failure. Part of the difficulty is semantic, because we tend to use the terms "heart failure" and "congestive heart failure" interchangeably. The adjective *congestive* refers to manifestations such as distended neck veins, peripheral edema, dyspnea, and orthopnea, which almost invariably indicate *elevated right or left ventricular filling pressures*. Such pressures may result from primary systolic failure, with passive backup of blood into the pulmonary and systemic venous beds, or from diastolic dysfunction, with increased *resistance* to filling of one or both ventricles (3). Thus, although there is some degree of diastolic dysfunction in most patients who present clinically with heart failure, as many as 40% of patients with heart failure do not have *congestion* but rather *normal systolic function* and thus *normal left ventricular systolic EFs* (4). These patients have one of many conditions associated with primary diastolic heart failure associated with virtually any form of heart disease. A partial list of these conditions is displayed in Table 6.10.1. Therefore, though patients with abnormal left ventricular EFs at rest (less than 50%) are suffering from left ventricular decompensation, we *cannot* assume that a *normal* left ventricular EF *excludes* heart failure. An unknown number of such patients with diastolic dysfunction and normal systolic EFs would in fact complain of dyspnea either at rest or on exertion.

Certain parameters of diastolic function such as peak filling rate and time to peak filling rate can be obtained with the gated radionuclide study, and often give a clue to the presence of unsuspected diastolic dysfunction in the presence of a normal systolic EF. These noninvasive special computer techniques can be used in any nuclear medicine department equipped with suitable software. Such methods have proved extremely useful in assessing diastolic function in hypertrophic and anthracycline-induced cardiomyopathies, hypertension, and coronary artery disease. A good example of these techniques is illustrated in Figure 6.10.1 showing a prolonged time to

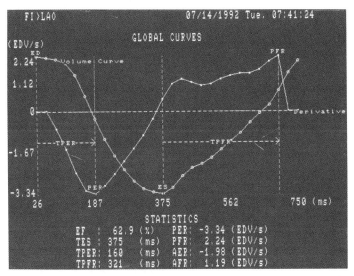

Figure 6.10.1. Various computer-derived physiological parameters of a ventricular volume curve in a patient with normal systolic function and abnormal diastolic function.

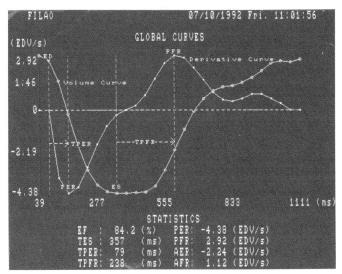

Figure 6.10.2. Another example of diastolic dysfunction in the presence of a normal systolic ejection function (EF = 84%).

peak filling rate (TPFR) of 321 msec (normal <180 msec) and a reduced PFR of 2.24 end diastolic volumes/sec (EDV/sec) (normal >2.5 EDV/sec). Note this patient had a systolic EF of almost 63%. The cause of diastolic dysfunction was thought to be moderately severe hypertension. In Figure 6.10.2 a subject on adriamycin therapy was found to have diastolic dysfunction with a prolonged TPFR in the presence of a systolic EF of 84%. The subject has been well summarized in a thorough review by Clements and the Mayo group (5) and by Soufer and Day (6).

Braunwald (7) has thoroughly summarized the relevant physiology in his classic textbook. In heart failure dilatation and hypertrophy are the principal compensatory mechanisms to an increased load. Thus, hypertrophy may have "the adverse effect of slowing relaxation and increasing the stiffness . . . of the ventricle. While these two aspects of cardiac function, e.g., relaxation and diastolic stiffness, are often considered together, they actually describe different properties of the heart."

Summary of Dyspnea

1. The principal etiological categories of dyspnea in order of importance are first pulmonary, followed by cardiac, psychogenic, anemic, and neurological.

2. Clinical assessment of the patient should enable the physician quickly to identify or exclude any one of the last three causes, in particular psychogenic. In these settings, investigation of dyspnea per se is not indicated.

3. Most remaining patients with dyspnea will have a pulmonary cause or suffer from heart failure. The important distinction between a pulmonary vs. a cardiac etiology of dyspnea again rests primarily on clinical history and physical examination of the patient, which should suffice in most cases.

4. The only routine studies indicated in pulmonary dyspnea are the posteroanterior (PA) and lateral chest radiograph and pulmonary function testing.

5. In patients with pulmonary dyspnea in whom clinical findings and chest radiography are equivocal or nondiagnostic, gallium scintigraphy has an important place in the diagnosis of unsuspected hilar disease and subradiographic interstitial fibrosis or pneumonia. This is of particular importance in Pneumocystis disease in patients with AIDS.

6. In patients with unexplained dyspnea with or without other symptoms, and at high risk for PE, pulmonary ventilation and perfusion imaging are always indicated. Most of these patients, especially the postoperative ones, will prove to have abnormalities of ventilation rather than PE.

7. The most helpful routine imaging study in suspected cardiac dyspnea is the PA and lateral chest radiograph, which may indicate the likelihood of subclinical heart failure. In most cases, however, *congestive* heart failure is a clinical diagnosis.

8. Radionuclide ventriculography or MUGA is an invaluable test in cardiac disease, whether or not heart failure is present. This study is unsurpassed in defining and following the course of chamber enlargement, right and left ventricular function, and wall motion abnormalities, among other parameters. In difficult cases, the MUGA study can be useful in determining the presence or absence of diastolic dysfunction in the presence of normal systolic function. Combined systolic and diastolic dysfunction are usually both present in *congestive* heart failure.

9. A normal systolic EF does not exclude heart failure per se, (without congestion), however, because up to 40% of such patients will have only diastolic dysfunction and normal systolic ejection fractions.

REFERENCES

1. Loge RB, Rogers Jr JV, Gray BBH. Subtle roentgenographic signs of left heart failure. Am Heart J 1963;65:464.
2. Harrison MO, Conte PJ, Heitzman ER. Radiological detection of clinically occult cardiac failure following myocardial infarction. Br J Radiol 1971;44(520):265–272.
3. Grossman W. Diastolic dysfunction in congestive heart failure. N Engl J Med 1991;325(22):1557–1564.
4. Soufer R, Wohlgelernter D, Vita NA, et al. Intact systolic left ventricular function in clinical congestive heart failure. Am J Cardiol 1985;55(8):1032–1036.
5. Clements IP, Sinak LJ, Gibbons RJ, Brown ML, O'Connor MK. Determination of diastolic function by radionuclide ventriculography. Mayo Clin Proc 1990;65(7):1007–1019.

6. Soufer R, Dey H. The radionuclide assessment of left ventricular diastolic filling: methodology and clinical significance. Echocardiography 1992;9(3):339–347.
7. Braunwald E. Heart Disease: A Textbook of Cardiovascular Medicine. 3rd ed. Philadelphia: W.B. Saunders 1988:434.

11/ Jaundice

> *The whole world looks yellow to the jaundiced eye.*
> *William Shakespeare*
> *The field cannot well be seen from within the field.*
> *Ralph Waldo Emerson*

General Discussion

Although Shakespeare talks of cynicism, Emerson, referring to the narrow view, was unwittingly speaking to us about medical myopia. Jaundice, both the sign and the symptom, should cause far less diagnostic insecurity than it often elicits. Common sense based on epidemiological facts is the key in deciding whether to image, and if so, what procedures to perform.

The competent clinician after performing a thorough history and physical examination should be able to determine the cause of jaundice in more than 80% of cases. Taken together with the clinical findings, the diagnostic yield of liver chemistries and antibody tests is said to be better than 90% (1, 2). Clinicians, however, do not consistently do as well as this, quite possibly because medical teaching still tends to stress disease descriptions and differential diagnosis to the neglect of disease prevalence. The thrust of this text continues to be that, given major symptoms or findings, the likelihood of specific disease can be predicted with considerable accuracy. Only in this way, *with a diagnosis in mind*, can investigation be conducted on a rational basis.

Table 6.11.1 lists the approximate frequencies of the principal causes of jaundice by age and is the basic key to any meaningful diagnostic approach. Table 6.11.2 lists the individual diagnostic possibilities in jaundiced patients (3). Contrast the two presentations and note the obvious superiority of the first table in dividing the major etiologies into categories. A simplified taxonomy is the best antidote to the perils of classical lists of "differential diagnosis." Because the causes of jaundice turn out to be so few and the incidence so age dependent, the imaging strategy becomes relatively straightforward.

To summarize the tabular findings, in 85% or more of jaundiced patients in the under 30 age group, the cause is some form of hepatocellular dysfunction secondary to hepatitis, either infectious or drug or alcohol induced. Imaging is almost never indicated in this group. In the 30- to 60-year age range the percentage of hepatocellular disease drops to 65%, but it is still by far the most common cause of jaundice. Only after the age of 60 do stones and malignancy become statistically dominant, and it is only in these latter two conditions that imaging is required. Hemolytic disease, which is usually obvious from the hematological findings, is not an indication for imaging and therefore will not be discussed.

For convenience, we will adhere to the useful division of jaundice into two major etiological categories, hepatocellular and obstructive disease, at one time erroneously classified as "medical" and "surgical" jaundice. This classification has the merit of

Table 6.11.1. Probable Cause of Jaundice in Different Age Groups (Adapted from Baer and Belsey, 1988; 3)

Diagnosis	Age (%)		
	1–30	30–60	≥60
Hepatitis	80	30	5
Drug toxicity	2	5	10
Alcoholic liver disease	3	30	10
Carcinoma	<1	10	45
Stones	5	15	25
Other (hemolysis sepsis, shock, etc.)	10	10	5

Table 6.11.2. Differential Diagnostic Considerations in Jaundiced Patients

Increased bile production	Intrahepatic cholestasis
Hemolytic anemias	Drug induced
	Carcinomatosis
Decreased conjugation of bile	Granulomatous hepatitis
Gilbert's disease	Cholangitis
Crigler-Najjar syndrome	Hepatitis
	Alcohol-induced cirrhosis
Hepatocellular disease	Primary biliary cirrhosis
Hepatitis A	
Hepatitis B	Extrahepatic cholestasis
Hepatotoxicity	Carcinoma
Alcoholic	Head of the pancreas
Toxic chemicals	Other tumors
Infectious mononucleosis	Biliary tree stones
	Primary sclerosing cholangitis

Reprinted by permission from *Medical Laboratory Products* (1988;Jan:16).

simplicity and logic. In terms of management it clearly divides patients into those for whom therapy is largely limited and those for whom therapy is largely mandatory.

Although this section is about imaging patients given the presence of jaundice, our overview has important implications for imaging patients with abnormal liver function tests. Individuals with hepatocellular dysfunction but without the clinical sign or symptom of jaundice will be discussed in the next chapter under presentation by abnormal laboratory findings.

Principal Imaging Studies in Obstructive Jaundice
ULTRASOUND

Ultrasonography is an imaging technology which has revolutionized the anatomical study of the biliary tract. Although it is generally poor in imaging the liver itself, sonography is extremely reliable in detecting dilatation of the biliary ducts, especially the common bile duct. The technique has its greatest utility however, in making the diagnosis of gall stones, where it is 93–95% sensitive and specific, an achievement few tests can claim (4). The rapid, convenient, and inexpensive detection of major ductal dilatation and changes in ductal size with time are further invaluable applications of ultrasound in the biliary tract. Ultrasonography is less consistently reliable for the detection of common duct stones but has a sensitivity of 70–75% for pancreatitis. In the technically adequate examination it has a proven accuracy of 85% in the detection of pancreatic cancer (5, 6).

How does one interpret the presence or absence of common bile duct (CBD) dilatation as determined by sonography? First and foremost, in the presence of jaundice, ductal measurement beyond the normal value of 6 mm for the common hepatic duct and 7–8 mm for the proximal CBD should usually be attributed to extrahepatic biliary obstruction. The only exceptions are in some normal older and perhaps a few postcholecystectomy patients, where normal distal duct size may range from 7–10 mm. In the clinical context of jaundice with no prior surgery, however, the false-negative rate of CBD dilatation is exceedingly low, i.e. a significantly dilated CBD (larger than 8–10 mm) implies obstruction in more than 95–97% of cases. The combination of dilated intrahepatic ducts and a normal common bile duct implies a hilar obstruction. Common duct dilatation followed distally to a mass in the pancreatic head or associated with sonographic findings of pancreatitis is an almost infallible sign of a pancreatic cause.

In the patient with a prior cholecystectomy and mild or transient jaundice suspected of having stones, almost one-third will have a normal-sized common duct, frequently because a stone has already passed. Even in the two-thirds of patients who have a dilated common duct, ultrasound is successful in detecting stones in only a minority of those patients (7). These patients, therefore, may benefit from scintigraphy.

HEPATOBILIARY SCINTIGRAPHY

The importance of radionuclide studies in diseases of the biliary tract, particularly in obstruction, has occasionally been ignored because of a misplaced confidence in invasive studies characteristic of today's medical climate. This probably has more to do with the enthusiasm of invasive specialists and the circulation of journals to which they contribute rather than with any dearth of nuclear medicine talent.

The use of radiolabeled iminodiacetic acid analogs (the IDA in HIDA) in hepatobiliary imaging has its highest success rate in the diagnosis of acute cholecystitis. When the criterion for a positive study is nonvisualization of the gall bladder up to 2–3 hours past injection, the test has been shown to be 97% sensitive in the presence of stones, and to be 90–100% specific for acalculous cholecystitis (8, 9). It is in this latter group of patients, when stones are not found on sonography (5–10% of patients with cholecystitis have the acalculous variety), that a positive scintigraphic study is critical in making the diagnosis. Moreover, scintigraphy is also useful in a fair number of patients between attacks, when delayed visualization indicates the presence of chronic cholecystitis. A normal scintigram between attacks of clinically suspected acute biliary colic, however, by no means rules out intercurrent acute attacks. The optimal timing for hepatobiliary scintigraphy is therefore the time of the attack itself or as close in time to the attack as possible. Normal scintiscans are often seen in patients with an obvious acute attack of cholecystitis that was permitted to subside for as little as 48 hours before scanning.

A useful test in patients suspected of having chronic acalculous cholecystitis with normal scintiscans, is the so-called gall bladder EF using cholecystokinin (CCK)-augmented scintigraphy. A significant number of patients without gall stones who have recurring attacks of postprandial right upper quadrant pain and who show normal gall bladder filling between attacks have abnormalities in function pointing to the presence of chronic disease. After CCK injection, using a gamma camera and a computer, the normal radionuclide-filled gall bladder reduces its volume by at least

35–40%. When this fails to occur, the diagnosis of chronic cholecystitis can be made with a high degree of confidence. Fink-Bennett and colleagues (10, 11) have reported a large series of such patients, 84% of whom experienced complete and 13% partial relief of recurring symptoms with cholecystectomy.

A recurring problem is the widespread neglect of hepatobiliary scintigraphy and its bizarre substitution by ERCP of the pancreatic duct in the attempt to diagnose extrahepatic obstruction. This is only one example of uncritical enthusiasm for complicated invasive procedures. A recent publication on the diagnosis of jaundice by members of the Patient Care Committee of the American Gastroenterological Association (12) states that ". . . if a clinical impression of extrahepatic obstruction persists despite negative results of noninvasive studies (CT and ultrasound), direct cholangiography is warranted." Hepatobiliary scanning is dismissed with the following remark, "(Cholescintigraphy) has little or no value in the differential diagnosis of jaundice, is expensive, and may be a serious source of confusion." The same article included an algorithm that completely omitted the use of scintigraphy for biliary obstruction (12). The operative phrase *differential diagnosis* obfuscates the issue, because the clinician first and foremost wishes to confirm the *presence* of extrahepatic obstruction by the easiest, safest, and most noninvasive method. The classic textbook on GI endoscopy also fails to mention radionuclide studies in biliary tract diagnosis (13). Yet numerous studies have shown the usefulness of scintigraphy alone or combined with sonography and occasionally CT in making the diagnosis of obstruction (8, 9, 14–18). Thus, sonography and scintigraphy are studies which help establish or *eliminate the need* for invasive studies. Some surgical writers have even stated that in patients subsequently shown to have periampullary carcinomas in whom distal common obstruction was confirmed with ultrasonography that "no further tests are necessary in most patients and the operation should be carried out promptly" (19). A classic study of 400 patients undergoing hepatobiliary scintigraphy demonstrated that the procedure is probably the most accurate means of identifying high-grade extrahepatic obstruction, with a 100% sensitivity, 99.5% specificity, and a PPV of 92% in the population studied (20).

CT AND MRI SCANNING

Because the place of MRI compared with CT in biliary tract diagnosis has yet to be established with confidence, we will assume for this discussion the two techniques are roughly comparable. Both modalities are expensive (approximately three to six times more than sonography), and CT carries with it some risk because of the remote possibility of contrast media reactions. Furthermore, because of the 79% sensitivity of CT for detection of gall stones (21), compared with 93% or better for ultrasound, it is generally agreed that CT is generally inferior to ultrasound in the diagnosis of cholelithiasis. Combined hepatobiliary sonography and scintigraphy almost always suffice for the diagnosis of gall bladder disease and extrahepatic obstruction due to stones and pancreatitis. However, in three principal categories of obstructive jaundice CT/MRI find application:

1. The patient with major ductal dilatation in whom pancreatic or gall bladder disease cannot be demonstrated by a combination of sonography and cholescintigraphy. CT should be considered a complementary procedure to sonography in visualizing the pancreas. This is especially true when the rates of technically unsatisfactory sonograms is high, as is often the case in obesity or excessive bowel gas.

2. The patient with dilatation of the intrahepatic ducts or patients in whom major ductal dilatation is absent in the presence of high grade obstruction demonstrated by hepatobiliary scintigraphy. This small but important subset includes patients with suspected obstruction proximal to the common bile duct due most commonly to metastatic disease of the porta. Rare causes include sclerosing cholangitis, cholangiocarcinoma (Klatskin tumor), and hepatic artery aneurysms.

3. Patients in whom a pancreatic tumor is suspected on clinical grounds but not seen on ultrasound.

In each of the above settings, CT/MRI are invaluable in determining the presence, location, and extent of a mass lesion, and equally important, in detecting adjacent organ and regional lymph node involvement. The precise place of CT in postoperative choledocholithiasis undetected by ultrasound remains unclear because of the wide range of accuracy reported, 60–90% (22), and because many of these patients will ultimately come to ERCP. However, CT is indeed valuable in this situation because it is noninvasive and in some cases may save the patient further investigation.

ERCP AND THC

To paraphrase Clausewitz, most invasive studies are far too important to leave them up to the generals. Transhepatic cholangiography (THC) and ERCP are two complicated and costly imaging techniques that are technically difficult with a *substantial failure rate—particularly ERCP*. ERCP requires considerable technical skill and experience and is performed with "conscious sedation," a euphemism for general anesthesia, and both ERCP and THC carry risks of complications and death (23).

Despite these statistics, there is a limited but essential place for these two invasive modalities. They make possible the direct opacification of the ductal system. Nevertheless, it is far preferable for the general physician, the surgeon, or the radiologist to call in the endoscopist only after deciding for themselves on the appropriateness of the procedure. Either ERCP or THC may be indicated *when and only when it becomes necessary to visualize the anatomy of the extrahepatic ductal system for therapeutic reasons*. The use of ERCP and THC for management of biliary tract obstruction has been strongly questioned in a series of 157 patients studied by Rothschild et al. (24). Elective, even early surgery may be preferred over ERCP in pancreatitis associated with stones (25). Except for severe hepatocellular dysfunction, where scintigraphy is not always diagnostic, it is difficult to envision any situation where either ERCP or THC would be required for the *diagnosis* of obstructive jaundice. The question of stone removal by ERCP, i.e. its use as a therapeutic procedure, calls for a different line of approach and is discussed here only because therapeutic appropriateness of both THC and ERCP are the prime indications for their diagnostic employment.

In the patient with stone disease and no prior surgery, hepatobiliary scintigraphy is the only available method for functional and anatomical visualization of the ductal system. In the postcholecystectomy patient with obstruction demonstrated by scintigraphy, and where therapeutic stone removal would be chosen over reoperation, ERCP is the procedure of first choice. On the other hand, the issue of endoscopic stone removal in patients with an intact gall bladder with stones who will ultimately require cholecystectomy continues to provoke controversy between surgeons and endoscopists. In older patients and those unfit for subsequent surgery, the endoscopic approach has much to offer. But a large number of patients are now being subjected

Table 6.11.3.   Published Results of Percutaneous Stone Extraction via T-Tube Tracts with Radiological Guidance

Author	Ref.	No. of Patients	Success (%)	Complications (%)	Deaths (%)
Mazzierello	13	1,086	1,043 (96%)	86 (8%)	1 (0.1%)
Burhenne	14	661	628 (95%)	27 (4%)	0
Caprini	15	219	210 (96%)	11 (5%)	2 (1%)
Brough	16	58	48 (83%)	0	0
Nussinson	17	204	158 (77%)	6 (4%)	0
Burhenne	19	612	557 (91%)	27 (4%)	0

Reprinted by permission from Cotton PB. Retained bile duct stones: T-tube in place, percutaneous or endoscopic management. *American Journal of Gastroenterology* (1990;85(9):1075–1078). Copyright 1990 by The American College of Gastroenterology.

Table 6.11.4.   Treatment Options and Success Rate for Retained Common Bile Duct Stones

Method	Success rate (%)
Extraction via T-tube tract	90–95
Endoscopy papillotomy	85–90
Reoperation	80–90
Dissolution	60–85
Fragmentation	50–80
Spontaneous passage	20–33

Reprinted by permission from Surgical Clinics of North America (1991;71(1):93–108) (29).

to endoscopic stone removal only to have the procedure followed by laparoscopic or open cholecystectomy, when common duct exploration could have been performed at the the same sitting. Certainly, a large proportion of common duct stones pass spontaneously, possibly 50–80% depending on size. Despite the 15–25% complication rate in patients with retained stones, a convincing case can be made for a limited period of watchful waiting in most of these patients (26, 27). The problem is enormously complicated because of the rapid introduction of laparoscopic cholecystectomy combined with new techniques of percutaneous transhepatic cholangioscopic lithotomy. Furthermore, the older technique of percutaneous stone removal via T-tube still enjoys an average success rate close to 94% with a low complication rate and negligible mortality as shown in Table 6.11.3. The subject has been extensively reviewed by Cotton (28), who points out that large series of sphincterotomies indicate significant complications occur in 10% of patients, and about 1% die. Gadacz (29), another outstanding surgical writer, has recorded the success rate with various treatments for retained common duct stones. This is shown in Table 6.11.4. Convincing contrary opinions, however, continue to be expressed (30), and we need to remind ourselves that the biliary tract continues to be a dangerous place to work no matter which modality is employed.

In patients in whom complete obstruction is expected above the level of the pancreas or distal common duct, THC is the only reliable way to image the duct above the obstruction and is an essential preliminary step before embarking on therapeutic percutaneous biliary drainage (22).

To summarize, either ERCP or THC are indicated in the following major categories of jaundice:

1. Patients with primary or secondary obstructing carcinoma of the biliary tract, from the pancreas and ampulla to the porta, in whom therapeutic intervention will be

required for palliation, or in whom ductal visualization is requested by the surgeon. Intervention would include surgical, endoscopic, or transcutaneous relief of obstruction. There is still controversy over the therapeutic advantages of ERCP vs. THC in distal common duct obstruction, but THC is to be preferred in any proximal lesions.

2. Patients with previous biliary tract surgery and retained or recurrent stones in whom either the surgeon desires to know ductal anatomy before anticipated surgery, or endoscopic stone removal is contemplated. Today, the majority of surgeons want some security and wish to avoid surprises in the operating room before reoperating on the biliary tract because of the high complication rate of repeat biliary tract surgery. Overall, the endoscopic approach to retained stones is now preferred to reoperation.

3. The rare patient with such severe hepatocellular dysfunction that scintigraphy cannot reliably diagnose extrahepatic obstruction, and in whom ultrasonographic findings are nonspecific.

4. Patients with biliary-enteric anastomoses. Here, ultrasonography is of virtually no help, but scintigraphy may sometimes be helpful. In this instance when direct opacification of the ducts is desired by many surgeons, ERCP has limited value because of technical problems, and if scintigraphy does not satisfy the surgeon, THC should be the study of choice.

Hepatobiliary scintigraphy is the only reliable method available for the detection of bile leaks occurring as a complication of trauma, surgery of the biliary tract, or instrumentation, in particular ERCP. Common bile duct perforations with bile leaks and bile peritonitis secondary to ERCP manipulation for stone extraction are especially dangerous and carry a significant mortality if unrecognized early.

To be fair, one wonders how often surgeons are anxious to avoid repeat surgery on the biliary tract and are only too glad to hand over the responsibility to the endoscopist. On the other hand, we are not aware of any careful long-term studies comparing the results of endoscopic sphincterotomy and stone removal with reoperation. A few will recall the brief enthusiasm for (operative) sphincterotomy back in the mid-1950s, when enthusiasts were recommending the operation for everything from the prevention of recurrent obstruction to the treatment of pancreatitis (31). Still, we will not know for many years the long-term effects of sphincterotomy and the overall results of endoscopic stone removal compared to surgical methods.

OTHER IMAGING METHODS

In addition to the above procedures, other imaging methods are available for the detection of biliary tract disease and obstruction, but these are of extremely low sensitivity and therefore outmoded. For example, plain films of the abdomen, though occasionally demonstrating gall stones serendipitously, will miss them more than 85% of the time.

The oral cholecystogram is still used in some centers but has been largely supplanted by ultrasound and hepatobiliary scintiscanning. There is a high percentage of false-negative tests (low sensitivity), and because of this, more than 15–25% of studies have to be repeated with a double dose (32). Still, there is almost 100% certainty of gall bladder disease or stones in the presence of nonvisualization after a double dose (and in the absence of liver disease). This suggests a limited place for the study, where both sonography and radionuclide studies are still unavailable.

A final word on an outmoded and highly dangerous test, the intravenous cholangiogram. Because of extremely poor visualization of the ductal system compared with scintigraphy and because of the risk of severe reactions (1 in 1600) and death (1 in 5000) (33), the procedure has been completely discredited. With the availability of hepatobiliary scintigraphy, the continued use of intravenous contrast cholangiography no longer can be justified.

Hepatocellular Jaundice

Referring to Table 6.11.1, from the prior probability of disease (prevalence) we can outline a useful diagnostic strategy for hepatocellular or medical jaundice:

1. Except for infants where biliary atresia must be a prime consideration, the great majority of patients under age 30 with jaundice have some type of hepatocellular dysfunction. Imaging is almost never indicated in this group with a confirmatory history and findings indicating hepatitis. Because almost all patients with drug-induced hepatitis, most patients with non-A infectious hepatitis, and a subset of patients with alcoholic hepatitis go through a phase of intrahepatic cholestatis, when the alkaline phosphatase is usually elevated at some time during the course of hepatocellular disease. This is not universally appreciated in hepatitis, where a majority of patients go through an "obstructive" phase fairly early in the course of their illness, and where there is a tendency to equate elevations of this enzyme with extrahepatic obstruction.

2. Persistent elevations of alkaline phosphatase, of course, are troubling chemical signs, but in most cases of non-A hepatitis, they start returning to normal usually before other hepatic enzymes have peaked. Elevations of serum alkaline phosphatase up to one and one-half to two times normal may be seen in growing children, pregnant women, patients over age 50, some subjects with blood groups O and B, after eating, and in other patients without known cause (34, 35). The clinical history along with liver function and hepatitis antibody tests should obviate the use of imaging in almost all such patients. With intrahepatic cholestatis due to drugs, the diagnosis is generally easy because of the temporal relation of jaundice to exhibition of the causative drug and the rapid subsidence of hepatic functional abnormalities with discontinuance of the drug. Particular offenders include the following classes of drugs: (a) chlorpromazine and its derivatives; (b) antithyroid drugs; (c) gold preparations; (d) steroids, such as methyl testosterone, anabolic compounds, and especially birth control drugs (and pregnancy); (e) chlorpropamide and tolbutamide; and (f) isoniazid. The unlikelihood of extrahepatic obstruction in this group should provide the best guide to avoiding unnecessary imaging procedures. It is safe to conclude that in the young patient with jaundice anatomical obstruction occurs in less than 3–5% of cases.

3. Already mentioned is the fact that right upper quadrant pain and tenderness in a young person is more likely to be caused by nonspecific pain or hepatitis than by gall stones. However, the younger jaundiced patient with prolonged elevations of alkaline phosphatase often causes concern that a common duct stone is being missed. In this situation, sonography of the gall bladder almost always settles the issue, because the combined presence of ductal dilatation and stones invariably indicates obstruction, whereas the absence of stones and ductal dilatation excludes the diagnosis. The mere presence of stones, of course, does not confidently indicate obstruction because of the frequent occurrence of this finding in asymptomatic individuals. Dilatation of the

common bile duct may not always be present on ultrasound, particularly with early or partial obstruction or after a stone has passed. Still, the *combined absence of stones and major ductal dilatation on sonography* rules out the presence of gall bladder disease with more than 95% accuracy.

4. Similarly, in jaundiced patients from age 30–60 with typical prodromal symptoms accompanied by fever and tender hepatomegaly, imaging is not needed in the presence of laboratory signs of hepatocellular dysfunction. In all other patients with jaundice, especially those over age 45 without significant enzyme elevations other than alkaline phosphatase, proceed to investigate for extrahepatic obstruction.

Obstructive Jaundice

In all patients with or without pain and without a confirmatory history or laboratory findings to suggest hepatocellular disease and in all those with *intermittent jaundice*, the most likely diagnosis is some type of obstructive jaundice due to extrahepatic obstructive disease, i.e. choledocholithiasis, carcinoma or inflammatory disease of the bile duct, ampulla, or head of the pancreas, or metastatic disease of the liver or porta hepatis. In this setting we advise the following:

1. First, perform ultrasonography of the gall bladder, common duct, and pancreas. If gall stones are found with dilatation of the common duct consider the diagnosis of choledocholithiasis almost certain whether or not stones are seen in the duct. We have frequently seen common duct stones pass within 1 or 2 days after onset of colic or jaundice, often by the time the patient is studied. In these cases, the common bile duct may or may not be dilated, depending on how long the acute obstruction has lasted and how recently the stone has passed. A dilated common bile duct may revert to normal size within 24–48 hours after passage of a stone. This may be one of the reasons, as mentioned above, that sonography has a low detection rate for choledocholithiasis. In the rare young patient with intermittent painless jaundice and a palpable right upper quadrant mass, ultrasonography may disclose a choledochal cyst.

2. If cholelithiasis or pancreatic disease is suspected or diagnosed by ultrasonography, it may or may not be necessary to proceed to hepatobiliary scintigraphy. If the patient has compelling clinical findings of acute cholecystitis associated with cholelithiasis, there is no reason to delay surgery for the purpose of further testing. Specifically, in a large series referred to previously (14), with gall stones associated with: (a) pain on pressure of the transducer over the right upper quadrant (a positive "ultrasound Murphy" sign); and (b) a thick-walled gall bladder, the diagnosis of acute cholecystitis was almost 100% certain, and no further imaging tests before cholecystectomy were indicated. This combination of findings, however, occurs less than 60% of the time.

The authors stated that even if stones were present, if all three of these criteria were not met, 23% of their 497 patients might have required hepatobiliary scintiscanning (14). We do not regard the absence of gall bladder wall thickening on sonography as a necessary indication for delaying surgery, but certainly scintigraphy should be performed in all patients without physical findings sufficient to justify surgical exploration. This is reasonable, considering the 2–12% of asymptomatic cholelithiasis in the general population (36–38). We emphasize again that given only acute right upper quadrant pain and tenderness, less than one-third of such patients will have acute cholecystitis (14).

3. Hepatobiliary scintigraphy, therefore, is mandatory in the following two groups of patients with suspected acute or chronic cholecystitis: (a) those with stones in whom clinical findings of cholecystitis are not convincing enough to enable the surgeon to proceed; and (b) those patients without stones suspected of having acalculous cholecystitis.

In either setting, hepatobiliary scintigraphy will be virtually 100% diagnostic for cystic duct obstruction, which is seen in almost all patients with acute cholecystitis. A positive test, therefore, is one in which the gall bladder fails to visualize within 2–3 hours. Chronic or subacute cholecystitis, whether calculous or noncalculous, as demonstrated by delayed gall bladder visualization (more than 1 hour, less than 2–3 hours), also will be detected with almost 95–100% sensitivity (8, 9). Many patients with acute but *subsiding* cholecystitis often have normal scintigraphic gall bladder visualization (within 20–60 minutes) if the cystic duct is no longer obstructed. This may sometimes occur as soon as 2 or 3 days after an acute attack. It follows, therefore, that in a high suspect for acute cholecystitis without stones or with subsiding physical findings, cholescintigraphy should be performed without delay. Because a significant number of patients with chronic (nonacute) acalculous cholecystitis may show normal visualization (less than 45–60 minutes) but a low EF (less than 35%), in all questionable cases this index should be determined by combining the scintigraphy with injection of CCK.

4. Cholescintigraphy also should be used to estimate the functional degree and approximate site of extrahepatic obstruction, i.e. main hepatic, proximal, or distal common bile duct, in cases where surgery has been delayed. This becomes important in properly timing surgery, because partial or complete relief of obstruction can be reliably predicted up to 1 week or more before changes are seen in hepatic function tests. Thus, the decision to intervene may be made much sooner in the case of either early stone passage or persistent obstruction.

5. In the rare patient with jaundice in whom results of gall bladder ultrasonography are discordant, i.e. ductal dilatation without identifiable gallstones, or vice versa, hepatobiliary scintigraphy will be required to exclude obstruction. CT is rarely indicated in this situation unless there is clinical evidence suggesting malignancy.

6. The indications for CT, MRI, ERCP, and THC have already been discussed but will be summarized here. In the absence of clear-cut gall bladder disease or inflammatory disease of the pancreas, particularly in the older patient, cancer of the biliary tract remains the most likely diagnosis. This is the situation where CT or MRI is called for and where their accuracy is unparalleled.

Predicting the Outcome of Imaging Studies in Jaundice

Some simple mathematical calculations using conditional probability help in comparing the efficacy of imaging studies in jaundice. The prevalences are derived from the original Table 6.11.1 for the respective patient age group. Each test is listed in a separate table for comparison. All sensitivities are derived from the literature or are clinical estimates. The most important columns are labeled as previously in the text: PPV, the positive predictive value of a test is the likelihood of disease given a positive test; and 1-NPV, the likelihood of disease given a negative test. With careful study of these charts the reader may confirm in his mind the reason why certain tests are indicated in specific clinical settings and at the same time appreciate the limitations of medical testing under certain conditions.

For example, using combined antigen/antibody testing (*assumed to be a single test only, with high sensitivity and low nonspecificity*), Tables 6.11.5 and 6.11.6 show tests for hepatitis that are highly predictive in the younger age group because of the high prevalence of hepatitis but are poorly predictive in the older age group. In a kind of circular reasoning we may conclude that hepatitis testing is useful for diagnosing hepatitis but useless for other conditions causing jaundice. Analyzing the utility of sonography for the diagnosis of jaundice becomes somewhat more complex, because we no longer can assume a binary test outcome. Tables 6.11.7 and 6.11.8 show hypothetical results with sonography with the same sets of disease prevalence representing younger and older patients. Causes of hepatocellular disease are combined. Here, however, the initial probabilities are given for different test results, because upper abdominal sonography will have different possible outcomes depending on the condition studied. Moreover, when a test has more than two possible outcomes, test sensitivity and nonspecificity are undefined. These tables are more complex than the ones constructed for hepatitis testing and require separate analysis of each outcome. In fact, the possible outcomes are combined so the permutations of combinations of outcomes are reduced. However, they again show what our knowledge of sonography could have told us, without even looking at the initial disease prevalences, i.e. upper abdominal sonography is a good test for biliary tract conditions.

There is no way to overcome the problem of disease prevalence when blindly choosing a test. When disease prevalence rises, obviously, the test should be appropriate for the diseases most likely to occur. However, without significant differences in sensitivity for certain conditions, the results are apt to be disappointing *unless prior probability or prevalence of various conditions is sufficiently high*.

Summary

1. In suspected hepatocellular jaundice, imaging is almost never indicated. The overwhelming number of patients under age 30 with jaundice, with the exception of infants, have hepatocellular jaundice.

2. Obstructive or surgical jaundice always calls for imaging to determine the site and probable cause of the obstruction (stone or cancer).

3. Ultrasonography of the gall bladder, common bile duct, and pancreas should always be the first imaging study performed in suspected obstructive jaundice. Because gall stones are present in 90–94% of all patients with cholecystitis, *the absence of stones on sonography rules out this diagnosis with a very high degree of confidence*.

4. In the presence of cholelithiasis and strong clinical findings of acute or subacute cholecystitis, no further imaging is usually necessary to confirm the diagnosis.

5. With suspected acalculous cholecystitis or with some clinical uncertainty about the presence of acute or subacute cholecystitis, hepatobiliary scintigraphy with or without the gall bladder EF is indicated.

6. Serial measurements of common bile duct diameter are extremely helpful in determining the course of obstruction due to stone, but scintiscanning is much more reliable in detecting the degree of obstruction and in establishing whether it has been completely or partially relieved by passage of calculi. In the setting of fluctuating jaundice due to stone, hepatobiliary scintiscanning gives the best functional estimate

Table 6.11.5. Calculated Predictive Values for Liver Function/Antibody Tests in Under-30 Age Group

Disease	Prevalence	Sensitivity	Nonspecificity	PPV	1-NPV
Hepatitis	80	85	10	97	40
Drug toxicity	2	10	71	<1	6
Alcoholic liver disease	3	10	72	<1	9
Carcinoma	1	10	71	<1	3
Stones	5	10	73	<1	15
Other	9	10	76	1	27

Table 6.11.6. Calculated Predictive Values for Liver Function/Antibody Tests, in Over-60-Age Group

Disease	Prevalence	Sensitivity	Nonspecificity	PPV	1-NPV
Hepatitis	5	85	10	31	<1
Drug toxicity	10	10	14	7	10
Alcoholic liver disease	10	10	14	7	10
Carcinoma	45	10	17	33	47
Stones	25	10	15	18	26
Other	5	10	14	4	5

Table 6.11.7. Test: Sonography: Estimated Probabilities of Various Test Results for Each Disease in Under-30 Age Group

Disease	Normal	Stones/Dilated CBD	Pancreatic Mass/Dilated CBD
Hepatocellular	96	4	0
Stone	5	95	0
Carcinoma	5	10	85
Other	96	4	0

Prior Probability (Prevalence) and Posttest Probability of Disease for Each Test Result

Disease	Prevalence	Posttest Probabilities		
		Normal	Stones/Dilated CBD	Pancreatic Mass/Dilated CBD
Hepatocellular	85	90	39	<1
Stone	5	<1	55	<1
Carcinoma	1	<1	1	>99
Other	9	10	4	<1

Table 6.11.8. Test: Sonography: Estimated Probabilities of Various Test Results for Each Disease, Over-60 Age Group

Disease	Normal	Stones/Dilated CBD	Pancreatic Mass/Dilated CBD
Hepatocellular	96	4	0
Stone	5	95	0
Carcinoma	5	10	85
Other	96	4	0

Prior Probability (Prevalence) and Posttest Probability of Disease for Each Test Result

Disease	Prevalence	Posttest Probabilities		
		Normal	Stones/Dilated CBD	Pancreatic Mass/Dilated CBD
Hepatocellular	25	74	3	<1
Stone	25	4	81	<1
Carcinoma	45	7	15	>99
Other	5	15	<1	<1

of the degree of obstruction. It provides quicker and more accurate information than does liver chemistries for determining the optimal time of surgery.

7. Hepatobiliary scintigraphy is the principal imaging method for making the diagnosis of extrahepatic and certain cases of intrahepatic obstruction. Invasive studies such as ERCP should *never* be used for this purpose except in the presence of severe hepatocellular dysfunction.

8. If sonography demonstrates a pancreatic tumor or there is absence of clinical or sonographic/scintigraphic evidence of stone, suspect malignancy and proceed to CT or MRI.

9. *Reserve ERCP and THC for patients in whom it is necessary to directly opacify the extrahepatic ductal system for therapeutic reasons.* This would be applicable in the following three categories:

(a) patients with malignant involvement of the biliary tract or ampulla in whom surgical, endoscopic, or transcutaneous intervention for relief of obstruction is required.
(b) patients with previous biliary tract surgery in whom endoscopic removal of stones has been decided upon or the surgeon desires to visualize the anatomy before reoperation.
(c) patients in whom reoperation is contemplated for complications involving biliary-enteric anastomoses. THC is indicated if scintigraphy fails. ERCP is usually not indicated in this situation.
(d) ERCP for endoscopic stone removal is preferred in the older patient or poor surgical candidate. The use of ERCP for sphincterotomy with endoscopic stone removal in patients who will ultimately require cholecystectomy is still considered controversial by many authorities.

10. ERCP should be avoided in nonmalignant pancreatic disease. This includes pancreatitis and complications thereof, in particular pseudocysts, where the procedure is contraindicated.

REFERENCES

1. Ottinger LW. Evaluation of jaundiced patients—a surgeon's perspective. Semin Ultrasound 1984; V(4):399–400.
2. Bourke JB, Cannon P, Ritchie HD: Laparotomy for jaundice. Lancet 1967;2(515):521–523.
3. Baer DM, Belsey RE. Clinical Problems in the office lab: Evaluating jaundice. Med Lab Prod 1988; Jan:16–18.
4. Sample WF, Sarti DA, Goldstein LI, Weiner M, Kadell BM. Gray-scale ultrasonography of the jaundiced patient. Radiology 1978;128(3):719–725.
5. Pollack D, Taylor KJW. Ultrasound scanning in patients with clinical suspicion of pancreatic cancer: a retrospective study. Cancer 1981;47(6)[suppl 1]:1662–1665.
6. Kamin PD, Bernardino ME, Wallace S, Jing BS. Comparison of ultrasound and computed tomography in the detection of pancreatic malignancy. Cancer 1980;46(11):2410–2412.
7. Cronan JJ, Mueller PR, Simeone JF, et al: Prospective diagnosis of choledocholithiasis. Radiology 1983;146(2):467–469
8. Fink-Bennett D, Freitas JE, Ripley SD, Bree RL. The sensitivity of hepatobiliary imaging and real-time ultrasonography in the detection of acute cholecystitis. Arch Surg 1985;120(8):904–906.
9. Swayne LC. Acute acalculous cholecystitis: sensitivity in detection using technetium-99m iminodiacetic acid cholescintigraphy. Radiology July 1986;160(1):33–38.

10. Fink-Bennett D, DeRidder P, Kolozsi WZ, Gordon R, Jaros R. Cholecystokinin cholescintigraphy: detection of abnormal gall bladder motor function in patients with chronic acalculous gall bladder disease. J Nucl Med 1991;32(9):1695–1699.

11. Misra Jr DC, Blossom GB, Fink-Bennett, Glover JL. Results of surgical therapy for biliary dyskinesia. Arch Surg 1991;126(8):957–960.

12. Frank BB, and members of the patient care committee of the American Gastroenterological Association. Clinical evaluation of jaundice. A guideline of the Patient Care Committee of the American Gastroenterological Association. JAMA 1989;262(21):3031–3034.

13. Wurbs DFW. Calculus disease of the bile ducts. In: Sivak MV, ed. Gastroenterologic Endoscopy. Philadelphia: W.B. Saunders Co., 1987:296–306.

14. Laing FC, Federle MP, Jeffrey RB, Brown TL. Ultrasonic evaluation of patients with acute right upper quadrant pain. Radiology 1981;140(2):449–455.

15. O'Connor KW, Snodgrass PJ, Swonder JE, et al. A blinded prospective study comparing four current noninvasive approaches in differential diagnosis of medical versus surgical jaundice. Gastroenterology 1983;84(6):1498–1504.

16. Lane RJ, Coupland GAE. Ultrasonic indications to explore the common bile duct. Surgery 1982; 91(3):268–274.

17. Honickman SP, Mueller PR, Wittenburg J, et al. Ultrasound in obstructive jaundice: prospective evaluation of site and cause. Radiology 1983;147(2):511–515.

18. Lieberman DA, Krishnamurthy GT. Intrahepatic versus extrahepatic cholestasis: discrimination with biliary scintigraphy combined with ultrasound. Gastroenterology 1986;90(3):734–743.

19. Olen R, Pickleman J, Freeark RJ. Less is better: the diagnostic workup of the patient with obstructive jaundice. Arch Surg 1989;124(7):791–795.

20. Lecklitner ML, Austin RA, Benedetto AR, Growcock GW. Positive predictive value of cholescintigraphy in common bile duct obstruction. J Nucl Med 1986;27(9):1403–1406.

21. Barakos JA, Ralls PW, Lapin SA, et al. Cholelithiasis: evaluation with CT. Radiology 1987;162:415–418.

22. Cronan JJ. The imaging of biliary obstruction. Semin Ultrasound 1984;5:379–398.

23. Ferguson AR, Sivak Jr MV. Indications, contraindications and complications of ERCP. In Sivak Jr JV, ed. Gastrointestinal Endoscopy. Philadelphia: WB Saunders Co., 1987:581–598.

24. Rothschild JG, Kaplan MM, Millan VG, Reinhold RB. Management of biliary obstruction: a comparison of percutaneous, endoscopic, and operative techniques. Arch Surg 1989;124(5):556–560.

25. Kourtesis GJ, Wilson SE, Williams RA. Safety of operation in biliary pancreatitis during the same hospitalization. Aust NZ J Surg 1990;60(2):103–107.

26. Johnson AG, Hosking SW. Appraisal of the management of bile duct stones. Br J Surg 1987;74(7): 555–560.

27. Wenckert A, Robertson B. The natural course of gallstone disease: eleven-year review of 781 nonoperated cases. Gastroenterology 1966;50(3):376–381.

28. Cotton PB. Retained bile duct stones: T-tube in place, percutaneous or endoscopic management? [editorial]. Am J Gastroenterol 1990;85(9):1075–1078.

29. Gadacz TR. Reoperation versus alternatives in retained biliary calculi. Surg Clin N Am 1991;71(1): 93–108.

30. Sivak Jr MV. Endoscopic management of bile duct stones. Am J Surg 1989;158(3):228–240.

31. Doubilet H. Section of the sphincter of Oddi. Surg Clin North Am 1956;36:865–882.

32. Berk RN, Clement AR. Radiology of the gall bladder and bile ducts. Philadelphia: W.B. Saunders Co., 1977.

33. Ansell G. Adverse reactions to contrast agents. Scope of problem. Invest Radiol 1970;5(6):374–391.

34. Chopra S, Griffin PH. Laboratory tests and diagnostic procedures in evaluation of liver disease. Am J Med 1985;79:221–229.

35. Rubenstein LV, Ward BA, Greenfield S. In pursuit of the abnormal serum alkaline phosphatase: a clinical dilemma. J Gen Intern Med 1986;1(1):38–43.

36. Friedman GD, Kannel WB, Dawber TR. The epidemiology of gall bladder disease: observations in the Framingham study. J Chronic Dis 1966;19(3):273–292.

37. Gracie WA, Ransohoff DF. The natural history of silent gallstones: the innocent gallstone is not a myth. N Engl J Med 1982;307(13):798–800.

38. Incidence of gallbladder disease in "normal" men. Gastroenterology 1959;36:251–255.

12/ Constipation and Diarrhea

*We forget ourselves and our destinies in health, and the chief use of
temporary sickness is to remind us of these concerns.*

Ralph Waldo Emerson
Journals, *1821*

General Discussion

Constipation and diarrhea, as everyone knows, are extremely common and generally innocent symptoms. In former times, most sufferers would endure such complaints without seeking medical advice, knowing they would, for the most part, subside spontaneously with time. Today the situation has changed, in part because of
international travel and the reappearance of an old public health problem, the infectious diarrheas. Moreover, there is an increased tendency of people in affluent socie-
ties to seek medical attention for self-limiting complaints, particularly in an era of
overconcern about cancer and other diseases.

It is useful in this connection to review hospital and outpatient statistics dealing
with some principal causes of diarrhea, constipation and other bowel complaints.
Figure 6.12.1 depicts the all-listed discharge diagnoses for the United States in 1990
for major serious and benign conditions likely to cause these symptoms and includes,
among others, alactasia (including malabsorption) and the functional digestive disorders, specifically constipation and irritable bowel syndrome (ICD 564). Colon malignancies (ICD 153), however, accounting for 179,000 discharges in 1990, were omitted (1). Table 6.12.1 lists discharge data for the principal infectious diarrheas in 1990,
omitting statistically insignificant cholera, shigellosis, and protozoal infections. Note
the preponderance of not elsewhere classified (NEC) diagnoses and "ill-defined" in-

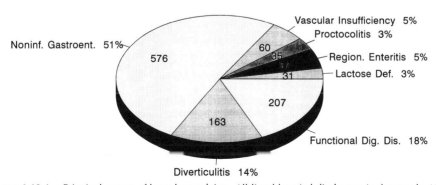

Principal Causes of Bowel Complaints
All-Listed Hospital Discharges In Thousands
1990 NHDS Data (1)

Figure 6.12.1. Principal causes of bowel complaints. All-listed hospital discharges in thousands, 1990
NHDS data (1).

Table 6.12.1. Principal Infectious Diarrheas, All-Listed Discharges in Thousands, U.S. Hospitals, 1990 (NCHS Data) (1)

All-listed ICD-9-CM	Total	Male	Female	Age <15	Age 15–44	Age 45–64	Age 65+
003. Salmonella infection[a]	18	8	10	7	5	0	0
005. Other food poisoning	6	0	0	0	0	0	0
008. Intestinal Infection NEC	176	73	103	58	38	24	57
009. Ill-defined intest infection	28	14	14	11	10	0	0

NEC, Not elsewhere classified.
[a]Excludes typhoid.

testinal infection. The frequency of outpatient visits for these conditions has been recorded by the NAMCS (2). In 1985, almost 90% of all such visits for the diagnoses tabulated in Figure 6.12.1 and Table 6.12.1 were for noninfectious gastroenteritis and colitis (ICD 558).

Again, what is striking on reviewing these statistics is the enormous preponderance of benign conditions. This is a common thread in the practice of medicine, emphasized throughout this book. Medical diagnostic strategy is nothing more than a variation on this major theme; always look first for the common conditions, not the exotic. For example, in Figure 6.12.1 the two ICD rubrics, 558, "other non-infectious gastroenteritis and colitis," and 564, "functional digestive disorders," together account for 783,000 discharge diagnoses or 69% of the total. Functional intestinal disorders alone, *including only those for which patients were hospitalized* in fact well exceeded the total estimated 151,000 new cases of colorectal cancer for 1989 (3). (The age-adjusted death rate for colon and rectal cancer has not changed significantly in the United States over the past 50 years, despite extensive screening and the increasingly widespread use of colonoscopy; 3).

Diarrhea

> *To avoid delay, please have all your symptoms ready.*
> *Anonymous*
> *Notice in an English physician's waiting room*

By far the most common causes of acute diarrhea are various identifiable and unidentifiable infectious agents. A large variety of organisms may cause acute diarrhea, but even with extensive investigation, pathogens are identified in only 60–80% of cases (4). (Thus, the ICD designation "other *noninfectious* gastroenteritis" may be a misnomer.) Principal infectious causes of acute diarrhea in the general population and among patients with AIDS have been listed in the literature and include a wide variety of bacterial (*Campylobacter, Salmonella, Escherichia coli, Shigella, Clostridium*) protozoal (*Entamoeba*), viral (rotavirus, Norwalk agent, adenovirus), and other agents (5).

Drugs are the second most common cause of acute diarrhea. Of all drugs, however, laxatives especially, followed by diuretics, antacids, and antibiotics, are the worst offenders.

Other important chronic diarrheal disorders are caused by a variety of dietary factors, especially lactose, coffee, colas, and fructose- and sorbitol-containing foods.

Table 6.12.2. Causes of Constipation by Estimated Frequency of Presentation

Most Common (95–99%)

1. Chronic constipation
    a. Emotional, (stress, grief, anger, fear)
    b. Early training or conditioning
    c. Voluntary delay in defecation, i.e. job-related, travel, combat, etc.
    d. Age
    e. Pregnancy
    f. Obesity
    g. Idiopathic, etc.
2. Laxative abuse

Much Less Common (<1–5%)

1. Mechanical
    a. Bowel obstruction (neoplasm, volvulus, diverticulitis, adhesions, etc.)
    b. Rectal lesions (hemorrhoids, fissure, abscess)

Rare (<0.1%)

1. Neurogenic
    a. Cortical
    b. Postganglionic disorders (Hirschsprung's, Chagas' disease)
    c. Central nervous system lesions (multiple sclerosis, tabes, spinal cord lesions)
2. Metabolic
    a. Hypokalemia (may include laxative abuse)
    b. Hypothyroidism
    c. Hypercalcemia
    d. Porphyria
    e. Malnutrition

A large number of clinically rare causes of diarrhea are always listed under "differential diagnosis," conditions such as pancreatic disease and malabsorption, GI neoplasms, dysautonomia, idiopathic secretory diarrhea, etc. In an interesting study of 27 patients with longstanding, previously investigated chronic diarrhea, investigation disclosed the most common causes to be surreptitious ingestion of drugs in 9 (laxatives in 7, diuretics in 2), followed by irritable bowel syndrome in 8. Only two patients had ulcerative colitis, the same number diagnosed as having anal sphincter dysfunction (6).

Constipation

Judging by the dollar volume of laxatives, stool softeners, suppositories, and prune juice sold annually in this country, we would seem to be suffering from a national preoccupation with our bowels. Certainly, laxative abuse is as common a cause of constipation as it is of diarrhea, and psychological factors have to be considered a major cause of this prevalent symptom. A list of possible etiologies of constipation, in order of prevalence, is given in Table 6.12.2.

For practical purposes almost all chronic constipation results from early training or conditioning, inhibition of defecation because of situational factors (work, travel, etc.) laxative abuse, obesity, pregnancy, or other causes of abdominal distension affecting voluntary musculature. This latter cause may be in part responsible for the enormous increase in constipation with age.

Imaging in Diarrhea and Constipation

Most patients suffering from diarrhea or constipation, of course, do not require investigation, but clearly when the history and physical findings suggest a clinically significant condition, testing must be initiated. In the severe diarrheas, estimates of fecal leukocytes and examination and culture of the stool should be the first diagnostic tests. The three mainstays of diagnostic imaging have not changed for the small and large bowel over the years: the upper GI series with small bowel follow-through, the barium enema, and flexible sigmoidoscopy (flex-sig).

In all patients with bloody diarrhea, flex-sig is mandatory to assess mucosal integrity. In some infections, such as toxigenic *E. coli* or cholera, the mucosa may be completely normal, whereas *Shigella* and *Campylobacter* may give an appearance similar to that of ulcerative colitis. Amebiasis and pseudomembranous colitis are other conditions in which typical mucosal abnormalities may be directly visualized (5). Diagnostic management of patients with frank blood in their stools without bowel dysfunction will be discussed in the next chapter.

When are barium studies or flex-sig indicated other than in rectal bleeding and bloody diarrhea? Manifestly, patients should be studied if one entertains the diagnoses of obstructive disease resulting from malignancy and other causes and complications of inflammatory bowel disease (diverticulitis, Crohn's disease, and ulcerative colitis). Patients with any unexplained anemia or change in bowel habits, particularly those over age 45 with a family history of bowel cancer, or those with lower GI symptoms and weight loss are considered prime cancer suspects. There is no question these patients also must be studied with barium enema (preferably with air contrast, the double contrast study) and flex-sig. Colonoscopy, that is, direct visualization of the entire colon, is rarely required in most cases, for several reasons which have been discussed in Chapters 5 and 6 (Sections 1 and 2).

The presence of active ulcerative colitis almost always can be suspected with a classic history of abdominal pain, bloody stools, frequent fever, and, in severe cases, weight loss. More than 96% of patients with active disease pass blood and mucus in their stools every day, and more than 80% of patients defecate more than three times a day as well as at night. Moreover, urgency (85%), a feeling of incomplete evacuation (78%), and tenesmus (63%) were strong diagnostic indicators in an important study (7). Yet 27% of patients with inactive disease at times had hard stools suggesting constipation (7). It has been suggested that because some of these complaints, particularly increased bowel frequency, pain relieved by defecation, and mucus, are commonly seen in irritable bowel, the distinction cannot be reliably made on the basis of these symptoms alone. We do not share this viewpoint, but strongly agree that flex-sig and double contrast barium enema should be done if there is any clinical question aroused by a history of changing bowel complaints. The overwhelming majority of patients with irritable bowel disease in this country, however, almost certainly will have had these investigations at least once. It is important not to make this a repetitive affair, particularly in the patient with long-standing complaints. This is the very type of patient who is at risk for iatrogenically induced cancer phobia.

Inflammatory bowel disease of the small intestine, i.e. regional enteritis or Crohn's disease, presents more often with systemic complaints, i.e. fever and generalized fatigability, abdominal pain, and diarrhea, than bowel complaints per se.

Summary

1. Most patients with acute diarrhea or chronic constipation do not require imaging.

2. All patients with bloody diarrhea should have flex-sig. If the diagnosis of nonspecific ulcerative colitis or other idiopathic noninfectious colitis is made, a barium enema should also be performed.

3. All patients with unexplained rectal bleeding should also have flex-sig. If a cause such as hemorrhoids or fissure is found, no further study is indicated in the young or low-risk patient. However, double contrast barium enemas should be performed in all other patients with the first rectal bleeding episode and patients with hemorrhoids over 40 years of age.

4. All patients with unexplained or new constipation, change in bowel habits, or *character* of the stools, including ribbon-like stools and diarrhea, and older patients with unexplained anemia should have a double contrast barium enema followed by flex-sig. Complete colonoscopy is not generally an alternative to these studies, except in those patients in whom a lesion is demonstrated proximal to the splenic flexure.

REFERENCES

1. U.S. Department of Health and Human Services, U.S. Public Health Service, Centers for Disease Control, and the National Center for Health Statistics. National Hospital Discharge Survey (NHDS). Detailed diagnoses, procedures, days of care, diagnoses-related groups for patients discharged from short-stay hospitals. Public Use Data Diskettes, 1985–1990.
2. McLemore T, DeLozier J. National Center for Health Statistics, 1985 Summary: National Ambulatory Medical Care Survey. Advance Data from Vital and Health Statistics, No. 128 DHHS Pub. No. (PHS) 87-1250. Hyattsville, Md: Public Health Service, Jan. 23, 1987.
3. Cancer Facts and Figures—1989. American Cancer Society, 1989. Atlanta. (derived from mortality statistics of the National Center for Health Statistics Department of Health and Human Services).
4. Fordtran JS. Speculations on the pathogenesis of diarrhea. Fed Proc 1967;26(5):1405–1414.
5. Lopez WC, Ferrante WA. Acute Diarrhea. Emerg Decis 1988;4(3):22–27.
6. Read NW, Krejs GJ, Read MG, SantaAna CA, Morawski SG, Fordtran JS. Chronic diarrhea of unknown origin. Gastroenterology 1980;78(2):264–271.
7. Rao SS, Holdsworth CD, Read NW. Symptoms and stool patterns in patients with ulcerative colitis. Gut 1988;29(3):342–345.

13/ Anorexia, Nausea, and Vomiting

The patient was a 19-year-old freshman college student admitted for recurrent nausea and vomiting of 4 days duration. She was started on antiemetic medication and intravenous fluids, but her symptoms persisted, and on the third hospital day she underwent upper GI endoscopy with gastric biopsy. The results of the study were reported as negative, but the patient continued to suffer severe nausea and vomiting, requiring significant fluid and electrolyte replacement. After being examined by several consultants, on the eighth hospital day she finally had a pregnancy test which proved positive.

To paraphrase Orwell, some symptoms are equal, but some are more equal than others. The symptoms of anorexia, nausea, and vomiting are, by themselves, generally too nonspecific to be of much diagnostic help. When they are unaccompanied by other major complaints, they seldom point to the presence of serious disease—and therefore rarely call for investigation.

The most common causes of solitary anorexia with or without accompanying nausea and vomiting would include, in addition to pregnancy and febrile illnesses, anxiety, depression, and various other psychophysiological states including the much rarer but serious condition, anorexia nervosa. Other common causes easily disclosed by history would, of course, include drugs, chemicals, and toxic agents, in particular alcohol, amphetamines, narcotics, digitalis, antibiotics, and the wide variety of chemotherapeutic agents.

It is obvious, however, that because anorexia, nausea, and vomiting are usually secondary or subsidiary symptoms, they can be seen in almost any category of disease, e.g. neurological, infectious, cardiac, pulmonary, neoplastic, metabolic (uremia, ketoacidosis, hypoadrenalism, hypercalcemia, etc.), as well as in the wide spectrum of intraabdominal disease.

Many of these latter conditions already have been discussed in this chapter under abdominal pain, a much more specific and important clinical symptom. It is appropriate merely to remind the reader that most of these conditions causing acute, recurrent, or chronic abdominal or pelvic pain or the gamut of other intraabdominal symptoms will be accompanied during some part of their clinical course with varying degrees or combinations of anorexia, nausea, or vomiting.

Summary

1. Anorexia, nausea, and vomiting *by themselves* are nonspecific and generally poor indicators of serious conditions. Major causes to be considered in this setting are pregnancy, psychophysiological conditions, exposure to drugs, or acute viral or other infectious illness. A good history and clinical assessment of the patient will generally obviate the need for imaging or other studies in patients without other significant complaints.

2. Because anorexia, nausea, and vomiting are principally subsidiary symptoms, the strongest clues to a diagnosis and therefore possible indications for imaging investigation are given by accompanying signs and symptoms. Among these coexistent clinical findings, the most important would include abdominal pain, chest pain, headache, and neurological findings.

14/ GI Bleeding: Hematemesis and Melena

> *Words are like leaves, and where they most abound,*
> *The fruit of sense beneath is seldom found.*
>
> *Alexander Pope*

Many words indeed have been written about GI bleeding. GI hemorrhage presents a recurring diagnostic challenge, but unlike most other symptoms, a much more urgent one. The vomiting of blood or the passage of blood in the stools may occur in patients with preexisting GI symptoms or may appear with dramatic suddenness in asymptomatic patients. For immediate management of the GI bleeding patient, because we already know *what*, the appropriate questions should be *where* and *how fast*. Thus, aside from bleeding disorders, the treatment and outcome of GI bleeding depend more on determining the site and rate rather than the precise etiology of hemorrhage.

Because treatment depends on whether bleeding arises in the upper or lower GI tract, it is crucial at the outset to determine this as soon as possible. The ligament of Treitz, at the junction of the lower duodenum and jejunum, is the landmark that divides the upper intestinal tract from the lower. Clinical differentiation between upper and lower GI hemorrhage calls for some remarks on terminology.

Hematemesis, the vomiting of blood, whether fresh and red or "coffee grounds," always indicates upper GI bleeding and occurs in about one-third of such patients. The appearance of vomitus, whether coffee grounds or bright red, is of little value in determining whether the actual site of bleeding is esophageal, gastric, duodenal, or, rarely, oro-nasopharyngeal.

Melena, of course, indicates the passage of black, usually tarry, often gummy stools. *Hematochezia* is the correct term to describe passage of red blood in the stools, though *melena* is occasionally used inaccurately to describe any bleeding in the stool regardless of color. True melena most often indicates a lesion distal to the pylorus, usually a duodenal ulcer, but lesions as low as the distal colon may rarely cause melena in the presence of delayed bowel motility.

Bright blood in the stool usually means a bleeding point relatively low in the intestinal tract, generally in the jejunum or below, but this too is not an infallible sign (1). It has been demonstrated, for example, that fresh blood introduced into the stomach may appear as bright red blood in the stool. The color of the stool, whether tarry, bright, or dark red, is thus more dependent on the time blood remains in the intestinal tract than on the level from which it arises (2). To the extent that motility is not significantly altered, however, time in the GI tract *is* dependent on the level of bleeding. Certainly, the appearance of the stool is not as invariable an indicator of bleeding site as is the presence of hematemesis or coffee grounds vomitus, but one will be right more than 90% of the time if he regards bright or dark red stools as signifying lower GI and tarry stools upper GI bleeding. A review of the prevalences of major causes of upper and lower GI hemorrhage is appropriate here.

Causes of Upper GI Bleeding

Table 6.14.1 gives the site of upper GI bleeding in 1500 patients studied by Palmer (3) with the so-called "vigorous diagnostic approach" using ice water lavage of the stomach promptly after the history and physical examination, followed immediately by upper EGD. The author claimed a "diagnostic accuracy" of 87% in a subset of 650 patients. It is important to note that more than 93% of patients with upper GI bleeding had duodenal or gastric ulcers, esophageal varices, gastritis, esophagitis, or Mallory-Weiss syndrome, whereas only 2.5% had malignancies. These percentages are in close agreement with other series, for example, the 1981 survey of the American Society of Gastroenterology (Fleischer, 4) and the even larger series of Sugawa (Table 6.14.2) (5). From these published series and others, the reader should be satisfied that the combined rare causes of all upper GI hemorrhage including neoplasms listed in Palmer's (3), Fleischer's (4), and Sugawa's (5) series averaged less than 3–5% of all cases.

Table 6.14.1.   Bleeding Sources Among 1500 Patients with Active Bleeding Studied by the Vigorous Diagnostic Approach

Source	Number of patients
Duodenal ulcer	406
Esophagogastric varices	295
Erosive gastritis	193
Gastric ulcer	186
Erosive esophagitis	109
Mallory-Weiss syndrome	77
Stomal (anastomotic) ulcer	47
Gastric carcinoma	21
Esophageal ulcer	10
Rendu-Osler-Weber disease	8
Gastric sarcoma	7
Esophageal carcinoma	5
Gastric leiomyoma	5
"Cirsoid" aneurysm into stomach	3
Gastric leukemia	2
Gastric and duodenal ulcer	2
Mucosal prolapse into esophagus	2
Duodenal leiomyoma	2
Liver, posttraumatic	2
Aortoesophageal fistula	2
Gastric biopsy site	2
Adenoma at gastroenteric stoma	2
Ulcer in duodenal diverticulum	1
Metastasis to stomach	1
Duodenal ulcer to varices	1
Gastric sarcoidosis	1
Aortic aneurysm into duodenum	1
Splenic artery aneurysm into gastric stump	1
Splenic artery aneurysm into duodenum	1
Pancreatic pseudocyst into stomach	1
Undetermined or wrong	104

Reprinted by permission from Palmer ED: *Upper Gastrointestinal Hemorrhage*. Springfield, Ill: Charles C Thomas (1970: 399).

Important historical features of the six most common conditions and two rare conditions causing upper GI bleeding are listed in Table 6.14.3 (6).

Causes of Lower GI Bleeding

In lower GI tract hemorrhage, the principal causes are also few in number. In Table 6.14.4 are listed the etiologies in an earlier series of *angiographic* studies (1). In recent years the situation has changed markedly. Angiodysplastic lesions, really arteriovenous malformations (AVMs), more properly "vascular ectasias" of the colon, now appear to be much more common in some series than bleeding diverticulae (7). Other authors claim each condition causes an equal number, about 40%, of all cases of lower intestinal bleeding. A list of common and uncommon causes of lower GI bleeding in the elderly is presented in Table 6.14.5 (8). Important and obvious diagnoses which should not be missed are anorectal conditions and the rare cases of infectious diarrheas presenting with brisk bleeding. Table 6.14.6 lists historical features helpful in diagnosing various rare causes of lower GI bleeding. In fact, clinical infor-

Table 6.14.2. Endoscopic Observations on 3549 Patients with Upper Gastrointestinal Bleeding

Source	Total no. of lesions	(%)	No. of patients	(%)
Erosive gastritis (acute mucosal lesions)	1813	(35.4)	1174	(33.1)
Gastric ulcer	723	(14.1)	637	(17.9)
Duodenal ulcer	607	(11.8)	520	(14.5)
Varices	712	(13.9)	448	(12.6)
Mallory-Weiss tear	404	(7.9)	362	(10.2)
Esophagitis	322	(6.3)	184	(5.2)
Marginal ulcer	60	(1.2)	56	(1.6)
Tumor	68	(1.3)	55	(1.5)
Duodenitis	304	(5.9)	51	(1.4)
Miscellaneous	115	(2.2)	62	(1.7)
Totals	5128	100	3549	100

Reprinted by permission from *Surgical Clinics of North America* (1989;69(6):1169).

Table 6.14.3. Upper GI Bleeding: Historical Features

Feature	Possible cause or source
ASA, NSAID use	Gastric or duodenal ulcer, gastritis
Epigastric burning, pain	Peptic ulcer
Vomiting	Mallory-Weiss tear
Alcohol use	Gastritis
Ingestion of K+, iron, vitamin C, quinidine, tetracycline	Esophagitis or esophageal ulcer
Liver disease	Varices, congestive gastropathy
Aortic graft	Aorto-enteric fistula
Epistaxis	Osler-Weber-Rendu

Reprinted by permission of *Geriatrics* (1989;44(2):25–40).

Table 6.14.4. Causes of Lower GI Bleeding When Extravasation Is Noted at Angiography

Cause	Percentage of patients
Diverticulosis	70
Angiodysplasia	10
Peptic ulcer	5
Meckel's diverticulum	3
Neoplasms	3
Vascular-enteric fistula	2
Jejunal diverticulum	2
Other	5

Courtesy of Walter Pederson, MD, Medical Grand Rounds, Southwestern Medical School, September 17, 1981.
Reprinted by permission from Blacklaw. *Signs and Symptoms*. Philadelphia: J. B. Lippincott (1983:399).

Table 6.14.5. Differential Diagnosis of Lower GI Bleeding in the Elderly

Common	Uncommon
Diverticula	Inflammatory bowel disease
Vascular ectasias	Infectious colitis
Ischemia	Radiation colitis
Polyps	Rectal fissures
Cancer	Rectal ulcers
Hemorrhoids	

Reprinted by permission from *Geriatrics* (1989;44(3):49–60).

Table 6.14.6. Lower GI Bleeding: Historical Features

Feature	Possible cause or source
Diverticulosis	Diverticulum
Aortic stenosis	Vascular ectasias
Change of bowel habits	Colon cancer, inflammatory bowel disease
Vascular disease	Ischemia
Abdominal pain followed by bloody diarrhea	Ischemia
Inflammatory bowel disease	Inflammatory bowel disease flare
Diarrhea with mucus, scant blood	Inflammatory bowel disease
Radiation colitis	Radiation therapy
Rectal pain	Rectal fissure, thrombosed hemorrhoid
Dripping blood	Perirectal
Bright red blood, streaks on stool	Left colon

Reprinted by permission from *Geriatrics* (1989;44(3):49–60).

Table 6.14.7. Final Diagnosis for 80 Patients with Severe Hematochezia

Lesion Site		No. of patients (%)	
Colonic			59 (74)
Angiomata		24 (30)	
Diverticulosis		13 (17)	
Active bleeding	6 (8)		
Adherent clot	7 (9)		
Polyps or cancer		9 (11)	
Focal colitis or ulcers		7 (9)	
Rectal lesions		3 (4)	
Bleeding polyp stalk		2 (2)	
Endometriosis		1 (1)	
Upper gastrointestinal			9 (11)
Small bowel[a]			7 (9)
No site found			5 (6)

[a]A diagnosis of presumed small bowel site of bleeding was made when panendoscopy and colonoscopy were negative, but fresh blood or clots or both were coming through the ileocecal valve.
Reprinted by permission from Jensen DM, Machicado GA. Diagnosis and treatment of severe hematochezia: the role of urgent colonoscopy after purge. *Gastroenterology* (1988;95:1569).

mation usually is not helpful in distinguishing the two principal causes of bleeding, diverticulae and vascular ectasias, but this has little practical relevance in management. Final diagnoses for 80 patients with severe hematochezia are listed in Table 6.14.7 (9). Note that in 11% the bleeding was from the upper GI tract and 9% from the small intestine, whereas in 6% no site was found.

Risk Factors and Management of the GI Bleeder

A crucial fact should be kept in mind when treating patients presenting with acute GI hemorrhage: *In approximately 85% of all patients the bleeding will stop spontaneously* (10). For this reason, it is essential to distinguish the low- from the high-risk patient. In the latter case, the diagnostic and therapeutic approach depend critically on identifying the one patient out of seven likely to bleed or rebleed massively and who requires urgent intervention.

Upper GI bleeding is a common problem and was reported in 1981 to have resulted in more than 300,000 hospitalizations annually in this country (11). The total all-listed diagnoses of both upper and lower GI hemorrhage in the NCHS statistics

Table 6.14.8. Causes of Bleeding on 73 Examinations in 64 Patients

Erosive gastritis		23	32%
Chronic peptic ulcer		18	25%
Gastric ulcer	13		
Duodenal ulcer	5		
Esophagitis		17	24%
Carcinoma		6	8%
Mallory-Weiss tear		2	3%
Duodenitis		1	1%
Normal		6	7%
Total		73	100%

Reprinted from Ref. 14.

amounted to approximately 769,000 in 1990 (12). The most significant indices of risk are the rate of bleeding reflected clinically in the amount of blood replacement required and the combination of patient age and presence of chronic medical disease. The typical high-risk patient would be over age 65 and, in the vernacular, with a "comorbid" condition, i.e. cardiovascular, kidney, lung, or other major organ system disease, likely to be acutely compromised by sudden blood loss.

Surprisingly, the incidence of bleeding ulcer in the elderly is twice that in the young and accounts for more than half of all deaths in the older group (6). Yet more than half of these patients have no history of previous peptic ulcer disease. Bleeding from the upper GI tract, because it is more often severe, is usually a more serious clinical problem with a higher overall mortality rate than lower tract bleeding.

Greatly increased risk is seen with gastric (as opposed to duodenal ulcer) site of hemorrhage, with a mortality rate of 41% in the elderly (in whom it is much more common), compared with 14% for bleeding gastric ulcer in younger patients. Bleeding from esophageal varices also has an extremely high mortality rate in the 50% range (6). The need for surgery, a reflection of the seriousness of the bleeding, is associated with a vastly increased mortality rate from GI bleeding. Moreover, there is a striking increase in mortality when massive upper GI bleeding first occurs after a patient is hospitalized. In this setting, the mortality rate was reported as 70% compared to 22% in outpatients who were seen because of bleeding (13). It is not surprising that in this same study mortality was higher in those patients with more rapid bleeding; among patients who presented with acute bleeding for less than 12 hours, 37% died, compared to 22% of those whose bleeding was present longer than 12 hours.

In the elderly, erosive mucosal lesions, either gastritis or esophagitis, are even more common than ulcer as a cause of hematemesis and melena. In Tables 6.14.8 and 6.14.9 the causes of bleeding and chemical agents associated with erosive gastritis and bleeding from any site are displayed. Alcohol, aspirin, and other nonsteroidal and steroidal analgesic and antiinflammatory drugs were the principal offenders (14). In Danne et al.'s study (15) predisposing factors for GI bleeding in the elderly were alcohol (56%), smoking (42%), and medication (29%) (steroidal and nonsteroidal antiinflammatory drugs).

A brief but useful clinical guide is given by Cootout (10) in his excellent review. The typical high-risk profile bleeder ". . . would be an elderly hospitalized patient in whom unexpected bleeding develops or an outpatient with acute bleeding of short duration and accompanying symptoms of volume depletion."

Table 6.14.9.   Chemical Agents Associated with Bleeding from Erosive Gastritis

Alcohol	6
NSAID	6
Aspirin	5
Bile	4
Steroids	1
Nil	1
Total	23

Chemical Agents Associated with Bleeding from Any Site in 43 Patients

NSAID	17
Aspirin	13
Alcohol	8
Bile	4
Heparin	1
Warfarin	1
Steroids	1

Reprinted from Ref. 14.

Medical Imaging in GI Bleeding: General Remarks

Acute GI bleeding is a difficult problem in medical imaging precisely because it must be "seen" at its source to be identified. But this is indeed the dilemma: GI hemorrhage is unpredictable and capricious in its behavior, speeding up, slowing down, stopping, or starting without warning. Thus, how or when to investigate the low-risk patient who has had only moderate bleeding that has already stopped is only one of several controversial issues to consider.

Conventional radiological studies with barium have little, if any, place in the diagnosis of acute GI hemorrhage. However, there are three other principal imaging approaches to the problem of acute upper or lower GI bleeding: endoscopy, arteriography, and bleeding scintigraphy using labeled red cells, each with advantages and disadvantages. The choice of these modalities, alone or in combination, raises difficult questions over their utility, timing, and effectiveness. Diagnostic precision is like Somerset Maugham's remark about the perfection Americans expect in a wife but the British want only in a butler—unrealistic at best. Our efforts should be concerned less with discovering an etiology than in establishing as soon as possible the source and rate of bleeding. It is axiomatic that the immediate treatment of the GI bleeder, i.e. replacing blood loss and maintaining the circulation, always takes precedence over any imaging investigation with the possible exception of urgent arteriography before emergency surgery.

We have two related questions to address: What study or studies are most effective in what clinical setting, and the important corollary, what are the comparative merits—and risks—of various methods of imaging specifically in terms of patient outcome?

Endoscopy in Acute GI Bleeding
UPPER GI BLEEDING

Upper EGD has been advocated for all patients with upper GI bleeding on the assumption that early diagnosis will improve patient outcome. A careful randomized, controlled trial suggests this is not the case (16). When two groups of 100 and 106 upper GI bleeding patients were assigned to routine vs. nonroutine endoscopy, there were no significant differences in overall hospital deaths, bleeding recurrences, number of transfusions required, deaths after recurrent bleeding, or duration of hospital stay. Furthermore, when the two groups were followed for 12 months after discharge, there was no difference in the incidence of further GI bleeding, number of hemorrhage-related deaths, and frequency of surgery.

Since this study was done, there has been increasing interest in the therapeutic use of endoscopic techniques to control bleeding. A recent Consensus Development Conference on therapeutic endoscopy and bleeding ulcers was sponsored by the NIH to consider several questions, among which were the following (17):

1. Which patients with bleeding ulcers are at risk for rebleeding and thus emergency surgery?
2. How effective and how safe is endoscopic hemostatic therapy?
3. Which bleeding should be treated?

The conclusions, as with many such consensus meetings, were convoluted and qualified, reflecting the uncertainty and disagreements of literally dozens of experts. The answer to question 1 was that "both clinical and endoscopic features are predictive" of the risk of rebleeding and thus emergency surgery. The crucial question 3, which bleeding patients should be treated, was discussed in vague terms of the high-risk bleeder, but the risk and effectiveness of endoscopic vs. surgical intervention were not addressed. This is because requisite controlled, randomized studies have not been done and are unlikely to be undertaken in the immediate future. Clearly, therapeutic endoscopy for massive GI bleeding, like surgery, is fraught with unavoidable risk and requires endoscopists highly skilled in the technique. At the present time, the risk of precipitating bleeding with therapy "is variable but has been as high as 20%" (17).

Although EGD continues to be widely accepted as the principal diagnostic approach in the upper GI bleeder, medical authorities still recognize areas of controversy (18). First, do all bleeders need endoscopy? This is doubtful in those 85% of patients who stop bleeding within the first few hours. Yet, which patients will rebleed, and which of these massively? Another question is whether EGD should be performed in the acutely bleeding patient. Most studies suggest that the diagnostic accuracy of EGD remains high for the first 12–24 hours after a bleeding episode, so that generally there should be no urgency in performing EGD until the clinical status can be determined and the patient stabilized. Certainly, EGD, because of its risk, is generally contraindicated in the unstable patient, and most authorities agree that it should be delayed until vital signs have been stabilized after adequate blood replacement. Massive bleeding is another setting where controversy abounds. If the patient is exsanguinating, endoscopy can follow induction of anesthesia just before surgery, but it is in the massively bleeding patient that endoscopy is most often unsuccessful in identifying a bleeding source. Emergency endoscopy in this circumstance is not for the inexperienced. With experienced endoscopists the procedure is accompanied by 0.5% major complications (perforation, aspiration, and bleeding) 0.4% minor complications, and significant fatality (one in 773 in the ASGE series) (19). Furthermore, if the bleeding is severe and surgery seems likely, angiography is the more accurate, safer, and therefore preferable study.

Again, to address the main question, *does endoscopy affect the clinical outcome*, we can only quote Peterson and his colleagues (16): "Current studies suggest that it does not. This may be more a reflection on the inadequacies of medical therapy and the dangers of nonelective surgical treatment of bleeding patients who are severely ill than on the usefulness of more accurate endoscopic detection of the bleeding source. *If endoscopic or pharmacologic methods of stopping bleeding prove to be safe and effective in controlled trials, more accurate endoscopic diagnosis may indeed affect the outcome favorably*" (emphasis added). These studies, to our knowledge, have yet to be done.

LOWER GI BLEEDING

With acute lower GI bleeding arising from the colon, colonscopy is the most direct and effective means of visualizing hemorrhaging mucosal lesions. Furthermore, therapeutic colonoscopy is more established, technically easier, and more effective than endoscopic treatment in the upper GI tract. Colonoscopy, however, like EGD, suffers unavoidable limitations. If the bleeding ceases or continues slowly, colonoscopy is the procedure of choice, but in the presence of brisk lower intestinal bleeding, the method often fails, because it is difficult to visualize the colonic mucosa through a blood-filled field. Moreover, in a significant number of patients with lower GI bleeding the source is proximal to the cecum, usually in the small bowel, and therefore not visualizable with the colonoscope. In addition, a large number of patients with vascular ectasias will be missed by colonoscopy. Even those ectasias visualized by angiography, however, cannot be said to be a source of bleeding unless they demonstrate extravasation (vide infra). Because upper GI bleeding is said to be the third most common cause of brisk rectal bleeding (after diverticulae and vascular ectasias), it is incumbent in doubtful cases to exclude an upper GI source of bleeding with nasogastric aspiration (8). Yet, in one series of 100 patients with 144 episodes of lower GI bleeding, in 58 the bleeding was bright red in color, whereas in 42 it was black and tarry (20).

Arteriography in Acute GI Bleeding
UPPER GI BLEEDING

Angiography is diagnostic of a bleeding source *only in those patients in whom active bleeding is occurring during the actual procedure*. Because each contrast injection lasts only 20–30 seconds and GI bleeding is intermittent, changing from minute to minute, angiography can monitor bleeding only during a brief period of time. Furthermore, angiography will identify areas of bleeding in about 65% of patients and then only in those *with active hemorrhage occurring at greater than 1 ml/minute* (21, 22). We stress that convincing proof of a bleeding source rests on the identification of a lesion *which shows extravasation during angiography*. The demonstration of angiodysplasia, for example, can be an incidental finding and may occur in patients with other hemorrhagic lesions such as Meckel's diverticulum and small bowel tumors. Experience also has shown it is impossible to be certain about the source of GI hemorrhage when there is more than one likely lesion (23).

In summary, celiac, superior, or inferior mesenteric angiography for GI bleeding is indicated *only when there is convincing clinical evidence of rapid and continuing hemorrhage*, and with the expectation that *identification of a bleeding site will determine type of therapy*, either embolic or surgical intervention. Many angiographers will not perform the study unless the nuclear GI bleeding study is done first.

The Radionuclide Study for GI Bleeding

In order to employ invasive methods such as endoscopy and arteriography effectively, the clinician must determine whether active GI bleeding is occurring at the time of the study. Because GI hemorrhage, even massive hemorrhage, as we have pointed out, is usually intermittent, *an effective imaging method should allow the acquisition of information over a significant period of time*. This became possible with the development of radionuclide studies for GI bleeding. Technetium-99m-labeled sulfur colloid or autologous Tc-99m-labeled red blood cells (RBCs) have been used for more than a decade in the imaging of both upper and lower GI bleeding (24, 25). The labeled RBC method is now preferred by most workers because of persistence of the labeled cells in the circulation over long periods of time, permitting sequential imaging of patients up to 24 hours.

This means effectively that a "physiological window" is now provided through which the occurrence of bleeding can be followed for periods of time sufficient to identify the source and presence of active hemorrhage. One of the most useful applications of the GI bleeding scintiscan is in demonstrating that bleeding has ceased, i.e. *in excluding the presence of active bleeding*. In the significant group of presumed active GI bleeders with a negative scintigraphic study, one can conclude that bleeding has stopped and predict that neither angiography nor endoscopy is likely to show active hemorrhage.

This was confirmed in an important study of 100 patients with a history of melena or maroon or bright red stools. Among 62% with abnormal studies the Tc-RBC study accurately located the site of hemorrhage in 83% of patients. When the test was carried out for only 1 hour, only 15% were positive, but 90% were positive between 4 and 14 hours, with a small number requiring 24 hours to visualize. Figure 6.14.1 shows the cumulative positive scintiscans with time, clearly demonstrating the intermittent nature of acute GI bleeding, and demonstrates why the procedure was more sensitive than angiography in detecting bleeding sources. Winzelberg et al. (26) stated that "a negative radionuclide study . . . with presumed active bleeding is good evidence that angiography will not detect the site of hemorrhage. Thus, emergency angiography can be deferred and elective angiography or endoscopy can be performed after the patient is adequately prepared." The greater the transfusion requirements the sooner the study became positive. Serial sequential images are required to establish a bleeding site, because intestinal blood may move from areas of extravasation either proximally or distally. However, "the finding of increasing intensity and distal movement of extravasated labeled red cells are criteria for active bleeding" (26). The labeled RBC method is extremely sensitive, because colonic bleeding rates of less than 0.04 ml/minute have been detected within 55 minutes in dogs (27).

Although the usefulness of the bleeding scintiscan is unquestioned in the lower GI tract, its application in upper GI bleeding has been limited. There are many reasons for this. First, because so few acute upper GI bleeders are referred for bleeding scintiscans, to our knowledge no comparative controlled studies have been performed. This is due as often to the enthusiasm of the endoscopist as to the unavailability of emergency nuclear studies in many hospitals. Furthermore, if the bleeding scintiscan is to be done correctly, it is a time-consuming procedure, and it is not always desirable—let alone safe—to keep the acute GI bleeder in the nuclear medicine depart-

Time Interval to Positivity of Tc-99m Labeled RBC's
In Patients with Positive GI Bleeding Scans (26)

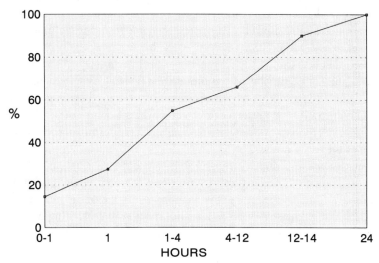

Figure 6.14.1. Time interval to positivity of Tc-99m labeled RBCs in patients with positive GI bleeding scans (26).

ment or transfer him back and forth from the clinical unit over a period of several hours. For the unstable patient imaging is seldom possible; few intensive care units are equipped with a gamma camera.

For the above reasons, GI bleeding scintigraphy remains sadly underused in today's invasive climate. The procedure is probably the single most helpful imaging study available for most acute GI bleeding patients, and under ideal conditions should be the procedure of first choice in all but the massive bleeder. But the ingrained habits of clinicians and persistent logistical problems make it unlikely the situation will improve in the near future. An encouraging note has been the establishment of specialized units for the care of acute GI bleeders in Europe and Australia, a development that may lead to similar changes in this country.

Summary of Diagnostic Approach to Acute GI Bleeding

Tables 6.14.10–6.14.13 summarize principal advantages and disadvantages of the three major imaging studies for massive and nonmassive upper and lower GI bleeding. The tables are our subjective estimates, and we make no claim for precision, particularly for the derived arithmetical "scores." Nevertheless, they may be used as guides to choice of procedure. Because even in massive GI bleeding it is not always possible to decide clinically whether the bleeding has indeed stopped, the row "determination of active bleeding" has been included in each chart. As previously outlined in the text, labeled RBC scintigraphy, *when logistically feasible*, is the best overall method for establishing whether GI hemorrhage is active.

Table 6.14.10. Imaging in Moderately[a] Severe Upper GI Bleeding: Comparative (Theoretical) Advantages and Disadvantages of Upper Endoscopy, Arteriography, and Labeled-RBC Scintigraphy Graded on a Scale of −2 to 4+

	Upper GI Endoscopy (EGD)[b]	Arteriography	Scintigraphy
Sensitivity for active bleeding	1–2 +	1–2 +	3–4 +
Specificity (bleeding site)	1–3 +	3–4 +	3–4 +
Risk	− 2	− 1	0
Therapeutic applications	1–2 +	1–2 +	0
Theoretical score	1–5	4–7	6–8

[a]With *any* severe or massive upper or lower GI bleeding, the patient should be sent immediately for arteriography.
[b]Endoscopy useless in detecting small bowel bleeding source.

Table 6.14.11. Imaging in Less Severe Upper GI Bleeding: Comparative (Theoretical) Advantages and Disadvantages of Upper Endoscopy, Arteriography, and Labeled RBC Scintigraphy

	Upper GI Endoscopy (EGD)[a]	Arteriography	Scintigraphy
Sensitivity for active bleeding	1–2 +	0–1 +	3–4 +
Specificity (bleeding site)	2–3 +	3–4 +	3–4 +
Risk	− 2	− 1	0
Therapeutic application	1–2 +	1–2 +	0
Theoretical score	2–5	3–6	6–8

[a]Endoscopy useless in detecting small bowel bleeding source.

Table 6.14.12. Imaging in Moderately Severe[a] Lower GI Bleeding: Comparative (Theoretical) Advantages and Disadvantages of Colonoscopy, Arteriography, and Labeled RBC Scintigraphy

	Colonoscopy[b]	Arteriography	Scintigraphy
Sensitivity for active bleeding	2–3 +	1–2 +	3–4 +
Specificity bleeding site	1–3 +	3–4 +	3–4 +
Risk	− 1	− 1	0
Therapeutic applications	1–2 +	1–2 +	0
Theoretical score	3–7	4–7	6–8

[a]With *any* severe or massive upper or lower GI bleeding, the patient should be sent immediately for arteriography.
[b]Colonoscopy useless in detecting small bowel bleeding source.

Table 6.14.13. Imaging in Less Severe Lower GI Bleeding: Comparative (Theoretical) Advantages and Disadvantages of Colonoscopy, Arteriography, and Labeled RBC Scintigraphy

	Colonoscopy[a]	Arteriography	Scintigraphy
Sensitivity for active bleeding	1–2 +	0–1 +	3–4 +
Specificity	1–3 +	0–1 +	3–4 +
Risk	− 1	− 1	0
Therapeutic applications	1–2 +	1–2 +	0
Theoretical score	3–6	0–3	6–8

[a]Endoscopy useless in detecting small bowel bleeding source.

Sensitivity of scintigraphy in the detection of active GI bleeding is superior to both angiography and endoscopy. Furthermore, scintigraphy has better overall specificity than endoscopy (in determining site of bleeding) simply because the entire GI tract can be visualized, not just the proximal and terminal portions. However, unlike angiography of endoscopy, scintigraphy has no therapeutic application in treating the GI bleeder. Regardless of one's emphasis or prejudice, the charts are meant to give a general perspective on the approach to imaging the acute GI bleeder. They cannot be used as a recipe, that is, as an algorithm, because each patient at the outset has an unpredictable bleeding pattern. It might be possible, however, to do better than create subjective scores, that is, calculate a figure of merit for each study in each of the four tables—if only it were possible to get a consensus from unbiased studies and experts. What follows is our best effort to summarize a reasonable diagnostic strategy in the GI bleeder.

MASSIVE UPPER AND LOWER GI BLEEDING

1. The patient must be stabilized clinically by blood replacement before embarking on any diagnostic studies. Emergent upper or lower GI endoscopy is seldom indicated diagnostically in massive bleeding but may well be vital if the endoscopist is trained and equipped to undertake therapeutic procedures.

2. If the bleeding is not massive clinically, Tc-RBC scintigraphy is unsurpassed in determining an uncertain source of bleeding and, most important, in establishing if bleeding may have actually have ceased.

3. All patients who remain unstable for more than 4 hours, who require more than 4–6 units of blood in 6 hours, or in whom bleeding is massive and continuing, i.e. any patient in whom emergency surgery is contemplated, should immediately be sent for *arteriography, not endoscopy.* An alternative strategy, only in the event of nondiagnostic arteriography in an exsanguinating patient, is to perform upper and/or lower endoscopy after anesthesia is induced just before surgery.

NONMASSIVE UPPER AND LOWER GI BLEEDING

The bleeding scintiscan is the preferred first study in order to establish the presence or absence of nonmassive active bleeding. Second, scintigraphy can provide a road map for the angiographer, i.e. indicate which vessel is to be cannulated, should angiography subsequently become necessary.

Summary

1. With massive, life-threatening GI hemorrhage, the patient should go directly to arteriography for determination of the source of bleeding and possible therapeutic intervention (Pitressin or gelfoam embolization). A few patients may be candidates for therapeutic upper or lower GI endoscopy when the source of bleeding is obvious and in centers where suitably trained therapeutic endoscopists are available.

2. With moderately or less severe upper or lower GI bleeding, that is, in all other cases of GI bleeding, the best initial imaging study is the Tc-RBC scintiscan, if this is available. The bleeding scintiscan should be used before arteriography in all cases of nonmassive bleeding, because it establishes two facts: (a) whether in fact there is active GI bleeding; and (b) if there is bleeding, its source in the GI tract. Only in light of this knowledge can the arteriographer decide whether arteriography is necessary, and if so, which vessel to cannulate.

3. In general, EGD, except where therapy is contemplated, is of doubtful use in upper GI bleeding. Colonoscopy may be useful in the occasional case of acute lower GI bleeding. Overall, the GI bleeding scintiscan is the imaging procedure of first choice in all nonmassive GI bleeding.

REFERENCES

1. Schiff L. Hematemesis and Melena. In: Blacklow RS, ed. MacBryde's signs and symptoms. 6th ed. Philadelphia: J. B. Lippincott & Co., 1983:393–394.
2. Hilsman JH. The color of blood-containing feces following instillation of citrated blood at various levels of the small intestine. Gastroenterology 1950;15:131.
3. Palmer ED. Diagnosis of Upper Gastrointestinal Hemorrhage, Pub. 443, American Lecture Series. Springfield, Ill: Charles C. Thomas, 1961.
4. Fleischer D. Etiology and prevalence of severe persistent upper gastrointestinal bleeding. Gastroenterology 1983;84(3):538–543.
5. Sugawa C. Endoscopic diagnosis and treatment of upper gastrointestinal bleeding. Surg Clin North Amer 1989;69(6):1167–1183.
6. Rosen AM, Fleischer DE. Upper GI bleeding in the elderly: diagnosis and management. Geriatrics 1989;44(2):25–40.
7. Spencer J. Lower gastrointestinal bleeding. Br J Surg 1989;76(1):3–4.
8. Rosen AM, Fleischer DE. Lower GI bleeding: updated diagnosis and management. Geriatrics 1989;44(3):49–60.
9. Jensen DM, Machicado GA. Diagnosis and treatment of severe hematochezia: the role of urgent colonoscopy after purge. Gastroenterology 1988;95(6):1569–1574.
10. Gostout CJ. Acute gastrointestinal bleeding—a common problem revisited. Mayo Clin Proc 1988;63(6):596–604.
11. Cutler JA, Mendeloff AI. Upper gastrointestinal bleeding: nature and magnitude of the problem in the U.S. Dig Dis Sci 1981;26(suppl 7):90S–96S.
12. U.S. Department of Health and Human Services, U.S. Public Health Service, Centers for Disease Control, and the National Center for Health Statistics. National Hospital Discharge Survey (NHDS). Detailed diagnoses, procedures, days of care, diagnoses-related groups for patients discharged from short-stay hospitals. Public Use Data Diskettes, 1985–1990.
13. Chojkier M, Laine L, Conn HO, Lerner E: Predictors of outcome in massive upper gastrointestinal hemorrhage. J Clin Gastroenterol 1986;8(1):16–22.
14. Booker JA. Haematemesis and melaena in the elderly. Age Ageing 1983;13(1):49–54.
15. Danne PD, Gray BN, Bennett RC. Haematemesis and melaena at St. Vincent's hospital, Melbourne. Aust NZ J Surg 1984;54(3):257–263.
16. Peterson WL, Barnett CC, Smith HJ, Allen MH, Corbett DB. Routine early endoscopy in upper-gastrointestinal-tract bleeding. A randomized, controlled study. N Engl J Med 1981;304(16):925–929.
17. Anonymous. Therapeutic endoscopy and bleeding ulcers. Consensus conference. JAMA 1989;262(10):1369–1372.
18. Silverstein FE, Rubin CE. Gastrointestinal endoscopy. In: Petersdorf RG, Adams RG, Braunwald E, Isselbacher KJ, Martin JB, Wilson JD, eds. Harrison's Principles of Internal Medicine. 10th ed. New York: McGraw-Hill Book Co., 1983:1683–1685.
19. National ASGE Survey on upper gastrointestinal bleeding. Complications of endoscopy. Dig Dis 1981;26(suppl 7):55s–59s.
20. Ramanath HK, Hinshaw JR. Management and mismanagement of bleeding colonic diverticula. Arch Surg 1971;103(2):311–314.
21. Best EB, Teaford KA, Rader Jr FH. Angiography in chronic recurrent gastrointestinal bleeding: a nine-year study. Surg Clin North Am 1979;59(5):811–829.
22. Bar AH, DeLaurentis DA, Parry CE, Keohane RB. Angiography in the management of massive lower gastrointestinal tract hemorrhage. Surg Gynecol Obstet 1980;150(2):226–228.
23. Steger AC, Galland RB, Hemingway AP, Wood CB, Spencer J. Gastrointestinal haemorrhage from a second source in patients with colonic angiodysplasia. Br J Surg 1987;74(8):726–727.
24. Winzelberg GG, McKusick KA, Strauss HW, Waltman AC, Greenfield AJ. Evaluation of gastrointestinal bleeding by red blood cells labeled in vivo with technetium-99m. J Nucl Med 1979;20(10):1080–1086.
25. Alavi A, Dann RW, Baum S, Biery DN. Scintigraphic detection of acute gastrointestinal bleeding. Radiology 1977;124(3):753–756.

26. Winzelberg GG, McKusick KA, Froelich JW, Callahan RJ, Strauss HW. Detection of gastrointestinal bleeding with 99m-Tc-labeled red blood cells. Semin Nucl Med 1982;XII(2):139–146.
27. Thorne DA, Datz FL, Remley K, Christian PE. Bleeding rates necessary for detecting acute gastrointestinal bleeding with technetium-99m-labeled red blood cells in an experimental model. J Nucl Med 1987;28(4):514–520.

15/ Ascites and Effusions

> *It is the drawback of all sea-side places that half the landscape is unavailable for purposes of human locomotion, being covered by useless water.*
>
> *Norman Douglas*

Etiology

The causes of peritoneal and pleuropericardial fluid collections are so diverse as to defy listing, because they would include literally hundreds of conditions. Any broad etiological classification would have to include virtually all the main categories of disease such as metabolic, infectious, neoplastic, inflammatory, collagen-vascular, traumatic, etc., whereas an anatomical classification of causes would be virtually hopeless.

A few generalizations, however, may suffice. For example, in the younger age group, the most common causes of effusion in the thoracic cavity are infections, specifically the pneumonias, including tuberculosis and various forms of pleurisy. In the older patient neoplasia, congestive heart failure, and pulmonary embolism predominate.

In the abdomen, ascites is most commonly associated with portal hypertension, particularly in the patient with jaundice where the most common cause is hepatic cirrhosis. Other causes include the gamut of inflammatory or neoplastic conditions involving any intraabdominal organ, the peritoneum, or the lymphatics, plus mechanical problems such as bowel obstruction.

Diagnosis

Physical examination is an insensitive method for diagnosing the presence of pleural or abdominal fluid collections; ultrasonography is unsurpassed. Chest radiography is said to be capable of detecting less than 50 ml fluid in the thoracic cavity, but this is not always borne out in practice. Small amounts of fluid frequently can be detected on ultrasound that were completely missed on chest X-ray. The typical peritoneal haze seen on plain abdominal films of patients with ascites does not occur before significant accumulations of fluid, perhaps 1–2 liters, yet on abdominal ultrasound, it is possible to detect considerably less than the 300 ml fluid that was claimed for the method back in 1976 (1).

Because the prognosis of ascites or pleural effusion is dependent on the etiology, it is rare that the early diagnosis of these conditions contributes materially to overall clinical outcome. Still, because fluid has such a characteristic appearance on sonography, it is easy to recognize fluid in the gutters, subhepatic or hepatorenal space (Morrison's pouch), pelvis, or pleural cavity in patients undergoing ultrasonography. For example, in seriously ill patients one often finds early fluid collections at the lung bases or in the abdomen during sonography of the gall bladder or kidneys. The finding of unsuspected pleural or peritoneal fluid, therefore, comes as a clinical surprise and may lead to changes in diagnosis and management. Because small collections of pleural fluid or ascites can be so routinely detected on sonography, the *absence or disappearance* of fluid in the abdomen or lung bases is itself important clinical information.

Thoracentesis and Paracentesis

Ultrasound is enormously useful in assisting the physician performing diagnostic or therapeutic pleural and peritoneal taps. The depth, angle, and direction of the needle is accurately determined so that difficult and thus repeat taps can be largely avoided. This is particularly true in the thorax when fluid frequently becomes loculated, and it is difficult to locate a "pocket." Pleural biopsies also can be more safely performed when small effusions can be located and the risk of lung puncture is thereby avoided.

In the abdomen, ultrasonic guidance for ascites is less frequently required except in the presence of chronic disease or adherent bowel loops when blind paracentesis should be avoided. It goes without saying that ultrasonic guidance is useful in tapping *any* fluid collection in the abdominal, pelvic, or thoracic cavities, be it transudate, exudate, or pure pus.

In times past, of course, most pleural and peritoneal taps were done blindly and successfully without the help of ultrasonic guidance, but how many of these were technically unsuccessful or had to be repeated we have no way of knowing. Certainly, in the face of a significant pleural effusion or ascites, sonographic guidance would not be called for. In today's climate of litigation, however, it would seem prudent to use ultrasound in the questionable case.

REFERENCES

1. Goldberg BB. Ultrasonic evaluation of intraperitoneal fluid. JAMA 1976;253(22):2427–2430.

16/ Fever of Unknown Origin

The approach to the patient with FUO is not to bring on yet another barrage of tests, . . . nor to douse (him) with antimicrobials or to subject him to exploratory surgery, (without) clinical clues and only as a last resort. There is no substitute for observing the patient, talking to him and thinking about him.

Louis Weinstein (1)

Since antiquity, fever has been recognized as a cardinal sign of disease, but the measurement of temperature had to wait for the invention of the thermometer by Fahrenheit in 1720. Much later, in 1868 the classic treatise "On the temperature in disease" was published by Wunderlich, who recorded temperature variations in nearly 25,000 patients with more than 20 conditions.

Many differing criteria have been offered for fever of unknown origin (FUO), but we propose either of two definitions, one each from world authorities, differing literally in degree only. We leave the choice up to the reader. Louis Weinstein (1) defines

FUO as the presence of a rectal or oral temperature of 37.7 C (99.6–100 F) or greater that persists for 3 weeks or longer and adds ". . . the cause of which has not been elucidated by a searching historical inquiry, a minutely detailed physical examination, laboratory studies of blood and urine, and radiograph of the chest." Dr. Robert Petersdorf (2), who also has written extensively on the subject, defines FUO as "daily temperature elevations of at least 101, presence of fever for at least three weeks, and failure to make a diagnosis after one week of intelligent investigation, usually in the hospital."

The more rigid criteria of Petersdorf (2, 3) restricts his two major series to patients with significant organic diseases, whereas Weinstein and others include a large number of clinically benign fevers of unknown cause such as "steroid fever" of the late menstrual cycle, "essential oral hyperthermia," psychogenic and exercise fever, and cases of sensitization, "polymer" and zinc fume fever.

The clinical encounter always takes precedence over testing, and perhaps in no other category of signs and symptoms does it assume so much importance, a fact that both authors repeatedly emphasize in their writings. Yet today, patients continue to be subjected to staggering workups when a combination of common sense and clinical acumen might have avoided needless expensive, painful, and frequently hazardous testing. For example, the need for further investigation may be nullified by the finding of a mass or lymph node for biopsy, the discovery of old imaging studies, or the successful search for a wound infection in a postoperative patient. Still, FUO remains a difficult and frustrating clinical problem that can and usually does challenge our most spectacular diagnostic skills.

It is virtually impossible to estimate the prevalences of the various causes of FUO, particularly because the previously reported series were by necessity limited in numbers (2, 3). True FUO fulfilling the classic criteria of Weinstein or Petersdorf is decidedly a rare clinical occurrence. The changing relative incidence of various causes of FUO has been well documented (4). Five major diagnostic classifications were originally proposed in Petersdorf's original 1961 report of 100 patients (2), and 20 years later the same criteria, categories, and nearly the same number of patients were again studied (3). There were 5 diagnostic categories: infections, neoplasms, collagen and granulomatous disease, and a miscellaneous group of febrile illnesses, including among others, multiple pulmonary emboli, drug fever, and factitious fever.

In the 1961 report (2) the largest category was infectious followed by neoplastic and collagen disease, which made up 70% of the series. This changed in some significant respects in the 1980 series, which is summarized in Table 6.16.1, and in the 1961 series, Table 6.16.2. Table 6.16.3 shows diseases that were rare or not seen in 1960. In both 1960 and in 1980 about 10% of the patients remained undiagnosed.

Of particular interest is that in both series there were 11 cases with intraabdominal abscess, and that in the later series the only three deaths attributable to infection were in this category. Most deaths, of course, occurred in the group with malignancy. In the 1961 series the authors felt that almost 40% of those who recovered did so only because the exact causes of their diseases were discovered. A surprising fact, however, was that despite the unavailability of present day imaging technologies in the early study, the combination of tissue biopsy and laparotomy was required just as often in the second series 20 years later to make a diagnosis. It is interesting to speculate on the likely incidence of disease were a large series of FUO patients to be studied today. Undoubtedly, we are seeing a changing spectrum of disease, but AIDS

Table 6.16.1. Diagnostic Categories

	1980 Series		1960 Series	
	No.	%	No.	%
Infections	32	30	36	36
Neoplasms	33	31	19	19
Collagen diseases	9	9	15	15
Granulomas	8	8	4	4
Miscellaneous	10	10	19	19
No dx	13	12	7	7
Total	105	100	100	100

Reprinted by permission from Larson EB, Featherstone HJ, Petersdorf RG. Fever of undetermined origin. *Medicine* (1982; 61(5)269–291).

Table 6.16.2. Diseases Prominent in 1960 but Sharply Decreased or Absent in 1980

Tuberculosis
SBE
Rheumatic fever
SLE
Familial Mediterranean fever

Reprinted by permission from Larson EB, Featherstone HJ, Petersdorf RG. Fever of undetermined origin. *Medicine* (1982; 61(5):269–291).

Table 6.16.3. Disease Not Seen or Rare in 1960 but Prominent in 1980

CMV
Osteomyelitis
Sinusitis
Malignant histiocytosis
Still's disease
Crohn's disease
Hematomas

Reprinted by permission from Larson EB, Featherstone HJ, Petersdorf RG. Fever of undetermined origin. *Medicine* (1982; 61(5):269–291).

largely accounts for many of the bizarre and formerly almost unknown conditions of a decade ago. Because the HIV test is available, however, it is doubtful whether most cases of secondary *Pneumocystis* pneumonia, avian tuberculosis, and other rare infectious or neoplastic syndromes seen in patients with AIDS today would fulfill the criteria of FUO.

Imaging the Patient with FUO

Unlike other signs/symptoms categories we have discussed, the fact of disease prevalence is difficult to take into account with FUO. Despite the small number of principal categories, the large number of possible conditions and disease sites make any facile generalizations about diagnosis of doubtful value. We are left with the usual admonition about the proven value of the clinical approach. Yet despite the best of intentions, in FUO possibly more than in any other category of illness, laboratory testing can escalate to the point of mindlessness.

In Larson's and Petersdorf's series (3, 4), for example, they described a variety of blood tests, chemistries, immunological tests, and even blood cultures as "notoriously unhelpful." Not a single blood culture turned out to be positive in their series (though in a kind of circular reasoning, one must exclude the diagnosis of bacteremia before the patient fulfills the criteria of FUO).

The most helpful imaging study, according to the investigators, was the chest radiograph, especially when it was possible to review previous or serial films. Upper GI studies or IVP were also helpful, but only when clinical findings pointed to the GI tract or kidney. Certain other imaging approaches would be appropriate, but again only when clinically justified, for example, when localized bone pain would call for radiographs or bone scintigraphy, etc. The foundation of diagnostic strategy rests in categorizing the patient into one of the major etiological groups. We will even deal with the question of whether it is permissible to employ certain types of imaging as a form of limited screening.

INFECTIONS

Abscess in the abdominal cavity was the most common infectious cause of FUO in both major series and the main cause of mortality in the infectious category. Imaging assumes its most important role here, but of course, a working diagnosis is invaluable. Collections in the subphrenic region occurred in three patients and would have been expected to result in physical and radiographic findings. Other upper abdominal collections might be anticipated to produce clinical findings, but obviously it is the occult abscess, particularly in the abdominal cavity, that most commonly presents as FUO in the first place. In females, the pelvis is another likely site of a collection.

Prolonged fever from urinary tract infections is uncommon without anatomical abnormalities such as caliectasis, hydronephrosis, parapelvic cyst, etc. As an intriguing clinical aside contradicting the conventional medical wisdom, Petersdorf (4) has observed that in patients who have lived for long periods in foreign countries, esoteric causes of FUO are unusual. He quotes his old professor as observing that in New England people do not die of tsutsugamushi disease; they die of cardiovascular disease.

Judging by the second series, one would expect a low diagnostic yield in imaging for infections outside the abdominal cavity, with the probable exception of osteomyelitis and sinusitis. This is true particularly because tuberculosis and cytomegalovirus accounted for 9 of the remaining 12 cases of extraabdominal infectious disease. Wound infections are often missed in the postoperative patients, particularly when physicians invoke other less likely causes such as drug fever and urinary tract infection.

The obvious imaging choices in suspected intraabdominal collections would include ultrasonography, CT/MRI, and radionuclide studies, often in that order.

NEOPLASM

The three H's, Hodgkin, hepatoma, and hypernephroma, are classic causes of cryptogenic fever caused by neoplasms. To this triad we should add leukemia and a heterogeneous variety of solid abdominal tumors, especially colorectal carcinoma, which has been reported to cause fever in almost 30% of preoperative patients (5).

The imaging method of first choice in the patient with suspected malignancy is radiogallium scintigraphy because of its high sensitivity in many tumors commonly causing FUO, particularly lymphomas. The yield in the leukemias is very low, however, with sensitivity virtually nil. Moreover, radiogallium has a low sensitivity for tumor of the urinary and GI tract and female pelvis, specifically neoplasms of renal, colonic, and gynecological origin.

COLLAGEN VASCULAR, GRANULOMATOUS, AND MISCELLANEOUS CAUSES OF FUO

We should not expect imaging to be very helpful in these three categories, which make up about 40% of the remaining cases of fever of undetermined cause. Well-known among the expects is the rare patient with ulcerative colitis or regional ileitis who presents with fever and anemia but without abdominal pain, diarrhea, or other bowel symptoms. Such patients would not usually have a diagnostic gallium scan but might well be diagnosed with 111-indium WBC scintigraphy, flex-sig, and small bowel series/barium enema.

Summary of Imaging Approach in FUO

To use CT/MRI, radionuclide scintigraphy, or other imaging procedures in an undirected fashion is to misunderstand the meaning of what one may casually dismiss as an unproductive clinical encounter. For example, such routine knowledge as the age, sex, and history of the most puzzling patient often gives a clue to the probable category with which one is dealing. Thus, it is obvious that young women are more likely to have collagen disease than neoplasm, postoperative patients to have infection, and older patients solid intraabdominal tumors, etc.

However, given the usual situation in which clinical information is of limited help, we must reluctantly admit that, in contrast to almost any other clinical category, imaging may occasionally have a useful role as a region-oriented screening procedure. Having stated this, how does one proceed without the slender lead of a skin rash, the valuable clue of a palpable mass, or localizing findings such as pain or tenderness? Although perhaps fewer than half of all FUO patients are likely to have an imageable condition, the following schema, following the routine PA and lateral chest radiograph, seems to be the most practical approach:

1. The initial imaging approach involves ultrasonography of the kidneys, gall bladder, subdiaphragmatic space, and in females, the pelvis. The yield may be low without localizing signs, but ultrasound allows the scanning of several important areas and is quickly and easily accomplished. The clinician at this stage must have formed some impression as to the relative likelihood of an inflammatory vs. a neoplastic or other cause.

2. In the case of suspected abdominal sepsis, the most frequent location in FUO, proceed with CT or MRI (7). If CT/MRI is unrevealing, proceed with indium-111 WBC scintigraphy (6).

3. If neoplastic disease is a strong consideration, proceed first with total body gallium scintigraphy. Gallium, though far from perfect, is the best tumor imaging agent available and has the additional advantage of detecting infection, though it is less reliable than indium in the abdomen. (Gallium scintigraphy should be the last radionuclide study to be performed, however, because it causes interfering radioactivity for up to 1 week or 10 days.)

4. Because gallium rivals indium for revealing infections extraabdominally and is the most effective tumor screening agent available, a negative gallium scintiscan is helpful in *excluding* an impressive number of tumors and extraabdominal infections.

Table 6.16.4. Summary of Gallium Scans Patient True Positive Rate

Less than 50% positive	50% to 70% positive	Over 70% positive
Myeloma	Liver metastases	Hodgkin's disease
Thyroid carcinoma	Leukemia	Non-Hodgkin's lymphoma
GI tract cancer	Head and neck cancer	Brain tumors
Bladder cancer	Breast cancer	Lung tumors
Gyn cancer	Wilm's tumor	Melanoma
	Prostate cancer	Hepatoma
	Hypernephroma	Bone tumors (excluding myeloma)
		Neuroblastoma
		Soft tissue sarcomas
		Testicular tumors

Table 6.16.4 summarizes the sensitivity of gallium for detection of various tumors (8). Many of these neoplasms are known to cause FUO, in particular lymphomas, hepatomas, and hypernephromas.

5. If indium and gallium scintigraphy along with abdominal CT or MRI are nondiagnostic, CT or MRI of the thorax should be performed next.

What To Do When Conventional Investigation Is Indeterminate or Negative

What is to be done when thorough, conventional diagnostic investigation is exhausted? Many studies have discussed this problem, and though there is considerable disagreement about when to explore, there is general consensus as to its ultimate value in the difficult case (9–11). Because the greater percentage of patients with FUO have diseases diagnosable and *treatable* in the abdominal cavity, and because a significant number of undiagnosed patients will succumb to their diseases, the most effective approach when all other avenues have been exhausted remains the exploratory laparotomy, formerly a refuge for the diagnostically destitute.

In a different context, Groucho Marx once commented, "I met my wife in a travel agency. I was looking for a vacation, and she was the last resort."

REFERENCES

1. Weinstein L. Fever of unknown origin. In: Branch WT, ed. Office Practice of Medicine, Philadelphia: W.B. Saunders Company, 1987:1098–1111.
2. Petersdorf RG, Beeson PB. Fever of unexplained origin: report on 100 cases. Medicine 1961;40:1.
3. Larson EB, Featherstone HJ, Petersdorf RG. Fever of undetermined origin: diagnosis and follow-up of 105 cases, 1970-1980. Medicine, 1982;61(5):269–292.
4. Petersdorf RG. FUO. How it has changed in 20 years. Hosp Pract 1985;20(4):84I–84M,84P,84T–84V passim.
5. Aderka D, Hausmann M, Santo M, Weinberger A, Pinkhas J. Unexplained episodes of fever: an early manifestation of colorectal carcinoma. Isr J Med Sci 1985;21(5):421–424.
6. Froelich JW. Indium-111 opens new era for labeled blood products. Diagn Imaging 1987;9:138–142.
7. McNeil BJ, Sanders R, Alderson PO, et al. A prospective study of computed tomography, ultrasound, and gallium imaging in patients with fever. Radiology 1981;139(3):647–653.
8. Teates CD, Bray ST, Williamson BR. Tumor detection with 67 Gallium citrate: a literature survey (1970–1978). Clin Nucl Med 1978;3(12):456–460.
9. Baker RR, Tumulty PA, Shelley WM. The value of exploratory laparotomy in fever of undetermined etiology. Johns Hopkins Med J 1969;125(3):159–170.
10. Geraci JE, Weed LA, Nickols DR. Fever of obscure origin—the value of abdominal exploration in diagnosis. JAMA 1959;169:1305.
11. Rothman DL, Schwartz SI, Adams JT. Diagnostic laparotomy for fever or abdominal pain of unknown origin. Am J Surg 1977;133(3):273–275.

17/ Palpable Lymphadenopathy

I'd rather be well for a whole day than sick for an entire year.
Professor Irwin Corey

Introduction

Adenopathy is classified etiologically in Table 6.17.1 (1), but it is also useful to designate lymph node enlargement in anatomical terms, either generalized or regional, deep or superficial. The table does not indicate the relative frequency of the forms of lymphadenopathy, but when examining a patient with enlarged nodes, it is always helpful to recall the rarity of hereditary adenopathy and the enormous preponderance of inflammatory (and usually benign) compared with neoplastic causes. Table 6.17.2 shows the frequency and rates per 100,000 population for the all-listed diagnoses of the major lymphomas and leukemias for 1990 (2). Table 6.17.3 is a simplified classification which also includes estimated frequencies.

Medical imaging of solitary groups of enlarged or abnormal superficial lymph nodes per se sonographically is hardly relevant, because it can only tell the clinician what he already knows. (We exclude from this discussion scintigraphic study of regional nodes for investigating cancer spread.) Yet, we are being asked increasingly by inexperienced clinicians to *identify* nodes sonographically. Some of these lymph nodes are obviously enlarged, cystic, or suppurated. The decision for needle aspira-

Table 6.17.1. A Classification of the Causes of Lymphadenopathy

Hereditary
Immunodeficiency diseases
   All systems—Swiss-type combined deficiency
   T-cell defects—DiGeorge's syndrome
   B-cell defects—Bruton-type agammaglobulinemia; selective deficiencies
Lysosomal storage diseases
   Mucopolysaccharidoses
   Lipoidoses
   Carbohydrate abnormalities

Acquired
Inflammatory
   Acute lymphadenitis
   Follicular hyperplasia
   Paracortical hyperplasia
   Histiocytic patterns
   Granulomatous patterns
   Miscellaneous reactions
Neoplastic
   Malignant lymphoma/leukemia
     Hodgkin's disease
     Non-Hodgkin's lymphoma
       Nodular lymphomas
       Diffuse lymphomas
       Other patterns of lymphoma
   Metastatic neoplasms

Reprinted by permission from Blacklow RS, ed. *MacBryde's Signs and Symptoms.* Philadelphia: J. B. Lippincott Co. (1983:481).

Table 6.17.2.   Discharge Diagnoses, Lymphomas and Leukemias, Rates/100,000 population, U.S. Hospitals, 1990

	Total	Male	Female	Age <15	Age 15–44	Age 45–64	Age 65+
200. Lymphosarc/reticulosarc	11	13	10	0	6	19	35
201. Hodgkin's disease	7	8	6	0	8	11	0
202. Oth mal NEO lymph/histio	42	44	40	13	14	64	161
203. Multiple myeloma et al.	24	28	19	0	0	34	127
204. Lymphoid leukemia	32	42	23	36	8	26	120
205. Myeloid leukemia	16	18	15	0	9	21	54
208. Leukemia-unspecif cell	4	5	0	0	0	0	0

Discharge Diagnoses, Lymphomas and Leukemias, Frequency in Thousands, U.S. Hospitals, 1990

All-listed ICD-9-CM	Total	Male	Female	Age <15	Age 15–44	Age 45–64	Age 65+
200. Lymphosarc/reticulosarc	28	16	13	0	7	9	11
201. Hodgkin's disease	18	10	8	0	9	5	0
202. Oth mal NEO lymph/histio	104	53	51	7	16	30	51
203. Multiple myeloma et al.	59	34	25	0	0	16	40
204. Lymphoid leukemia	80	51	29	20	9	12	38
205. Myeloid leukemia	41	22	19	0	10	10	17
208. Leukemia-unspecif cell	10	6	0	0	0	0	0

Table 6.17.3.   A Simplified Classification of Adenopathy with Estimated Frequencies of Occurrence

Etiological category	Estimated frequency (%)
Acquired (inflammatory)	>95
Neoplastic (primary and metastatic)	<5
Hereditary	>0.01

tion almost always can be made solely on clinical grounds, and whether aspiration or biopsy becomes a therapeutic or diagnostic decision depends more on the look, feel, extent, and clinical history of superficial adenopathy rather than the results of any sonographic studies. Where metastatic disease, intrathoracic, or intraabdominal adenopathy is suspected, of course, imaging has a crucial place in diagnosis. The subject of imaging strategy given the presence of deep adenopathy is discussed in Chapter 7.

Generalized Lymphadenopathy

A wide variety of systemic illnesses or syndromes may be associated with generalized lymphadenopathy. Some of these conditions are listed in Table 6.17.4. Clinical assessment combined with straightforward testing usually suffice to make the diagnosis of the most commonest causative conditions, usually viral or infectious diseases. An increasingly prevalent cause of generalized adenopathy is infection with HIV and the AIDS syndrome in its many guises. Given a patient with generalized adenopathy, causes such as metastatic malignancies, the lympho-proliferative syndromes, lymphomas, and leukemias are distinctly uncommon. The most crucial diagnostic question in any type of adenopathy is whether or not to biopsy a lymph node. It is disturbing to note that errors in lymph node diagnosis are made more often than with any other tissue. In a well-known series already quoted (3), a nationally known pathologist disagreed with the diagnosis of Hodgkin disease made by colleagues in almost half the cases. Needle aspiration biopsy of suspicious nodules and lymph nodes is a productive exercise only if the pretest probability of disease is significant. An example is a

Table 6.17.4. Causes of Generalized Adenopathy

1. Viral
    A. AIDS
    B. Mononucleosis and mononucleosis-like syndromes
    C. Hepatitis
    D. Rubella
    E. Cytomegalovirus
    F. Cat scratch disease
    G. Other acute or chronic viral diseases or syndromes
2. Bacterial/spirochetal/fungal
    A. Tuberculosis
    B. Secondary syphilis
    C. Tularemia, plague, brucellosis
    D. Various tropical diseases
3. Autoimmune/unknown etiology (neoplastic)
    A. Serum sickness
    B. Sarcoidosis
    C. Rheumatoid arthritis
    D. Diffuse skin disorders
    E. Drug reactions, etc.
    F. Lymphoma, etc.

series of such biopsies performed on 130 patients which yielded 84 positive findings (65%), 40 benign (31%), and six suspicious (4%). We can only infer most of these patients were high cancer suspects, because 77 out of the 84 positive biopsies or 87% showed metastatic malignancy. Yet almost all those *without* histological verification were known to have primary carcinoma and evidence of metastatic disease (4).

Thus, adenopathy in cancer does not always indicate involvement of the enlarged nodes. Superficial adenopathy is a physical finding, not a diagnosis, but there is seldom a place for medical imaging, with the important exceptions discussed below.

Regional Adenopathies: Cervical, Axillary, and Inguinal

Our purpose is not to be exhaustive, but rather to lump together the regional adenopathies for the purposes of simplifying the diagnostic approach. Localized adenopathies of the neck, axilla, and groin are almost always the result of inflammatory responses resulting from antigenic stimuli to the lymph nodes, rather than from infiltration by a lymphoma or metastatic tumor. Chronic skin irritations, bacterial, fungal, or viral infections in both children and adults are the most common causes of adenopathy, but other conditions occasionally must be considered, in particular, foreign body reactions, granulomatous, and collagen vascular diseases. None of these conditions, of course, is amenable to medical imaging.

In the case of neoplastic causes, there are so many clinical clues to the presence of malignancy, we can provide the reader with only a few simple generalizations. Given significant adenopathy (or significant *anything* in the way of signs or symptoms), diagnosis begins with the clinical history and examination. The most difficult problem remains the identification of adenopathy itself, because as lymph nodes enlarge or become fixed they may be indistinguishable from other subcutaneous masses. Another problem is the identification of the normally palpable node (usually less than 1 cm in size) and the ability to differentiate it from the abnormal. Clinical determination of suspicious adenopathy is something that cannot be taught but can only be acquired with long clinical experience. Certain features are suspicious for malignant involvement:

1. The *absence* of a history of infection, in particular ear, nose, and throat infections in cervical adenopathy, or the absence of systemic or localized infections of the extremities or the absence of skin lesions (rashes, dermatophytosis, or scalp conditions).

2. Constitutional or systemic complaints such as weight loss, fever, or night sweats (in the absence of a diagnosis of systemic infection), unexplained anemia, or other blood abnormalities and abnormal findings on chest radiography.

3. New cervical adenopathy in an adult smoker. This should always make one concerned about metastatic oro-pharyngeal or laryngeal cancer.

4. Most significant of all, adenopathy associated with the finding of a regional mass or other unexplained lesion should raise the possibility of metastatic cancer. Prime examples are: axillary adenopathy in the presence of a breast mass, cervical adenopathy associated with a thyroid mass, and any regional adenopathy seen with suspicious melanotic or other skin lesions.

Medical imaging when undertaken for suspicious malignancy should be done only in a *directed* approach. Thus, we continue to emphasize that choosing the appropriate study depends on having a *diagnosis in mind*. It is essential not to embark on fishing expeditions, as is so often done, in patients with unexplained regional adenopathy. Specific approaches to the diagnosis of malignancy will be discussed in subsequent sections.

REFERENCES

1. Jeghers H, Clark SL, Templeton AC. Lymphadenopathy and disorders of the lymphatics, In: Blacklow RS, ed. MacBryde's *Signs and Symptoms*. 6th ed. Philadelphia: J. B. Lippincott Co., 1983:481.
2. U.S. Department of Health and Human Services, U.S. Public Health Service, Centers for Disease Control, and the National Center for Health Statistics. National Hospital Discharge Survey (NHDS). Detailed diagnoses, procedures, days of care, diagnoses-related groups for patients discharged from short-stay hospitals. Public Use Data Diskettes, 1985–1990.
3. Symmers Sr WS. Survey of the eventual diagnosis in 600 cases referred for a second histological opinion after an initial biopsy diagnosis of Hodgkin's disease. J Clin Pathol 1968;21(5):650–653.
4. Kline TA, Neal HS, Holroyde CP. Needle aspiration biopsy: diagnosis of subcutaneous nodules and lymph nodes. JAMA 1976;235(26):2848–2849.

18/ Breast Masses

> *Dost thou not see my baby at my breast*
> *That sucks the nurse asleep?*
> > William Shakespeare
> > Antony and Cleopatra, *V:2*
> > *(Cleopatra holding the asp to her breast)*

Breast cancer is the most common malignancy in women (excluding skin cancer) and the second most frequent cause of female cancer deaths, just after lung cancer. Its incidence of 28% makes it the highest of all malignancies in females at 109 cases per 100,000 women. In 1990 it is estimated that 150,000 women in this country will have been diagnosed with primary invasive breast cancer, and almost 30% or 44,300

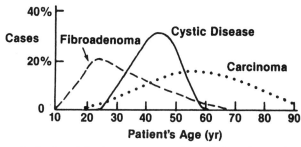

Figure 6.18.1.   Age distribution of the three commonest breast lesions that produce masses. (Adapted from Donegan WL, 1979.)

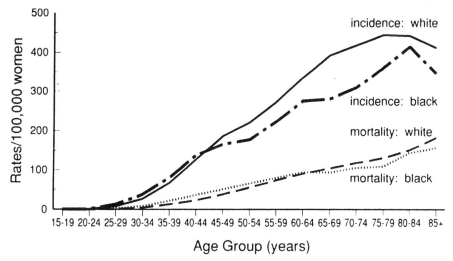

Figure 6.18.2.   Average annual age-specific SEER incidence and U.S. mortality rates, by race, 1983–1987.

will die of the disease. The lifetime risk of developing breast cancer is 1 in 11 women in the United States or 9% (1, 2).

Despite popular enthusiasm for breast screening tests, primarily X-ray mammography for the detection of nonpalpable, asymptomatic lesions, more than 90% of breast cancers are discovered by palpation, the overwhelming number by patients themselves (3). When one tallies both the signs and symptoms of breast cancer by frequency of presentation, almost 75% of patients have a palpable mass, 7% have nipple changes (discharge, retraction, or erosion), and, contrary to general opinion, 6% have pain (3). *In young women under 25 years of age, 99% of all dominant breast masses will be benign, usually a fibroadenoma.* In the reproductive years, the majority will be due to fibrocystic changes, whereas in postmenopausal women the incidence of cancer rises precipitously. There is considerable overlap by age group over 30, which is shown in Figure 6.18.1, showing the distribution of these three most common causes by age. The age-specific incidence of breast cancer by race in Figure 6.18.2 shows the extremely low incidence in young women, less than 1 case per 100,000 under age 20, rising to almost 450 cases per 100,000 at age 75. Figure 6.18.3 shows breast cancer mortality rates from 1973–1987 by age group and race (4). Less than 900 cases of breast cancer were recorded in U.S. males in 1989 (5, 6).

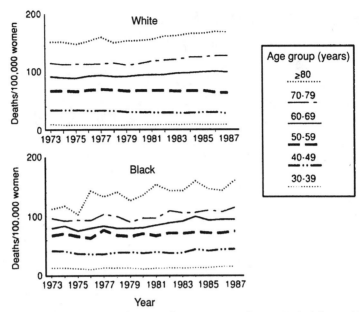

Figure 6.18.3. Breast cancer mortality rates, by age group and race—United States, 1973–1987.

When we come to risk factors in breast cancer, issues of screening and diagnosis take on a new perspective. For example, a history of breast cancer in the immediate family or a first-degree relative places a woman at *two to three times excess risk*, especially if the relative was premenopausal or the disease was bilateral. Other less important but validated risk factors include obesity, early menarche, women who first conceive over age 30, late menopause, and nulliparity. Fibrocystic changes remain doubtful as an index of breast cancer risk, because to some extent they are seen in the large majority of women, whereas oral contraceptives have not been shown to increase the risk of the disease in premenopausal women (7).

Other than palpation, demonstrably the *most important* of all diagnostic tests for breast masses, there remain two imaging modalities used for breast cancer, mammography and ultrasonography, the former for both screening and diagnosis, the latter for diagnosis only. *Diagnosis* in this context means excluding or establishing the need for biopsy or fine needle aspiration.

Diagnostic Mammography

Because it is both impossible and unnecessary to biopsy every palpable breast abnormality, the physician must depend on history and clinical findings to guide his management. In all clinically suspicious breast masses, the patient should have mammography for the principal purpose of excluding coexistent malignancy in the contralateral breast and then proceed directly to biopsy. When the patient is in the over-30 to 35-year age group, if clinical findings or sonography (see below) indicate other than a pure cyst, and especially if the patient is in one of the high-risk groups, mammography should be performed, followed by fine needle aspiration cytology or open biopsy if mammographic findings are suspicious or inconclusive.

In an important Italian study of 14,000 women over age 30 referred to a breast clinic (8), a total of 2,102 breast masses were seen and divided into three classes:

Table 6.18.1. Type of Response and Sensitivity of the Physical, Mammographic and Cytological Examination in 285 Lumps

Examination	No. of cases	Unsatisfactory	Negative or benign	Suspect	Malignant	Sensitivity
Physical	285	—	48	148	89	0.83
Mammographic	285	18	60	76	131	0.73
Cytological	285	67	46	41	131	0.50

Reprinted by permission from *European Journal of Surgical Oncology* (1987;13:335–340).

Table 6.18.2. Specificity of the Diagnostic Triad in 346 Benign Lumps

Result	No. of cases	%
No test positive	117	51.1
One test positive	118	34.1
Two tests positive	51	14.8
All three tests positive	0	

Reprinted by permission from *European Journal of Surgical Oncology* (1987;13:335–340).

Class 1 included 942 patients (45%) with cystic masses confirmed by needle aspiration and clinically benign lumps unchanged in size for more than 2 years.

Class 2 included 529 patients (25%) with clinically advanced cancers, i.e. those with nipple change, skin retraction, and/or axillary node involvement.

Class 3, the focus of their study, included 631 patients (30%) with solid breast masses and clinical characteristics of varying degree ranging from apparently benign to suspicious features, but not evident malignancy. Five hundred twenty-five of these patients had surgical removal of their masses. The other 105 patients or about 5% of the series showed spontaneous regression of their lesions within 2 months (confirmed by subsequent follow-up) and hence were not subjected to surgery.

Thus, about 15% of patients (2,102 out of 14,000) over age 30 referred to a surgical oncology breast unit had palpable masses. Of these, 50% had benign, generally cystic masses, and 25% had obvious cancer. The remaining 25% (525 patients) subsequently had their lumps removed surgically after the diagnostic triad of physical examination, mammography, and fine needle aspiration biopsy. Two hundred eighty-five of the 526 nodules removed (54%) were cancer (2% of the entire series), and 162 or 57% of these did not exceed 2 cm in size. The sensitivities and specificities of these tests singly and combined for cancer detection in 285 malignant, 346 benign, and 631 malignant and benign lumps are shown in Tables 6.18.1, 6.18.2, and 6.18.3 (8). The thrust of these tables is to show that examination of the breasts is the single most important test in the malignant group with the highest sensitivity, and that mammography and fine needle aspiration have significantly higher specificity in the benign group. Table 6.18.4 shows the PPV of each positive finding singly and combined. Note that the PPV of physical examination alone was almost equal to mammography (0.63 vs. 0.74). Clearly, in the author's words, "The systematic use of the diagnostic triad . . . allowed the clinicians to select malignant cases and plan inpatient/outpatient surgical treatment" (8). The value of mammography was clearly established in the high-likelihood group, and the importance of fine needle aspiration was obvious. The real problem remains in detecting early breast cancer, a goal not achieved either by detection of palpable abnormalities or, as pointed out below, with screening mammography.

Table 6.18.3. Overall Diagnostic Accuracy of the Three Examinations on 631 Malignant and Benign Lumps

Examination	No. correct/total	Accuracy
Physical	446/631	0.70
Mammographic	479/631	0.76
Cytological	513/631	0.81

Reprinted by permission from *European Journal of Surgical Oncology* (1987;13:335–340).

Table 6.18.4. Predictive Value of a Positive Response of the Three Examinations

Examination	No. positive responses	No. malignant cases	Predictive value
Physical	374	237	0.63
Mammographic	281	207	0.74
Cytological	177	172	0.97
All three tests positive with triplet	117	117	1.00
Two tests positive	163	112	0.69

Reprinted by permission from *European Journal of Surgical Oncology* (1987;13:335–340).

Screening Mammography

The limitations of mammography in screening are shared by all tests applied to disease detection in a population with low pretest probability. There is simply no way to avoid this basic fact of life in any clinical testing. If we accept the official average incidence rate of 109 cases of new breast cancers per 100,000 population (2), we must continue to take into account that this overall figure is still an average and changes significantly with age. Under age 40, the incidence rate is only 63 new cases per 100,000, rising to 227 per 100,000 at age 55. For screening mammography, if we assume a sensitivity of 0.8 and specificity of 0.9 for a binary outcome—either positive or negative—these incidence rates give PPVs of only 4% for an abnormal mammogram in a woman under 40 but 66% for a patient of 55.

Mammography, however, like clinical examination, has degrees of positivity, with findings suggesting cancer ranging from low suspicion to almost pathognomonic. In the 15-center randomized Canadian National Breast Screening Study (NBBS) (9) 44,718 women were studied by mammography and physical examination. Not surprisingly, the overall sensitivity of the technique was 0.75, and the specificity was 0.94 with a PPV for cancer of only 7%. The predictive value of disease given a negative test (1-NPV), as can be anticipated, was 0.2%, not significantly different from the prevalence of disease in the general population. Since the 1988 report of the Canadian study, criticism has been leveled at the methodology, particularly the mammographic techniques employed, but even with a higher sensitivity (it is difficult to find a better *specificity* for mammography), the results are not unexpected or surprising. These figures again demonstrate the obvious limitations of *any* diagnostic test used in a population of low disease prevalence.

This is confirmed in another important study in which biopsy was performed in 1,300 occult breast lesions discovered roentgenographically (10). Only 19% were found to be malignant. Biopsy results of mammograms from outside facilities yielded a lower PPV, 17% vs. 26% at the authors' institution. They concluded reasonably that "this statistically significant difference lends support to the value

Table 6.18.5. Percentage of Breast Biopsies with Cancer According to Patient Age Group[a]

Age group (yrs)	Biopsies with cancer (%)
10–19	0 (0/19)
20–29	1.2 (2/165)
30–39	9.0 (30/333)
40–49	19.7 (72/365)
50–59	36.8 (114/310)
60–69	59.9 (161/269)

[a]Data from reference 25.
Reprinted by permission from *American Surgeon* (1982;48:326–332).

of a second opinion in patients with biopsy recommendations for occult breast lesions, especially when findings are inconclusive" (10). Table 6.18.5 (11) further illustrates this point. Once again we see that, given the average sensitivities and specificities of *any* medical test, prevalence of disease is the most important determinant of test predictability.

Although the figures are disappointing, one finds it difficult to accept the reliability of screening mammography to predict the *presence* of breast cancer in patients with and without the condition (PPV of 41% and 59% only). Furthermore, negative or equivocal screening mammography disease, given a patient with cancer, is valueless. In other words, screening mammography is only of significant help in *excluding cancer in women without cancer*. This seems counterintuitive, yet numerous studies (11–14) point up the problem of false-negative and false-positive mammographic studies in the "normal" population, i.e. those women without palpable breast abnormalities.

Further documenting this is a superb epidemiological study by Eddy (15) with mathematical models demonstrating that *mammographic screening annually with breast physical examination* will decrease the probability of death from breast cancer by about 25 in 10,000 for women in the three major age groups and increase life expectancy by about 20 days. "If women are screened annually for 10 years with breast physical examination and mammography, the chance for a false-positive result over the 10-year period is approximately 2,500 in 10,000" (15). On the population level, the author estimated that if 25% of women are screened annually, cancer deaths would be reduced by 4,000 by the end of the century, an estimated reduction of 7–10% of total breast cancer deaths, at a cost of $1.3 billion or $325,000 per case (15). However, he does not estimate the potential medical costs as well as risks in a 25% false-positive rate. Although these figures appear to be depressing, they should not be taken to mean we do not urge mammographic screening in high-risk or older patients. Sensitivity, outcomes, and other types of mathematical analysis should provide rational guidelines for an effective approach to the problem of early breast cancer detection in an asymptomatic population.

The following recommendations of official organizations for mammographic screening in asymptomatic women are a reflection of the confusion abounding in this area (15):

American Cancer Society: All women between 20 and 40 years of age are advised to have breast examinations every 3 years, baseline mammograms for all women between 35 and 40, annual breast examinations from age 40–50, mammograms every 1–2 years from age 40–50 and yearly over age 50.

The National Cancer Institute recommends physical examination of the breast at every periodic examination, encourages mammography every 1–2 years beginning at age 40 and annual mammograms for women with a personal history of breast cancer.

The American College of Obstetrics and Gynecology recommends baseline mammograms for women between the ages of 35 and 50 and breast examinations in the same age group. Mammograms are recommended at any age in the presence of strong risk factors, i.e. family or personal history of breast cancer, breast augmentation implants, or first pregnancy over age 30.

The American College of Radiology recommends baseline mammograms before the age of 35–40 years and subsequently every 1–2 years.

The American Medical Association recommends mammographic screening and breast examination every 1–2 years in women between 40 and 49 years of age and yearly examination and mammography in women over 50.

The American College of Physicians does not recommend mammography for women under 50 years of age.

The U.S. Preventive Services Task Force recommends annual clinical breast examinations for women 40–49 years of age but does not recommend mammograms for this age group.

To summarize, the majority of breast cancers are found by physical examination. It may be convincingly argued that by the time a mass is felt, many cancers are not early, and therefore this is not the optimal way to find cancer. Still, there is no way to avoid the statistical drawbacks of mass screening; the efficacy of widespread screening mammography always will be poor because of the extremely low PPV in populations with low prevalence of disease. Nevertheless, screening mammography is of proven merit particularly in older patients and those in high risk groups. Because of this, we agree with Eddy (15) that a reasonable strategy is for a woman of average risk to have breast physical examinations annually after age 40 and mammography every 1–2 years after 50. For women in high-risk groups mammography is recommended annually beginning at age 40.

Breast Ultrasonography

Approximately 25% of all nonpalpable circumscribed masses studied by ultrasound are cystic, but the actual percentage of total palpable breast lesions that are cystic is probably considerably higher. Mammography cannot determine whether a mass is cystic or solid unless the mass contains fat or calcium. It is important to realize that although cystic changes (not "disease") as an index of cancer risk is controversial (16, 17); most authorities hold that cysts themselves are virtually never premalignant or malignant. Feig (12) states the issue strongly, ". . . The sonographic demonstration of a simple cyst implies that neither biopsy, aspiration, nor follow-up of the mass is necessary." He adds that strict sonographic criteria be applied in order to achieve close to 100% accuracy of diagnosis.

The place of ultrasound in diagnosis of breast disease other than cystic is still controversial, but in the hands of experts the modality has significant applications in several clinical settings. For example, in the assessment of localized breast pain and tenderness in the absence of clinical or mammographic findings, ultrasonography is often helpful. Although no figures are available on the fre-

Table 6.18.6.   Potential Roles of Breast Ultrasound

Indications
  Evaluation of a nonpalpable circumscribed breast mass
  Evaluation of a palpable mass that is indeterminate on mammography
  Evaluation of an asymmetric mammographic density that could be due to an underlying discrete
    mass
  Evaluation of a palpable or questionably palpable mass where the mammogram is negative
  Evaluation of localized breast pain and tenderness
  Primary imaging modality for all women below age 30 years and most women below age 35 years
  Localization of a lesion seen on only one mammographic projection
  Aspiration guidance for a nonpalpable cyst
Possible applications
  Biopsy localization of a nonpalpable mass seen on two perpendicular mammographic projections
  Evaluation of a breast with numerous nonpalpable masses
  Evaluation of the male breast
Non-indications
  Screening for breast cancer including screening subgroups of women with dense breasts or with
    breast implants
  Examination of patients who refuse mammography

Reprinted by permission from *Seminars in Ultrasound, CT, and MR* (1989;10(2):90–105).

quency of cystic disease as a cause of breast pain or tenderness, one series is revealing. Sickles et al. (18) found with ultrasound all 492 cysts disclosed by palpation and mammography in 15,000 women but also found 362 additional cysts undetected by the other methods.

Other areas where ultrasound has proven itself are listed in Table 6.18.6 (12). It is unfortunate indeed that supplementary breast ultrasonography has been neglected except in a few major centers, because, if expertly used, it is a diagnostic technique of significant importance with the potential of saving many patients the trouble and anxiety of biopsy. It certainly complements, and at times, outperforms mammography in some specific clinical settings. Breast sonography, however, does not have a place in screening.

Suggested Diagnostic Approach to Breast Masses

Once a breast mass is found on physical examination, the approach depends on two factors: the patient's age and presence of risk factors. Because only 3–6% of patients under age 35 undergoing biopsy for a breast mass will have cancer, ultrasonography is the preferred first imaging procedure. If a pure cyst is found, no further workup is required. Table 6.18.7 (12) gives an extremely useful guide to the use of mammography and sonography in evaluating a palpable breast mass.

All patients over age 20 with risk factors and breast masses, particularly those with family histories of breast cancer, and all other patients over age 35 with palpable breast masses should have mammography. Other patients between 20 and 35 with masses should have sonography first. Depending on the physical, sonographic, and mammographic findings, the patient would be a candidate either for fine needle aspiration or should go directly to surgery for open biopsy if a high cancer suspect.

With ultrasonography, up to half of all breast masses in patients under age 45 may prove to be benign cysts (8). With the combination of breast physical examination, mammographic, and needle biopsy findings, open or excisional biopsy can be avoided

Table 6.18.7. Use of Mammography and Sonography to Evaluate a Palpable Breast Mass

Patient age (yrs)	Imaging modalities
Younger than 20	Sonography only.
20–30	Sonography first.
	Mammography (usually a single oblique lateral view of one breast only) if sonography does not show a simple cyst and if breast cancer is a clinical consideration.
30–35	If no close family history of breast cancer, same as for age 20 to 30 years
	If mother or sister with breast cancer same as for age 35 and older.
35 and older	Bilateral two-view per breast mammogram first. Sonography if mammography negative or nonspecific.

Reprinted by permission from *Seminars in Ultrasound, CT, and MR* (1989;10(2):90–105).

in about half the remaining patients. The likelihood of a positive biopsy for cancer in any patient with an abnormal mammogram averages *only 15–20%*.

REFERENCES

1. Cancer statistics, 1990. Ca-A Cancer Journal for Clinicians. American Cancer Society, 1990;40(1):19–20.

2. Breast cancer risk factors and screening: United States, 1987. National Center for Health Statistics, Jan. 1990, Series 10, no. 172.

3. Onofrey D, Tartter PI, Iberti TJ. Breast mass evaluation. Emerg Decis 1988;May:19–25.

4. Qualters JR, Lee NC, Smith RA, Aubert RE. Breast and cervical cancer surveillance, United States, 1973–1987. CDC Surveillance Summaries. Apr 24, 1992. MMWR 1992;41(SS-2):1–16.

5. Cancer incidence and mortality in the United States. SEER. 1973–1981. U.S. Department of Health of Human Service. U.S. Public Health Service. National Institutes of Health.

6. Cancer statistics, 1989. Ca-A Cancer Journal for Clinicians. American Cancer Society, 1989;39(1):3–20.

7. Schlesselman JJ, Stadel BV, Murray P, Lai S. Breast cancer in relation to early use of oral contraceptives. No evidence of a latent effect. JAMA 1988;259(12):1828–1833.

8. DiPietro S, Fariselli G, Bandieramonte P, et al. Diagnostic efficacy of the clinical, radiological-cytological triad in solid breast lumps: results of a second prospective study on 631 patients. Eur J Surg Oncol 1987;13(4):335–340.

9. Baines CJ, McFarlane DV, Miller AB. Sensitivity and specificity of first screen mammography in 15 NBSS centres. J Can Assoc Radiol 1988;39(4):273–276.

10. Meyer JE, Eberlein TJ, Stomper PC, Sonnenfeld MR. Biopsy of occult breast lesions. Analysis of 1261 abnormalities. JAMA 1990;263(17):2341–2343.

11. Spivey GH, Perry BW, Clark VA, Coulson AH, Coulson WF. Predicting the risk of cancer at the time of breast biopsy: variation in the benign to malignant ratio. Am Surg 1982;48(7):326–332.

12. Feig SA. The role of ultrasound in a breast imaging center. Semin Ultrasound CT MR 1989;10(2):90–105.

13. Moskowitz M. The predictive value of certain mammographic signs in screening for breast cancer. Cancer 1983;51(6):1007–1011.

14. Hall FM, Storell JM, Silverstone DZ, Wyshak G. Non-palpable breast lesions: recommendations for biopsy based on suspicion of carcinaoma at mammography. Radiology 1988;167(2):353–358.

15. Eddy DM. Screening for breast cancer. Ann Intern Med 1989;111(5):389–399.

16. Dupont WD, Page DL. Risk factors for breast cancer in women with proliferative breast disease. N Engl J Med 1985;312(3):146–151.

17. Love SM, Gelman RS, Silen W. Sounding board. Fibrocystic "disease" of the breast—a nondisease? N Engl J Med 1982;307(16):1010–1014.

18. Sickles EA, Filly RA, Callen PW. Benign breast lesions: ultrasound detection and diagnosis. Radiology, 1984;151(2):467–470.

19/ Abdominal Masses

I come from a family of long-livers; my liver is about . . . this long.
Anonymous

It is one thing to discuss lumps and masses of specific organs, e.g. the lymphatics, breast, and thyroid, but quite another to deal with an entire body cavity containing numerous organs, all subject to a variety of enlargements and other distortions in size and shape. Epidemiological methods have been applied to well-defined, (*nameable*) categories, but not, sad to say, the poorly classifiable conditions or abnormalities that clinicians often encounter. This is not the fault of epidemiology but results from our failure to systematize and quantify the occurrence of clinical signs and symptoms as well as the varieties of normal findings. For example, *given only a mass in the abdomen*, where indeed is one to begin, with what organ or system, what region, what etiology? In this area we must rely solely on clinical experience.

We will limit this discussion to the most common masses and enlargements the physician is apt to encounter in the abdomen. Emphasis will be on the asymptomatic mass discovered incidentally on abdominal examination. Our knowledge of these findings is based on clinical experience in the practice of general medicine and with patients referred for sonographic and scintigraphic imaging. Deliberately omitted are the bizarre and the unusual. It is the failure to recognize the garden variety anatomical variation in the abdomen that all too often leads to inappropriate imaging and sometimes even disaster.

Because abdominal masses or enlargements are primarily identified by region, we will adhere to this classification scheme. A brief mention of the concept of organ enlargement is appropriate. Conventional wisdom holds that abnormalities of organ size can be reduced to considerations of measurement, as in: "the normal right kidney in the adult is 9.5–12.3 cm in length"; "the normal nulliparous uterus in premenopausal women is 5.5–9 cm. in length"; or worse, issues of palpability, as in, "the adult spleen is normally not palpable," or the now-discredited, "the normal liver is not palpable more than two and one-half fingerbreadths below the right costal margin," etc. Attempts at quantifying organ size by volume measurements, though mathematically more exact, also fail when one attempts to rely on them too rigidly.

This medical obsession with size measurement classically fails when we attempt to define *obesity*. Whether we use the height-weight tables compiled by the insurance companies, estimates of lean body mass with deuterium, or skin fold measurements, we frequently end up in a dilemma. Who, indeed, is fat, the "chunky" teen-age girl who weighs 120 lbs and is 5 ft, 2 in, the beefy 6-ft right guard who is 235 lbs and all muscle, the 55-year-old woman who appears normal but according to a life insurance table, is 12 pounds overweight? And what medical authority has yet defined *skinniness* or the thin body habitus?

Whether we try to define obesity or uterine size, it seems, we are limited by the accuracy of our methods and our range of normal, with no appeal except to statistical tables. But people vary so much in their "normality," we must be prepared to accept a certain amount of subjectivity in our assessment of human variation, be it liver, ovarian, or total body size. In the obvious case, someone is fat if he or she *looks* fat. We do not need height and weight tables except for quantification and for the questionable. This is not to deny the importance of measurement, but we may confidently conclude that the person who is defined as obese because of mild increases in skin fold thickness and who does not *look* obese is unlikely to have a serious weight problem. This raises other issues, many of which are unanswerable, such as, what is the clinical significance of borderline splenomegaly or questionable reduction in renal size or mass?

We face the same difficulty with stature. Is that 5 ft, 9 in man short? It depends. In northern Holland where many men are tall he may be described as short, whereas in the Philippines he might be regarded as tall. Without belaboring the point, we may conclude that large males are apt to have larger organs than small females, and young patients larger organs than older ones. Although tables of normal organ volumes and sizes have been constructed, they are not related consistently to body habitus, race, weight, age, and even sex. Important exceptions are the tables of crown-rump length, femoral length, biparietal diameter, abdominal circumference, and other measurements so relied upon for gestational age. Here, however, not only size but growth rate is determined, and the results are far more reliable.

As medical imagers, we certainly use tables of organ measurement, but always with some skepticism, hesitating to place undue emphasis on borderline size deviations from the "normal." As with obesity, we prefer to observe that if the spleen or the uterus or the kidney in a given patient *looks* or *feels* large, it probably *is* large. And if it doesn't look or feel enlarged, regardless of a borderline measurement, it probably isn't.

Right Upper Quadrant and Flank Masses

The single most common right upper quadrant mass, of course, is the liver, an organ whose size is often difficult to assess clinically. Although hepatomegaly is easily ascertained in the person of normal habitus, the obese patient and particularly the broad or barrel-chested individual with emphysema and depressed diaphragm frequently present problems. In such individuals, even with careful percussion of the upper liver border in the chest, the distance of hepatic descent below the right costal margin is often more than expected, perhaps up to 12 cm, yet the liver will prove to be of normal size.

An anatomical variant, much more common than most physicians appreciate, is the Riedel's lobe or variant thereof, a tongue-like elongation of the lateral aspect of the right hepatic lobe, which may extend as far down as the pelvic brim.

Another common normal finding in the right upper quadrant or flank is the anteriorly placed right kidney, which is often mistaken for a mass. The normal right kidney, especially in thin young patients, can be so close to the anterior abdominal wall it may be felt just underneath the liver margin. Ultrasonographic examination immediately establishes the diagnosis.

Abnormal right upper and right flank masses further include the palpable gall bladder, the hard, nodular liver of cirrhosis or metastatic cancer, and the enlarged right kidney secondary to hydronephrosis, cyst, or tumor. In infants and children with right or left flank masses, think first of hydronephrosis, Wilms tumor, and neuroblastoma, in that order.

Upper Abdominal and Left Upper Quadrant Masses

In infants the mass of hypertrophic pyloric stenosis may occasionally be felt in the upper or midabdomen. The most common periumbilical mass is, of course, due to umbilical hernia. In older patients the most common source of confusion is the abdominal aorta. Occasionally we are referred patients in their 30s for sonography for

Table 6.19.1.

All-listed ICD-9-CM	Total	Male	Female	Age <15	Age 15–44	Age 45–64	Age 65+
441. Aortic aneurysm	122	82	41	0	0	20	101

"possible aortic aneurysm." Table 6.19.1 shows the frequency of aortic aneurysms among all-listed hospital discharges in the United States for 1990 (1). Note that aortic aneurysm is virtually unknown in the under-44-year age group, with more than 82% of cases occurring in patients over age 65. Confusion arises because of the frequency of a normally palpable aorta. During ultrasonography of the abdomen, particularly in the thin patient, the upper abdominal aorta can be seen to take an extremely anterior course, frequently lying just underneath the upper anterior abdominal wall. It is sometimes difficult to identify enlargement of the normal pulsatile aorta, but if one keeps in mind the age distribution of aneurysm, and the fact that thin subjects as a rule have very anterior abdominal aortas from about 3–5 cm below the xiphoid to just above the umbilicus (at the bifurcation), most unnecessary referrals for aortic aneurysm can be avoided.

One of our mentors, a hematologist, once remarked, "there are two kinds of internists, spleen-feelers and nonspleen-feelers." As always, the habitus of the patient as much as the skill of the examiner determines whether splenomegaly is diagnosed on physical examination. The normal spleen tip is indeed palpable in up to 10% of normal thin subjects, and the enlarged spleen is often not palpable in the heavy-set patient, even by the skilled internist. We have had many disagreements with competent examiners over the presence of splenomegaly, but it is very difficult to argue with a scintiscan. Complicating this, as we have already observed, are questions as to the upper limits of normal spleen size in a patient of given habitus, sex, race, age, and weight. If there is a question of hepato- or splenomegaly, the issue can only be resolved, if at all, by scintigraphy, rarely by CT scans.

Lower Abdomen and Pelvic Masses Felt Abdominally

The *most common* palpable lower abdominal mass in both sexes, is the *distended bladder.* The most important masses in the female pelvis felt abdominally include the pregnant and the leiomyomatous uterus and large ovarian masses, almost always ovarian cysts. These will be discussed in the next section.

Fecal masses may sometimes mimic pathological entities anywhere in the abdomen, most often in the lower quadrants. However, their consistency, lobulation, migration, and especially disappearance with bowel cleansing should make identification easy. Many other important conditions, of course, will present as abdominal masses, especially inguinal hernias. Femoral hernias and other inguinal masses may be mistaken for abdominal masses. Other intraabdominal masses would include such important conditions as strangulated hernias, appendiceal and other abscesses, and distended bowel loops felt in small or large bowel obstruction. Much less common are palpable benign or malignant tumors of the kidney, adrenal, stomach, pancreas, bowel, and pelvis, etc.

With suspected intestinal obstruction, the plain abdominal film should be done first, usually followed by careful barium studies. CT and MRI are not indicated. In almost all other intraabdominal masses, *ultrasonography is the preferred first imaging examination.* It is not necessary, for example, to perform MRI or CT scanning, as one

Table 6.19.2.   Diagnosis of Common Abdominal Masses

Region	Organ	Condition	Imaging study
Upper abdomen	Liver/spleen	Enlargement	Physical exam (scintigraphy if phys. exam inconclusive)
	Liver mass(es) or	Tumor/cyst Metastatic dis	Sonography first followed by CT/MRI (if necessary)
	Gall bladder	Cholecystitis	Sonography
		Ca pancreas	Sonography
Flanks	Kidney	Enlargement	Sonography
	Kidney	Anterior position	Sonography
	Kidney	Cyst, tumor	Sonography followed by CT/MRI (if necessary)
	Kidney	Hydronephrosis	Sonography (if positive, followed by scintigraphy)
Mid/upper	Aorta	Aneurysm	Sonography
Pelvis/lower	Bladder	Distension	Sonography
	Uterus	Pregnancy	Sonography
	Uterus	Enlargement, leiomyomatous or tumor	Sonography
	Ovary	Cyst	Sonography
	Ovary	Non-cystic mass	Sonography followed by CT/MRI
Any abdominal or pelvic mass thought to be arising in bowel			Barium enema first; if nondiagnostic, follow with upper GI

of our patients was advised, for a simple hernia. Another patient with an obvious large irreducible inguinal hernia in the scrotal sac was referred for testicular ultrasound. Without physicians competent enough to perform physical examinations, we may as well start imaging patients' ears. The alternative is Zymurgy's law of evolving systems dynamics, "Once you open a can of worms, the only way to recan them is to use a larger can." One needless test almost always leads to another.

Summary: Diagnostic Approach to the Palpable Abdominal Mass, Including Questionable Enlargements of the Liver, Spleen, Kidneys, Uterus, and Bladder

1. For the estimation of liver and spleen size, physical examination should suffice for most cases.

2. For accurate determination of questionable hepatic or splenic enlargement, or to distinguish enlargement from localized masses involving these organs, liver-spleen scintigraphy is the procedure of first choice. Ultrasonography, CT, and MRI, because they give two-dimensional slices, are poor in assessing overall organ size. Moreover, scintigraphy gives functional data as well.

3. For the initial assessment of all palpable intraabdominal masses, upper abdominal or pelvic ultrasonography is the easiest, quickest, and most desirable first imaging procedure, and gives the most information. With sonography, two crucial facts about a mass in the abdomen can usually be discovered: (a) the probable organ from which the mass arises; and (b) whether the mass is cystic or solid.

4. When there is a question of aortic aneurysm, ultrasonography is indicated, but this diagnosis should almost never be considered in the patient under age 45–50.

5. Given any *abnormal* palpable abdominal mass, depending on location, do not perform CT or MRI unless the diagnosis cannot be made by ultrasonography, the

plain abdominal film, or occasionally scintigraphy. In the large majority of palpable intraabdominal masses, CT or MRI will prove to be unnecessary.

Table 6.19.2 gives recommendations for the diagnosis of common intraabdominal masses.

REFERENCES

1. U.S. Department of Health and Human Services, U.S. Public Health Service, Centers for Disease Control, and the National Center for Health Statistics. National Hospital Discharge Survey (NHDS). Detailed diagnoses, procedures, days of care, diagnoses-related groups for patients discharged from short-stay hospitals. Public Use Data Diskettes, 1985–1990.

20/ Pelvic Masses in Females

> For the nicely brought-up girl, there is something that is hard to reconcile with her genteel sensibilities about walking into the inner sanctum of a complete stranger, solomnly describing her symptoms, and at the end of her recital hearing the stranger say, "Will you please go into the next room and take off everything except your shoes and stockings?" It wouldn't seem so bad if it weren't for that shoes and stockings clause! To my impressionable mind it has always smacked of the more erotic refinements of Berlin during its decadence.
>
> *Cornelia Otis Skinner*

Palpable masses are frequently found on pelvic examination, but in many cases their significance cannot be determined. Except for the distended bladder more often discovered in a hospital setting, the most common mass in the female pelvis is an enlarged uterus. Pregnancy is probably the most frequent cause of uterine enlargement in the reproductive age group, but overall, leiomyomatous disease is the most common cause of uterine enlargement. It used to be taught that the fibroid uterus was a distinct rarity in the patient under age 30, but in practice we are seeing this condition with increasing frequency in younger patients, occasionally those even in their early 20s, especially in black women.

The next most common palpable pelvic mass in women is an ovarian cyst. A variety of other pelvic conditions involving the uterus, ovary, or adnexal structure tumors are encountered. A list of nonovarian adnexal masses is presented in Table 6.20.1 (1). However, the eight common gynecological conditions listed in Table 6.20.2 are the most frequent causes of abnormal pelvic masses.

Ultrasound

> The moral world of the sick-bed explains in a measure some of the things that are strange in daily life, and the man who does not know sick women does not know women.
>
> *S. Weir Mitchell*

Ultrasonography is so expeditious, accurate, and effective an imaging procedure in the female pelvis that it alone suffices in more than 95–99% of cases. Sonography

Table 6.20.1. Nonovarian Adnexal Masses

A. Uterine
   1. Pedunculated fibroids
   2. Bicornuate uterus
B. Nonovarian cysts
   1. Para-ovarian cysts
   2. Endometriomas
   3. Mesenteric cysts
C. Neoplasm
   1. Pelvic sarcomas
   2. Bowel tumors
   3. Sacral/pelvic girdle masses
   4. Adenopathy
   5. Peritoneal metastatis
D. Inflammatory disease
   1. Abscess
      a. Appendicitis
      b. Diverticulitis
      c. Inflammatory bowel disease
   2. Genital inflammation
      a. Tubo-ovarian abscess
      b. Hydrosalpinx
E. Postsurgical
   1. Abscess
   2. Hematoma
   3. Lymphocele
   4. Urinoma
F. Anatomical structures
   1. Pelvic musculature
   2. Pelvic kidney
   3. Bowel
   4. Genitourinary
      a. Bladder diverticula
      b. Dilated ureters
G. General peritoneal abnormalities
   1. Ascites
   2. Hemoperitoneum
   3. Pseudomyxoma peritonei

Reprinted by permission from *Seminars in Ultrasound* (1983;IV(3):193–205).

therefore should always precede any other imaging modality for the study of pelvic conditions or masses because it usually makes further studies, including the oft-used laparoscopy, unnecessary. Actual percentage by sonographic diagnoses of patients undergoing surgery are given in Table 6.20.3. That these percentages correspond closely to surgical diagnoses can be seen from Table 6.20.4, showing the respective sensitivities, specificities and the high PPVs for sonography by surgically confirmed diagnosis (2).

Ultrasonography of the female pelvis is so widely available and easily performed, it should be considered—perhaps more so than any other imaging study—an adjunct to the physical examination. The method is especially valuable in women who are difficult to examine because of obesity, anxiety, pain, or other problems, and can answer several important clinical questions. These have been nicely summarized by Zweibel (3) from which the following are condensed and adapted:

Table 6.20.2. Principal Causes of Pelvic Masses in Females in Order of Frequency

1. Pregnancy (under age 35)
2. Leiomyomatous uterus
3. Ovarian cysts
4. Pelvic inflammatory disease
5. Ectopic pregnancy
6. Endometriosis
7. Ovarian tumors
8. Uterine cancer

Table 6.20.3. Distribution of Sonographic Diagnoses in a Group of 705 Gynecological Patients Undergoing Surgery (Adapted from Loutradis; Ref. 2)

Diagnosis	Percent of Total	Cumulative Percent
Ovarian cyst	39	
Leiomyomatous uterus	33	72
Ectopic pregnancy	13	85
Tubo-ovarian abscess inflammatory disease inc. hydrosalpinx	4	89
Endometriosis	2	91
Miscellaneous (polycystic ovary luteohematoma, ascites hematoma, etc.)	8	99
Ovarian carcinoma	1	100

Table 6.20.4. Sensitivity, Specificity, and PPV of the Sonographic Evaluation in the Diagnosis of the Gynecological Conditions Where the Total of Patients Was More Than 10 in the Group of Consecutively Examined Gynecological Patients Undergoing Surgery

Diagnosis	Sensitivity (%)	Specificity (%)	PPV (%)
Leiomyoma	94.5	95.3	91.0
Ovarian cyst	95.3	93.8	89.7
Ectopic pregnancy	89.2	99.8	98.9
Tubo-ovarian abscess	88.9	100.0	100.0
Endometriosis	78.9	99.8	93.8
Leuteohematoma	75.0	100.0	100.0

Reprinted by permission from *Gynecologic and Obstetric Investigation*. Basel: S. Karger AG (1990;29(1):47–50).

Is the Pelvis Normal or Abnormal? A negative pelvic ultrasound study is a strong indication of normality, because the method has an overall sensitivity of 90% for the detection of abnormal conditions (4).

What Anatomical Structures Are Involved? Uterine, tubal, and ovarian masses are frequently indistinguishable on examination. A pedunculated uterine myomata, for example, may mimic an ovarian mass in a middle-aged woman. Although sonography does not always distinguish a pedunculated fibroid from an ovarian neoplasm adherent to the uterus, or endometriosis from other disease, the method has an overall specificity of 93–100%.

What Are the Characteristics of the Mass? Specifically, is it *solid, cystic,* or *mixed?* Once a purely cystic lesion is demonstrated, for example, in the ovary of a premenopausal female, the benign nature of the mass is absolutely established. (This is not always true in a postmenopausal woman, however.)

Is a Given Pelvic Mass Regressing or Enlarging? Sonography is highly accurate in measuring changes of size and character of pelvic masses with time. It is therefore invaluable in deciding on therapy, particularly whether surgical intervention is necessary for a given patient.

How Reliable Is Pelvic Ultrasound in Making a Diagnosis?   In the impressive series quoted above, ultrasound established the correct diagnosis in an average of 95% of cases (Table 6.2.4) (2).

CT and MRI in the Pelvis

Despite the superiority of ultrasonography over all other imaging methods in the pelvis, the modality fails to provide adequate information in at least two specific instances: in cancer staging, and in examining the posthysterectomy pelvis for cancer recurrence.

The relative advantages of CT vs. MRI have yet to be established in these clinical settings, but certain guidelines can be given. It has been stated that CT (and ultrasound) are inaccurate compared to MRI for staging of endometrial and cervical cancer (5, 6), but that CT is more accurate than MRI in staging ovarian carcinoma (7, 8).

Pelvic Laparoscopy

There has occurred an almost 50% decline in diagnostic laparoscopies performed in U.S. hospitals since 1985 (9), an encouraging—and surprising—development in the annals of modern invasive procedures. Pelvic, like abdominal, laparoscopy has an important place in diagnosis in a specific but limited group of patients, those in whom the diagnosis remains in doubt, i.e. when *after careful examination and pelvic ultrasonography* the decision to operate *cannot otherwise be made*. The potential for laparoscopic surgery enormously enhances the usefulness of the procedure in this group of patients.

Summary

Ultrasonography is so effective, reliable, and accurate, it should be considered virtually an adjunct to the gynecological pelvic examination. Sonography should *always* be used as the *premier imaging modality* in the female pelvis. Principal indications are:

1. Examination of female patients in whom pelvic examination is difficult, e.g. infants, children, and uncooperative, nervous, or obese patients;
2. As a screening test in symptomatic female patients without pelvic findings to confirm the presence of a normal pelvis;
3. When a mass is found, to determine what anatomical structures are involved;
4. To determine the characteristics of a pelvic mass, specifically whether it is solid, cystic, or mixed; and
5. To determine whether a given pelvic mass is regressing or enlarging.

CT and MRI in the pelvis are indicated only after ultrasonography is performed, and generally only in the following categories:

1. Initial or preoperative gynecologic cancer staging;
2. Postoperative cancer staging or staging in the posthysterectomy pelvis; and
3. When ultrasound is unsuccessful in determining the extent, location, or character of a mass, e.g. pelvic collection or deep, lateral, or posterior masses.

Some authorities hold that MRI is superior to CT in staging of endometrial and cervical cancer, but that CT is more accurate than MRI in staging ovarian carcinoma.

Laparoscopy is useful only in patients in whom surgery is contemplated when the diagnosis cannot be made sonographically, or in whom laparoscopic biopsy or surgery is indicated.

REFERENCES

1. Ralls PW, Rotter AJ, Halls JM. Non-ovarian adnexal pathology. Semin Ultrasound 1983;IV(3):193–205.
2. Loutradis D, Antsaklis A, Creatsas G, et al. The validity of gynecological ultrasonography. Gynecol Obstet Invest 1990;29(1):47–50.
3. Zweibel WJ. The problem of pelvic sonography [Letter from the Editor]. Seminars Ultrasound 1983; 4(3):143–144.
4. Lawson TL, Albarelli JN. Diagnosis of gynecologic pelvic masses by gray scale ultrasonography: analysis of specificity and accuracy. AJR 1977;128(6):1003–1006.
5. Choyke PL, Thickman D, Kressel HY, et al. Controversies in the radiologic diagnosis of pelvic malignancies. Radiol Clin North Am 1985;23(3):531–549.
6. Hricak H. MRI of the female pelvis: a review. AJR 1986;146(6):1115–1122.
7. Fishman-Javitt MC, Lovecchio JL, Stein HL. MR imaging of ovarian neoplasms. Radiology 1987; 165(P):123,432.
8. Fishman-Javitt MC, Lovecchio JL, Stein HL. Imaging strategies for MRI of the pelvis. Radiol Clin North Am 1988;26(3):633–651.
9. U.S. Department of Health and Human Services, U.S. Public Health Service, Centers for Disease Control, and the National Center for Health Statistics. National Hospital Discharge Survey (NHDS). Detailed diagnoses, procedures, days of care, diagnoses-related groups for patients discharged from short-stay hospitals. Public Use Data Diskettes, 1985–1990.

21/ Thyroid Masses and Enlargements

> *Writing to his father about Simon Bolivar in his final illness, Colonel Wilson mentioned that his "rejection of doctors was the result of lucidity, not contempt."*
>
> Gabriel Garcia Marquez
> The General in His Labyrinth

Thyroid Masses
GOITER

The most common thyroid disease throughout the United States and large parts of the world is colloid nodular goiter, occurring in 300 million people, or more than 5% of the human population (1–3). In the United States the second most common thyroid condition is Hashimoto's struma (4). Scrimshaw (5) records that endemic goiter was so common in parts of this country in World War I that thousands of men from the Great Lakes westward into the far western states of Montana, Idaho, Utah, Oregon, and Washington were rejected for military service because they could not button the collars of their military tunics. It is difficult to believe today that in goitrous areas of the United States during those years, rates of 20–80% were commonly reported.

Within a few years of the introduction of iodine prophylaxis in the late 1920s, the prevalence of goiter had dropped to a fraction of its earlier value (6). Yet by the mid 1960s goiter was on the upswing. Among other places, it was found in 10–16% of women 20–40 years of age in Tecumseh, Mich (7) and in 33% of school children in a county in Kentucky (8). In both series there was proof of adequate iodine uptake.

Although the geographical prevalence of goiter still varies widely, goiter remains one of the world's major public health problems.

It is curious indeed that endemic goiter, formerly, in Stanbury's words, "the adaptation of man to iodine deficiency," and which virtually disappeared in this country after iodized salt was introduced in 1926, has had such an enormous resurgence in the past 60 years. In the opinion of many, this may well be due to the effects of environmental pollutants, both natural and man-made. Beierwaltes (4) tells us the incidence of goiters in Great Lakes fish in the 1970s increased 2- to 6-fold without any change in water iodine content. He also states that "not everyone exposed to iodine deficiency or to goitrogenic chemicals in the environment develops a goiter ... (indicating) that a considerable portion of the population has an inherited or acquired biochemical defect that predisposes to these environmental stresses on the thyroid gland."

THYROID CANCER

In contrast to endemic goiter, thyroid cancer is extremely rare, with one of the lowest incidence rates of all malignancies; 12,000 new cases of thyroid cancer were estimated for the United States in 1990, an incidence of 4 per 100,000 (9). Total all-listed discharge diagnoses of thyroid malignancy in U.S. hospitals in 1990 were only 8 per 100,000 (10). The age-specific prevalence rates for thyroid cancer in Connecticut in 1982 varied from 4 cases under age 30 to 49 cases at age 70 in males with corresponding rates of 15 and 107 cases per 100,000, respectively, for females (11). These relatively high prevalences (the number of individuals *with* the condition) compared with the low incidence (the number of people *developing* the condition) are explained by the extremely long survival rates for most patients with thyroid cancer and consequent low mortality rate, estimated at 1,000 deaths in 1990 (9).

Another interesting fact can be gleaned from autopsy studies carried out on thyroid glands obtained from patients from various countries throughout the world. A Swedish study of 430 thyroid glands obtained at autopsy showed occult papillary thyroid carcinoma occurred in about 8% of all patients with an even distribution in all age groups over 20 (12). In an oft-quoted study (13) the prevalence of occult papillary thyroid cancer ranged from 5.5% in Colombia to 9.1% in Poland to 28.4% in Japan, prompting the authors to remark that, *"Most papillary thyroid carcinomas grow slowly and probably remain occult for the life of the patient"* (13) (our emphasis).

THE SOLITARY NODULE

> *Whoever named it necking was a poor judge of anatomy.*
> *Groucho Marx*

Selwyn Taylor has shown that the frequency of malignant nodules is fairly constant throughout life, and benign nodules show their highest incidence in the ages between 20 and 60, peaking at 40 as shown in Figure 6.21.1 (14). The graph shows that because total solitary nodules are distinctly uncommon in the age groups under 20 and over 60, it is logical to conclude solitary nodules are much more likely to be cancerous in these two age groups. These clinical data are consistent with the epidemiology of thyroid cancer quoted above. Taylor's series (14) also shows that a preponderance of nodules thought to be solitary are indeed proven not to be at surgery. This is shown in Table 6.21.1. The figures are still subject to strong surgical bias,

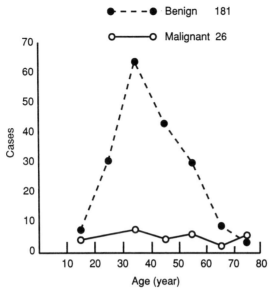

Figure 6.21.1. Age distribution of 207 benign and malignant nodules. Reprinted by permission from Werner SC, Ingbar SH, eds. *The Thyroid*. Philadelphia: J. B. Lippincott Co. (1978;4:510).

Table 6.21.1. Nodules Found Solitary by Clinical, Surgical, and Histologic Criteria

	No.	%
Clinically	207	100
Surgically	124	60
Histologically	108	52

Reprinted by permission from Werner SC, Ingbar SH, eds. *The Thyroid*. Philadelphia: J.B. Lippincott Co. (1978;4:510).

being a select group because they represent high tumor suspects. Table 6.21.2 shows the pathology of 207 clinically solitary nodules from Taylor's series (14). Indeed, the actual percentage of *all* solitary nodules that are malignant is estimated to be 0.1–0.2% (15). Thus, given any unselected patient with a thyroid nodule, the chance of cancer is less than 1 in 1000. Yet an autopsy study of patients with clinically normal thyroids showed 50% with one or more nodules (16). This suggests that the true incidence of thyroid cancer in nodules is probably even lower. Nodules, however, are 4 to 5 times more common in women than men, and because thyroid cancer is fairly equally common in both sexes, the finding of a nodule in a male patient has much more significance than in a female.

The frequency of thyroid cancer in series of operated patients with palpable solitary nodules has ranged from 8–33% with a median of 20%, figures which are so highly inflated because of selection bias as to be almost meaningless (15, 17).

Because of the foregoing, it should be obvious that nodules or lumps discovered in palpating the thyroid gland generally have far less significance than lumps discovered elsewhere in the body, particularly in the breast. The overall chance of an unselected single thyroid nodule being cancer is less than 1 in 1000 (though the chance of a dominant nodule in a multinodular goiter being malignant is somewhat higher). Nevertheless, because many physicians are fearful of missing a malignancy, they feel compelled to investigate every palpable thyroid "abnormality."

Table 6.21.2.   Pathology of 207 Clinically Solitary Nodules

| Classification | Nodularity | | Total |
	Single	Multiple	
Benign	94	87	181
Malignant	14	12	26
Total	108	99	207

Overall incidence of carcinoma, 12.6%.
Reprinted by permission from Werner SC, Ingbar SH, eds. *The Thyroid*. Philadelphia: J.B. Lippincott Co. (1978;4:510).

EXAMINING THE THYROID: PLATITUDES, PERILS, AND PITFALLS

Because of the high frequency of goiter in the general population, there is obviously a significant chance of finding a palpable thyroid abnormality in the average patient. Like most endocrinologists, however, we often encounter patients who are referred to us with "phantom" thyroid abnormalities. This is not surprising in view of the neglect of the thyroid gland in medical school physical diagnosis courses. Four normal findings rarely mentioned in textbooks are frequent sources of confusion.

1. The soft, symmetrical, normally palpable thyroid gland, usually seen in young females, is often mistaken for thyromegaly. Sometimes one or both thyroid lobes may be quite easily palpable and discrete, perhaps even firm. Although some of these glands may represent a *forme fruste* of Hashimoto's disease, they are more often variations of the normal.

2. In the patient with a thin neck, particularly males, a prominent band-like cricoid cartilage lying in the midline above the thyroid just below the thyroid cartilage is often mistaken for a nodule or enlargement, especially because the cricoid moves with swallowing.

3. A frequent source of confusion can be seen and felt in the obese or plump female patient who presents with a prominent pretracheal fat pad overlying the region of the gland, the so-called "Collière de Venus." This, of course, does not move with swallowing.

4. Not uncommonly, a prominent sternocleidomastoid muscle, often with fatty infiltration, can be mistaken for an abnormal thyroid gland.

Once encountered, these four variants are seldom forgotten. If every medical student or intern could spend 2 hours of his training examining 50 thyroids with an experienced clinician, the potential annual savings to the health care system would probably be staggering.

Palpable thyroid abnormalities come in different types and sizes, but essentially they can be categorized into four principal findings:

A. Diffuse enlargement;
B. A single nodule;
C. Multiple nodules; and
D. Multiple nodules with a dominant nodule.

B, C, and D may or may not be associated with A.

THE THYROIDAL RADIOIODINE UPTAKE

The 24-hour thyroidal radioiodine uptake (RAI) first introduced in the early 1940s immediately became the most successful and popular test of thyroid function.

Because of the increasing ubiquity of stable iodine in the environment over the past thirty years, e.g. iodates used widely in baking, iodine in antiseptics, vitamins, douches, and cleaners, etc., the normal 24-hour uptake range has declined from an average of 20–50% in the 1960s to 10–35% today. (This list does not even include radiographic contrast material, which is the most common cause of spuriously low uptakes.) This means that the sensitivity of the RAI for detection of *hypothyroidism* is now too low to make the test reliable for this condition. The iodine-131 uptake is still helpful in confirming hyperthyroidism, however, especially in patients with borderline thyroxine (T_4) levels, and in studying the occasional patient with subacute thyroiditis. In some obviously thyrotoxic patients a high normal or borderline elevated uptake often suggests the possibility of triiodothyronine (T_3) toxicosis and the need for obtaining free T_3 values. In addition, there is the rare thyrotoxic patient who has a very low RAI in the presence of high T_4, a combination which is diagnostic of factitious hyperthyroidism or subacute thyroiditis.

Practice habits have a way of lingering on, but despite some suggestions that thyroid uptakes are usually unnecessary in clinically euthyroid patients we continue to perform them routinely with scintigraphy. The reasons for this are multiple. First, when patients present themselves, their thyroid functional status is not always clinically obvious, and sometimes the serendipitous diagnosis of thyrotoxicosis or *forme fruste* hyperthyroidism can be made on the RAI. Much more frequent, however, is the finding of an extremely low uptake in a euthyroid patient. This indicates either thyroid blockade with iodides, suppression with thyroid hormone, which was missed in the initial interview, or an unsuspected thyroiditis. In these cases the low uptake saves patients the expense and trouble of undergoing scintigraphy, which is useless in this event, and allows rescheduling radionuclide imaging for a later date. If the patient indeed has subacute or acute thyroiditis, scintigraphy is not necessary and generally futile anyway because of a spuriously low iodine uptake. Furthermore, performing the RAI initially obviates the difficulty of interpreting thyroid scintigrams without knowing thyroid functional status. Last, when the uptake is low or borderline, we can increase the usual dose of technetium-99m to obtain a more optical scintiscan. In some older patients with a borderline low RAI and unimpressive but palpable, low-lying nodular thyroid enlargement, one should be alerted to the possibility of a substernal goiter.

THYROID SCINTIGRAPHY

When thyroid imaging is indeed appropriate, and it is not always so in the patient with goiter, the modality of first choice is always radionuclide scintigraphy using either technetium-99m or iodine-123. Ultrasonography of the thyroid may occasionally be helpful, but only in a small subset of patients, to be discussed below. CT with contrast has been rightly called the "scourge" of thyroid imaging because, usually performed with contrast, it prevents reliable thyroid scintigraphy for 6 weeks or longer due to iodine blockade. (Ironically, it is usually unnecessary to use contrast material with thyroid CT, because the iodine-containing thyroid gland normally shows up so well.) In fact, CT and MRI are seldom indicated in thyroid imaging, particularly in patients with upper mediastinal masses suspected of being substernal goiter where these studies are most inappropriately applied. In these cases, scintigraphy, which is a functional as well as anatomical imaging method, is unexcelled because it *unequivocally identifies functioning thyroid tissue*. Scintigraphy, therefore, should always be performed before any other modalities are used to image the thyroid. In the overwhelming majority of cases, sonography and CT/MRI will prove to be superfluous or unnecessary once the radionuclide scan is interpreted.

The issue of technetium-99m vs. iodine-123 scintigraphy is periodically raised because of occasional reports of discordant findings with the two radionuclides, particularly with functioning, i.e. "warm" or "hot" nodules on technetium scanning turning out to be nonfunctioning or "cold" with iodine. The controversy is complicated by the fact that the availability of cyclotron-produced iodine-123 is limited and the price high. Furthermore, the 13-hour half-life of the radionuclide forces undue rigidity in scheduling thyroid scintigraphy, often to 2 or 3 days a week. In a careful study of 316 cases (18), discrepancies between technetium-99m and iodine-123 images were found in 5–8% of cases, but most of these were in multinodular goiters. "Twelve cancers were found (4%), but none in nodules showing a discrepancy." It was concluded that "*routine* reimaging of 99m-Tc hot nodules with radioiodine for cancer detection does not appear to be necessary" (18) (our emphasis).

FINE-NEEDLE ASPIRATION (FNA) OF THE THYROID

The combination of history, especially rapid growth, physical examination, maleness, young and older age, and a history of radiation to the head or neck in childhood always provide the most powerful predictors of thyroid cancer in patients with nodules. Clinical assessment together with thyroid scintigraphy is more than 95% sensitive in diagnosing the presence of thyroid enlargement, multinodular goiter, and dominant nodules, either those that are nonfunctioning and take up little or no radionuclide (cold) or those that function and take up radionuclide (hot). In the presence of a single or dominant cold nodule, i.e. one that is nonfunctioning and does not take up radioiodine, usually more than 2–3 cm, in a multinodular gland, FNA of the thyroid is indicated, because surgery can thus be avoided in the majority of cases. The incidence of false-positive diagnoses is very low, and false-negative diagnoses of 10% are seen in good hands (19, 20). Table 6.21.3, which gives the relative sensitivities and specificities of various thyroid diagnostic tests, shows why FNA is so important in thyroid cancer diagnosis (17). Note that, compared to FNA, scintiscanning, ultrasonography, and thyroid suppression have extremely poor specificities, which means their diagnostic usefulness is severely compromised (21). The number of false-positive results with these tests will be intolerably high, particularly because more than 80% of solitary thyroid nodules are cold. Because the specificity of FNA may range from 75–95% (15, 17, 22, 23), many authorities have even argued that a cost-effective strategy (presumably in the hands of an expert who can accurately palpate the thyroid) would dictate that FNA completely replace scintigraphy in the management of solitary thyroid nodules. If one is only interested in diagnosing cancer, this strategy makes sense. However, in the hands of the generalist or even the experiencd endocrinologist, without excluding the likelihood of other much more common thyroid diseases, especially Hashimoto's struma, with scintigraphy, serum antibodies and the thyroid-stimulating hormone (TSH) radioimmunoassay it is not possible in the case of a negative fine-needle aspiration to "decide whether a fine-needle aspiration result is representative as a cause of the goiter" (4). We once more stress that biopsy of a cold nodule smaller than 1.5–2.0 cm is seldom required unless enlargement under observation with or without suppression and/or patient anxiety warrant the procedure.

Table 6.21.3. Test Sensitivities and Specificities in the Diagnosis of Carcinoma of the Thyroid

Diagnostic test	Definition of positive result	Sensitivity (%)	Specificity (%)
Scintigraphic scan	Cold, solitary nodule		
Iodine-131		83	25
Technetium-99m		93	15
Ultrasonography	Solid or mixed lesion	95	18
Thyroid hormone suppression	No change in size or growth of the nodule	85	25
Fine-needle aspiration	Cytology suspicious or positive for malignancy	87	75
	Malignant	. . .	. . .
	Suspicious	. . .	. . .
	Benign	. . .	. . .

Reprinted by permission from Panzer RJ, Black EF, Griner PF, eds. *Diagnostic Strategies For Common Medical Problems.* Philadelphia: American College of Physicians (1991:388).

THYROID ULTRASONOGRAPHY

Sonographic examination of the thyroid is performed increasingly but has limited application in diagnosis. The value of sonography is generally overrated, and its use may only add confusion to the management of the average case. Clinicians occasionally request sonography of a solitary cold nodule to determine whether it is a simple cyst. The problem is that true ab initio thyroid cysts are extremely rare. When a cystic lesion of the thyroid is visualized it is almost invariably an older nodule that has undergone hemorrhage or central necrosis. Although most of these lesions are indeed benign, the sonographic characteristics are not sufficiently specific to exclude the presence of cancer. Thus, unlike the situation in the breast, most of these patients should have FNA regardless of the sonographic demonstration of a cystic lesion. Moreover, the ultrasound distinction of benign from malignant nodules is unreliable. Another problem is the exquisite sensitivity of ultrasound in detecting small, unsuspected lesions of the thyroid whose clinical significance is doubtful. Because of the prevalence of these unsuspected nodules in the normal population and despite (or because of) the known incidence of microscopic thyroid cancer discovered incidentally at autopsy, it seems prudent *not* to subject patients with clinically insignificant thyroid lesions to further investigation. In view of the wide variety of possible sonographic findings in diffuse thyroid disease, its value in this area is controversial (24). If a sonographically detectable nodule is not palpated or not seen on scintigraphy it is almost certainly of no significance.

There are legitimate indication for ultrasonography of the thyroid, however, which are shown in Table 6.21.4. Ultrasonographic guidance to determine the depth, angle, and direction of the needle for FNA is one of the most important reasons. Common sense suggests that sonography almost never would be indicated in FNA of the thyroid, because only palpable lesions are generally aspirated. Yet we have not found this to be true. Numerous failed biopsies of what seemed to be easily accessible lesions were later successfully performed after sonographic guidance. This is not surprising in view of the fact that up to 20% of FNAs in one series were cytologically indeterminate because of poor needle placement (24). Another important application is in detecting reduction in size of a solitary nodule treated with suppression. Although physical examination may suffice in these cases, small decrements in size may

Table 6.21.4.   Suggested Indications for Thyroid Ultrasonography

1. Guidance for fine needle aspiration or thyroid biopsy
2. To monitor more precisely than physical examination the change in size of a nodule treated with thyroid suppression
3. Determination of the presence or absence of a thyroid mass thought to be equivocal on physical examination
4. Determining the presence of multinodularity in a gland thought to be harboring a solitary nodule

Relative indications
1. Imaging pregnant women, infants, and patients who refuse scintigraphy
2. The detection of occult thyroid cancer in patients with metastatic disease of unknown origin
3. Screening high risk patients such as those with a history of neck irradiation in childhood
4. Mass localization when a clinical determination cannot distinguish between thyroidal and extrathyroidal origin, i.e. branchial cleft cyst, lymph node, etc.

Adapted from James (24), Simeone (25), and Wang (27).

not be appreciated for long periods of time. In addition, physical examination and scintigraphy do not have the high sensitivity in detecting the presence of small additional nodules less than 1–1.5 cm in size, which, if found, greatly lessen the chance of cancer in the patient thought to have a dominant *single* nodule. This is important because the likelihood of a *true* single cold nodule larger than 2 cm being malignant is considerably higher than that of an average-sized nodule (<1–2 cm) in a multinodular goiter (20, 25, 26).

PLAIN RADIOGRAPHY OF THE NECK

Plain soft tissue films of the neck, anterior and lateral, are sometimes taken in patients with large goiters, especially those with substernal extension. However, in practice, the compressed tracheal air column is almost always seen on the chest radiograph. According to the World Health Organization, the most common cause of death from goiter is strangulation from tracheal compression. It is sometimes difficult even with radiographs to determine if the degree of tracheal compression warrants thyroidectomy. In these cases, barium swallow is of little help, nor are the usual pulmonary function tests. The *only* reliable test is the *flow volume loop* when it can be shown that peak flow rates are *distinctly muted* in the presence of even early upper airway obstruction.

Summary of the Diagnostic Approach to Palpable Thyroid Abnormalities

DIFFUSE ENLARGEMENT

In order of likely diagnoses:

1. If the gland is firm and "rubbery" (and often with irregular surface nodularity) think first of Hashimoto's struma;

2. If the gland is less firm or soft, think next of simple goiter.

3. Consider hyperthyroidism with diffuse, usually symmetrical enlargement. Here, the gland may be soft with relatively recent onset of disease, and more firm with long-standing thyrotoxicosis.

4. With true diffuse enlargement in the absence of nodules, cancer is essentially excluded.

5. Perform the radioiodine uptake and do scintigraphy in all cases in which there is clinical uncertainty as to the presence of nodularity.

6. If the radioiodine uptake is elevated or borderline, regardless of clinical findings, always follow with T_4, TSH, and thyroid antibody studies to help identify hyperthyroidism and Hashimoto's disease. It is always advisable to perform scintigraphy in hyperthyroidism for confirming gland size, to exclude the presence of toxic nodular goiter, and thus for estimating an appropriate therapy dose of iodine-131.

MULTINODULAR GOITER WITHOUT A CLINICALLY DOMINANT NODULE

1. In multinodular goiters in women, scintigraphy is advisable if only to exclude the unsuspected dominant nodule and to provide a baseline if the patient subsequently develops further thyroid enlargement. (Parenthetically, thyroid suppression therapy prevents further enlargement of goiter, and often results in regression. Examination, TSH level, and sometimes subsequent scintiscans indicate whether the patient is taking her medication.)

2. Perform scintigraphy in all males with multinodular goiters.

THE SINGLE NODULE OR THE DOMINANT NODULE IN A MULTINODULAR GLAND

Always perform the RAI and radionuclide scintigraphy to determine the functional status of the nodule and appearance of the rest of the gland, particularly the presence and function of other nodules.

The Functioning (Warm) or Hyperfunctioning (Hot) Nodule

1. Because the incidence of cancer in hyperfunctioning nodules is well under the 1% range, further study is generally not necessary except when clinical indicators such as increasing size, hardness, fixation, adenopathy, etc., are found. Be wary, however, of the warm or normally functioning nodule, which raises slightly the probability of malignancy. Most of these warm nodules are actually cold nodules with "shine-through" from underlying normal thyroid tissue.

2. In solitary hot nodules when the rest of the gland or the contralateral lobe is not visualized, do not assume the presence of an autonomous nodule with suppression. The most common cause is a "hot nodule in a dying thyroid" secondary to an old goiter or chronic thyroiditis (Beierwaltes, W. H.), or less common, regenerative tissue after thyroidectomy. In either event, specific treatment is not called for except in the rare instance when coexistent hyper- or hypothyroidism is diagnosed.

The Single Dominant Poorly or Nonfunctioning (Cold) Thyroid Nodule

1. Short of surgery, which is unnecessary in most patients, scintigraphy, TSH/ antibody studies, and FNA form the diagnostic triad for thyroid cancer. Even in the single cold nodule, the chance of thyroid cancer is probably less than 3–5%.

2. If a representative FNA or large needle thyroid biopsy is negative for malignancy, there is less than 5–10% chance of malignancy. A trial of thyroid suppression for 3–6 months is usually indicated. If the nodule diminishes in size during this period, the likelihood of cancer is almost nil. To complicate management, however, many benign nodules may not decrease in size.

3. Early thyroid surgery or open biopsy for single cold dominant nodules is indicated in the following categories:

A. Males;

B. Patients with a history of radiation therapy to the head and neck before age 20;

C. Patients under the age of 20 and older patients over 60, especially those in whom the nodule is hypercellular on FNA;

D. Patients whose nodules enlarge under thyroid suppression for 3 months or fail to decrease in size in 6 months;

E. If the nodule is hard or fixed; and

F. If there is associated lymphadenopathy or nerve dysfunction (recurrent laryngeal, phrenic, etc.)

REFERENCES

1. Beierwaltes WH. The most common thyroid disease in the state of Michigan is endemic goiter not due to iodine deficiency. Wash County Med Soc Bull 1987;39:3–10.

2. Beierwaltes WH. The diagnosis and treatment of endemic goiter. The most common thyroid disease in the United States: a challenge to physicians. Wash County Med Soc Bull 1987;39:2–11.

3. Gaitan E, Nelson NC, Poole GV. Endemic goiter and endemic thyroid disorders. World J Surg 1991; 15(2):205–215.

4. Beierwaltes WH. Comparison of technetium-99m and iodine-123 nodules: correlation with pathologic findings [Editorial]. J Nucl Med 1990;31(4):400–402.

5. Scrimshaw NS. The geographic pathology of thyroid disease. In: Hazard JB, Smith DE, eds. The Thyroid. Baltimore: Williams and Wilkins, 1964:102.

6. Kimball OP. Prevention of goiter in Michigan and Ohio. JAMA 1937;108:860–864.

7. Matovinovic J, Hayner NS, Epstein FH, Kjelsberg MD. Goiter and other thyroid diseases in Tecumseh, Michigan. JAMA 1965;192:234.

8. London WT, Koutras DA, Pressman A, Vought RL. Epidemiologic and metabolic studies of a goiter endemic in eastern Kentucky. J Clin Endocrinol Metab 1965;25:1091.

9. Cancer Statistics, 1990. Ca-A Cancer Journal for Clinicians, American Cancer Society, 1990;40(1):19–26.

10. U.S. Department of Health and Human Services, U.S. Public Health Service, Centers for Disease Control, and the National Center for Health Statistics. National Hospital Discharge Survey (NHDS). Detailed diagnoses, procedures, days of care, diagnoses-related groups for patients discharged from short-stay hospitals. Public Use Data Diskettes, 1985–1990.

11. Feldman AR, Kessler L, Myers MH, Naughton MD. The prevalence of cancer—estimates based on the Connecticut Tumor Registry. N Engl J Med 1986;315(22):1394–1397.

12. Bondeson L, Ljungberg O. Occult papillary thyroid carcinoma in the young and the aged. Cancer 1984;53(8):1790–1792.

13. Fukunaga FH, Yatani R. Georgraphic pathology of occult thyroid carcinomas. Cancer 1975;36(3): 1095–1099.

14. Taylor S. Sporadic nontoxic goiter. In: Werner SC, Ingbar SH, eds. The Thyroid. 4th ed. New York: Harper and Row, Inc., 1978:510.

15. Dolan JG. Thyroid nodules. In: Griner PF, Panzer RJ, Greenland P, eds. Clinical Diagnosis and the Laboratory—Logical Strategies for Common Medical Problems. Chicago: Year Book Medical Publishers, 1986:573–577.

16. Mortensen JD, Woolner LB, Bennett WA. Gross and microscopic findings in clinically normal thyroid glands. J Clin Endocrinol Metab 1955;15:1270.

17. Dolan JG. Thyroid nodules. In: Panzer RJ, Black EF, Griner PF, eds. Diagnostic Strategies for Common Medical Problems. Philadelphia: The American College of Physicians, 1991:388.

18. Kusic Z, Becker DV, Saenger EL, et al. Comparison of technetium-99m and iodine-123 imaging of thyroid nodules: correlation with pathologic findings. J Nucl Med 1990;31(4):393–399.

19. Meinders AE. The role of fine-needle aspiration biopsy cytology in the management of thyroid neoplasms [Editorial]. Neth J Med 1983;26(8):213–214.

20. Klonoff DC, Greenspan FS. The thyroid nodule. Adv Intern Med 1982;27:101–126.

21. Ashcraft MW, Van Herle AJ. Management of thyroid nodules: II. Scanning techniques, thyroid suppressive therapy, and fine needle aspiration. Head Neck Surg 1981;3(4):297–322.

22. Gharib H, Hay ID, Beahrs OH. Cancer of the thyroid. In: Ariyan S, ed. Cancer of the Head and Neck. Baltimore: Williams & Wilkins, 1985.

23. Straub WH, Watson CG. Solitary thyroid nodule. In: Straub WH, ed. Manual of Diagnostic Imaging. Boston: Little, Brown & Co, 1989:72–75.

24. James EM, Charboneau JW. High-frequency (10MHz) thyroid ultrasonography. Semin Ultrasound CT MR 1985;6(3):294–309.
25. Simeone JF, Daniels GH, Mueller PR, et al. High resolution real-time sonography of the thyroid. Radiology 1982;145(2):431–435.
26. Brown CL. Pathology of the cold nodule. Clin Endocrinol Metab 1981;10(2):235–245.
27. Wang CA. Management of thyroid disease based on needle biopsy pathology. Clin Endocrinol Metab 1981;10(2):293–298.

22/ Pregnancy

Religion has done love a great service by making it a sin.

Anatole France

When obstetrical ultrasonography was first introduced in the 1950s (1), no one could have foretold the consequences of this extraordinary medical advance. Although one easily can make a case against the routine use of sonography in pregnancy, in today's affluent society and amidst the fear of litigation, many physicians are opting for at least one ultrasound examination during gestation, despite the fact that only 4% of pregnancies are abnormal (2). The discussion that follows does not deal with indications for sonography in fertility problems, patients on fertility drugs, and those with repeated first trimester miscarriages.

At the present time, it is estimated that more than half of all pregnant women in the United States undergo diagnostic ultrasonography during their pregnancies. This figure will almost certainly rise significantly in the next decade. Because of exaggerated and frequently ill-founded public fears over the risks of various environmental and man-made hazards, a brief refutation of medical "risks" of sonographic imaging is in order. Extremely low energies are employed in diagnostic ultrasound with "spatial/temporal averages" of 2.7–60 mW/cm^2 on the radiating surface of automatic sector scanners (3). In a recent summary article, reviews of various studies of insects, plants, cell suspensions, and even small mammals failed to provide any consistently reliable data for application to human populations. In more than 30 years no epidemiological evidence in human beings has demonstrated *any ill effects* from levels of acoustic energies used in ultrasonic diagnosis. The authors' summary (3) concluded: "Current data indicate that there are no confirmed biologic effects on patients and their fetuses from the use of diagnostic ultrasound and that the benefits . . . of ultrasound *outweigh the risks, if any*" (4) (emphasis added). (It should be added, however, that the safety of pulsed Doppler ultrasound of the umbilical cord in late pregnancy is still under study.)

Ultrasonography of the Pregnant Uterus: Specific Indications

The question remains: is there life after birth?

Anonymous

Important questions arise concerning ultrasonography during gestation. What is the place of sonography in the normal and abnormal pregnancy? If sonography is to be performed, when is the optimal time during gestation? Should the examination be repeated, and if so, when and under what circumstances?

Table 6.22.1.   General and Relative Indications for Ultrasonography of the Pregnant Uterus

1. Determination of gestational age, and its corollary, detection of fetal growth disorders
2. Determination of fetal presentation
3. Detecting the presence of congenital anomalies
4. Evaluation of multiple pregnancies
5. Assessment of placental normality and in particular the diagnosis and grading of placenta praevia
6. Determination of amniotic fluid volume, i.e. the diagnosis of oligo- or polyhydramnios
7. Ultrasonic guidance for amniocentesis and other invasive procedures, etc.

Clear-cut indications for sonographic examination in pregnancy are obvious and include such situations as the diagnosis of suspected ectopic pregnancy, the determination of fetal viability, and the status of the fetus in threatened abortion. General and relative indications for performing fetal sonography are shown in Table 6.22.1.

Because it is possible to diagnose gestation by the 8th to 10th day after fertilization with the urinary urinary chorionic gonadotropin (UCG) or the blood β-subunit human CG (HCG) test, but impossible before the 4th or 5th week by sonography, it is obvious that *sonographic imaging is never appropriate for the diagnosis of pregnancy*. Yet it is employed all too often for this purpose. The predictable result is confusion if sonography is done too early and, invariably, repetition of the study in later pregnancy when it should have been performed in the first, not the second, place.

Sonography of the pregnant uterus is therefore performed in two situations, either as: (a) for estimation of gestational age or to detect the presence of a fetal anomaly, optimally between the 16th and 18th weeks of gestation; or (b) for well-defined obstetrical indications at any time during pregnancy.

Antenatal Detection of Fetal Anomalies

Well over 150,000 children with congenital anomalies are born annually in the United States, representing 3–5% of all live births (5). A relatively new debate has surfaced with regard to the fetus *defined as a patient*. This has given rise to increasingly strident discussions regarding such moral dilemmas as conflicting rights between the fetus and the mother, specifically at what point in pregnancy do they occur, and whose rights take precedence.

An important issue is the use of ultrasound in pregnancy to make the antenatal diagnosis of congenital anomalies. Zweibel (6) observes that some members of society regard prenatal diagnosis of congenital anomalies as the medical equivalent of a "search and destroy mission." As he aptly points out, the purpose of a diagnostic procedure in pregnancy is to diagnose and not to dictate a course of action, which only can be chosen by the patient and her family. Indeed, in this situation, termination of pregnancy would never be an issue if anomalies could not be diagnosed in the first place. But patients have a right to know, and this knowledge cannot be denied to those whose moral beliefs may differ from others.

Zweibel (6) points out that many women, particularly in high-risk categories such as the older age group, want to be reassured as to fetal normality. In addition, large numbers of patients who otherwise would not even consider having children may be enabled, through antenatal sonographic diagnosis, to become pregnant. These women are known or potential carriers of hereditary defects who claim a right to know whether their fetuses are likely to be afflicted, and if so, to act on this knowledge based on their own convictions.

For those women who choose to carry abnormal fetuses to term, we are reminded that antenatal diagnosis helps them prepare emotionally, physically, and economically for the future, and aids the physician in managing the pregnancy, especially in making crucial decisions over timing and method of delivery (6). Finally, the detection of lethal fetal anomalies may dramatically alter obstetric management. For example, Cesarean section may not be performed for fetal distress if it is known that the fetus will not survive outside the uterus. Common fetal anomalies that are predictably fatal are reviewed in a useful paper (7).

When and Under What Conditions Is Fetal Ultrasound Appropriate?

> *My mother loved children—she would have given anything if I had been one.*
>
> *Groucho Marx*

Experience suggests that first trimester ultrasonography in a normal pregnancy is largely a waste of time. In the case of bleeding during early pregnancy, sonography does help indicate whether there is threatened, incomplete, missed, or complete abortion and is therefore helpful in obstetrical management. However, most patients with mild first trimester bleeding or spotting have subchorionic bleeding; more than 80% go on to normal term pregnancies (8). If it is uncertain whether miscarriage has occurred, then sonography is indicated. Even here, however, if the pregnancy is less than 4–5 weeks, the study usually will not add anything.

Threatened Abortion More Than 6 Weeks Gestation

If gestation is thought to be more than 5–6 weeks (though this cannot always be certain) and no sac is seen in the uterus, complete or incomplete abortion can be assumed, usually the former. Ultrasound can help establish the completeness of miscarriage, but it is not infallible. Formerly, most women with miscarriages were followed for a few days and if bleeding ceased were not subjected to D&C. Today in certain centers, far too many patients with early miscarriage receive early, routine D&Cs without waiting to see if bleeding subsides spontaneously.

The use of ultrasound in suspected ectopic pregnancy is, of course, mandatory, but we emphasize that even in the patient with a high clinical suspicion, i.e. amenorrhea, pelvic pain, and vaginal bleeding, the pregnancy test always should be done first, because *a negative UCG or β-subunit test absolutely rules out pregnancy* (beyond 8–10 days). We stress that ultrasonography with a vaginal probe (transvaginal study; TVS) should be performed along with the routine transabdominal study, if there is any question of ectopic pregnancy. Furthermore, TVS should be used in all cases of early pregnancy or if a sac cannot be seen in a gestation thought to be more advanced than 5–6 weeks. As an aside, transvaginal ultrasonography should always be used if adnexal disease is suspected, whether or not the patient is pregnant. TVS is now "state-of-the-art" pelvic sonography, and no department can be considered adequately equipped without a transvaginal probe or transducer.

Suspected Fetal Anomalies

For the detection of congenital fetal anomalies, the first sonogram should ideally be obtained by 16–18 weeks gestation. Serial scanning may be necessary before a

Table 6.22.2. Incidence of Significant or Major Congenital Malformation[a]

Condition	Approximate incidence (%)	
	of malformations/1,000 live births	of all defects
GU predominantly hydrocoele, 16/1,000 live male births	10	42
Cardiovascular	6	25
Skeletal, fetal tumors, and miscellaneous	3.2	13
Central nervous system incl spina bifida, hydrocephaly anencephaly, encephalocoele microcephaly, etc.	2.4	10
GI	1.3	5
Head and neck cleft lip or cleft palate	1	4
Chest	0.1	>0.5
Total	24	100%

[a]Data taken from Hill et al. (5).

definitive diagnosis can be made or a particular anomaly is excluded. Only then can the patient be advised and appropriate options considered (5). It is unfortunate indeed that our diagnostic capability far too often exceeds our therapeutic abilities in fetal, as in adult, medicine. Table 6.22.2 gives a summary of the major fetal malformations and their relative incidence.

Determination of Gestational Age

Every physician who has attended a pregnant patient knows that estimation of gestational age based on maternal recollection of the last normal menstrual period (LNMP) can be inaccurate, sometimes seriously so. In a careful Canadian study, early second-trimester ultrasound biparietal diameters were compared with maternal LNMP estimates in more than 11,000 women (9). Sensitivities, specificities, PPV, and 1-NPV for term, preterm, and postterm gestations were calculated. The probability that an infant born at term based on the LNMP was actually a term infant was 95%. However, the probability that a preterm infant, based on menstrual dating, was indeed preterm dropped to 78%. Based on the last normal menses the probability that a baby born postterm was actually postterm plummeted to 12%. The authors concluded that "these systematic errors in menstrual (gestational age) estimates have profound implications for unnecessary induction, dysfunctional labor and Caesarean section, and resultant neonatal and maternal morbidity."

This brings us full circle back to the question of routine ultrasound examination of the pregnant patient. In a profession—and a society—which have permitted the Cesarean section rate to rise to more than 1 in 4 live births and where *Cesarean section is the most frequently performed abdominal surgical operation* (almost 1 million performed in 1990) (10), we must assume that routine sonographic examination is becoming virtually mandatory. In regions or countries where rational (old-fashioned) obstetrical practices still prevail, and where the tort system has not hypertrophied, sonography during pregnancy is probably not needed for the majority of patients.

Summary

1. Sonography should never be used to make the diagnosis of uncomplicated pregnancy.

2. In present-day America, routine ultrasonography during pregnancy is probably advisable because of the spectacularly high Cesarean section rate.

3. Sonography is rarely indicated in first trimester threatened abortion with mild bleeding but is indicated in patients at more than 6 weeks gestation in whom gestational status is in doubt, i.e. question of fetal demise or complete or incomplete abortion.

4. During normal pregnancy and for the antenatal detection of fetal anomalies, the optimal time of sonographic study is between 16–18 weeks gestation. This is only because, even though small structures may be difficult to see, if termination of pregnancy is an option, waiting beyond this point carries increasing risk.

5. Any suspicion of ectopic pregnancy (usually before 5–6 weeks) or any suspected abnormality in pregnancy after the first trimester calls for immediate (transvaginal and transabdominal) sonography.

Among indications for early, late, or repeat sonography during pregnancy are the following:

1. The high-risk obstetrical patient, particularly diabetics, cardiacs, teen-agers, those with multiple pregnancies, and women in the over 30–35 age group (between 16–18 weeks and again at 28–30 weeks);
2. Clinically suspected abnormal presentations such as breech or transverse, after 36 weeks; and
3. Presence of placenta praevia. In these cases, repeat sonography usually need not be done before the 36th week, by which time normal placental migration usually will have taken place in more than 95% of patients with low-lying placentas found earlier in pregnancy.

REFERENCES

1. Donald I, MacVicar J, Brown TG. Investigation of abdominal masses by pulsed ultrasound. Lancet 1958;1:1188–1195.
2. Powledge TM, Fletcher J. Guidelines for the ethical, social and legal issues in prenatal diagnosis. N Engl J Med 1979;300(4):168–172.
3. AIUM/NEMA Safety Standard for Diagnostic Ultrasound Equipment. AIUM/NEMA Standards Publication UL1-1981. J Ultrasound Med 1983;2(suppl):S1–S50.
4. Reece EA, Assimakopoulos E, Zheng XZ, Hagay Z, Hobbins JC. The safety of obstetric ultrasonography: concern for the fetus. Obstet Gynecol 1990;76(1):139–146.
5. Hill LM, Breckle R, Gehrking WC. The prenatal detection of congenital malformations by ultrasonography. Mayo Clin Proc 1983;58(12):805–826.
6. Zweibel WJ. The fetus as a patient—broader considerations [Letter from the editor]. Semin Ultrasound CT MR 1984;5(3):211–212.
7. Sanders RC, Blakemore K. Lethal fetal anomalies: sonographic demonstration. Radiology 1989;172(1):1–6.
8. Bloch C, Altchek A, Levy-Ravetch M. Sonography in early pregnancy: the significance of subchorionic hemorrhage. Mt Sinai J Med 1989;56(4):290–292.
9. Kramer MS, McLean FH, Boyd ME, Usher RH. The validity of gestational age estimation by menstrual dating in term, preterm, and postterm gestations. JAMA 1988;260(22):3306–3308.
10. U.S. Department of Health and Human Services, U.S. Public Health Service, Centers for Disease Control, and the National Center for Health Statistics. National Hospital Discharge Survey (NHDS). Detailed diagnoses, procedures, days of care, diagnoses-related groups for patients discharged from short-stay hospitals. Public Use Data Diskettes, 1985–1990.

23/ Anxiety, Nervousness, Fatigue, and Depression

I don't do any invasive procedures; I just have language.
James Coane, PsyD

The patient, described by his family and friends as a "card-carrying neurotic," spent much of his time and money discussing a staggering variety of complaints with various physicians, including a number of specialists. One day he returned home after seeing a new consultant who reported an abnormal test result and announced triumphantly to his wife, "Thank God, it's organic!"

When physicians order medical imaging or other tests for patients with symptoms of anxiety, nervousness, fatigue, or depression, the approach usually reflects a futile attempt to rule out some highly unlikely diagnosis. Patients suffering from metabolic disease, especially hyperthyroidism, certain toxicities, infections, and a variety of other conditions may, of course, present with any of the above neuropsychiatric symptoms. But recall that Chapter 6 in its entirety addresses the question, given *only this specific sign or symptom*, what is the likely diagnosis?

Faced with such a patient complaining only of anxiety or nervousness, fatigue, depression, conversion, or other psychiatric symptoms or combinations thereof, and without significant physical findings, the competent physician *must be able to make the diagnosis of psychoneurosis on clinical grounds*. Medical imaging and other types of clinical testing in this situation are to be condemned. The pursuit of clinical investigations may fix in the patient's mind that he has, like the man in the case study above, "organic" disease, or worse, enable him to deny the true nature of his problem. Furthermore, when inappropriate tests are abnormal, more tests are usually ordered, and proper treatment may be unduly delayed. Phillip's Law states, "Four-wheel-drive just means getting stuck in more inaccessible places."

The most prevalent psychiatric problem in medical practice is depression, which presents with many faces, both somatic and psychic. Not all patients are so obvious as the esteemed writer Samuel Beckett, who was taking a walk with a friend one bright spring Sunday morning in a London park. The friend could not restrain his enthusiasm and exclaimed, "what a glorious day to be alive." Beckett replied cautiously, "I wouldn't go that far."

Another story comes to mind if only because it illustrates the therapeutic value of a psychiatry seasoned and made rational by old-fashioned common sense. Alfred Adler in his early, more psychoanalytic days, would ask the patient at the end of the first consultation, "What would you do if you were cured?" The patient would answer, and then Adler would say, "Well, go and do it then."

7

Imaging by Abnormal Laboratory Findings

1/ Abnormal Urinalysis: Renal Dysfunction

> *What is man, when you come to think upon him, but a minutely set, ingenious machine for turning, with infinite artfulness, the red wine of Shiraz into urine.*
>
> *Isak Dinesen*

A reductionist approach lets us simplify conventional disease classification schemes. Thus, for the GU tract as with the hepatobiliary tract, we can divide etiologies into two fundamental categories, medical and obstructive. Despite the obvious condensation, this dichotomous grouping of urinary tract conditions determines the logical basis not only for diagnosis but for management as well.

For example, conditions such as upper or lower urinary tract obstruction, malformations, and tumors often call for surgical treatment, sometimes urgently. Other conditions, which can be lumped together as medical urinary tract disease, comprise most of the remaining disease entities such as lower and upper tract infections and inflammatory conditions, the nephritides, secondary renal disease, and the like. The only condition classifiable in either category is calculous disease, which, unlike most GU tract disease, usually presents as a characteristic pain syndrome and is therefore discussed elsewhere.

It is in the diagnosis of obstructive urinary tract disease that the anatomical study, ultrasonography, plays a central role. Functional tests such as scintigraphy or pyelography are generally indicated after the demonstration of sonographic abnormalities. In established medical renal disease of known etiology imaging usually can be omitted or deferred, but in new parenchymal renal disease or renal failure, functional imaging, particularly renal scintigraphy with flow studies, provides the most useful clinical information in a wide variety of conditions. Obstructive urinary tract disease in adult males is secondary, for all intents, to urolithiasis and prostatic disease, in females, to stone, pelvic surgery, and cancer (uterine, ovarian, or cervical), or radiation. In children, clinically significant obstructive problems are rare and most often related to ureteral reflux and other congenital problems.

Analysis of the urine may disclose one or more cardinal abnormalities: proteinuria, pyuria (with and without bacteriuria), hematuria, and various types of casts. The responsibility of the clinician, as always, is to estimate the likelihood of specific conditions, given the clinical, urinary, and blood chemical findings. This "working" diagnosis is well named; it always must come before the ordering of any imaging or other extensive diagnostic studies. *Diagnosis always precedes investigation, and not vice versa.* Without one or two working diagnoses (not a list of differential diagnoses) it is impossible to decide whether imaging is indicated, let alone choose among the bewildering array of available and often competing procedures.

Internists, nephrologists, and urologists differ in their favorite imaging repertoires, the urologists for historical reasons strongly favoring the IVP. Yet thoughtful specialists should pose the same questions as the generalist: Is imaging indeed necessary in this patient, and if so, which study should be ordered as the initial procedure? When is ultrasound superior to scintiscanning or pyelography? When is pyelography to be preferred to both? For what suspected conditions is it desirable to order CT or MRI, and when are invasive procedures such as cystoscopy, retrograde pyelography, or arteriography called for? Far too often, the availability of so many complementary imaging procedures leads to diagnostic overkill. Today, it is not unusual to see patients subjected to multiple imaging and even invasive studies when one, or rarely two, would have sufficed. This is not the fault of technology, but too often the result of medical teaching, which stresses a "ruling out" rather than a "ruling in" strategy. Furthermore, there seems to be a growing kinship between medical testing and mountain climbing: we do it because it's there. And, like mountain climbing, testing proves to be expensive and sometimes even hazardous to your health.

Because of significant differences in GU disease prevalence by age and sex, we will concentrate on these aspects in the discussion that follows. The imaging of renal and other types of organ trauma is covered in other more specialized literature.

Renal Imaging: General Remarks

The six principal indirect methods for imaging the urinary tract are, *in order of general applicability:*

1. Renal ultrasonography;
2. Radionuclide scintigraphy;
3. IVP;
4. CT;
5. MRI; and
7. Renal arteriography.

The direct imaging techniques are urethro-cystoscopy, retrograde pyelography and cystography.

For visualization of the kidneys for nontraumatic conditions, *ultrasonography* should be the *first* imaging procedure to be ordered. If the study is *normal*, it may suffice as the *sole* imaging study for evaluating renal structure.

Renal Ultrasonography

Ultrasound is the procedure par excellence for differentiating medical from obstructive renal disease. Furthermore, it remains an acceptable initial screening test for tumors of the kidney and bladder. Ultrasound is painlessly and quickly performed, inexpensive, and without risk. What do we look for in ultrasonography of the kidney? Of primary importance are the normal tightly clustered central renal echoes. If these echoes are "split" or widened it indicates varying degrees of dilatation of the collect-

Table 7.1.1.   Some Clinical Indications for the Use of Transrectal Prostatic Ultrasound

1. Evaluation of a palpable mass, an area of induration or asymmetry of the prostate on digital rectal examination
2. Assessment of a palpable prostatic mass with a negative, conventional digitally guided biopsy
3. Assessing the prostate in patients with elevations of prostatic specific antigen (PSA) without palpable abnormality on digital rectal examination
4. Guidance for transrectal biopsy in small lesions
5. Radiation seed implantation guidance
6. Evaluation of prostatic cancer recurrence

Adapted from Rifkin (4).

ing system. This finding is virtually pathognomonic of present or past obstruction. It occasionally may represent regional caliectasis from obstruction within the collecting system but most often is due to obstruction at or distal to the ureteropelvic junction. The reliability of this finding cannot be overestimated. Failure to find dilatation of the renal collecting system in ureteric obstruction is seen in only 4–5% of all cases (1). In a series of patients with normal renal function, ultrasound had a sensitivity of 90% and a specificity of 85% in the diagnosis of hydronephrosis (2).

Of less importance in renal ultrasound are changes in the character or amplitude of the normal parenchymal/cortical echoes with or without changes in renal size. These findings, *when present*, are strong indicators of acute or chronic medical renal disease. However, the renal parenchyma may be sonographically *normal* in up to 40% or more of patients with medical renal disease, including those with acute or chronic renal failure. Nor is the frequency of sonographic findings in medical renal disease necessarily related to severity or chronicity (3). Thus, an abnormal collecting system on ultrasound is the crucial finding in distinguishing obstructive from nonobstructive (medical) renal disease regardless of the presence or absence of renal parenchymal changes.

If bladder or prostatic conditions are suspected, bladder ultrasonography should be performed, because the diagnosis of bladder neoplasm, stone, or occasionally chronic cystitis can be made. Moreover, postvoiding sonography of the bladder is an excellent noninvasive screening test for urinary retention due to neurogenic causes or lower tract outlet obstruction due to prostatism. One usually can detect as little as 25–35 ml residual urine by this method.

Ultrasonography of the prostate transabdominally is of little value, but in recent years transrectal ultrasonography has gained significant clinical acceptance. Rifkin (4) has enumerated several suggested indications for the use of prostatic ultrasound, some of which are listed in Table 7.1.1 (4). We emphasize, however, that prostatic sonography is not at present established or accepted as a screening test for prostatic cancer. The method, however, is extremely valuable in the assessment of palpable abnormalities of the gland or elevations of the prostate-specific antigen. Neither ultrasonography nor MRI is highly accurate in staging early prostate cancer (5).

IVP and Radionuclide Studies

Contrast pyelography and renal scintigraphy are the only studies that give physio-logical as well as anatomical information, with pyelography distinctly superior in de-lineating anatomy, particularly of the collecting systems, ureters and bladder. Radio-nuclide studies are clearly superior in the quantification of renal perfusion, function, and obstruction, and in the study of the patient in renal failure where pyelography is not only useless but contraindicated. With radionuclide scintigraphy using DTPA and other agents such as the newer MAG-3, it is usually possible to obtain functional and anatomical information of the urinary tract when the blood urea nitrogen is as high as 150–200 mg/dl. Radionuclide renography, for all intents, is risk-free and should be used in preference to repeat intravenous urography to follow the clinical course of patients with previously diagnosed obstructive disease. Plain radiographs should not be neglected, however, because they may well show antegrade migration of ureteral stones.

Pyelography, more often with high osmolar contrast, but even with low osmolar agents, *always* entails some risk and should generally not be used if sufficient information can be obtained with sonography, scintigraphy, or a combination of the two. One of the most common clinical blunders, already stressed, is to perform pyelography in the presence of obvious medical renal disease. Intravenous contrast used in the IVP or with CT is generally contraindicated in the following patients: juvenile or adult diabetics with proteinuria or renal disease, any patient with known or potential renal functional impairment, those with multiple myeloma, and patients with known allergy to contrast media (see Chapter 4). Contrast material is relatively contraindicated in infants and children and should be used with extreme caution in patients with an allergic history, especially asthmatics. Contrary to many patients' fears, radionuclide studies are completely safe in the patient with a known history of reaction to contrast material, and, in fact, this is one of the important indications for radionuclide renography.

On the other hand, in the absence of contraindications, pyelography remains the best overall imaging method for the investigation of hematuria of uncertain etiology and in patients with renal or ureteral stone.

CT and MRI

Because of pervasive and uncritical enthusiasm, MRI and CT continue to be enormously overused compared with older imaging techniques; in fact, they are rarely needed for most medical diagnoses. In the urinary tract the only appropriate indications for CT or MRI are the study of abscesses and noncystic or mixed masses of the kidney (intra, para-, and perirenal) and bladder and in the staging of renal and bladder carcinoma. These will be discussed in the next chapter.

Imaging in Patients with Abnormalities on Urinalysis

> *I have Bright's disease and he has mine.*
>
> S. J. Perelman

PROTEINURIA ASSOCIATED WITH OTHER ABNORMALITIES SUGGESTING PARENCHYMAL RENAL DISEASE

Isolated, variably occurring proteinuria is most often benign. Idiopathic, transient, or benign proteinuria is usually associated with fever, exercise, dehydration, or postural changes. Protein excretion is usually minimal and in patients with orthostatic proteinuria rarely exceeds 1 g urinary protein daily. The key to diagnosis is the demonstration of normal protein excretion on awakening in the morning. Systemic causes of persistent proteinuria are numerous, as noted in Table 7.1.2 (6). To simplify the presentation, proteinuria is frequently associated with hematuria and casts,

Table 7.1.2. Systemic Conditions and Other Causes of Persistent Proteinuria

Common in clinical practice
  Congestive heart failure
  Hypertensive nephrosclerosis
  Diabetic benign nephrosclerosis
  Drug side effect, allergy, or toxicity: nonsteroidal antiinflammatory agents, probenecid, captopril,
    trimethadone, penicillins, aminoglycosides, etc.
Unusual causes, sometimes associated with the nephrotic syndrome
  Vesicoureteral reflux
  Diabetic intracapillary glomerulosclerosis (Kimmelstiel-Wilson disease)
  Amyloidosis
  Allergic reactions (bee stings, pollen, poison ivy, insect repellents)
  Heavy metal toxicity (mercury, bismuth, gold)
  Renal vein thrombosis
  Multiple myeloma
  Hodgkin's disease and other neoplasms
  Systemic lupus erythematosus
  Chronic active hepatitis
  Secondary lues
  Quartan malaria
  Other chronic infections
  Hereditary nephritis (Alport's syndrome)
  Homograft rejection
  Myxedema
  Constrictive pericarditis

Reprinted by permission from Branch WT, ed. *Office Practice of Medicine.* Philadelphia: W. B. Saunders Co. (1987: 505).

with or without white cells, and is associated with almost the entire spectrum of GU tract disease, i.e. one or more of the following:

1. Pyelonephritis, renal tuberculosis, or other infections of the urinary tract;
2. Hydronephrosis or vesicoureteral reflux;
3. Nephrolithiasis;
4. Renal or other GU tumors; and
5. Focal, membranous, or diffuse glomerulonephritis.

In patients showing persistent isolated proteinuria or the nephrotic syndrome, imaging procedures are seldom helpful. In practice, however, ultrasound is often ordered because of unjustified anxiety over missing the rare treatable surgical condition. In almost all such cases, sonography will be normal. With the possible exception of renal calculi, *cystoscopy or other invasive procedures, though necessary in unexplained hematuria, are never indicated in medical renal disease.* In young patients with proteinuria associated with an "active urine sediment" containing red and white blood cells and coarsely granular or red cell casts with the syndrome of acute glomerulonephritis, urinary tract imaging again is not indicated. Renal ultrasonography, however, is still an essential study if renal biopsy is contemplated, because the nephrologist always wants to know beforehand if there are two kidneys. These are the only principal indications for renal imaging in established or diagnosed medical renal disease. IVP, CT, or other studies using contrast should be *strenuously avoided* in patients with acute or chronic medical renal disease.

In patients, particularly adults, with previously undiagnosed or new renal disease, sonography suffices to exclude clinically significant obstructive conditions. This often

Table 7.1.3. Final Diagnosis In Selected Patients with Hematuria

	1000 Adults with gross hematuria (%)	500 Adults with asymptomatic microhematuria (%)
Bladder	39.5	9.6
Cystitis	22.0	3.4
Vesical neoplasm	15.0	1.8
Miscellaneous: trigonitis, diverticulum, varices, calculi, trauma, irradiation, chemical injury, foreign body	2.5	4.4
Prostate	23.6	25.4
Benign hyperplasia	12.5	23.6
Miscellaneous: varices, prostatitis, stricture, calculus, carcinoma	11.1	1.8
Kidney	15.2	6.4
Renal neoplasm	3.5	0.4
Glomerulonephritis	1.6	0[a]
Calculi	2.7	3.4
Pyelonephritis	3.0	0.2
Miscellaneous: renal cyst, hydronephrosis, horseshoe kidney, renal agenesis, trauma, polycystic kidneys, ptosis, infarct, nephrosclerosis, drug toxicity	4.4	2.4
Ureter	6.5	2.2
Calculus	5.3	0.4
Miscellaneous: tumor, stricture, ureteritis cystica, ureterocele	1.2	1.8
Urethra	4.3	22.6
Urethritis	1.3	21.2
Miscellaneous: stricture, calculus, tumor, foreign body, trauma, diverticulum, polyps	3.0	1.4
Other causes	2.4	0.8
Tuberculosis	0.7	0
Miscellaneous: hemophilia, sickle cell disease, thrombocytopenia, sodium warfarin (Coumadin) overdose	1.7	0.8
Essential hematuria	8.5	34.4

[a]Excluded all with RBC casts or proteinuria.
Adapted from Kurdish GC. Determining the cause of hematuria. Postgrad Med 1975;58:118 and Greene LF, et al. Study of 500 patients with asymptomatic microhematuria. JAMA 1956;161:610.

needs to be followed with radionuclide studies. Contrast material frequently exacerbates medical renal disease and may lead to acute renal failure and death.

The importance of renal biopsy in the diagnosis and management of patients with various forms of medical renal disease tends to fluctuate with therapeutic advances but has declined somewhat in recent years. At present its main value is in systemic lupus and in the nephrotic syndrome. If biopsy is indeed indicated, ultrasonic guidance has proved invaluable, though some nephrologists still continue to prefer CT.

GROSS AND MICROSCOPIC HEMATURIA IN ADULTS

We already have implied that definitions of biological "abnormality" such as stature, weight, and anemia represent statistical deviations from a continuum of values. Microscopic hematuria in males has been defined previously as the presence of more than one RBC per hpf in a midstream urine specimen (7). Yet vigorous exercise is known to cause hematuria. In a survey of asymptomatic military recruits, two to four or more RBC per hpf were present in more than 5% of

Table 7.1.4. Nature and Incidence of Significant Lesions in 500 Selected Patients with Asymptomatic Microhematuria

Urologic lesion	Number of patients	Percentage
Carcinoma of the bladder	9	1.8
Renal calculus	4	0.8
Renal cyst	4	0.8
Renal neoplasm	2	0.4
Ureteral calculus	2	0.4
Hydronephrosis	1	0.2
Occlusion of renal pedicle	1	0.2
Urethral stricture	1	0.2
		4.8

Adapted from Greene LF, et al. Study of 500 patients with asymptomatic microhematuria. JAMA 1956;161:610.

urinalyses performed and more than eight RBC per hpf in 1% (8). Clearly, the upper normal limit might better be set greater than two to four RBCs, at least in the young and physically active, and three to five WBCs in urinary infection. However, there is no way to avoid the pervasive problems of the ROC curve discussed in Chapter 1. No matter where we place the level of normality, we will have to accept a trade-off between sensitivity and specificity. If we place the normal number of red cells too low, we exclude some normal patients; if we place it too high, we will miss some abnormals.

Another problem arises when urine specimens are picked up at physician's offices or clinics for examination in outside laboratories. In the intervening hours before microscopic examination is performed, the cellular elements, red and white blood cells, may undergo significant lysis. This problem may be circumvented, at least for hematuria, by chemical tests for hemoglobin, particularly the Hemastix or Dipstix test. However, for the determination of pyuria, it would seem prudent to ensure proper microscopic examination of all urine specimens while they are still fresh. Every physician's office or clinic obtaining urine specimens should be equipped with microscopes.

Since gross hematuria *in adults* not resulting from cystitis, is much more likely than microscopic hematuria to be caused by a serious condition, the diagnostic approach in hematuria must take this and age factors into account. Tables 7.1.3 and 7.1.4 are extremely important because they indicate the likelihood of various diagnoses given the findings of either gross or microscopic hematuria. Final diagnoses are listed for 1000 patients with gross and 500 adults with asymptomatic microhematuria, all of whom had complete urological investigation (9–11). Table 7.1.4 (10) shows the incidence of significant conditions in the 500 patients with microscopic hematuria. From the tables we note that of 1000 patients referred for urological investigation, more than 18% had carcinoma of the kidney or bladder, whereas in patients with microscopic hematuria the total incidence of cancer was only 2.2%. Because this was a selected series of older patients, we can readily explain the extremely high occurrence of neoplasms. Other authors have dealt with the problem of hematuria in adults (12), and various algorithms have been proposed based on the presence but not the frequency of specific findings (13). We remain skeptical about such deterministic recipes, because they perpetuate the "differential diagnosis" approach while ignoring the concept of pretest probability of disease. The study of patients with hematuria secondary to renal trauma is a separate issue and is discussed elsewhere (14).

GROSS AND MICROSCOPIC HEMATURIA IN CHILDREN AND YOUNG ADULTS

In young adults and children, the incidence of GU tract neoplasms is so low as to be negligible. For example, below the age of 35 the incidence of bladder cancer is only about 1 per 100,000, rising to 1 in 1000 over age 65 (15, 16). Renal cancer is less common than bladder neoplasia and was found in only 3.5% of those with gross hematuria and only 0.4% of those with microscopic hematuria in Kudish and Greene et al.'s series (9, 10). In Froom et al.'s series of Israeli military recruits (8), almost 50% with microhematuria had calculous disease, more than 25 times the incidence reported by Greene et al. (10) in adults. This is not unexpected because of the high incidence of calculous disease in warm climates. The observed cumulative incidence of neoplasms at age 15 was comparable to that of Israeli men age 18–40 with microhematuria, only 0.1%. The authors concluded that "microhaematuria detected during a screening examination probably should not be regarded as a specific sign of a significant lesion and *does not of itself warrant urological investigation in adults aged 40 or less*" (emphasis added) (8). In a series of more than 128,000 patient visits to an outpatient pediatric clinic, gross hematuria was proven in only 158 patients under age 18 (1.3 per 1,000 visits), only one of whom had a tumor (17).

The tables again underscore the critical importance of disease prevalence in determining predictive values of specific tests. In Table 7.1.5 PPVs for cystoscopy are estimated for bladder neoplasm, given two groups of patients with gross hematuria, those over or under age 40. Note the extremely poor PPV for a younger patient who typically has an extremely low prevalence of bladder cancer. Table 7.1.6 shows the PPV and 1-NPV values for cystoscopy in various conditions shown in Table 7.1.3 causing asymptomatic microhematuria. Note in Table 7.1.6 that essential hematuria, benign prostate, urethral, and bladder conditions account for 91% of cases. The low prevalence of bladder neoplasm indicates that cystoscopy might be justified as a ruling out procedure, but its diagnostic usefulness in the setting of overwhelmingly benign disease, at least in the young patient, is doubtful. A more careful analysis shows that cystoscopy has different possible outcomes for each possible condition. With a negative cystoscopy the possibility of an upper tract condition such ureteral stone or renal tumor might well increase to 20–30%. Predicting the PPV of, say retrograde pyelography or IVP in this setting becomes a much more difficult mathematical problem. This is precisely where computer-assisted analysis of test performance would be of great help in patients requiring complicated diagnostic strategies.

PYURIA AND BACTERIURIA IN ADULTS

Pyuria means the presence of leukocytes in the urine. In Wright's study (18), 90% of males had less than two WBCs per hpf, and 76% of noncatheterized females had less than five WBCs per hpf (18). Again, the physician and not the laboratory must decide on common-sense grounds where to establish normality. If one were to accept the upper limit of five WBCs for women, this means that more than 24% of female patients would be defined as having pyuria. Thus, contamination of urine specimens in females always should be taken into account. However, precise quantification of pyuria, particularly the definition "per hpf," is subject to

Table 7.1.5.   Calculated Predictive Values for the Test: Cystoscopy in the Presence of Gross Hematuria

Disease	Age	Prevalence	Sensitivity	Nonspecificity	PPV	1-NPV
Bladder neoplasm	>45	15	95	2	89	<1
Bladder neoplasm	<40	0.05	95	2	2	<1

Table 7.1.6.   Test: Cystoscopy: Estimated Probabilities of Various Test Results for Each Group of Conditions Causing Asymptomatic Microhematuria

Disease	Prevalence	Sensitivity	Nonspecificity	PPV	1-NPV
Essential hematuria	35	0	0	0	0
Prostate	25	70	10	70	90
Urethral	23	70	10	68	91
Other bladder cond	8	95	5	62	>99
Kidney	7	0	0	0	0
Bladder neoplasm	2	95	5	28	>99

the vagaries of centrifugation and resuspension techniques, and these should, if possible, be standardized (7).

Solitary pyuria means infection or inflammation and therefore always should be regarded as a sign of medical GU disease. Urinary tract infections (UTIs) are much more common than other inflammatory disease. Pyuria always requires bacteriological studies first, and in the case of unresponsive infections, a search for site of involvement, either upper or lower tract. In the absence of positive cultures, however, look for lower tract involvement. If hematuria accompanies pyuria, various conditions of the lower tract, cysts, calculi, or tumors may be responsible. In young patients glomerulonephritis is the most likely cause.

Acute infections of the urinary tract are a significant health problem, affecting from 10–20% of women at some time during their lives (19). Women account for more than 30 million and men about 9 million ambulatory care physician office visits annually for GU problems, most of which are for UTIs (20). In the unobstructed male, upper tract infections are rarely seen.

Various combinations of pyuria and bacteriuria occur.

1. Pyuria without a positive urine culture for the more common pathogens ("sterile" pyuria) can be seen in early pyelonephritis, often up to 48 hours after onset of illness or until infection breaks through into the nephron or collecting system. It is more often noted in lower tract disease. In males the most common cause of sterile pyuria is prostatitis or urethritis caused by *Chlamydia*, viruses, or mycoplasma. In females, sterile pyuria is usually the result of urethritis, occasionally vaginitis and cystitis, particularly the interstitial type in elderly patients. Patients with urethral or vaginal discharge, dysuria, urgency, and frequency with or without suprapubic tenderness are prime suspects for lower tract disease, and here imaging is seldom needed. The three- or four-glass or Stamey-Meares test is often helpful in urethral/prostatic localization of infection in males. Initial pyuria signifies a urethral or prostatic source, and white cells in the terminal specimen indicate prostatitis, but the only reliable method for diagnosing prostatitis employs comparison of bacterial counts in the first three specimens with those after prostatic massage (fourth speci-

men). Pyuria and comparable bacterial counts in all three specimens sometimes indicate a source in the bladder or above, but according to Stamey (21), make interpretation impossible.

If lower tract disease is unlikely or excludable, persistent, unexplained sterile pyuria in symptomatic younger or immunocompromised patients calls for special bacteriological studies, such as cultures for tubercle bacilli, fungi, anaerobes, even parasites. Because asymptomatic bacteriuria in elderly men and women does not require treatment, investigation in these patients is rarely indicated (22).

Some patients with various urinary findings and developing renal impairment may have another problem. Medical texts of late make much of "tubulo-interstitial nephropathy," previously called interstitial nephritis, a large group of chronic renal disorders of varying etiologies (7).

If pyuria is accompanied by positive cultures, the source often can be determined on the basis of the clinical presentation, i.e. lower tract symptoms of dysuria, frequency, urgency, and voiding of small volumes, vs. upper tract symptoms and signs of high fever, flank pain, and tenderness, etc. However, there remains a group of patients in whom the distinction between pyelonephritis and urethro-cystitis is difficult. *Very rarely are imaging studies other than ultrasonography indicated in UTIs, particularly of women* (23). Pyelography or renal scintigraphy are indicated when sonography shows obstruction, but whether these studies are ultimately of clinical benefit in patients with *negative* sonography with recurrent or chronic pyelonephritis remains doubtful. Various studies report that up to one-third of bacteriuric young men without recurrent infections have pyelographic abnormalities (24), and one-third of men and women hospitalized for febrile UTIs have previously unrecognized findings on sonography (25). However, there is widespread clinical skepticism over the prognostic and therapeutic implications of such findings. Despite the demonstration of radiographic and urodynamic abnormalities in adults with UTIs, the information obtained almost never causes clinicians to alter their therapy (22, 23, 26).

If renal sonography, however, shows a dilated collecting system or stone in the presence of recurrent UTI, it remains incumbent to visualize the anatomy and functional status of the excretory tract with urography or scintigraphy. One has to choose between good delineation of anatomy in the upper tract and collecting system but limited functional information with the IVP, and much less anatomical detail but good dynamic assessment of obstruction with radionuclide scintigraphy. Thus, both techniques enjoy advantages in certain clinical situations. Unfortunately, few controlled studies are available for comparing the sensitivity and specificity of IVP and radionuclide scintigraphy in various conditions, and pyelography continues to be the mainstay in these patients. Specific applications of renal scintigraphy are discussed below.

As already mentioned, clinicians face a therapeutic dilemma in asymptomatic bacteriuria with or without pyuria and chronic UTI in older patients, particularly females. In the absence of symptoms most physicians do not treat. Others use Macrodantin or sulfa drugs in chronic low doses as prophylactic treatment. Such treatment usually results in a sterile culture for only a transient period of time, after which urine cultures again become positive. In these patients, sonography is helpful in excluding an obstructive problem.

PYURIA AND BACTERIURIA IN YOUNG PATIENTS

Infections of the urinary tract are the second most common bacterial infections in infants and children, after respiratory and middle ear diseases. Cystitis is much more common than pyelonephritis, particularly in girls. Between 1.5–2% of all children between 1–5 years of age will develop symptomatic UTIs, and perhaps as many as 5–10% of healthy girls will have UTIs (27–30). Because of the extremely short female urethra and the almost routine colonization of the perineum with colonic bacteria, it is not surprising that the great majority of UTIs occur in girls and females in general (especially elderly women). Eighty percent of girls experiencing UTIs can expect to have at least one more episode (31). But contrary to popular medical belief, congenital anomalies of the GU tract are *rarely* the cause of isolated UTIs either in children or adults.

Although pyuria is much more common with bacteriuria, the latter may be present without pyuria, because pyuria is often intermittent or absent, especially in chronic pyelonephritis. In acute hematogenous pyelonephritis (now referred to as tubulointerstitial nephropathy) bacteriuria and pyuria can be absent during the first 24–48 hours, for the reasons mentioned above. Because of the ubiquity of GU infections in children, the great majority of which are benign cystitis in girls, the question of investigation becomes paramount. Because only a small fraction of infants and children with UTIs have correctable urological lesions, perhaps 98–99% of unselected patients will not benefit from medical imaging. A reasonable approach is to identify those young patients likely to have such lesions on the basis of age, sex, response to therapy, and recurrences. These are among the patients at highest risk for repeated pyelonephritis and progressive loss of renal function.

First infections of the urinary tract in children seldom justify investigation except in the rare case when there is failure to respond to appropriate therapy. Repeated or recurrent UTIs, however, do require investigation, though again, therapeutic benefit is achieved in only a small subset of these patients. What are the best initial GU imaging procedures in this younger age group? Controversy continues to dominate discussion. Many authorities insist on an initial voiding cystoureterogram (vide infra) followed by sonography. This seems extreme and unwarranted.

Our first preference is for renal ultrasonography, which remains the easiest, most acceptable, and effective screening procedure. Without dilatation of the collecting system, potential surgically correctable lower tract disease is so unlikely as to be excluded with an exceedingly high degree of certainty. If sonographic study does show dilatation of the collecting system, radionuclide scintigraphy with DTPA or the newer agents such as MAG 3 is indicated.

Many cases of hydronephrosis in children and adults are due to *functional* and not fixed mechanical obstruction. These patients can be distinguished with "diuretic renography" or radionuclide scintigraphy performed during the administration of intravenous Lasix. With this test many patients will be shown to have diuretic-responsive emptying of a dilated collecting system, which effectively rules out a mechanical cause. Patients with this type of functional obstruction virtually never develop loss of kidney function. This observation is consonant with the more clinically meaningful definition of hydronephrosis enunciated by Dr. James Conway of Children's Hospital in Chicago: "True hydronephrosis results in the progressive loss of renal function with time."

IVP has little place in studying renal infection in children for several reasons. Pyelographic images are of poor quality in the younger age group, particularly infants. This is because of poor renal concentrating ability and interference from overlying bowel gas, which renders pyelography of little value in visualizing the renal parenchyma, nor is it capable of distinguishing between functional and mechanical obstruction as is diuretic renography. Furthermore, the radiation dose (if you're phobic about it) of pyelography is significantly higher than with scintigraphy, and, last, there is increased risk of allergic and hyperosmolar reactions in children.

Therefore, with recurrent upper tract infections in children, scintigraphy is vitally important. In the patient with acute pyelonephritis, either hematogenous or from the lower tract, who has responded poorly to therapy or who has suffered recurrent infections or relapses within 1–2 months after adequate therapy, the decision to change antibiotics, prolong treatment, or resort to long-term prophylaxis may depend on the results of renal scintigraphy. In these patients glucoheptonate or dimercaptosuccinic acid (DMSA) imaging is indicated for the detection of cortical defects or scarring. Outside of bacteriological studies, cortical changes in the kidney revealed by scintigraphy provide the best correlation with the activity and degree of acute or chronic pyelonephritis.

UPPER VS. LOWER TRACT SOURCE OF UTIs IN CHILDREN

The ureterovesical junction acts as a one-way valve in the normal urinary tract, which allows urine to enter the bladder but prevents bladder contents from refluxing, or backing up the ureters toward the kidneys. This normal protective mechanism, unfortunately, is often faulty or incompetent in infants and children and is seen in 20–30% of patients referred to pediatric urology clinics for recurrent infection. It becomes less of a problem with age, because only about 5% of the patients are over 10 years of age (32). The condition is detected by the voiding cystoureterogram performed by instilling either radiographic contrast or radionuclide in the bladder and looking for the presence or absence of ureteral reflux during voiding. Nuclear cystoscopy is more sensitive than the X-ray study and generally preferred for several reasons. First, the nuclear study gives less radiation to the child and is easier to perform. Furthermore, it may show reflux during bladder filling, at maximal filling, or during voiding. Finally, the radionuclide study may be recorded on a computer for dynamic viewing and enhancement of images; image timing is not a problem as with fluoroscopic spot films.

We must assume, therefore, on the basis of the above-quoted percentage of pediatric urological referral (33), that at least 70% of pyelonephritis in children is hematogenous in origin. Because we can image reflux, and in a few cases specific therapy is available, urinary tract imaging in children is also concerned with the detection and study of this structural/functional urological problem.

VESICOURETERAL REFLUX (VUR)

VUR probably occurs in less than 1% of normal children, but for unknown reasons is limited almost entirely to the white race. Children with VUR have asymptomatic siblings suffering the same condition up to 40% of the time. There appears to be some correlation with renal parenchymal abnormalities. For example, only 3% of patents with normal voiding cystoureterograms but 18% of those with reflux have parenchymal scarring (33). Clearly, reflux, according to Asscher et al. (28), "may theoretically hamper the ability of the urinary tract to maintain sterility, (but) it is doubtful that reflux causes infection (or that infection causes reflux). . . .”

An international grading system for reflux is used to describe severity. Grade 1 reflux extends into the proximal ureter and spares the collecting system. This degree of reflux is often intermittent and is therefore frequently missed or not reproducible on X-ray voiding cystoureterogram. Grade 2 reflux extends and fills but does not dilate the collecting system. It is rare indeed that either grades 1 or 2 are clinically significant. Grades 3, 4, and 5 progress from distension of the collecting system only, to progressive ureteral and calyceal distortion. The severity of VUR has been studied in large numbers of patients and has been found to correlate well with renal scarring (34). In an important retrospective study by Strife and colleagues (34), of 455 girls who had nuclear cystography and sonography for proven UTI, VUR was seen in only 31% of patients, of whom only 12% had renal parenchymal scarring. Only 7% (10 of 142) of these patients had Grade 3 or 4 VUR. Abnormal sonograms were found in only 17%. This study makes clear the generally good prognosis of reflux grades lower than 3.

Most patients with *severe* reflux ultimately will require surgical reimplantation of the ureters in order to avoid chronic renal damage. This is usually postponed until the early teens, because the majority of patients with grades less than 4 or 5 will improve spontaneously. But out of the millions of children with recurrent UTIs we can anticipate an extremely poor predictive value of positive cystography. Judging from the study of Strife et al. (34), only a tiny percentage of such children would ultimately be candidates for late corrective surgery. On the other hand, in a carefully selected population of patients with repeated UTIs and especially with sonographically demonstrable dilatation of the collecting system, cystography would indeed have an important diagnostic role.

OLIGURIA AND RENAL FAILURE

This subject has been touched upon in the preceding sections but deserves a few additional paragraphs. Because renal transplant imaging is a topic of interest primarily to the nephrologist, we will not discuss it here.

If the patient is suffering from acute or chronic renal failure, oliguria, or anuria, the abdominal plain film occassionally will be of help but by itself is of limited value. The only two appropriate studies in cases of urinary failure remain renal ultrasonography and the radionuclide flow and scintigraphic study. The sonograph will detect or exclude obstructive or surgical renal disease with a high degree of confidence, and scintigraphy will indicate the adequacy of renal perfusion and the severity and progress over time of functional impairment.

Radionuclide renal scintigraphy is the only study that can yield useful physiological and anatomical information in the presence of renal functional impairment from any cause. For example, in the rare patient with unilateral or bilateral complete renal arterial obstruction, the flow study is diagnostic. Radionuclide studies are also invaluable in the patient with unilateral renal artery stenosis, small vessel renal disease, transplant rejection, and acute tubular necrosis. Demonstration of renal dysfunction secondary to chronic ureteral obstruction due to stone, tumor, or previous surgery is critical because the documentation of such potentially treatable conditions provides the only hope for therapy, but almost all of these patients would be first discovered with sonography.

Scintigraphy is the most useful study in patients presenting for the first time with renal failure or in following patients postoperatively for renal complications related to pelvic surgery. In particular, women with any history of recent pelvic surgery, whether it be a hysterectomy for a leiomyomatous uterus or radical pelvic surgery for carcinoma of the cervix, endometrium, or ovaries *should be studied at least once with radionuclide renal scintigraphy to detect early mechanical or functional obstruction.*

GU PROBLEMS AND THE POSTSURGICAL FEMALE PELVIS

The majority of postabdominal hysterectomy patients have varying degrees of functional urinary tract obstruction postoperatively secondary to direct trauma or edema of the distal ureters. Though this phenomenon does not appear to have been studied systematically, its degree and severity obviously bear a direct relationship to the extent of surgery, with significantly more protracted problems in patients undergoing radical pelvic operations. In the average case, functional obstruction is temporary, lasting less than 3–10 days. Yet, particularly in some radical hysterectomy patients, partial obstruction as evidenced by hangup of radiopharmaceuticals in the renal collecting systems may be seen, often with calyceal dilatation, for up to 1–3 months or longer postoperatively. The majority of these patients ultimately will have normal scintigrams, but careful renal studies have not been reported in large series. It is not clear how often these patients develop permanent renal damage from unsuspected partial obstruction. Certainly, in recurrent pelvic cancer where involvement of the ureters and bladder is common and where death is usually from renal failure, this outcome is the rule. The question remains, however, to what degree are all posthysterectomy patients at risk for the late development of renal damage secondary to ureteral injury?

For this reason, it is advisable to study all such patients with renal sonography 2–4 weeks postoperatively, and to follow up all abnormal patients with serial scintigraphic studies in order to avoid the possibility of delayed renal damage due to obstructive uropathy.

Summary of Imaging Approaches Given Abnormal Urinary Findings or Renal Functional Impairment

The immediate thrust of urinary tract diagnosis should be to distinguish medical from obstructive conditions. This always can be accomplished most expeditiously with renal ultrasonography. The following summarizes the approach to imaging of the GU tract in the presence of urinary findings or renal failure.

1. Renal ultrasonography should be the initial study in virtually all patients. Failure to demonstrate dilatation of the renal collecting system with ultrasonography almost always excludes clinically significant obstructive (surgical) conditions.

2. If lower tract disease such as bladder or prostatic conditions are suspected, bladder ultrasonography may be helpful. Although bladder tumors are extremely rare in patients under age 40, hypertrophic cystitis or even unsuspected stones may be detected.

3. Postvoiding sonography of the urinary bladder is the best noninvasive study for detecting urinary retention due to the presence of lower tract obstruction, i.e. prostatic enlargement or neurogenic bladder.

4. In patients with functional impairment, if ultrasonography shows a normal renal pelvocalyceal echo pattern *with or without changes in renal size or parenchymal echogenicity*, medical urinary tract disease of some type is present. Further GU imaging studies

are seldom indicated in cases of acute noninfectious medical renal disease such as the nephritides.

5. In the following medical urinary tract diseases, appropriate imaging studies are listed:

(a) Persistent proteinuria associated with medical renal disease, nephrotic syndrome and systemic causes: none or ultrasonography only;
(b) Proteinuria with an "active urinary sediment" indicating glomerulonephritis in its various forms and stages: none or ultrasonography only;
(c) Pyuria with or without bacteriuria and source in the lower tract in adults: renal radionuclide scintigraphy and sonography; and
(d) Asymptomatic bacteriuria in patients over age 60: sonography only.

6. All other patients with urinary tract conditions should have renal and occasionally bladder ultrasonography as their first imaging studies, including patients presenting with gross and microscopic hematuria, pyuria with or without bacteriuria, and suspected renal and bladder masses.

7. All patients with renal sonography showing dilated collecting systems should have functional urinary tract studies, starting with radionuclide scintigraphy or IVP. If previous pyelography has been performed or contraindications to pyelography are present, radionuclide renography should be done.

8. Patients under age 40 with microscopic hematuria and children with gross hematuria almost *never* have cancer or surgical GU disease, and this urinary finding by itself rarely justifies cystoscopy. Sonography and, rarely, pyelography or scintigraphy may be indicated. Most of these patients will have urolithiasis, lower tract inflammatory disease, or congenital abnormalities.

9. Patients between the ages of 15–40 with *gross* hematuria may have surgical renal disease, though GU cancer is extremely rare. These patients should have pyelography, but urological investigation including cystoscopy is indicated *only* with suspicion of surgically treatable disease based on clinical and pyelographic findings. The *routine* use of cystoscopy for gross hematuria in this age group is *not* encouraged.

10. Patients over age 40–45 with gross or microscopic hematuria should have ultrasonography followed by excretory urography and/or radionuclide studies. All such patients without an obvious diagnosis such as stones should have urological investigation including cystoscopy. If a cause is not established, retrograde pyelography is indicated.

11. Pyuria with or without bacteriuria in adults rarely requires further imaging studies in the presence of a normal collecting system on renal ultrasonography. The potential clinical benefit of pyelography or scintigraphy in such patients is doubtful.

12. The first attack of UTI in infants and children does not justify investigation unless the infection fails to respond promptly to treatment. More than two-thirds of such attacks are due to hematogenous pyelonephritis. Second attacks occur in a large number of females; therefore, their significance is much greater in males. In both sexes repeat UTIs call for ultrasonography. Renal scintigraphy also should be done in those patients who have responded poorly to treatment or who have suffered recurrences in 1–2 months after adequate antibiotic therapy.

If sonography is negative, a conservative approach in girls is to treat and wait. In boys with second and girls with third UTIs or in all UTIs responding poorly to treatment, a voiding cystoureterogram preferably with radionuclides should be performed. If there is less than grade 3 VUR, ultimate surgical treatment rarely will be indicated. It should be anticipated that less than 1% of all girls and probably less than 5% of all boys with recurrent UTIs will end up with a surgically correctable problem.

REFERENCES

1. Naidich JB, Rackson ME, Mossey RT, Stein HL. Nondilated obstructive uropathy: percutaneous nephrostomy performed to reverse renal failure. Radiology 1986;160(3):653–657.
2. Dalla-Palma L, Bazzocchi M, Pozzi-Mucelli RS, Stacul F, Rossi M, Agostini R. Ultrasonography in the diagnosis of hydronephrosis in patients with normal renal function. Urol Radiol 1983;5(4):221–226.
3. Chang VH, Cunningham JJ. Efficacy of sonography as a screening method in renal insufficiency. J Clin Ultrasound 1985;13(6):415–417.
4. Rifkin MD. Prostate ultrasound. Semin Ultrasound CT MR 1988;9(5):352–369.
5. Rifkin MD, Zerhouni EA, Gatsonis CA, et al. Comparison of magnetic resonance imaging and ultrasonography in staging early prostate cancer. N Engl J Med 1991;323(10:621–626.
6. Branch WT. Abnormal urinalysis. In: Branch WT, ed. Office Practice of Medicine. Philadelphia: W. B. Saunders Co., 1987:505.
7. Brenner BM, Rector FC. The Kidney. 4th ed. Philadelphia: W. B. Saunders Co., 1991:948.
8. Froom P, Ribak J, Benbassat J. Significance of microhematuria in young adults. Br Med J 1984; 288(6410):20–22.
9. Kudish HG. Determining the cause of hematuria. Postgrad Med 1975;58(6):118–122.
10. Greene LF, O'Shaugnessy Jr EJ, Hendricks ED. Study of 500 patients with asymptomatic microhematuria. JAMA 1956;161:610.
11. Lee LW, Davis E. Gross urinary hemorrhage: a symptom, not a disease. JAMA 1953;153:782–784.
12. Carson III CC, Segura JW, Green LF. Clinical importance of microhematuria. JAMA 1979;241(2): 149–150.
13. Sutton JM. Evaluation of hematuria in adults. JAMA 1990;263(18):2475–2480.
14. Benson GS, Brewer ED. Hematuria: algorithms for diagnosis II. Hematuria in the adult and hematuria secondary to trauma. JAMA 1981;246(9):993–995.
15. Doll R, Payne P, Waterhouse J, eds. International Union Against Cancer: Cancer Incidence in Five Continents. vol 1. New York: Springer-Verlag, 1966.
16. Morrison AS, Cole P. Epidemiology of bladder cancer. Urol Clin North Am 1976;3(1):13–29.
17. Ingelfinger JR, Davis AE, Grupe WE. Frequency and etiology of gross hematuria in a general pediatric setting. Pediatrics 1977;59(4):557–561.
18. Wright WT. Cell counts in the urine. Arch Intern Med 1959;103:76.
19. Kass EH, Savage W, Sanatamarina BA. The significance of bacteriuria in preventive medicine. In: Kass EH, ed. Progress in Pyelonephritis. Philadelphia: F. A. Davis Co., 1965:3–10.
20. Nelson C, McLemore T. National Center for Health Statistics. The National Ambulatory Medical Care Survey. United States, 1975-1981 and 1985 Trends. Vital and Health Statistics. Series 13, No. 93. DHHS Pub. No. (PHS)88-1754. Public Health Service. Washington: U.S. Government Printing Office, 1988.
21. Stamey TA. Pathogenesis and Treatment of Urinary Tract Infections. Baltimore: Williams and Wilkins, 1980.
22. Lipsky BA. Urinary tract infections in men: epidemiology, pathophysiology, diagnosis, and treatment. Ann Intern Med 1989;110(2):138–150.
23. Fair WR, McClennan BL, Jost RG. Are excretory urograms necessary in evaluating women with urinary tract infections? J Urol 1979;121(3):313–315.
24. Pead L, Maskell R. Urinary tract infection in adult men. J Infect 1981;3(1):71–78.
25. Simons RJ. Genitourinary tract abnormalities in patients with urinary tract infection [Abstract]. Clin Res 1988;36:749A.
26. Corrado ML, Grad C, Sabbaj J. Norfloxacin in the treatment of urinary tract infections in men with and without identifiable urologic complications. Am J Med 1987;82(suppl 6B):70–74.
27. Ogra PL, Faden HS. Urinary tract infections in childhood: an update. J Pediatr 1985;106(6):1023–1029.
28. Asscher AW, Fletcher EWL, Johnston HH, et al. Sequelae of covert bacteriuria in school girls: a four-year follow-up study. Lancet 1978;1(8090):889–893.
29. Kunim CM, Zacha E, Paquin AJ. Urinary tract infection in school children. 1. Prevalence of bacteriuria and associated urologic findings. N Engl J Med 1962;266:1287–1296.

30. Newcastle Asymptomatic Bacteriuria Research Group. Asymptomatic bacteriuria in school children in Newcastle-upon-Tyne. Arch Dis Child 1975;50(2):90–102.
31. Gillenwater JY, Harrison RB, Kunin CM. Natural history of bacteriuria in schoolgirls: A: A long-term case control study. N Engl J Med 1979;301(8):396–399.
32. Mason Jr WG, Stevens PS. Options in the evaluation of pediatric urinary tract infections: the role of radiography and ultrasound. Semin Ultrasound CT MR 1986;7(3):234–245.
33. Gelfand MJ. Radionuclide cystography and vesicoureteral reflux. Lecture on continuing medical education. Society of Nuclear Medicine Meeting, Washington, DC, June 1990.
34. Strife JL, Bisset III GS, Kirks DR, et al. Nuclear cystography and renal sonography: findings in girls with urinary tract infection. AJR 1989;153(1):115–119.

2/ Hepatocellular Dysfunction

> LIVER, n. *A large red organ thoughtfully provided by nature to be bilious with. . . . It was at one time considered the seat of life; hence its name—liver—the thing we live with.*
>
> Ambrose Bierce
> The Devil's Dictionary

Medical Causes

Investigation of the patient with abnormal liver chemistries shares many similarities with that of jaundice. For example, the division of etiologies into hepatocellular and obstructive categories, as in jaundice, provides the most logical conceptual approach. Furthermore, the spectra of conditions causing abnormal liver chemistries and jaundice display considerable overlapping. Salient differences, however, between these two categories should be noted. For example, in hepatocellular dysfunction, medical causes will predominate over surgical to a much greater extent than in jaundice, even in the older age group.

Given a patient with abnormal liver function tests, what is the likelihood of making a diagnosis on the basis of clinical findings alone? If we include the results of hepatitis antibody tests, the diagnostic yield in good hands should approach that already quoted, in the 90% range (1, 2). Certainly, the capable clinician should be able to distinguish between medical and obstructive causes with an exceedingly high degree of confidence. Because medical causes of hepatocellular dysfunction account for the large majority of cases and do not call for diagnostic imaging, a ruling-out strategy is seldom justifiable except in the older patient, where some doubt may exist as to the presence of stone or cancer. Medical imaging, otherwise, should be limited to those patients with clear-cut clinical indications of surgical disease.

As the reader should now be ready to acknowledge, given significant symptoms, signs, or abnormal laboratory findings, the likelihood of a specific condition can be predicted with considerable accuracy. Thus, *a reasonable diagnostic hypothesis inevitably precedes and therefore guides investigation.* The use of any laboratory or imaging test must be seen simply as a tactic to reduce the uncertainty of a clinical diagnosis. Attempting to increase one's confidence in an already highly probable diagnosis with tests of even good sensitivity and specificity is one route to confusion if not disaster. Ordering more tests is usually not the best policy.

Extrahepatic vs. Hepatic Causes

The diagnostic approach to hepatocellular dysfunction will be far less confusing if we keep in mind that elevations in liver enzymes, with or without mild abnormalities in bilirubin, are often nonspecific and may reflect the presence of nonhepatic disease. For example, it is obvious that imaging is not needed in patients with cardiac failure, sepsis, and systemic illness where hepatic dysfunction is secondary to an extrahepatic cause. Significant elevations of various enzymes, e.g. aspartate aminotransferase (AST/SGOT), alanine aminotransferase (ALT/SGPT), lactic dehydrogenase, and even alkaline phosphatase (ALP), as well as bilirubin, are encountered in such a wide variety of conditions it is merely necessary to apply clinical common sense to avoid the pitfalls of a mindless diagnostic segue.

Mildly "abnormal" liver enzyme tests are frequently reported by laboratories, and one should learn to be wary of them. One interesting study was carried out on almost 700 patients, 54 or 9% of whom presented with unexplained elevations of ALP on health screening (3). *The PPV of an abnormal test was only about 5% among patients who were not pregnant and who had no prior diagnosis of cancer or liver or bone disease.* Thus a solitary, modest elevation of ALP hardly ever calls for investigation in an otherwise well patient. We already have mentioned that ALP is normally elevated in growing children, elderly patients, patients with fractures, and even after a meal, because of an increase in the intestinal isoenzyme in some patients belonging to type O or B blood groups.

Another source of needless investigation involves patients with mild increases in the other common enzymes, i.e. AST/SGOT, lactic dehydrogenase, and SGPT. The laboratory estimation of hepatic enzyme levels, especially with testing kits, is often misleading, and even in laboratories regarded as reliable poor quality control of assay conditions, particularly temperature, may lead to errors. In addition, factors of patient variability and meals frequently account for results outside the normal range. As a rule, it is wise to ignore mild or minimal enzyme elevations in patients who were unfortunate enough to have had an SMA 12 done as a "screening." Most patients with hepatocellular disease have AST activity at least two to three times normal, and those with obstruction usually have ALP three to four times the reference level. We do not suggest that mild enzyme abnormalities be ignored; obviously, they may point to some form of chronic or active hepatitis. However, these patients usually can be identified by further follow-up and hepatitis antigen/antibody testing.

One occasionally will encounter cases of congestive failure or severe sepsis with impressive elevations of AST/SGOT and especially ALP in which the question of accompanying obstructive disease is raised. In almost all of these cases, the preceding medical history and the presence or absence of abdominal findings are much more reliable clues to the presence of obstructive disease than the derangement of blood chemistries. Because we are all fearful of missing a common duct stone or a malignancy, if there is concern it is not unreasonable in this setting to perform ultrasonography of the biliary tract. If the study is normal, i.e. in the absence of cholelithiasis, common bile duct dilatation, and abnormalities in the pancreas, obstructive liver disease is excluded with more than 95% certainty, and further medical imaging can be omitted. When abnormalities are indeed found, one should proceed as outlined in the summary for the investigation of jaundice, Chapter 6, Section 11. Recall, however, that 4–8% or more of the population have asymptomatic cholelithiasis, so

Table 7.2.1. Estimated Raw Percentages of Medical vs. Obstructive Causes of Abnormal Liver Function Tests in Different Age Groups, Corresponding Estimated Percentages in Jaundiced Patients given in Parentheses

Diagnosis	Age		
	1–30	30–60	>60
Medical conditions (including spurious elevations due to lab error), congestive failure, systemic disease, sepsis, shock, hemolysis, hepatitis (viral, alcohol, drugs), etc	98% (95%)	85% (75%)	60% (30%)
Obstructive conditions Primary/metastatic cancer biliary tract Stones, etc.	2% (5%)	15% (25%)	40% (70%)

Adapted from Baer and Belsey, 1988 (4).

Table 7.2.2. Test: Sonography: Estimated Probabilities of Various Test Results for Each Disease

Disease	Normal	Stones	Dilated CBD	Stones/dil. CBD
Hepatocellular	95	4	1	0
Cholecystitis/obstruction	5	60	5	30

Prior Probability (Prevalence) of Disease and Posttest Probability of Disease for Each Test Result

Disease	Prevalence	Posttest probabilities			
		Normal	Stones	Dilated CBD	Stones/dil. CBD
Hepatocellular	95	>99	56	<1	<1
Cholecystitis/obstruction	5	<1	44	>99	>99

that the solitary finding of gall stones without changes in ductal measurements does not prove the presence of cholecystitis. In this event, obviously, hepatobiliary scintigraphy should be done only if cholecystitis is suspected clinically.

Table 7.2.1 is adapted from Chapter 6, and Section 11 on jaundice, and gives hypothetical frequencies of various causes of hepatocellular dysfunction by age. The numbers represent reasonable clinical estimates of the incidence of medical vs. obstructive conditions, given abnormal hepatic function tests (without hyperbilirubinemia) in the three major age groups.

To summarize the tabular findings, it is clear that in patients under age 60 with abnormal hepatic function tests, the great majority will prove to have some nonsurgical cause. The significance of abnormal liver chemistries does change markedly in the older age groups, as is the case with hyperbilirubinemia. Given only abnormal liver function tests and no other clinical information in a patient over age 60 there is probably less than 40% chance of an obstructive cause. Sonography is clearly the first study of choice in suspected obstructive disease in the hepatobiliary tract.

When one examines the predictive value for sonography, it becomes obvious that a binary outcome cannot be assumed. Various test outcomes must be considered, a problem we have touched upon. For example, in Table 7.2.2, lumping

Table 7.2.3.   Test: Sonography: Estimated Probabilities of Various Test Results for Each Disease

Disease	Normal	Stones	Dilated CBD	Stones/dil. CBD
Hepatocellular	95	4	1	0
Cholecystitis/obstruction	5	60	5	25

Prior Probability (Prevalence) of Disease and Posttest Probability of Disease for Each Test Result

Disease	Prevalence	Posttest probabilities			
		Normal	Stones	Dilated CBD	Stones/dil. CBD
Hepatocellular	80	99	21	44	<1
Cholecystitis/obstruction	20	1	79	56	>99

Table 7.2.4.   Test: Sonography: Estimated Probabilities of Various Test Results for Each Disease

Disease	Normal	Stones	Dilated CBD	Stones/dil. CBD
Hepatocellular	95	4	1	0
Cholecystitis/obstruction	5	60	5	25

Prior Probability (Prevalence) of Disease and Posttest Probability of Disease for Each Test Result

Disease	Prevalence	Posttest probabilities			
		Normal	Stones	Dilated CBD	Stones/dil. CBD
Hepatocellular	70	98	13	32	<1
Cholecystitis/obstruction	30	2	87	68	>99

extrahepatic and hepatocellular causes together and comparing them with the diagnoses of cholecystitis and/or obstruction, we note several interesting findings. Because gall stones are present on average in about 4% of the population compared with an estimated 60% of patients with cholecystitis (90% of patients if we include those with or without ductal dilatation), the posttest probability of cholecystitis/obstruction with a prevalence of 5% in the sole presence of stone, is in the 44% range. With a dilated CBD and stones, however, the posttest probability is greater than 99%. Note in Tables 7.2.3. and 7.2.4. the effect of increasing the prior prevalence of cholecystitis/obstruction to 20% and 30%. Although the sensitivity figures for these outcomes are hypothetical estimates, it is clear that the problem of interpreting test results cannot always be approached in a simple fashion. *Most tests have multiple outcomes*, at the minimum, three: positive, negative, and indeterminate or equivocal. Many imaging tests, including the example of sonography above, have seven or more possible outcomes. We could have, for example, included "thick walled gall bladder" in the normal, with or without stones and dilated CBD.

It is important to consider once again the implications of high disease prevalence for the use of these and other imaging studies. Like an old refrain, the melody lingers on—if we only would pause to listen. A ruling out strategy is almost always counterproductive, and only when obstructive or other biliary tract disease is *suspected* should imaging be performed. If, for example, the patient is a 40-year-old woman, has a history of fat intolerance and attacks of right upper quadrant postprandial distress, pain, and tenderness, along with abnormal liver function, then the probability of an obstructive problem is obviously not 2%, but closer to 90%.

Summary

1. In suspected hepatocellular disease, imaging is *almost never* indicated; the large majority of patients with abnormalities in liver function under age 40–50, with the exception of infants, have hepatocellular disease.

2. Obstructive or surgical liver disease *always* calls for imaging to determine the site and probable cause of the obstruction, i.e. stone or cancer. Abdominal ultrasonography (gall bladder, common bile duct, and pancreas) is the imaging study of first choice in all such patients, followed if necessary by hepatobiliary scintigraphy.

3. If ultrasonography of the biliary tract is negative, surgical liver disease has been excluded with more than 90–95% confidence. Further imaging studies are almost never indicated.

4. If ultrasonography is abnormal, showing changes in the liver, bile ducts, or pancreas, imaging should proceed as outlined in Chapter 6, Section 11.

5. Unexplained liver functional abnormalities, especially painless or *intermittent*, in any patient, are ample justification for general use of ultrasonography as a screening test for obstructive liver disease.

REFERENCES

1. Schenker S, Balint J, Schiff L. Differential diagnosis of jaundice: a report of a prospective study of 61 proved cases. AM J Dig Dis 1962;7:449–463.
2. O'Connor KW, Snodgrass PJ, Swonder JE, et al. A blinded prospective study comparing four current noninvasive approaches in the differential diagnosis of medical versus surgical jaundice. Gastroenterology 1983;84(6):1498–1504.
3. Rubenstein LV, Ward NC, Greenfield S. In pursuit of the abnormal serum alkaline phosphatase: a clinical dilemma. J Gen Intern Med 1986;1(1):38–43.
4. Baer DM, Belsey RE. Clinical problems in the office lab: evaluating jaundice. MLP/Med Lab Prod 1988;Jan:16–18.

3/ Endocrine Dysfunction

> *What we think and feel and are is to a great extent determined by the state of our ductless glands and our viscera.*
>
> *Aldous Huxley*

General Remarks

Despite its widespread availability, medical imaging does not qualify as a hunting expedition. This applies notably in endocrine disease, where diagnosis begins with clinical suspicion and proceeds to laboratory confirmation. Given the presence of a biochemically validated endocrine disorder, when is imaging required, and which studies are appropriate? The answer is straightforward and unequivocal: Medical imaging is indicated for management decisions in thyroid, pituitary, parathyroid, adrenal, and some types of gonadal dysfunction, but *not* for primary diagnosis.

For example, adrenal scintigraphy is often ordered to rule out suspected pheochromocytoma or Cushing disease, or imagining of the parathyroids may be sought in patients with hypercalcemia of uncertain etiology before the necessary laboratory testing has been completed. These requests arise from a fundamental misconception, i.e. failure to realize that the diagnosis of endocrine dysfunction rests finally on chemical verification, and that imaging, when applicable, is important only to guide therapy. Adrenal, pituitary, and parathyroid hyperfunction cannot be diagnosed per se with radionuclide studies, CT, or MRI.

THE THYROID

> *Worry affects circulation, the heart and the glands, (and) the whole nervous system. . . . I have never known a man who died from overwork, but many who died from doubt.*
>
> Charles H. Mayo

The principal indication for thyroid imaging, namely the presence of palpable abnormalities of the gland, has been discussed in Chapter 6, Section 21. Thyroid hypofunction usually does not require scintigraphy, but in the case of hyperthyroidism, there are good reasons for performing it. Thyrotoxicosis comes in several anatomical varieties, the common, diffuse type with a uniformly enlarged gland, hyperthyroidism arising in nodular goiter (toxic multinodular goiter), and, exceedingly rare, thyrotoxicosis resulting from a single toxic nodule, true Plummer's disease. It is generally possible to distinguish these categories on a clinical basis, but the thyroid scintiscan is more consistently reliable. Because therapeutic radioiodine is at present the safest and most effective treatment for adult patients with thyrotoxicosis, the identification of the type of goiter is anything but academic; the treatment dose of iodine-131 is based on the radioiodine uptake and the size and type of gland. Diffuse hyperthyroidism in an average-size gland may require only 6–12 mCi iodine-131 depending on the 24-hour iodine-131 uptake, whereas in a large multinodular gland or in true toxic nodular goiter the dose could well be in the 20–30 mCi range.

Thus, the 24-hour thyroidal iodine uptake should be considered part of the thyroid imaging procedure for thyrotoxicosis when it is used to help determine the iodine-131 therapy dose. As many as 18% of women attending one clinic were taking estrogens (1), and in Nolan and Tarsa's series (2), which included an even higher number of patients taking a variety of drugs affecting thyroid function, the specificity of the total T_4 (TT_4) was only 91%. This is not sufficiently high for this single test to justify radioactive iodine therapy for hyperthyroidism in a clinically questionable patient. In addition, the clinical spectrum of Graves ranges from the subtle to overt. Because the causes of spuriously abnormal thyroid function tests are legion, the thyroidal iodine uptake was at one time considered useful in documenting hyperfunction, though it too can be spuriously abnormal. The principal use of the RAI other than in estimating treatment dose of iodine-131 is in identifying factitious disease and in distinguishing thyroiditis from other forms of hyperthyroidism. At present the sensitive TSH assay is the preferred test to confirm biochemical hyperthyroidism.

HYPERPARATHYROIDISM

Hyperparathyroidism rarely presents as a clinical problem but is usually found serendipitously with the discovery of an elevated serum calcium. Diagnosis thus becomes a matter of distinguishing parathyroid hyperactivity from other much more common causes of hypercalcemia. The diagnosis of normocalcemic hyperparathyroidism is obviously a much more difficult task for the skilled endocrinologist, so the place of imaging in this variant remains as controversial as its management.

Causes of hypercalcemia other than parathyroid disease are multiple and range from various malignancies to vitamin D intoxication, milk-alkali syndrome, hypervitaminosis A, sarcoidosis, adrenal insufficiency, thiazide diuretics, hyperthyroidism, etc. It is important for the clinician to keep in mind that by far the most common cause of elevated serum calcium is some type of malignancy. This may be a tumor metastatic to bone, especially breast cancer, lymphoma/myeloma, or a malignancy without bony metastases, such as hypernephroma, pancreatic cancer, or various squamous cell tumors arising in the lung, esophagus, and cervix (3).

The low incidence and prevalence of primary hyperparathyroidism has been reported from a Mayo Clinic study (4) and also can be estimated by the NCHS data derived from the National Hospital Discharge Summary (5). The average annual incidence of hyperparathyroidism in Rochester, Minn, more than tripled from 8 to 28 cases per 100,000 between 1965–1974 after the availability of routine measurement of serum calcium. If we attempt to equate discharge data with incidence the all-listed NHDS data for the hospitalized population in 1990, 7 cases per 100,000 agrees more closely with the lower figure (5). The discordancy may be explained by failure to diagnose hyperparathyroidism outside of Rochester, Minn, but like other epidemiological data, there are many confounding and unmeasurable statistical biases. We may at least conclude that hyperparathyroidism, like other examples of nonthyroidal endocrine hyperfunction, is an exceedingly rare condition.

Only when the diagnosis of primary hyperparathyroidism is established with reasonable biochemical certainty does the issue of parathyroid imaging arise. Despite countless reports in the literature, the value of preoperative localization of parathyroid adenomas remains controversial because of an inescapable paradox: when the tumor is of adequate size, larger than 2 cm, the success rate of parathyroid exploration in good surgical hands is exceedingly high, just as is the sensitivity of most imaging methods. When the tumor is small, as is often the case, surgical as well as imaging failures occur with increasing frequency. Still, because ectopic or multiple tumors occur in 5–10% of cases, imaging maintains an important role.

Four principal modalities are available for parathyroid visualization: computer-assisted thallium-201/technetium-99m scintigraphy (TTS), ultrasound, CT, and MRI. In scintigraphy, thallium-201, which is taken up nonpreferentially by the normal thyroid and most parathyroid tumors, is injected, and serial images are acquired and stored on a digital computer. After this, technetium, which is used in thyroid imaging, is then injected so that the thyroid uptake of thallium can be "normalized" and therefore subtracted from the thallium image. This is similar to the subtraction of the "mask" image in digital subtraction angiography. If the study is carefully performed with no patient motion, the presence of a radioactive thallium focus in *or outside* the thyroid bed, including the mediastinum, is assumed to be due to parathyroid adenoma or hyperplasia, because the normal parathyroids do not visualize with technetium-99m pertechnetate.

How do these methods compare? One prospective blinded study was undertaken on 40 patients with primary hyperparathyroidism (6). The sensitivities of TTS and CT were much superior to ultrasound (72%, 72%, and 57%, respectively). For tumors in the superior mediastinum, CT was very poor (29% sensitivity), whereas TTS was excellent (86% sensitivity), and for smaller tumors weighing less than 250 mg TTS was most sensitive (60% vs. 0% for CT). Sonography compared poorly with both TTS and CT even in larger tumors. For patients with prior neck exploration, TTS was clearly superior to CT and ultrasound.

In our experience with a much smaller series, TTS has been helpful in a fair number of cases. Several colleagues anecdotally report finding approximately 50–60% of parathyroid tumors, usually those easily located at surgery. A nihilistic and somewhat extreme approach has been expressed by an excellent neck surgeon at an unnamed medical center, i.e. don't bother to image unless the first exploration is unsuccessful.

Even though parathyroid scintigraphy may not have the high sensitivity we would like, it is at present the best imaging method for parathyroid tumors. It would therefore seem prudent to perform routine thallium/technetium scintigraphy in patients undergoing neck exploration for parathyroid tumors. Ultrasound and CT have little or no place in first-time parathyroid localization. However, in patients undergoing reexploration, where every attempt should be made to locate a tumor previously missed, if TTS fails, then certainly CT or perhaps MRI is indicated. The patients most likely to benefit from TTS will be those with multiple or ectopic, particularly mediastinal, parathyroid tumors. Those undergoing reexploration with a negative TTS scan will benefit principally from CT or MRI.

THE ADRENAL

Effective medical imaging of the adrenal gland is limited to the use of scintigraphy, CT, and MRI. Sonography, despite occassional claims, has such poor sensitivity for adrenal disease as to be virtually without merit. Of the three other methods, scintigraphy is by far the most reliable technique in directing patient management, the only drawback being limited availability of the required radiopharmaceuticals in some centers (vide infra).

Clinically significant adrenal syndromes resemble those of the parathyroid and pituitary in their rarity, but like most endocrinopathies—and unlike many other chronic conditions—treatment is much more consistently rewarding and effective. Three principal adrenal endocrine disorders require imaging. All of them represent specific types of hyperfunction and result respectively from excess production of cortical steroids or androgens, cortical mineralocorticoids, and medullary catecholamines, i.e. Cushing syndrome/androgen excess, hyperaldosteronism or Conn Syndrome, and pheochromocytoma. Malignant tumors of the adrenals, pituitary, and parathyroids (ICD 194) occur in only 3 and benign neoplasms in only 8 individuals per 100,000 population. The NHDS hospital discharge data of 1990 for major endocrine conditions are presented in Table 7.3.1 and demonstrate their extremely rare occurrence. The rate for hyperaldosteronism (ICD 255.1) was only 2 cases per 100,000 population in 1990, and the rate for pheochromocytoma (ICD 255.6) is too low even to be listed (5).

ADRENAL SCINTIGRAPHY

A quiet revolution begun at the University of Michigan in the early 1970s under Dr. William H. Beierwaltes and his colleagues, Sisson, Shapiro, Gross, Wieland and others (7–11), has contributed enormously to our understanding, diagnosis, and therapeutic approach to Cushing disease, hyperaldosteronism, pheochromocytoma, and a spectrum of other endocrine and hypertensive disorders. Two outstanding adrenal imaging agents, the radiopharmaceuticals, NP-59 and metaiodobenzylguanidine (MIBG), have been developed at Michigan and are now used throughout the world.

Table 7.3.1.   Major Pituitary, Parathyroid and Adrenal Endocrinopathies, Discharge Rates/100,000 Populations, U.S. Hospitals, 1990, NHDS Data (5).

All-listed ICD-9-CM		Total	Male	Female	Age <15	Age 15–44	Age 45–64	Age 65+
252.0	Hyperparathyroidism	6	0	10	0	0	11	25
253.	Pituitary/hypothalm dis	20	18	23	0	4	32	85
253.2	Panhypopituitarism	2	0	0	0	0	0	0
253.5	Diabetes Insipidus	2	0	0	0	0	0	0
253.6	Neurohypophysis dis NEC	13	10	16	0	0	15	73
255.0	Cushing's syndrome	5	0	7	0	0	17	0
255.1	Hyperaldosteronism	2	0	0	0	0	0	0
255.4	Corticoadrenal insufficiency	9	8	11	0	0	15	35

It is because of the different *functional* forms of adrenal disease that scintigraphic procedures are usually so much more crucial than CT, an anatomical method, in the management of various adrenal endocrinopathies.

ADRENOCORTICAL DISEASE: CUSHING'S SYNDROME

NP-59, the short name for I-131-iodo-6-β methylnorcholesterol, is the principal radiopharmaceutical used in imaging the adrenal cortex in both Cushing's disease and hyperaldosteronism. Again we stress that the diagnosis of adrenocortical hyperfunction, like other endocrinopathies, first must be established clinically and chemically before the need for scintigraphy is determined. It is only the *functional form* of the disease that is established by imaging and upon which therapy is so dependent. In other words, adrenal scintigraphy is appropriate *only when the diagnosis of hypercorticism already has been made.*

The majority of patients with cortisol excess have secondary or adrenocorticotropin (ACTH)-dependent Cushing's syndrome with bilateral adrenal hyperplasia. Imaging is seldom indicated in these subjects, and then only in the unusual case when ACTH or steroid excretion and suppression patterns are equivocal. This occurs most frequently in those unfortunate patients with malignant tumors and the ectopic ACTH syndrome. In patients with secondary hypercorticism, of course, therapy is not directed to the adrenal, but rather to the pituitary or the causative malignancy, e.g. oat cell tumor of lung or lymphoma.

Primary adrenocortical hyperfunction, on the other hand, is usually a surgical condition. Hypercorticism arising in the adrenal is much less common than ACTH-dependent disease and is seen in only 20–30% of patients with Cushing's. Most cases of primary disease are caused by a benign unilateral cortical adenoma; the next most likely etiology is bilateral cortical nodular hyperplasia; and the least likely cause is adrenocortical carcinoma. At least four typical patterns of adrenal visualization with NP-59 have been described in Cushing's disease. In ACTH (pituitary)-dependent disease, bilaterally symmetrical and intense adrenal visualization is seen. In unilateral adenoma the tumor is intensely visualized with nonvisualization of the other adrenal, because of contralateral suppression due to endogenous ACTH inhibition. In bilateral nodular hyperplasia, asymmetric adrenal visualization is noted. In adrenal carcinoma there is almost always nonvisualization of both adrenals secondary to unilateral adrenal destruction and contralateral suppression. In a series of 24 cases of primary adrenal hypercorticism referred to the University of Michigan (12) all 14 patients with adenomas showed focal unilateral uptake, and 3 of 4 patients with carcinoma showed the typical pattern of nonvisualization. CT during the study depicted anatomically abnormal adrenals in all of these patients, but no functional information was obtained. CT demonstrated abnormal adrenals in only one patient with nodular hyperplasia, whereas scintigraphy showed a typical pattern in all six cases of nodular disease (12). These findings indicate that adrenal scintigraphy is the initial imaging method of choice in all forms of primary adrenal hypercorticism and some forms of secondary or ACTH-dependent disease. CT and MRI are most effective in detecting significant adrenal enlargement but present some problems in displaying borderline enlargement and in comparing size of the two adrenals. Their principal drawback, however, is that they are only anatomical studies; neither CT nor MRI can assess comparative functional status of the hyperfunctioning gland. One must conclude, therefore, that CT if used alone, at the very least would result in diagnostic and therefore therapeutic errors in the treatment of many patients with adrenal dysfunction.

Other indications for adrenal cortical scintigraphy include the study of hyperandrogenism in women, some of whom turn out to have diseases of adrenal rather than ovarian origin (13). Many of these cases are examples of Cushing's disease with androgen excess; a few are pure androgen-producing tumors of the adrenal cortex, ovary, or testis (in men) (14); and an undetermined percentage represent newly discovered forms of bilateral adrenal hyperfunction. In addition to virilizing syndromes, a spectrum of new adrenal abnormalities now has been described thanks to adrenal scintigraphy, including certain cases of low renin hypertension (vide infra) and rare types of "Pre-Cushing's syndrome" or functional adrenal nodules (15, 16). Beierwaltes, Gross, and others feel there exists a spectrum of nodular adrenal disease analogous to that found in the thyroid. Thus, some functional adrenal nodules may be suppressible, whereas others are nonsuppressible and may become autonomous, just as in the case of functioning thyroid nodules, some of which go on to overt hyperthyroidism. Gross has emphasized that the definition of "endocrinopathy" should be broadened to include this assortment of clinically indeterminate syndromes (Gross, M., personal communication). Although most of these patients will be discovered incidentally and never develop clinical disease, the study of these experiments in nature nonetheless will bring needed insight into the pathogenesis of more obvious examples of endocrine dysfunction.

Twenty-five years ago, before the reintroduction of transsphenoidal surgery for the removal of pituitary tumors and microadenomas, the accepted mode of treatment for Cushing's disease was bilateral adrenalectomy. Persistent cortisol excess after adrenalectomy is still seen in the rare patient, and adrenal scintigraphy has proved to be an effective technique to locate an adrenal remnant before exploration. In fact, scintigraphy is the *only* method of localization in these patients. Freitas et al. (17) visualized adrenal remnants in five of nine patients with persistent Cushing's disease after bilateral adrenalectomy. Scintigraphic visualization of the remnant enabled surgical localization in all five patients. No other localizing procedures, including adrenal venous sampling, arteriography, or venography, were successful in identifying an adrenal remnant.

HYPERALDOSTERONISM

Prevalence estimates for primary aldosteronism range from 0.05–2% of all hypertensive patients (18, 19). Yet the incidence of all primary and secondary hyperaldos-

Table 7.3.2.   Interpretation of DS Adrenal Scans[a]

Pattern	Days	Pathology correlate
Unilateral image	3–5	Adenoma
Bilateral image	<5	Hyperplasia
Bilateral image	>5	Nondiagnostic

[a]Four milligrams of DS for 7 days before and throughout the imaging interval.
Reprinted by permission from Gross MD, Thrall JH, Beierwaltes WH. The adrenal scan: a current status report on radiotracers. In: Freeman LM, Weissmann HS, eds. *Nuclear Medicine Annual.* New York: Raven Press (1980:147).

teronism, including Bartter's Syndrome (ICD 255.1) is so low in the 1990 NHDS survey of all-listed diagnoses as to be recorded as statistically unreliable, that is, less than 5,000 cases in the United States for an incidence, as noted above, of 2 cases per 100,000 population (5). From these figures, one may calculate, assuming a 20% prevalence of hypertension in the U.S. population, that 1 out of 250,000 Americans with high blood pressure is suffering from Conn syndrome. Still, hypertension due to excessive secretion of aldosterone can be caused by an adrenal tumor curable by surgery or bilateral micro- or macronodular hyperplasia, which should be treated medically. The biochemical distinction of these two forms of disease is far from reliable. Both CT and bilateral adrenal vein sampling leave much to be desired in detecting a unilateral tumor or differentiating a tumor from bilateral hyperplasia. Bilateral adrenal vein sampling for renin and aldosterone is costly, invasive, and sometimes unreliable, and catheterization of the right adrenal vein is frequently unsuccessful. We have seen a patient in whom an aldosterone tumor was correctly localized by scintigraphy after incorrect localization by venous sampling because the blood sample tubes were inadvertently switched by the technician and thus mislabeled. This proves only that human errors plague all testing, even the most "elegant."

In primary aldosteronism, the radiopharmaceutical required is again NP-59. In order to enhance the specificity of the test and inhibit visualization of the normal adrenal, scintigraphy is performed after 7 days of adrenal suppression with dexamethasone and thyroid blockade with stable iodine. Several patterns have been described and are depicted in Table 7.3.2. It should be noted that *on dexamethasone suppression* unilateral adrenal visualization 3–5 days after NP-59 injection usually indicates an aldosterone-producing tumor, bilateral faint visualization before the 5th day indicates hyperplasia, and bilateral visualization after the 5th day is nondiagnostic or "normal." In an earlier study the overall accuracy of the NP-59 suppression scintiscan in aldosteronism when patients with adrenal hyperplasia or adenoma were considered together was 80% (21). However, in 15 of 16 patients with lateralizing scans, adenomas were found at surgery, a specificity of 94% (22).

Thirty percent of hypertensive patients have been found to have subnormal plasma renin activity (22). Because the incidence of primary aldosteronism is so low, it can be assumed that an enormous number of patients with high blood pressure have what is now called low renin essential hypertension or (LREH). Suppression adrenal scintigraphy has been performed in a number of these patients, and functional abnormalities often have been demonstrated despite the failure to confirm pathological aldosterone excess (23). That these patients with abnormal adrenal visualization responded to spironolactone, an antialdosterone agent, "strongly supports the view that there are functional adrenal cortical abnormalities in patients with LREH. That hypertensives with normal imaging patterns did not respond to spironolactone therapy suggests that LREH is a heterogeneous disorder and adrenal scintigraphy can be used to identify a subset of patients with an adrenal cortical component to their disease" (23).

We do not suggest, of course, that the usual patient with essential hypertension have adrenal scintigraphy, but in certain cases plasma renin activity should be determined, particularly if the patient becomes hypokalemic on thiazides or normotensive on spironolactone. Very few of these patients will prove to have primary aldosteronism, but as is the case with functional nodules of the adrenal, we may be seeing examples of *forme fruste* adrenal mineralocorticoid dysfunction and, as Gross suggests, the concept of "endocrinopathy" may some day have to be broadened considerably to include a number of subclinical adrenal and other endocrine gland disorders.

ADRENAL MEDULLARY DISEASE: PHEOCHROMOCYTOMA

Pheochromocytoma (pheo), a catecholamine-producing tumor arising from neuroectoderm, is another extremely rare condition with an incidence of only 1 or 2 cases per 100,000 adults per year (24). Although 90% of pheos originate in the adrenal glands (25), the other 10% may arise anywhere from the base of the skull to the pelvic floor. These extraadrenal tumors are notoriously elusive when conventional imaging modalities such as plain CT or MRI are used to locate them (26). Furthermore, arteriography and venous sampling for catecholamines are invasive, technically difficult, often precipitate a hypertensive crisis, and should almost never be used. Consequently, in the late 1970s NP-59 scintigraphy was used with mild success to image pheochromocytomas by noting a defect in the adrenal on scintiscanning (27). This changed profoundly in 1980 when Wieland et al. (10) synthesized the enzyme inhibitor MIBG, an analog of guanethidine, which localizes in adrenergic tissue including the heart. Scintigraphic localization of pheochromocytomas with iodine-131- or -123-labeled MIBG has since become the first-line imaging procedure in this condition.

Various studies have confirmed the usefulness of MIBG in localizing adrenergic tumors. In a paper comparing the efficacy of MIBG, CT, and MRI in 19 patients (28), there was one false-negative MIBG study, two false-negative CT scans, and one false-negative MRI study. Because there were only 5 patients with extraadrenal tumor sites, the relative effectiveness of MIBG was underestimated. The authors, nevertheless, recommended that MIBG scintigraphy be used as the initial localizing study of choice, reserving CT or MRI as secondary procedures.

In their excellent paper, Sisson and Shapiro (29) discuss the important potential implication of MIBG in the study of heart failure and other types of adrenergic dysfunction. Additional mention is made of the wide range of neuroendocrine and other tumors in which MIGB may localize. These tumors include some cases of neuroblastomas, ganglioneuromas, medullary thyroid cancer, carcinoid tumors, etc. Cases of positive images have even been reported in, among other tumors, chemodectoma, metastatic choriocarcinoma, pancreatic islet cell tumor, oat cell carcinoma of the lung, and parathyroid adenoma. The unusual localization of MIBG in such a wide range of tumors raises fascinating possibilities for further research with this interesting agent. However, the apparent nonspecificity of MIBG by no means reduces its usefulness for its principal indication, anatomical localization of pheochromocytoma, because, as always, endocrine diagnosis is based on confirmatory biochemical testing. Cases of malignant pheochromocytomas have even been treated with some success with large doses of iodine-131 MIBG. If clinical findings are supported by the presence of excess urinary and blood catecholamine levels, one may assume that a positive MIBG scintiscan localizes a pheochromocytoma in the vast majority of cases. Sisson and Shapiro (29) also did a meta-analysis on the efficacy of MIBG scintigraphy from a total of 6 groups of investigators and a total of 1322 studies. They found a sensitivity of 79–91%.

HYPO- AND HYPERPITUITARISM AND DIABETES INSIPIDUS

Pituitary hyperfunction is represented primarily by the syndromes of acromegaly (growth hormone excess), ACTH-dependent Cushing's syndrome, and hyperprolactinemia, all caused by intracellular tumors, in the two latter conditions, usually microadenomas. Hypopituitarism, except in those rare cases of infarction or Sheehan's syndrome, may be "idiopathic" although most often is due to tumor. In a large series of 450 sellar/juxtasellar lesions, more than 36% were adenomas, and another 30% were fairly equally divided among gliomas, meningiomas, craniopharyngiomas, and aneurysms (30). Hypothalamic syndromes, particularly diabetes insipidus, may be associated with tumor less than half the time.

Given a patient who presents with signs, symptoms, and laboratory evidence of pituitary or hypothalamic dysfunction, skull X-rays may well show an abnormality of the sella, but the imaging procedure of choice is either CT or MRI. Which modality is used will rest on factors of availability and experience of the interpreter. Overall, however, it appears that MRI in experienced hands is generally superior to CT.

A Note on Adrenal Scintigraphy and Investigational New Drugs

The University of Michigan Department of Radiopharmacy has made NP-59 available to major medical centers throughout the world since 1975, and MIBG since 1981. The safety and effectiveness of these scintigraphic imaging agents has been attested to in thousands of patients and hundreds of published studies. Yet these important radiopharmaceuticals remain to this day investigational new drugs (IND) in the United States. This is all the more astounding, because NP-59 has been approved and commercially available for some time in Europe and Asia. The situation may change at least for MIBG, since the French company CIS has purchased the patent rights for the United States and is actively working with the Michigan group to obtain FDA approval. However, at present in this country, in order to use either MIBG or NP-59, the nuclear physician must not only possess an IND from the University of Michigan, the sole manufacturer, or the FDA, but be willing to file yearly forms with the FDA, obtain consent from his hospital institutional review board, and get signed informed consents from every patient he injects. In certain places, New York City, for example, local radiopharmaceutical regulations largely have prevented most institutions from using these drugs. Unless the present law is changed, it cannot be predicted when either NP-59 or MIBG will obtain an NDA (new drug) status from the FDA.

A historical digression may be of interest. In response to the Thalidomide disaster, Congress passed in 1962 the Kefauver-Harris amendments to the Food, Drug, and Cosmetic Act. This law, in many aspects a much needed improvement over the 1935 act, nevertheless extended an already powerful bureaucratic stranglehold over new drug development. According to pharmaceutical industry spokespersons, in 1985 it took an average of 12 years and $50–70 million from initial discovery of a drug until completion of required FDA studies (31–33). Today the average cost of developing a new drug is approximately $150–200 million. Parenthetically, the life of a U.S. patent is 17 years. Thanks to what has been described as regulatory malpractice by the FDA, the United States is rapidly becoming a pharmaceutical backwater among advanced countries. More and more new drugs are being developed, tested, and released abroad, often years before they are permitted to be used in this country.

In an attempt to remedy this situation and particularly to make available life-saving drugs which otherwise would not be developed, the Orphan Drug Act was passed in 1983 (34). This act focused on "rare diseases and conditions," which were defined as those affecting less than 200,000 persons [sic] in the United States and for which "there is no reasonable expectation that the cost . . . of making available in the U.S. a drug for such disease or condition will be recovered from U.S. sales of such drugs." The definition is quite broad when one considers that it includes, among at least 5,000 other conditions, Tourette syndrome, amyotrophic lateral sclerosis (ALS or Lou Gehrig's disease), adrenal hyperplasia, breast cancer, and AIDS, all of which afflict far fewer than 200,000 patients. The law provides for tax incentives, grants, and contracts for development and the granting of "exclusive approval for 7 years for a designated drug. . . ." This latter provision allows for at best an average 2 years extension on the effective patent life of a new drug, assuming usual development time. Although the law, like previous legislation, was well intentioned, its provisions have not proven to be of any significant help in obtaining new drug approvals (NDAs), nor has it had any discernible effect in stimulating drug research and development by the pharmaceutical industry. The FDA has come under increasingly effective attack from AIDS and other advocacy groups for the continuing logjam over the release of life-saving drugs. But lost in the furor has been any concerted effort to improve the situation with regard to diagnostic or "nonpolitical" drugs. IND status of NP-59, MIBG, *and other important pharmaceuticals* continues to punish innocent patients by causing severe logistical difficulties in obtaining adrenal scintigraphy. Nevertheless, these two agents have unique diagnostic efficacy in patients with adrenal tumors and various types of adrenal dysfunction. It would be a shame if their unavailability in the average community hospital discourages physicians from referring patients with these rare conditions to a center holding an appropriate IND.

Summary of Imaging Approach in Patients with Endocrine Dysfunction

1. Endocrine diagnosis is guided by clinical findings and confirmed with biochemical testing. The principal purpose of medical imaging in endocrine dysfunction is in guiding patient management.

2. The sensitive TSH essay is the best confirmatory test for biochemical hyperthyroidism. The 24-hour radioiodine uptake may be of diagnostic help in thyroiditis and factitious hyperthyroidism, but its principal value, along with the thyroid scintiscan, is in helping to estimate the required dose of radioactive iodine in the treatment of various forms of thyrotoxicosis.

Hypothyroidism usually requires neither an uptake nor thyroid scintigraphy for diagnosis or management.

3. In patients with chemically confirmed hyperparathyroidism, attempts at preoperative localization of tumors or hyperplasia should be made, especially because of the known occurrence of mediastinal and other ectopic or multiple tumors in 5–10%

of cases. The most effective method for localization is combined TTS. CT, MRI, and ultrasound are demonstrably inferior in the preoperative patient.

The patient most likely to benefit from preoperative localization studies has been subjected to previous unsuccessful parathyroid exploration. In these cases, TTS and CT are advised in order to maximize the chance of finding a tumor that already has been missed.

4. Approximately 70% of Cushing syndrome is secondary to pituitary ACTH excess, leaving about 30% of cases due to primary adrenal disease causing cortisol excess. This may result from unilateral adenoma, bilateral nodular hyperplasia, and, rarely, adrenocortical carcinoma. In all three examples, adrenal scintigraphy with NP-59, when available, is the preferred first imaging study to localize the involved gland or glands and to determine functional behavior in order to decide on appropriate therapy. In the rare case where results are equivocal, CT or MRI are indicated in all three adrenal conditions. Rarely, adrenal scintigraphy should be performed on suspected secondary or ACTH-dependent Cushing disease with equivocal chemical findings. This will occur mainly in patients with the ectopic ACTH syndrome resulting from malignant tumors. Adrenal venography and adrenal vein sampling are outmoded and should almost never be performed in these cases.

5. Rarely, patients with virilizing syndromes and low renin hypertension will benefit from adrenal scintigraphy with NP-59, because unsuspected adrenal, ovarian, and testicular abnormalities may be uncovered.

6. In cases of hyperaldosteronism, NP-59 scintigraphy with adrenal suppression is the best initial imaging procedure and averages 85% sensitivity and 90% specificity. In the rare case in which scintigraphy is equivocal or nondiagnostic, CT and MRI should be performed.

7. In cases of chemically confirmed pheochromocytoma, scintigraphy with MIBG *always* should be performed for localization before surgery and to identify the 10% of tumors which may be bilateral or extraadrenal. Although CT and MRI are usually also performed in cases of pheochromocytoma, their value in management is doubtful, especially in extraadrenal tumors. There is virtually no place for invasive studies in the localization of pheochromocytoma. Adrenal venography, arteriography, and venous sampling are useless and dangerous.

8. In cases of chemically confirmed hypothalamic dysfunction, the incidence of sellar and juxta/sellar tumors is high, and CT or MRI is indicated.

REFERENCES

1. Dos Remedios LV, Weber PM, Feldman R, Schurr DA, Tsoi TG. Detecting unsuspected thyroid dysfunction by the free thyroxine index. Arch Intern Med 1980;140(8):1045–1049.
2. Nolan JP, Tarsa NJ, DiBenedetto G. Case-finding for unsuspected thyroid disease; costs and health benefits. Am J Clin Pathol 1985;83(3):346–355.
3. Aurbach GD, Marx SJ, Spiegel AM. Parathyroid hormone, calcitonin, and the calciferols. In: Williams RH, ed. Textbook of Endocrinology. 6th ed. Philadelphia: W. B. Saunders Company, 1981.
4. Heath III H, Hodgson SF, Kennedy MA. Primary hyperparathyroidism. Incidence, morbidity, and potential economic impact in a community. N Engl J Med 1980;302(4):189–193.
5. U.S. Department of Health and Human Services, U.S. Public Health Service, Centers for Disease Control, and the National Center for Health Statistics. National Hospital Discharge Survey (NHDS). Detailed diagnoses, procedures, days of care, diagnoses related groups for patients discharged from short-stay hospitals. Public Use Data Diskettes, 1985–1990.
6. Krubsack AJ, Wilson SD, Lawson TL, Collier BD, Hellman RS, Isitman AT. Prospective comparison of radionuclide, computed tomographic and sonographic localization of parathyroid tumors. World J Surg 1986;10(4):579–585.

7. Beierwaltes WH, Lieberman LM, Ansari AN, Nishiyama H. Visualization of human adrenal glands *in vivo* by scintillation scanning. JAMA 1971;216(2):275–277.

8. Blair RJ, Beierwaltes WH, Lieberman LM, et al. Radiolabelled cholesterol as an adrenal scanning agent. J Nucl Med 1971;12:176–182.

9. Sarkar SD, Cohen EL, Beierwaltes WH, Ice RD, Cooper R, Gold EN. A new and superior adrenal imaging agent 131I-6-beta-iodomethyl-19-norcholesterol (NP-59). Evaluation in humans. J Clin Endocrinol Metab 1977;45(2):353–362.

10. Wieland DM, Wu J, Brown LE. Radiolabeled adrenergic neuron blocking agents: adrenomedullary imaging with [131I]iodobenzyl-guanidine. J Nucl Med 1980;21(4):349–353.

11. Shapiro B, Copp JE, Sisson JC, Eyre PL, Wallis J, Beierwaltes WH. Iodine-131 metaiodobenzylguanidine for the locating of suspected pheochromocytoma; experience in 400 cases. J Nucl Med 1985;26(6):576–585.

12. Fig LM, Gross MD, Shapiro B, et al. Adrenal localization in the adrenocorticotropic hormone-independent Cushing syndrome. Ann Intern Med 1988;109(7):547–553.

13. Freitas JE, Beierwaltes WH, Nishiyama RH. Adrenal hyperandrogenism: detection by adrenal scintigraphy. J Endocrinol Invest 1978;1(1):59–64.

14. Carpenter PC, Wahner HW, Salassa RM, Duick DS. Demonstration of steroid-producing gonadal tumors by external scanning with the use of NP-59. Mayo Clin Proc 1979;54(5):332–334.

15. Beierwaltes WH, Sturman MF, Ryo UY, Ice RD. Imaging functional nodules of the adrenal glands with 131-I-19-iodocholesterol. J Nucl Med 1974;15(4):246–251.

16. Charbonnel B, Chatal JF, Ozanne P. Does the corticoadrenal adenoma with "pre-Cushing's syndrome" exist? J Nucl Med 1981;22(12):1059–1061.

17. Freitas JE, Herwig KR, Cerny JC. Preoperative localization of adrenal remnants. Surg Gynecol Obstet 1977;145(5):705–708.

18. Lund JO, Nielsen MD, Giese J. Prevalence of primary aldosteronism. Acta Med Scand 1981;646:54–57.

19. Streeten DHP, Tomycz N, Anderson Jr GH. Reliability of screening methods for the diagnosis of primary aldsoteronism. Am J Med 1979;67(3):403–413.

20. Gross MD, Thrall JH, Beierwaltes WH. The adrenal scan: a current status report on radiotracers, dosimetry, and clinical utility. In: Freeman LM, Weissman HS, eds. Nuclear Medicine Annual. New York: Raven Press, 1980:127–175.

21. Thrall JH, Freitas JE, Beierwaltes WH. Adrenal Scintigraphy. Semin Nucl Med 1978;VIII91:23–41.

22. Seabold JE, Cohen EL, Beierwaltes WH, et al. Adrenal imaging with 131I-19-iodocholesterol in the diagnostic evaluation of patients with aldosteronism. J Clin Endocrinol Metab 1976;42(1):41–51.

23. Rifai A, Beierwaltes WH, Freitas JE. Adrenal scintigraphy in low renin essential hypertension. Clin Nucl Med 1978;3(7):282–286.

24. Beard CM, Sheps SG, Kurland LT, Carney JA, Lie JT. Occurrence of pheochromocytoma in Rochester, Minnesota, 1950 through 1979. Mayo Clin Proc 1983;58(12):802–804.

25. Manger WM, Gifford RW. Pheochromocytoma. New York: Springer-Verlag, 1972:31–37.

26. Gross MD, Shapiro B. Scintigraphic studies in adrenal hypertension. Semin Nucl Med 1989;19(2):122–143.

27. Sturman MF, Moses DC, Beierwaltes WH, Harrison TS, Ice RD, Dorr RP. Radiocholesterol adrenal images for the localization of pheochromocytoma. Surg Gynecol Obstet 1974;138(2):177–180.

28. Velchik MG, Alavi A, Kressel HY, Engelman K. Localization of pheochromocytoma: MIGB, CT, and MRI correlation. J Nucl Med 1989;30(3):328–336.

29. Sisson JC, Shapiro B. Metaiodobenzylguanidine for cardiac and tumor imaging. Current Opin Radiol 1989;194:485–491.

30. Osborne AG. MRI of the sellar/juxtasellar region. Part 1: Intrasellar and suprasellar masses. MRI Decis 1990;4(6):19–30.

31. Van Woert MH. Introduction. In: Cooperative Approaches to Research and Development of Orphan Drugs. New York: Alan R. Liss, Inc., 1985:3–6.

32. Stucki JC. The development of orphan drugs — a pharmaceutical company perspective. In: Cooperative Approaches to Research and Development of Orphan Drugs. New York: Alan R. Liss, 1985:95–104.

33. Crooks GM. The orphan products board of the Department of Health and Human Services. In: Cooperative Approaches to Research and Development of Orphan Drugs. New York: Alan R. Liss, 1985:19–23.

34. Orphan products development. Food and Drug Administration. U.S. Department of Health and Human Services, 1990.

8

Further Imaging Strategy Given an Abnormal Imaging Study

I smoked a cigarette the same day I experienced my first kiss. I never smoked a cigarette again.

Arturo Toscannini

1/ Lung: The Solitary Pulmonary Mass

Few incidental findings cause so much anxiety and potential mischief as the unexpected mass found on an imaging study. Single lung masses are discovered fortuitously once or twice in 1000 chest radiographs and are among the most common radiological findings in asymptomatic individuals (1). Seventy-five percent of these "spots" are found incidentally, the rest, usually more ominous, are discovered because of symptoms such as cough or hemoptysis (2). Most of these lung masses, first described as a "coin lesion" by Thornton et al. in 1944 (3), are in fact not malignant, but the approach to their management to this day continues to provoke controversy. The generally accepted term for a single lung mass is *solitary pulmonary nodule* (SPN), which is defined as a single, relatively well-circumscribed, rounded, or oval density surrounded by aerated lung (4). There is disagreement as to whether this definition should include masses larger than 4–6 cm or ones invading the chest wall or mediastinum, but we will follow Godwin's definition (4), which includes lesions of any size so long as a mass lesion is identifiable, and even when other disease is present in the lungs.

One of the largest collection of patients before the advent of CT was compiled by Bateson (5) in a meta-analysis of more than 3400 cases from 33 papers published between 1944 and 1960, the results of which are listed in Table 8.1.1. Bateson's own series of 155 cases is summarized in Tables 8.1.2 and 8.1.3, showing the age distribution in his patients and confirming the significant correlation of malignancy with increasing age. Toomes et al. (2) also have listed the histological findings in 955 resected coin lesions shown in Table 8.1.4, in which etiologies were equally divided between benign and malignant. These and other series of resected lesions report cancer frequencies ranging from 10–50% (6, 7), suggesting that far too many patients with benign disease are subjected to unnecessary thoracotomy. This may be attributable to poor selection criteria, a form of diagnostic failure, but more likely reflecting the fear of missing malignancy, first expressed by Clavell in 1911. "When in doubt, cut it out." This philosophy has been echoed by many writers over the past 5 decades, despite the fact that the overwhelming majority of SPNs in younger patients are benign, particularly in nonsmokers.

Table 8.1.1. Meta Analysis of 3478 Cases of Solitary Pulmonary Nodules, with Corrections for Percentage of Total Lesions, Rounded Off

Etiology	Percentage of cases
Primary carcinomas	31
Nontuberculous granulomas	31
Tuberculous granulomas	15
Other lesions	8
Solitary metastases	5
Mixed tumors	5
Cysts	3
Adenomas	2
Total	100

Adapted with permission from Bateson (5).

Table 8.1.2. Etiology of the 155 Solitary Lung Lesions

Nature of the lesion	No. of lesions	Nature of the lesion	No. of lesions
Malignant tumors	95 (61.3%)	Benign tumors	40 (25.6%)
Primary carcinomas	80 (51.6%)	Mixed tumours	23 (14.8%)
Solitary metastases	15 (9.7%)	Fibromas	3
		Neurogenic tumors	3
Inflammatory lesions	20 (12.9%)	Bronchial adenomas	3
Tuberculous lesions	15 (9.7%)	Parapericardial lipomas	1
Massive fibrosis	2	Benign lymphoma	1
Pyogenic abscess	1	Arterio-venous malformation	1
Granulation tissue	1	Bronchial cysts	4
Dilated bronchus	1	Unclassified	1

Reprinted by permission from Bateson (5).

This is further confirmed by Steele's VA series (6), a cooperative study of resected asymptomatic SPNs in males from 78 institutions demonstrating the single most important epidemiological fact about lung cancers, namely their increasing preponderance with age. In other quoted series, including Bateson's (5), the incidence of cancer in resected SPNs in patients under age 35 is also about 5%, rising to 50% or more in patients over age 60. This agrees closely with the NHDS hospital statistics (8), indicating that less than 4% of patients with a diagnosis of carcinoma of the lung or bronchus in the NHDS survey for 1990 were under 44 years of age. The cumulative yearly incidence of lung cancer by age and sex is indicated in Figure 8.1.1 (9).

Further statistical analysis is needed to help formulate a reasonable clinical approach to the single pulmonary nodule, because unnecessary procedures such as bronchoscopy, lung biopsy, and thoracotomies can be largely avoided in the low tumor suspect. There were 351,000 diagnostic procedures on the lung and bronchus in the United States in 1988, mostly bronchoscopies and open and closed biopsies (8). This is a large number, more than double the total estimated cases of bronchogenic carcinoma for the United States and more than six times the total number of operations performed on the lung and bronchus the same year.

The American Cancer Society estimated that in 1991 there will be 161,000 new cases and 143,000 deaths due to lung cancer in this country, making it the number-one cause of cancer deaths in both sexes, not only in this country but throughout the world (10). In starker terms this translates into the prediction that 89% of individuals *having*

Table 8.1.3. Clinical Features of the 155 Solitary Lung Lesions

Age and Sex Incidence	Primary carcinoma	Solitary metastasis	Tuberculous lesions	Non-tuberculous inflammatory lesion	Mixed tumors	Other benign tumors
Male	79	11	15	4	16	7
Female	1	4	0	1	7	10
0–9 years	0	0	0	0	0	1
10–19 years	0	0	1	0	0	1
20–29 years	0	0	1	0	2	1
30–39 years	3	2	4	0	3	2
40–49 years	10	1	4	1	5	3
50–59 years	35	5	3	2	12	5
60–69 years	27	5	2	2	0	3
70–79 years	5	2	0	0	1	1
Over 40 years	77	13	9	5	18	12
Percentage over 40 years	96.3	86.7	60.0	100	78.3	70.5
No. of patients without symptoms	32	7	8	2	16	11
No. of patients with symptoms due to the lesion	43	8	5	2	6	4
(No clinical details available)	5	0	2	1	1	2
Percentage without symptoms	42.6	46.7	61.5	50	72.7	73.7
No. with hemoptysis	20	3	1	0	3	1
No. with cough and sputum	27	6	4	1	3	3
No. with chest pain	15	2	1	1	4	1
No. with weight loss	11	1	1	0	3	1
No. with dyspnea	11	4	3	1	4	1
No. with finger clubbing	6	0	1	0	2	1
Blood sedimentation rate						
Normal	1	0	4	2	3	2
Raised	17	2	0	0	1	2
Bronchoscopic examination						
Negative result	55	7	10	2	14	11
Positive biopsy	2	0	0	0	0	0
Malignant cells found in the bronchial washings	5	1	0	0	0	0

Reprinted by permission from Bateson (5).

Table 8.1.4. Classification of 955 Coin Lesions as Malignant or Benign

Malignant lesions		479 = 49%
Bronchogenic carcinoma	364 = 38.1%	
Metastases	89 = 9.2%	
Others	16 = 1.8%	
Benign lesions		486 = 51%
Benign tumors	132 = 13.8%	
Tuberculosis	225 = 23.6%	
Others	129 = 13.5%	

Reprinted by permission from *Cancer* (1983;51:533).

lung cancer will die of it within the year. The actual mean (50%) survival rate supplied by the Epidemiology Branch of the National Cancer Institute is less than 8 months. This malignancy has now surpassed breast cancer in women, which for 50 years has been the major cancer killer in females. By far the most important risk factor for lung cancer, other than age, is tobacco use. More than 80% of all cases occur in smokers (9), and the incidence rates are 10 time higher in smokers than nonsmokers. Because only

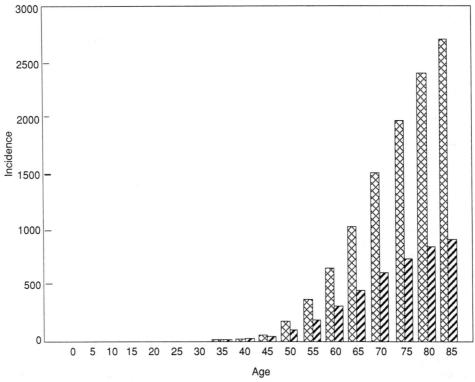

Figure 8.1.1. Incidence of lung cancer in men and women by age. Reprinted by permission from Ref. 9.

about one-third of the population are tobacco users, the incidence of lung cancer in nonsmokers is approximately 25% of that shown in Figure 8.1.1. Only 13% of unselected patients with lung cancer live longer than 5 years. Those patients detected in a localized stage belong to a subset representing only one-fourth of all cases discovered. Even in this most favourable group, however, the 5-year survival is only about 33% (11). Both the mortality and incidence rates for lung cancer in both sexes have continued to rise since 1973 despite the introduction of new therapies (12). This means we are *losing* the battle against lung cancer, i.e. prevalence is rising without any improvement in survival. We emphasize these depressing facts in the spirit of *primum non nocere* (first, do no harm), to bring some sense of perspective toward diagnostic and therapeutic approaches to this appalling malignancy.

Imaging Methods for Assessing the Solitary Nodule
RADIOGRAPHY

> *Two out of every three deaths are premature; they are related to loafer's heart, smoker's lung and drinker's liver.*
>
> *Thomas J. Bassler, M.D.*
> *Pathologist*

Plain chest radiography can reliably exclude lung cancer in an SPN on the basis of two radiographic features: calcification of the nodule in a characteristic benign pat-

Table 8.1.5. Significance of Radiographic Appearance of Solitary Pulmonary Nodule

Radiographic pattern		Favors benign disease	Favors malignant disease
Size	≤2 cm	+	
	≥4 cm		+ +
Margins	Sharp	+	
	Hazy or indistinct		+ +
Contour	Smooth	+	
	Lobulated or irregular		+
Presence of satellite lesions		+ + +	
Presence of cavitation		−	−

Reprinted by permission from Branch WT, ed. *Office Practice of Medicine*. 2nd ed. Philadelphia: W. B. Saunders Co. (1987:355).

tern and failure of the nodule to increase significantly in size over an extended period of time (11).

Calcification

Calcium is almost never present in lung cancers in amounts sufficient to be visualized by conventional radiography. Thus, diffusely calcified nodules, "target" lesions, and peripheral ring-shaped, laminated, or clump-like lesions described as "popcorn ball" calcifications are virtually always benign granulomas or hamartomas, a fact confirmed by enormous clinical experience over the past several decades. Eccentric or fine stippled calcification, however, cannot be relied on to exclude cancer. Special techniques can be used to highlight calcification, such as low kilovoltage, tomography, spot films, and the like. The best technique for screening patients over age 40 is probably the stereoscopic posteroanterior *and lateral* study, because up to 10% of SPNs are seen only on the lateral view (13).

Radiographic Stability

Lung cancers have a relatively constant exponential growth rate exhibited as a volume doubling time almost always less than 460 days (14). Translated into planar measurements, this means a lesion failing to increase in diameter by more than 26% in less than 15–16 months is almost invariably benign. At the other extreme, a nodule that doubles its volume in less than 10 days is usually benign, such as a "round" pneumonia or pulmonary infarct. This is rare, however. A conservative rule of thumb is: if a solitary pulmonary nodule has been present and stable in size on conventional radiographs for 18 months to 2 years or more, it can be presumed to be benign (15). Sometimes, the decision to watch and wait is a deliberate strategy in the presence of a lesion with a low probability of cancer; sometimes the decision already has been made, for example, in the patient with a "new" SPN, which ultimately proves in retrospect to have been present on a previous radiograph. About two-thirds of all solitary nodules will be accurately diagnosed as benign by this method.

Additional predictive features of the radiograph of a single pulmonary nodule include initial size, margins, contour, etc., and are indicated in Table 8.1.5 (11). These features, however, unlike growth rate and calcifications, are said to be only 75% accurate in predicting a benign etiology (16). Size, in particular, always has been thought to correlate with increased likelihood of malignancy, but the rule is violated at least for small lesions, less than 2 cm. Larger size, however, is a more reliable predictor.

The management of SPNs can be greatly improved by analyzing clinical and radiological findings mathematically using decision analysis and Bayes' theorem, techniques previously mentioned (17). In particular, using Bayes' theorem combining age, sex, smoking history, and other clinical information with radiographic findings, we can enormously amplify our ability to estimate the likelihood of cancer in a solitary pulmonary nodule.

CT

After plain radiography, CT retains its primacy in the diagnosis and management of solitary pulmonary nodules. Because CT is considerably more sensitive than radiography in detection of calcification, it *always* should be used when the presence of calcification by plain radiographic techniques is indeterminate (11). As with radiography, for the lesion to be considered benign on CT, calcification must be present in one of the three above-mentioned patterns: central, diffuse (solid), or laminar. Particular caution is urged in the patient with a known primary extrathoracic tumor, because metastatic cancer to the lung may in fact show calcification (osteogenic Ca) (15). Four to five percent of SPNs detected with conventional radiographs in patients with no known evidence of malignant disease eventually turn out to be metastatic foci (18). On the other hand, SPNs in patients with known cancer do not always represent metastatic disease. Among 707 such patients undergoing thoracotomy at Memorial Hospital between 1940 and 1975, 500 proved to have primary lung cancers, 196 were solitary metastases, and 11 were benign lesions (19). Overall, in 50–70% of patients with SPNs and histories of an extrathoracic primary lesion, the SPN represents a metastasis from the primary lesion (20). Parenthetically, because the 5-year survival rate in individuals with excised pulmonary metastatic lesions is 20–30%, resection may be indicated only in selected patients.

GALLIUM-67 SCINTIGRAPHY

Radiogallium is not taken up by the normal lung, but an average of 85% of lung cancers take up the radionuclide, though this is size related, the smaller tumors taking up radionuclide much less frequently (21). The PPV of an abnormal gallium-67 study for primary lung cancer is probably greater than 90%, though a negative gallium scintiscan predicts the *absence* of cancer in an SPN with considerably less reliability. Gallium scintigraphy has been reported to be more sensitive than mediastinal CT and chest roentgenography in assessing mediastinal metastases from a variety of lung cancers, especially squamous tumors (22).

MRI

In its present state of development, MRI is inferior to CT in the chest and should not be relied on. Spritzer et al. (23) state categorically, "Currently, MRI has little application in the assessment of pulmonary nodules, bronchogenic cancer, and diffuse parenchymal disease." However, the authors admit in certain settings MRI images may assist in tumor staging, because "... it may more clearly show tumor extension into the axilla, brachial plexus, and spinal canal in patients with superior sulcus neoplasms." The only other application for MRI at present would seem to be its use in assessing the hilum and mediastinum of patients who cannot receive contrast.

DIRECT DIAGNOSTIC PROCEDURES

Sputum cytology is of great value, but biopsy is the most reliable direct method, short of thoracotomy, of establishing the presence of malignancy. Biopsy usually is performed at bronchoscopy, mediastinoscopy, occasionally of scalene nodes, or as direct percutaneous needle aspiration biopsy of localized pulmonary lesions.

Bronchoscopy

In this country, bronchoscopy is almost invariably performed as a kind of diagnostic reflex in patients presenting with solitary pulmonary nodules. The value of flexible fiberoptic bronchoscopy with forceps and brush biopsy depends entirely on the size and location of the lesion. In nodules that are 2 cm or larger or ones that are contiguous with a visualized bronchus, the biopsy via bronchoscopy should be attempted initially (11). But the positive yield of bronchoscopic biopsy is less than 10% for malignant nodules 1–1.5 cm in diameter and only 20–27% for lesions smaller than 2 cm, central or peripheral (24, 25). In Bateson's series of 155 solitary malignancy lung tumors (5), only 8 of 107 bronchoscopic examinations were positive.

Biopsy of the Solitary Pulmonary Nodule

Transthoracic needle aspiration biopsy, when feasible as in peripheral and some more central lesions, is the most direct method of diagnosing lung cancer. The procedure must be properly performed, often with up to three attempts, and the results, as with any procedure, are dependent on the skill and experience of the operator. One group claimed a specificity of 95% in 486 malignant and 88% in 137 benign lesions (26, 27). The procedure is not without risk, because complications occur in a significant number of patients, and fatalities have been reported. Hemoptysis is common, and pneumothorax occurs in up to one-third of patients. One-third of these patients may require chest tubes (11, 27).

Staging of Lung Cancer: Invasive and Noninvasive Approaches

Because the only possible cure for lung cancer remains excision of the malignancy, the rationale for staging is to identify that subset of patients with resectable tumors. Unfortunately, more than 70% of all cases have metastases to regional nodes at the time of diagnosis (28). Moreover, extrathoracic metastases occur in another 20% of patients (29, 30). Thus, judging by these figures and the appalling 5-year survival rate, which has not changed over the last several decades, *it is likely that 85–90% of all patients with lung cancer are inoperable at the time of diagnosis.*

CT and CT/Mediastinoscopy

CT remains the principal noninvasive method for demonstrating spread of lung cancer to the hilar or mediastinal nodes, but it is far from ideal. The overall results are variable in different series and with different tumor types. For example, one authority states that the sensitivity of CT in predicting the absence of metastatic disease "is unacceptably low" (31), no doubt because of inability of any imaging modality other than microscopy to detect tumors in nodes that are not yet enlarged. Other authors question whether CT has any utility in assessing mediastinal lymph node involvement in nonsmall cell bronchogenic carcinoma (32). Some writers, however, claim a 70% sensitivity and 88% specificity for CT (33). One of the most disturbing reports is an important series (34) in which 25% of patients who had bronchogenic carcinoma but *no evidence of hilar or mediastinal adenopathy* on CT proved to have *extrathoracic metastases*. The brain was the most common site, followed by bone, liver, and adrenal glands.

Many writers feel that mediastinoscopy is the most reliable method to assess mediastinal node status in lung cancer patients, with other claiming a false-negative rate of 10% (35). Mediastinoscopy, like lung biopsy, is an invasive procedure with certain limitations, because it requires general anesthesia and has a finite morbidity and mortality rate, probably exceeding that of fine-needle lung biopsy. However, new techniques promise to enormously improve the safety and efficacy of lung biopsy. One of these methods is described by the Mayo group (36), which used thoracolaparoscopy in managing a patient with an SPN.

Gallium-67 Scintigraphy

Despite its proven value in detecting mediastinal and distant spread, gallium scintigraphy remains underused in the assessment of lung cancer operability. This is largely because of wide disparities reported in various studies. Many of these discordant findings can be blamed on the lack of scintigraphic standardization, for example, in failure to use an adequate dose of gallium-67 in earlier studies, and in the use of different diagnostic criteria for mediastinal involvement. As a result, in the detection of regional spread, several groups report a high sensitivity (21, 37, 38), others a high specificity (39), and still others poor overall accuracy (40). Several investigators have emphasized the improved detection of lesions with gallium SPECT imaging (a radionuclide technique described in Chapter 3). Alazraki et al. (37, 38) have even proposed that patients whose primary tumor displays gallium-67 uptake but who have no abnormal uptake in the hila and mediastinum should be spared mediastinoscopy and go directly to thoracotomy. Others stress the extremely high likelihood of metastatic disease with positive gallium-67 uptake in the mediastinum (39).

If the primary lung tumor takes up gallium-67, there is a better than 90% chance that an extrathoracic focus of gallium uptake represents a metastasis (39). Adrenal, liver, and brain secondaries often can be detected by this method. Most important, gallium scintigraphy is noninvasive, with no mortality or morbidity. *It should be used routinely to assess the operability of lung cancer*. Nevertheless, it must be admitted that neither gallium nor CT will detect microscopic tumors in involved nodes.

Summary
DIAGNOSTIC INDICATORS FOR OR AGAINST MALIGNANCY IN PATIENTS PRESENTING WITH A SOLITARY OR MULTIPLE PULMONARY NODULES

Age.   Lung cancer is rare in younger age groups with less than 4% of all lung cancers occurring in patients under age 45. If a solitary nodule is found in a patient under age 35, there is only 5% chance it is cancer, over age 60, better than 50% chance of cancer.

Smoking.   More than 80% of all lung cancers occur in smokers. A smoker with a solitary pulmonary nodule has more than four times the likelihood of cancer than a nonsmoker. In an older smoker with an SPN, the likelihood of cancer may exceed 90%.

Lesion Size.   Smaller SPNs, those less than 1.5–2 cm, are not highly correlated with the presence of malignancy, but lesions larger than 3 cm very likely represent cancer.

Calcification.   If calcium is present in an SPN in a characteristic benign pattern on the plain chest radiography, a benign lesion is present, and cancer is almost completely excluded.

Radiological Stability.   If the lesion does not increase in diameter by more than 26% in 18–24 months, that lesion is benign. This means, however, that an SPN only 1 cm in diameter increasing by 2.6 mm would have to be regarded with suspicion. Rare lesions increasing in size in *less than 10 days* are also benign.

Multiple Nodules.   Multiple noncalcified nodules on CT or the plain radiograph always raise the high likelihood of metastases. Multiple calcified nodules indicate granulomatous disease.

DIAGNOSTIC APPROACH TO THE SOLITARY PULMONARY NODULE DISCOVERED ON THE PLAIN RADIOGRAPH

1. If an SPN has a characteristic type of calcification—popcorn, central, solid, and diffuse or laminar, the diagnosis is a benign lesion, and further diagnostic imaging or invasive studies should not be performed. The most common benign lesions are hamartoma, calcified granuloma, and sometimes an arteriovenous malformation where feeding vessels are usually demonstrable.

2. When previous radiographs are available for comparison and no significant change in size can be demonstrated over an 18-month period, the lesion can be regarded as benign, and again, no further studies need be performed.

3. All patients with SPNs without calcification or with equivocal calcification on the plain chest radiographs should have CT. If characteristic calcification is found and benignity is established, no further studies should be performed.

All other patients can be divided into two categories: *high* (more than 10%) and *low* (less than 10%) pretest probability of cancer.

LOW PRIOR PROBABILITY OF CANCER

If probability is less than 10%, based on young age, lack of significant smoking history, size of lesion, and CT findings:

1. Perform Gallium scintigraphy. If this study is negative, i.e. no uptake in the lesion, the likelihood of cancer is reduced to 3–4%, and a watch-and-wait strategy is the best course.

2. If there is gallium-67 uptake in an SPN, the likelihood of cancer rises to more than 75%, and biopsy should be performed.

HIGH PRIOR PROBABILITY OF CANCER

1. In any SPN, whether or not CT shows mediastinal involvement, biopsy confirmation of malignancy should be obtained. This can be attempted first with sputum cytology. In the event the lesion is central and larger than 1.5–2 cm in size or contiguous with a visualized bronchus, bronchoscopy should be performed; otherwise bronchoscopy is of virtually no value.

2. In the case of smaller lesions, particularly peripheral lesions, percutaneous transthoracic needle aspiration may be performed first, recognizing the small but finite risks of the procedure.

3. If mediastinal involvement is seen on CT, and bronchoscopic biopsy fails to prove the presence of malignancy, the choice lies between mediastinoscopy with nodal biopsy and direct percutaneous needle biopsy.

4. Because small cell lung cancer is now almost never treated surgically, the precise microscopic diagnosis has significant implications for therapy and must be obtained in all patients.

THE DECISION FOR THORACOTOMY IN PATIENTS WITH DIAGNOSED LUNG CARCINOMA: SUMMARY OF DIAGNOSTIC APPROACH TO STAGING

Between 80–90% of lung cancer patients have metastatic disease at the time of diagnosis. Because surgery is not only fruitless, but life threatening, these patients must be considered inoperable, and every effort should be made to exclude the presence of regional or distant cancer spread before considering thoracotomy. Even if CT is negative for regional adenopathy, the possibility of macro- or microscopic mediastinal or hilar involvement is still 20–35% (28). Furthermore, asymptomatic distant tumor spread to the brain, bone, liver, adrenals, or soft tissue may be seen in another 25% of patients. The following routine studies are therefore *strongly advised before* attempting surgical resection of any biopsy-proven or suspected lung cancer:

1. 67-Gallium-67 scintigraphy should be done to exclude mediastinal involvement in CT-negative patients and simultaneously to exclude distant spread to brain, bone, adrenal, etc. If significant gallium uptake is seen in the lesion and also in the mediastinum or peripherally, the uptake can be assumed to be in metastatic foci.

2. If the gallium study is completely negative, the absence of metastatic disease cannot be assumed. All such patients should undergo brain and upper abdominal CT to include liver, kidneys, and adrenal.

3. In the event of an adrenal mass larger than 3–4 cm detected on CT, NP-59 scintiscanning should be done, because a large percentage of adrenal masses are incidentalomas and not metastases (vide infra).

4. Only in the event that all the above are negative for metastatic disease, and there are no medical contraindications, should exploratory thoracotomy be done in the hope of performing curative resection.

REFERENCES

1. Good CA, Wilson TW. The solitary circumscribed pulmonary nodule. Study of seven hundred five cases encountered roentgenologically in a period of three and one-half years. JAMA 1958;166:210–215.
2. Toomes H, Delphendahl A, Manke HG, Vogt-Moykopf I. The coin lesion of the lung: a review of 955 resected coin lesions. Cancer 1983;51(3):534–537.
3. Thornton Jr TF, Adams WE, Bloch RG. Surg Gynecol Obstet 1944;78:364.
4. Godwin JD. The solitary pulmonary nodule. Radiol Clin North Am 1983;21(4):709–721.
5. Bateson EM. An analysis of 155 solitary lung lesions illustrating the differential diagnosis of mixed tumours of the lung. Clin Radiol 1965;16:51–65.
6. Steele JD. The solitary pulmonary nodule: report of a cooperative study of resected asymptomatic solitary pulmonary nodules in males. J Thorac Cardiovasc Surg 1963;46:21–39.
7. Ray III JF, Lawton BR, Magnim GE, et al. The coin lesion story: update 1976. Chest 1976;70(3):332–336.
8. U.S. Department of Health and Human Services, U.S. Public Health Service, Centers for Disease Control, and the National Center for Health Statistics. National Hospital Discharge Survey (NHDS). Detailed diagnoses, procedures, days of care, diagnoses-related groups for patients discharged from short-stay hospitals. Public Use Data Diskettes, 1985–1990.
9. Eddy DM. Screening for lung cancer. Ann Intern Med 1989;111(3):232–237.

10. Boring CC, Squires TS, Tong T. Cancer statistics, 1991. CA 1991;41(1):19–36.
11. Fanta CH. Solitary pulmonary nodule. In: Branch WT. Office Practice of Medicine. 2nd ed. Philadelphia: W.B. Saunders Co., 1987:354.
12. Cancer incidence and mortality in the United States. SEER. 1973–1981. U.S. Department of Health and Human Service, U.S. Public Health Service, National Institutes of Health.
13. Swensen SJ, Jett JR, Payne WS, Viggiano RW, Pairolero PC, Trastek VF. An integrated approach to evaluation of the solitary pulmonary nodule. Mayo Clin Proc 1990;65(2):173–186.
14. Nathan MH, Collins VP, Adams RA. Differentiation of benign and malignant pulmonary nodules by growth rate. Radiology 1962;79:221.
15. Zerhouni EA, Stitik FP, Siegelman SS, et al. Computed tomography of the pulmonary nodule: a cooperative study. Radiology 1986;160(2):319–327.
16. Templeton AW, Jansen C, Lehr JL, Huff TR. Solitary pulmonary lesions. Computer-aided differential diagnosis and evaluation of mathematical methods. Radiology 1967;89(4):605–613.
17. Cummings SR, Lillington GA, Richard RJ. Estimating the probability of malignancy in solitary pulmonary nodules: a Bayesian approach. Am Rev Respir Dis 1986;134(3):449–445.
18. Coppage L, Shaw C, Curtis AM. Metastatic disease to the chest in patients with extrathoracic malignancy. J Thorac Imaging 1987;2(4):24–37.
19. Cahan WG, Shah JP, Castro EB. Benign solitary lung lesions in patients with cancer. Ann Surg 1978;187(3):241–244.
20. Neifeld JP, Michaelis LL, Doppman JL. Suspected pulmonary metastases: correlation of chest x-ray, whole lung tomograms, and operative findings. Cancer 1977;39(2):383–387.
21. Hayes RL, Edwards C. New applications of tumor-localizing radiopharmaceuticals, In: Medical Radioisotope Scintigraphy. Vienna: IAEA, 1973;II:531–552.
22. Fosburg RG, Hopkins GB, Kan MK. Evaluation of the mediastinum by gallium-67 scintigraphy in lung cancer. J Thorac Cardiovasc Surg 1979;77(1):76–82.
23. Spritzer C, Gamsu G, Sostman HD. Magnetic resonance imaging of the thorax: techniques, current applications, and future directions. J Thorac Imaging 1989;4(2):1–18.
24. Cortese DA, McDougall JC. Biopsy and brushing of peripheral lung cancer with fluoroscopic guidance. Chest 1979;75(2):141–145.
25. Stringfield JT, Markowitz DJ, Bentz RR, Welch MH, Weg JG. The effect of tumor size and location on diagnosis by fiberoptic bronchoscopy. Chest 1977;72(4):474–476.
26. Khouri NF, Meziane MA, Zerhouni EA, Fishman EK, Siegelman SS. The solitary pulmonary nodule: assessment, diagnosis, and management. Chest 1987;91(1):128–133.
27. Khouri NF, Stitik FP, Erozan YS, et al. Transthoracic needle aspiration biopsy of benign and malignant lung lesions. AJR 1985;144(2):281–288.
28. Swensen SJ, Brown LR. Conventional radiography of the hilum and mediastinum in bronchogenic carcinoma. Radiol Clin North Am 1990;28(3):521–538.
29. Hirleman MT, Yiu-Chiu VS, Chiu LC, Shapiro RL. The resectability of primary lung carcinoma: a diagnostic staging review. J Comput Tomogr 1980;4(2):146–163.
30. Matthews MJ, Kanhouwa S, Pickren J. Frequency of residual and metastatic tumor in patients undergoing curative resection for lung cancer. Cancer Chemother Rep 1973;4:83.
31. Aronchick JM. CT of mediastinal lymph nodes in patients with non-small cell lung carcinoma. Radiol Clin North Am 1990;28(3):573–581.
32. McKenna RJ, Libshitz HI, Mountain CF. Roentgenographic evaluation of mediastinal nodes for preoperative assessment in lung cancer. Chest 1985;88:206.
33. Patterson GA, Ginsberg RJ, Poon PY, et al. A prospective evaluation of magnetic resonance imaging, computed tomography, and mediastinoscopy in the preoperative assessment of mediastinal node status in bronchogenic carcinoma. J Thorac Cardiovasc Surg 1987;94:679–684.
34. Sider L, Horejs D. Frequency of extrathoracic metastases from bronchogenic carcinoma in patients with normal-sized hilar and mediastinal lymph nodes on CT. AJR 1988;151(5):893–895.
35. Goldberg EM. Mediastinoscopy in assessment of lung cancer. In: Strauss MJ, ed. Lung Cancer—Clinical Diagnosis and Treatment. New York: Grune and Stratton, 1977:113.
36. Miller DL, Allen MS, Deschamps C, Trastek VF, Pairolero PC. Video-assisted thoracic surgical procedure: management of a solitary pulmonary nodule. Mayo Clin Proc, 1992;67:462–464.
37. Alazraki NP. Usefulness of gallium imaging in the evaluation of lung cancer. CRC Crit Rev Diagn Imaging 1980;13:249.
38. Alazraki NP, Ramsdell JW, Taylor A, Fraiedman PJ, Peters RM, Tisi GM. Reliability of gallium scan chest radiography compared with mediastinoscopy for evaluating mediastinal spread in lung cancer. Am Rev Respir Dis 1978;117(3):415–420.

39. DeMeeseeseester TR, Golomb HM, Kirchner P, et al. The role of gallium-67 scanning in the clinical staging and preoperative evaluation of patients with carcinoma of the lung. Ann Thorac Surg 1979; 28(5):451–464.
40. Neumann RD, Merino M, Hoffer PB. Gallium-67 in hilar and mediastinal staging of primary lung carcinomas. J Nucl Med 1980;21:32.

2/ Kidney: Renal Masses

> *To a physician, each man, each woman, is an amplification of one organ.*
>
> Ralph Waldo Emerson

We continue to pose the paramount and quintessential clinical question, the principal litany repeated throughout this book: given only a finding, what are the *principal and most likely* diagnoses, *in the order of their likelihood?* Table 8.2.1, adapted from Pollack et al. (1), gives the final diagnosis for 206 patients referred for renal mass lesions. Note that cysts represented 70%, pseudotumors (fetal lobulation and compensatory hypertrophy) 15%, and tumors only 6.5% of all such masses. This series was compiled in 1974, before ultrasonography was widely used in diagnosis, and it is likely the percentage of benign cysts would be even higher in an unselected series today if patients also included those in whom sonography was the only imaging study. Obviously, the percentage of patients with tumor would be much higher in those with other findings, e.g. hematuria. However, we are speaking now only of the patient with the finding of a renal mass lesion. A much more extensive survey is Lang's study of 940 space-occupying masses of the kidney (2), which again shows the overwhelming percentage of benign lesions given this finding and almost the identical percentage of malignancies (5.5%) (Table 8.2.2).

Renal Cysts

Simple renal cysts varying in size from a few millimeters to several centimeters are found in at least *half* of all patients over age 50 (3, 4). Benign cysts are less common in the younger age groups and extremely rare in children. Sometimes the cyst is solitary, but more often cysts are multiple and bilateral. They may occur anywhere in the kidney, including the parapelvic region, where they rarely may cause symptoms such as pain or hematuria associated with bleeding or localized obstruction. Other less common forms of cystic, noncancerous conditions include multiloculated or infected cysts and polycystic and multicystic renal disease. All of these conditions may present as a mass or multiple masses.

In view of the wide prevalence of benign renal cysts and the low prevalence of renal tumor, 16 per 100,000 hospital admissions in 1990 (5), it is not surprising that when pyelography is performed as a first imaging study for GU disease, masses distorting the collecting system are found in a significant percentage of patients. Renal masses incidentally discovered on IVP *almost always* prove on sonography, to be *simple benign cysts*.

Various sonographic criteria are used to distinguish the "pure" or simple from the "mixed" renal cyst, a strategy that is more than 95% accurate in the hands of a com-

Table 8.2.1.   Final Diagnosis in 206 Patients Referred for Renal Mass Lesions

Diagnosis	Number	Percentage
Cysts	141	70
Pseudotumors	32	15
Tumors	13	6.5
Hydronephrosis	6	
Polycystic kidneys	5	
Abscess	4	
Hematoma	4	
Perirenal pseudocyst	1	
Total	206	

Adapted from Pollack HM, Goldberg BB, Morales J, et al. A systematized approach to the differential diagnosis of renal masses. *Radiology* 1974;113:153. Reprinted by permission from Branch WT, ed. *Office Practice of Medicine.* Philadelphia: W. B. Saunders Co. (1987:497).

Table 8.2.2.   Underlying Pathological Conditions in 940 Asymptomatic Space-Occupying Lesions of the Kidney

Type of lesion	No. of lesions	% of total no. of lesions
Cystic lesions		58
Benign cysts	515	
Benign hemorrhagic cysts	4	
Hydronephrosis	8	
Cystic dysplastic kidney	3	
Polycystic kidney	17	
Malignant neoplasms		5.5
Hypernephromas	21	
Other malignant neoplasms	31	
Benign neoplasms	40	4.2
Inflammatory lesions (pyelonephritis, abscess)	213	23
Intrarenal hematoma	7	0.7
Pseudotumors	81	8.6

Modified from Lang EK. Diagnosis of renal and parenchymal tumors. In: Skinner DG, deKernion JB, eds. *Genitourinary Cancer.* Philadelphia: W. B. Saunders (1978:42).

petent sonographer. There remain, however, the multilocular or septated cyst, the hemorrhagic, the calcified, and the inflammatory cyst. In only about 5% of cases when the sonographer is uncertain that a pure cyst is present is it necessary to resort to CT. Sagel et al. (6) found CT to be virtually 100% accurate in distinguishing between renal cysts and neoplasm (6). Thus, the practice of performing diagnostic cyst puncture in every questionable case no longer can be condoned. The concept of a tumor arising in the wall of a cyst is a controversial one, and it seems more likely that cysts are simply adjacent to a de novo tumor or a tumor becomes incorporated into a preexisting cyst. Because cystic renal tumors are extremely rare, the large majority of these lesions will prove benign even in the rare case when cyst puncture with examination of the fluid is felt to be indicated. Of course, difficulties sometimes arise, for example, in tumors or abscesses with central necrosis mimicking cysts. Another problem is the occasional peri or parapelvic cyst, which cannot always be distin guished sonographically from hydronephrosis.

In practice, however, it is only necessary for the clinician to note that *all* true or pure asymptomatic renal cysts are *benign* and *need not be studied further unless there is obstruction or bleeding.* Only when the radiologist expresses some doubt is CT required for a cystic lesion.

Tumors of the Urinary Tract

Small benign renal adenomas, though reported to occur in 10–20% of all autopsies, are clinically unimportant and rarely diagnosed during life (7). Other less common benign tumors include angiomata, angiomyolipomas (hamartomas), and the extremely rare but interesting hemangiopericytoma, a renin-secreting tumor. None of the benign renal tumors are common clinically, and for all intents, *any noncystic renal mass should be considered malignant until proven otherwise.*

The most common renal tumor is the renal-cell adenocarcinoma or so-called hypernephroma, occurring almost exclusively in patients over age 20. Unfortunately, hematuria occur in only about 60% of cases. This is more often microscopic than gross. Clinical signs and symptoms in advanced cases include fatigability, weight loss, fever, and, in half the cases, anemia. The classic triad of gross hematuria, flank pain, and a palpable abdominal mass probably occurs in less than 10% of cases (7).

The second most common malignancy of the kidney is nephroblastoma or Wilms tumor, usually diagnosed in children before 5 years of age and the most common pediatric GU malignancy. Lymphomas rarely involve the kidneys. Metastatic disease to the organ occurs in a small minority of cancer patients. In a large autopsy series of patients dying of cancer (8) only 12% of patients had metastatic involvement of the kidney. This represents a high figure, and the incidence of metastatic lesions among tumors discovered in the kidneys is probably well below 2–3%.

The relative advantages and indications for MRI vs. CT have yet to be established, but at present CT appears to be superior in primary tumor imaging. In one study evaluating MRI, the detection rate in renal cell carcinoma was 95% for larger tumors, but only 8 of 13 masses less than 3 cm were detected (9). MRI has an important place in patients allergic to contrast, but one group concluded, "CT should remain the primary imaging modality in patients with suspected renal mass, but MRI should be used in cases where CT results are equivocal" (10). However, we must concede the rapid development of MRI techniques could change its relative indications with respect to CT in medical diagnosis, not only in the urinary tract but elsewhere. It will take years of carefully controlled clinical studies before these issues are analyzed and resolved.

Summary

1. Because of its high sensitivity for detecting masses and its high specificity for distinction of cystic from solid lesions, ultrasound always should be the first imaging study performed in any patient suspected of having a renal mass lesion.

2. Because sonography is also the imaging study *par excellence* in distinguishing medical from surgical renal disease, pyelography rarely should be the first study performed for any kidney condition. If intravenous urography is performed first, expect to find a fair number of unsuspected "mass lesions," almost all of which will prove to be benign cysts on sonography.

3. For all renal mass lesions of the adult discovered incidentally, if sonography is not diagnostic of a benign cyst, always proceed to CT. With the availability of CT, pyelography has little place in the study of renal masses.

REFERENCES

1. Pollack HM, Goldberg BB, Morales J, Bogash M. A systematized approach to the differential diagnosis of renal masses. Radiology 1974;113(3):653–659.
2. Lang EK. Diagnosis of renal and parenchymal tumors. In: Skinner DG, deKernion JB, eds. Genitourinary Cancer. Philadelphia: W. B. Saunders, 1978:42.
3. Laucks Jr SP, McLachlan MSF. Aging and simple cysts of the kidney. Br J Radiol 1981;54(637):12–14.
4. Elyaderani MK, Gabriele OF. Ultrasound of renal masses. Semin Ultrasound 1981;2(1):21–43.
5. U.S. Department of Health and Human Services, U.S. Public Health Service, Centers for Disease Control, and the National Center for Health Statistics. National Hospital Discharge Survey (NHDS). Detailed diagnoses, procedures, days of care, diagnoses-related groups for patients discharged from short-stay hospitals. Public Use Data Diskettes, 1985–1990.
6. Sagel SS, Stanley RJ, Levitt RG, Geisse G. Computed tomography of the kidney. Radiology 1977; 124(2):359–370.
7. Brenner BM, Humes HD, Milford EL. Tumors of the urinary tract. In: Harrison's Principles of Internal Medicine. Petersdorf RG, Adams RD, Braunwald E, Isselbacher KJ, Martin JB, Wilson JD, eds. 10th ed. New York: McGraw-Hill Book Co., 1983:1679.
8. Abrams HL, Spiro R, Goldstein N. Metastases in carcinoma: analysis of 1000 autopsied cases. Cancer 1950;3:74–85.
9. Hricak H, Thoeni RF, Carroll PR, Demas BE, Marotti M, Tanagho EA. Detection and staging of renal neoplasms: a reassessment of MR imaging. Radiology, 1988;166(3):643–649.
10. Baumgartner BR, Chezmar JL. Magnetic resonance imaging of the kidneys and adrenal glands. Semin Ultrasound CT MR 1989;10(1):43–62.

3/ Incidentalomas: Hepatic, Pituitary, Adrenal, and Other Masses

Formerly, when religion was strong and science weak, men mistook magic for medicine; now, when science is strong and religion weak, men mistake medicine for magic.

Thomas Szasz, M.D.

In the startlingly strange world of modern imaging, we continue to be stunned by the unexpected. As new imaging techniques are used on ever larger numbers of patients, a plethora of serendipitous findings are discovered. If only we had the knowledge and wisdom to ignore most of these incidental findings, how many untold patients, their families, and physicians would sleep more soundly at night.

The typical surprise finding is that of an unexpected mass, the quaintly but appropriately named *incidentaloma*. These masses, occasionally as small as a few millimeters in size, are testimony to the sensitivity and resolution of modern CT and MRI scanners, but such structures also can be discovered on physical examination, by ultrasonography, and occasionally scintigraphy and conventional radiography. Strictly speaking, any incidentally discovered mass fits the definition of incidentaloma, for example, the ubiquitous renal cyst. We are now aware that innocent cysts can be seen not only in the kidneys and breast, but also in the liver, pancreas, adrenal, pituitary, spleen, and other organs. The most common clinical example of an incidentaloma is the thyroid nodule, 99% of which are clinically meaningless, but which cause inordinate concern. Because of the importance of these incidentally discovered thyroid masses, we have devoted virtually an entire chapter to them, but they are indeed prototypical examples of incidentalomas.

Adrenal Incidentalomas

> *The history of medicine is a story of amazing foolishness and amazing intelligence.*
>
> *Jerome Tarshis*

Aside from the thyroid, breast, and kidney, the adrenal is perhaps the most common site of incidentaloma. The frequency of endocrinologically "silent" adrenal masses discovered on high resolution abdominal CT ranges from 1–10% of patients (1). This should cause no surprise. In one important series of 114 consecutive necropsies, mild cortical nodularity was seen in 50%, and incidental macroscopic adrenal nodules were identified in 14% of subjects (2).

Because of these data, we stress at the outset the overwhelmingly benign nature of the adrenal incidentaloma. From epidemiological data on the incidence of Cushing's syndrome due to unilateral adenoma, pheochromocytoma, aldosterone-producing tumors, and adrenal carcinoma, one can estimate the probable prevalence of these adrenal conditions in patients with adrenal masses. For example, only about 30% of cases of Cushing's Syndrome are caused by adrenal adenomas. The annual incidence of the disease in Hokkaido, Japan, was only 0.138 per 100,000 from 1975–1984 (3). Reference already has been made to the 1990 NHDS rates for all-listed discharge data for Cushing, primary hyperaldosteronism, pheochromocytoma, and malignant adrenal tumors, all of which account for less than 1 case in 20,000–50,000 population (4). Considering these low prevalences, Ross and Aron (5) have estimated the PPV of an abnormal overnight 1-mg dexamethasone suppression test for Cushing to be only 3.0% in a patient with an adrenal mass. Copeland's review (1) of six series of adrenal carcinoma disclosed that 92% of all malignant adrenal tumors were larger than 6 cm in diameter, though many now feel that size larger than 2 cm is not predictable of malignancy.

In fact, annual incidence of adrenocortical carcinomas from cancer registries ranges from 0.0006–0.00017% (6, 7). Because of the poor survival rate of patients with these tumors, the incidence approaches the prevalence of the disease in the population, i.e. in the range of 1:59,000–1:167,000. Assuming conservatively only 5% of all patients have an adrenal incidentaloma, then less than 1 out of 3,000–8,300 would likely be malignant. However, as we will point out, in a patient with a history of cancer the presence of an adrenal incidentaloma has greater clinical significance and raises the possibility of adrenal metastasis, by far the most frequent cause of malignancy in the adrenal.

In an important detailed analysis of findings in a series of 119 euadrenal patients with previously unsuspected unilateral adrenal masses found incidentally on abdominal CT, the Michigan group (8) found 64% benign adenomas and 16% metastatic tumors. Diagnoses were established by needle aspiration biopsy, adrenalectomy, or extended follow-up with repeat CT scans.

Gross, Shapiro, and colleagues (8) studied this group of patients with adrenal scintigraphy using [^{131}I]6-β-iodomethyl-norcholesterol (NP-59). In *76 out of 76 patients* when activity of NP-59 lateralized to the abnormal adrenal seen on CT scans (concordant imaging), the diagnosis was *benign adenoma* (100% specificity). Twenty-six patients had discordant imaging, that is, greatly reduced or absent NP-59 uptake on the side of the CT abnormality. Nineteen or 73% of these patients had metastatic malignancies, and an additional 4 patients or 17% had primary adrenal neoplasms. Thus, discordant imaging is 90% specific for the presence of malignancy. Bilateral symmetric visualization of NP-59 was seen in 17 patients and had variable diagnostic implications. An almost equal number in this group of patients had either metastatic malignancies, adenomas, or pseudoadrenal masses.

In patients with a known malignancy, the presence of an adrenal mass obviously is more ominous. Yet, in a study of oncological patients again carried out by the Michigan group (9), concordant uptake with NP-59 still consistently indicated benign adenoma, whereas discordant uptake indicated metastatic disease in 9 of 11 patients, the other 2 having benign adrenal cysts. In 2 of 3 patients with symmetric uptake, adenomas were present. Thus, concordance on NP scintiscanning ruled out metastatic disease. The authors concluded that "adrenal masses with discordant or indeterminate uptake of NP-59 require further evaluation in oncologic patients *if the presence of metastatic neoplasm would alter subsequent therapy,*" (9) (our emphasis).

Pituitary Incidentalomas

An oft-quoted 1936 study of Costello (10) reported a series of 1000 pituitary glands obtained from unselected autopsies. Pituitary adenomas occurred with the astonishing frequency of 22.5%. This has been confirmed more recently with a report of subclinical pituitary adenomas in 4.8–27% of unselected autopsy subjects (11). Almost all of these tumors are benign microadenomas, usually endocrinologically "silent." Given the extremely low prevalence of ACTH-dependent Cushing disease, acromegaly, and functioning prolactinomas, it is doubtful that endocrine screening of asymptomatic patients with small pituitary incidentalomas is justified. Ross and Aron (5) make the point that even assuming an elevated serum prolactin level greater than 75 ng/ml is 100% sensitive and 90% specific for the diagnosis of prolactinoma, the likelihood that such a patient with an incidental pituitary mass harbored a prolactinoma would be only 8.7%. The same argument suggests the doubtful value of biochemical testing for other endocrinopathies when small, asymptomatic pituitary incidentalomas are discovered. Again, disease prevalence determines PPV much more so than sensitivity or specificity of a given test.

In a neurosurgical series of 18 patients (12) with an intrasellar mass of 5–25 mm incidentally discovered by CT or MRI imaging, 14 patients shown in Table 8.3.1 were treated conservatively and found to have no change in tumor size at the time of follow-up (median, 22 months). Of the 4 patients who underwent neurosurgical treatment, all had either uni- or bitemporal hemianopsia or proven endocrine hyperfunction before surgery.

Investigators at the NIH reported a 15% incidence of occult pituitary abnormalities on MRI in a series of asymptomatic young patients, and a Cleveland group has found that the size and configuration of the normal pituitary on MRI may mimic adenomas in some patients (13). Although the figure of 15% is not high for autopsy subjects, most of whom would be in the much older age group, the true incidence of asymptomatic adenomas in young subjects must be considerably lower. The authors suggested wisely that MRI studies of the pituitary need to be interpreted with care.

Hepatic Incidentalomas

A 35-year-old X-ray technician underwent abdominal sonography for vague GI symptoms. The study was negative except for the incidental discovery of a small

Table 8.3.1. Clinical, Radiological, and Biochemical Data of 14 Patients With an Incidentaloma of the Pituitary Gland Treated Conservatively

Patient/ age/ sex	Complaint (reason for CT)	Maximum tumor diameter, (mm)		Endocrine function	Follow-up, (mo)
		First CT	Last CT		
5/65/F	Concussion	22	25	Hypopituitarism (LH, FSH)	19
6/68/M	Cerebrovascular disease	20	20	Normal	20
7/61/F	Headache	16	15	Hypopituitarism (LH, FSH)	42
8/59/M	Cluster headache	14	20	Normal	20
9/56/M	Vertigo	14	14	Hypopituitarism (LH, FSH)	48
10/32/F	Psychiatric disorder	12	12	Normal	48
11/27/F	Headache	11	11	Normal	17
12/15/F	Epilepsy	9	9	Normal	29
13/19/F	Concussion	8	8	Normal	12
14/22/F	Syncope	8	4	Normal	14
15/24/F	Headache	8	8	Normal	17
16/43/F	Vertigo	8	8	Normal	24
17/37/F	Psychiatric disorder	5	5	Normal	20
18/44/F	Headache	5	9	Normal	96

CT indicates computed tomography; and LH (luteinizing hormone) and FSH (follicle-stimulating hormone), hormone deficiencies in patients with hypopituitarism. Reprinted by permission from *JAMA* (1990;263(20):2772–2776). Copyright 1990, American Medical Association.

hepatic "lesion." She was told, "it might be serious," and a biopsy was suggested. Over the next several weeks she developed a serious depression and finally underwent CT with contrast, which was "nondiagnostic." She delayed having further studies for several more weeks, during which time she consulted a psychiatrist in the belief she might have cancer. Ultimately, hepatic angiography was performed with the demonstration of a benign hemangioma. Later review of the sonographic study showed a typical pattern of a benign hemangioma. Review of the CT study disclosed that appropriately timed films had not been taken to exclude hepatic hemangioma. *Medical cost:* $6500 (including psychiatrist). *Emotional cost:* Impossible to estimate.

Among other lessons, the above clinical story demonstrates it is not unusual to encounter echogenic or benign cystic lesions of the liver while performing routine abdominal or renal ultrasonography. Almost all the echogenic lesions prove to be benign hemangiomas on further study, which is preferably carried out with SPECT hepatic blood pool scintigraphy or CT with contrast. As expected, this innocent tumor is commonly seen at postmortem. In addition, simple cysts of the liver occur in perhaps 0.5–1% of routine abdominal sonograms. These are usually under 2 cm in size.

In an important Australian study of 36 "unexpected filling defects" on liver scintigraphy (the authors excluded cystic lesions) 29 or 81% were benign, and the remaining 7 or 19% were malignant: 5 secondary tumors and two primaries (14). The most common lesion was hemangioma, found in 20 or 56% of all patients. The authors observed that an enlarging mass or an elevated alkaline phosphatase were strong indicators of malignancy. If one assumes these findings to be absent, more than 95% of hepatic incidentalomas would be benign tumors. On this basis, the average patient with a hepatic incidentaloma without known malignancy and with normal liver function tests would be ill-served by any further testing. We have seen patients such as the one described above undergo not only arteriography, but even biopsy, for benign solid hepatic masses. It goes without saying that any attempt to biopsy an hemangioma could prove disastrous.

If one recalls that hepatic hemangiomas are the most common benign liver neoplasm, occurring in up to 7% of the population, (15) most work-ups for hepatic incidentalomas could be eliminated completely.

Summary

Pure cystic lesions of the thyroid, liver, kidneys, breast, adrenal, spleen, and pancreas are almost never malignant and can, for all practical purposes, be clinically ignored. Do not succumb to anxiety over an incidentaloma in a well patient. Above all, reassure the patient, even in the rare instance when further imaging studies are indicated. As a general rule, careful follow-up studies are almost always preferable to needless and dangerous investigation. More than 99% of such patients will turn out to have no treatable disease.

ADRENAL INCIDENTALOMA

1. Asymptomatic patients with adrenal incidentalomas found on CT or MRI almost overwhelmingly will have benign disease. (Shapiro, B., personal communication). Except in those with unexplained abdominal pain, a history of malignancy, or a lesion larger than 3–4 cm, *nothing further should be done*. If there is any question, a repeat study in 6–12 months is the safest strategy. Even in lesions larger than 5–7 cm, the ratio of benign to malignant lesions was greater than 2:1. (Gross, M. D., personal communication).

2. Obviously, if there is any clinical suspicion of an endocrinopathy in a patient with an adrenal incidentaloma, biochemical studies should be carried out to exclude the rare case of subclinical (preclinical) adrenal dysfunction.

3. All patients with abnormal biochemical studies, a history of malignancy, or large lesions should have NP-59 adrenal scintiscanning.

4. In patients with concordant findings on scintigraphy and CT (uptake on the same side as the CT mass), more than 90–95% of all adrenal incidentalomas, the presence of a benign adenoma can be assumed, i.e. cancer has for all intents been excluded.

Those patients, however, who show lack of visualization of the contralateral adrenal should be studied with suppression testing. The reason for this is the possibility of finding the rare early case of autonomous adrenal adenoma with suppression. A positive 1-mg overnight dexamethasone suppression test (failure to suppress) indicates Cushing's syndrome due to a functioning adrenal adenoma, or "Cushing's to come." Gross recommends adrenalectomy in cases of documented hypersecretion or nonsuppressibility but adds that, "What we don't know here is the natural history of these incidental lesions with contralateral suppression on scintigraphy without documented nonsuppressibility. If we knew which ones were going to go on to develop autonomy with hyperfunction, then perhaps we would have a better handle on this situation." He stresses that suppressibility is a reliable sign that the lesion is not only benign, but also functioning normally. These patients may be followed by repeat suppression testing at yearly intervals but will not require further imaging studies. Probably less than 5–10% of patients with contralateral suppression on scanning but with normal suppressibility on dexamathasone go on to true Cushing's syndrome (Gross, M. D., and Shapiro, B., personal communication).

Table 8.3.2. Diagnostic Approach to Discovery of Hepatic Incidentaloma First Detected by Various Modalities (Assuming Suspected Malignancy, Enlarging Hepatic Mass, or Unexplained Abnormal Liver Function Tests)

If detected by:	Next step
A. Ultrasound	
1. Typical appearance of hemangioma	Stop
2. Typical cystic lesion	Stop
3. Possible hemangioma	SPECT liver scan (RBCs) or CT with timed images
4. Atypical solid lesion	CT
B. Liver spleen scintigraphy	
1. Solitary defect	Ultrasound for cyst or hemangiomata (if not typical for latter, proceed as in A, 3 and 4)
2. Multiple defects	CT
C. CT	
1. Solitary or multiple lesions	Proceed to ultrasound if CT pattern for hemangioma is atypical (if sonography nondiagnostic, proceed to SPECT liver scintigraphy)

Only if patient has one or more of the following indications: history or suspicion of malignancy, an enlarging hepatic mass, age over 45, or unexplained abnormal liver function tests. Note: Do not proceed to arteriography or biopsy unless a treatable lesion has been established with reasonable certainty on the basis of sonography and SPECT liver scintigraphy, or, if necessary with CT, i.e. unless a benign lesion has been excluded with a high degree of certainty.

5. A vanishingly small group of patients turn out to have discordant findings on NP-59 scintigraphy and CT, that is NP-59 adrenal uptake on the side contralateral to the CT abnormality. These individuals should be presumed to have a very high likelihood (greater than 80%) of metastatic or primary adrenal tumor and further diagnostic studies initiated, i.e. needle biopsy or exploration.

6. Patients with adrenal incidentalomas on CT and non-localizing (symmetrical) findings on NP-59 scintigraphy should be considered indeterminate, and appropriate further studies performed, as in (5) above.

7. Patients with adrenal incidentalomas and known malignancies, particularly cancer of the lung, breast, colon, or lymphoma, should be considered suspects for adrenal metastatic disease. However, even in known cancer patients, an NP-59 scintiscan showing concordant uptake rules out metastatic disease (and primary adrenal malignancy) with almost 100% certainty.

PITUITARY INCIDENTALOMAS

Neurologically intact patients with pituitary incidentalomas smaller than 2.0–2.5 cm in size almost always should be left alone, except for CT follow-up at yearly intervals initially, and less frequent subsequently. The only individuals likely to require neurosurgical treatment are those with hemianopsia or other neuroendocrine findings. Routine endocrine screening of such patients is not indicated unless there is clinical suspicion of an endocrinopathy.

HEPATIC INCIDENTALOMAS

Because more than 95% of unselected hepatic incidentalomas are benign, the largest number represented by simple hemangiomas, the following schema is advised.

1. In patients without a history of malignancy, clinical signs of an enlarging mass, and without abnormal liver function tests, the likelihood of a primary or secondary hepatic tumor is vanishingly small, and nothing further should be done.

2. When CT and ultrasound fail to indicate a likely diagnosis in hepatic incidentaloma, *and only if there is adequate clinical justification as outlined in 1*, proceed to

the nuclear flow study and blood pool image with technetium-99m in vivo-labeled RBCs, preferably using the SPECT technique, to exclude hemangioma. Otherwise, proceed as in Table 8.3.2.

3. When CT and ultrasound fail to indicate a likely diagnosis in hepatic incidentaloma, the nuclear flow study and blood pool image with technetium-99m in vivo-labeled RBCs, preferably using the SPECT technique, should be used to exclude hemangioma.

4. Except in high tumor suspects, diagnostic percutaneous biopsy is almost never indicated in hepatic incidentalomas and may be risky, especially in cases of unsuspected angioma.

REFERENCES

1. Copeland PM. The incidentally discovered adrenal mass. Ann Intern Med 1983;98(6):940–945.
2. Dobbie JW. Adrenocortical nodular hyperplasia: the ageing adrenal. J Pathol 1969;99(1):1–18.
3. Iimura O, Shimamoto K, Nakahashi Y, Nakamura Y. Actual incidence of adrenal tumors in Hokkaido. In: Takeda R, Miyamori I, eds. Controversies in Disorders of Adrenal Hormones: Proceedings of the Open Symposium of Disorders of Adrenal Hormones. Tokyo, Japan, 1988. New York: Elsevier Science, 1988:37–41.
4. U.S. Department of Health and Human Services, U.S. Public Health Service, Centers for Disease Control, and the National Center for Health Statistics. National Hospital Discharge Survey (NHDS). Detailed diagnoses, procedures, days of care, diagnoses-related groups for patients discharged from short-stay hospitals. Public Use Data Diskettes, 1985–1990.
5. Ross NS, Aron DC. Hormonal evaluation of the patient with an incidentally discovered adrenal mass [Current concepts]. N Engl J Med 1990;323(20):1401–1405.
6. Flannery JT. Connecticut Tumor Registry, 1976–1980. Hartford: Department of Health Services, 1980.
7. Surveillance, Epidemiology and End Results: Incidence and Mortality Data 1973–77. Bethesda: National Cancer Institute, 1981;NIH publication no. 81-2330.
8. Gross MD, Shapiro B, Bouffard JA, et al. Distinguishing benign from malignant euadrenal masses. Ann Intern Med 1988;109(8):613–618.
9. Francis IR, Smid A, Gross MD, Shapiro B, Naylor B, Glazey GM. Adreaenal masses in oncologic patients: functional and morphologic evaluation. Radiology 1988;166(2):353–356.
10. Costello RT. Subclinical adenoma of the pituitary gland. Am J Pathol 1936;12:205–216.
11. McComb DJ, Ryan N, Horvath E, Kovacs K. Subclinical adenomas of the human pituitary: new light on old problems. Arch Pathol Lab Med 1983;107(9):488–491.
12. Reincke M, Allolio B, Saeger W, Menzel J, Winkelmann W. The "incidentaloma" of the pituitary gland: is neurosurgery required? JAMA 1990;263(20):2772–2776.
13. Carswell H. MR of pituitary shows surprising variability. Diagn Imaging 1990;Nov:103–105.
14. Little JM, Kenny J, Hollands MJ. Hepatic incidentaloma: a modern problem. World J Surg 1990; 14(4):448–451.
15. Ishak KG, Rabin L. Benign tumor of the liver. Med Clin North Am 1972;59:995–1013.

4/ Abdominal Abscesses and Collections

Speaking of the importance of draining abscesses he referred to the time when he was called to Balmoral to operate upon Queen Victoria for an axillary abscess and playfully said, "Gentleman, I am the only man who has ever stuck a knife in the Queen."

J. R. Leeson
Referring to Sir Joseph Lister

Abdominal abscesses, infections, or localized collections may present in bewildering variety and develop in a spectrum of clinical settings. Although commonplace conditions are stressed throughout this text rather than the unusual, the abdomen is one region where one may anticipate diagnostic surprises. Imaging principles, however, remain the same for the investigation of all intraabdominal collections, rare or common, septic or nonseptic.

The most frequently encountered simple infections in the abdominal cavity are seen in the GI, GU, or hepatobiliary tract. Diagnoses of gastroenteritis or pyelonephritis, for example, are made clinically or on the basis of simple laboratory tests, whereas problems in the hepatobiliary system require investigation with ultrasound and scintigraphy. Intraabdominal abscess or collections, however, either of the visceral organs, the peritoneum, or retroperitoneum, present special diagnostic problems. *Trauma and prior abdominal surgery remain the two most common causes of intraabdominal collections.* Moreover, it is common knowledge that abscesses or collections may occur locally or at distant sites in conditions such as appendicitis, diverticulitis, or salpingitis. Localized or generalized abdominal sepsis is also seen in immunocompromised patients, e.g. those on chemotherapy or with cancer or AIDS. The risk of death from intraabdominal abscess is considerable and directly related to factors such as age, concurrent disease, organic system failure and, most important, *delayed diagnosis*. The importance of prompt diagnosis can be inferred from the statistics showing mortality in untreated patients approaching 100% (1). Even in treated patients the death rate ranges from 11–39% (2–4). Not surprisingly, predisposing operations are the ones most commonly performed, such as those on the colon, appendix, stomach, and biliary tract.

When intraabdominal infection occurs in the postoperative patient, clinical findings and laboratory studies are highly sensitive for the presence of sepsis but nonspecific as to location. Plain abdominal radiography, though highly specific in the detection of gas patterns, is less than 50% sensitive for abscess detection, and errors in interpretation of plain films are reported to be frequent (1, 5). Because the use of contrast studies for identifying suspected sites of perforation or sinus tracts is applicable in few patients, our discussion is limited to the three established localizing methods: ultrasound (US), CT and radionuclide scintigraphy using either gallium-67 or WBCs labeled with indium-111 or technetium-99m HMPAO.

Postoperative Complications in the Abdomen

> *Medical education is not completed at the medical school: it is only begun.*
>
> *William H. Welch*

Approximately 5 million general abdominal, 4 million female pelvic, and 1.5 million urological operations were performed in the United States in 1985. Table 8.4.1 lists the 13 most frequently performed abdominal/pelvic/GU operations in that year. (Only about 10% were, strictly speaking, diagnostic procedures.) These comprised about half of all such operations performed in the United States in 1985 (6). Table 8.4.2 shows the figures for 1990. Note that over half of these operations, four out of the first five, are performed exclusively on females. Allowing for the preponderance of cholecystectomies in females, this means that *more than 80% of all patients undergoing the most frequently performed pelvic and abdominal operations in this country are women.* Again, note the appalling frequency as well as the increase in number of Ce-

Table 8.4.1. Most Frequently Performed Abdominal, Pelvic, and GU Operations in the United States, 1985 Adapted from Rutkow (6)

	Number	Percentage
1. Cesarean section (74)	879,000	16.4
2. Hysterectomy (68.3–68.6)	669,000	12.4
3. Unilateral or bilateral open destruction or occlusion of fallopian tubes (66.3–66.6)	531,000	9.8
4. Inguinal herniorrhaphy (53.0–53.1)	476,000	8.9
5. Cholecystectomy (51.2)	475,000	8.8
6. Unilateral or bilateral salpingo-oophrectomy (65.4–65.6)	472,000	8.8
7. Prostatectomy (60.2–60.6)	367,000	6.8
8. Diagnostic dilatation and curettage of uterus (69.09)	349,000	6.5
9. Lysis of peritoneal adhesions (54.5)	309,000	5.7
10. Appendectomy (47.0)	283,000	5.3
11. Large bowel resection and/or colostomy (45.7, 45.4)	249,000	4.6
12. Diagnostic laparoscopy (54.12)	212,000	4
13. Exploratory laparotomy (54.1)	104,000	2
Total	5,375,000	100

Figures in parentheses are ICD-9-CM codes. Adapted from Rutkow (6).

Table 8.4.2. Most Frequently Performed Abdominal, Pelvic, and GU Operations in the United States, 1990

	Number	Percentage
1. Cesarean section (1989 figures) (74)	944,000	19.6
2. Hysterectomy (68.3–68.6)	582,000	12.1
3. Cholecystectomy (51.2)	522,000	11
4. Unilateral or bilateral open destruction or occlusion of fallopian tubes (66.3–66.6)	472,000	9.8
5. Unilateral or bilateral salpingo-oophrectomy. (65.4–65.6)	436,000	9.1
6. Prostatectomy (60.2–60.6)	357,000	7.4
7. Lysis of peritoneal adhesions (54.5)	323,000	6.7
8. Appendectomy (47.0)	274,000	5.7
9. Diagnostic dilatation and curettage of uterus (69.09)	220,000	4.6
10. Inguinal herniorrhaphy (53.0–53.1)	205,000	4.3
11. Large bowel resection and/or colostomy (45.7, 45.4)	204,000	4.2
12. Diagnostic laparoscopy (54.12)	161,000	3.4
13. Exploratory laparotomy (54.1)	102,000	2.1
Total	4,802,000	100

Figures in parentheses are ICD-9-CM codes. From U.S. Department of Health and Human Services, U.S. Public Health Service, Centers for Disease Control, and the National Center for Health Statistics. National Hospital Disease Survey (NHDS). Detailed diagnoses, procedures, days of care, diagnoses-related groups for patients discharged from short-stay hospitals. Public Use Data Diskettes, 1985–1990.

sarean sections performed in the United States. Of interest is the drop in total procedures performed, especially herniorrhaphies, a reflection of increasing outpatient procedures. An assortment of postoperative complications occur, of which the major ones are listed in Table 8.4.3 (7–11).

Diagnosing common, generally benign complications of the abdominal wall should be a straightforward clinical exercise, but all too frequently physicians overlook the obvious. We are often asked to image patients with a suspected intraabdominal collection only to find that a wound abscess has been missed. Delay in diagnosing these superficial collections may be serious in view of the risk for subsequent wound dehiscence, incisional hernia, deep extension of infection, and septicemia. Ul-

Table 8.4.3. Various Principal Postsurgical Complications with Frequencies

Generally benign complications	Occurrence (%)
Wound infection and dehiscence (7–9)	5–10
Abdominal wall hematomas	15–25 (est)
Incisional hernias (8–10)	up to 14
Peritoneal effusions (11)	19 at 4 days
	6 at 8 days
	2.5 at 12 days
Serious complications	
Intraabdominal abscess	20–25[a]
Bile Leak (postcholecystectomy)	5–10 (10)
Anastomotic leakage (lower colon resections) (10)	5–10 (10)
Intraabdominal bleeding	

[a]In emergent cholecystectomy, appendectomy, and GI operations for inflammatory or neoplastic problems.

trasound is an extremely useful method in identifying these collections, but scanning in the region of a recent operative incision or a draining wound presents technical problems and requires the presence of the physician sonographer, who should be prepared to assist the technologist in the examination. This should present no problem if, as in good medical practice, the ultrasound examinations are physician witnessed. In difficult cases CT is also helpful, but ultrasound generally suffices for the diagnosis of these superficial or extraperitoneal (abdominal wall) collections and can also provide guidance for percutaneous drainage.

In Search of a Collection: Ultrasonography vs. CT vs. Scintigraphy

> *Among the arts, medicine, on account of its eminent utility, must always hold the highest place.*
>
> *Henry Thomas Buckle*

The optimal approach for imaging abdominal abscesses remains controversial. Some writers stress certain studies because of their specialization in a given area and unfamiliarity with competing techniques. Frustrated or anxious clinicians often follow the line of least resistance by ordering every available test. Imaging strategy must be neither "scattershot" nor routine, but rather individualized on the basis of clinical severity, suspected location of the collection, etc. There is no such thing as the typical case in abdominal abscess. Many patients are subjected to multiple studies when one would have sufficed, whereas others are denied the appropriate examination out of ignorance or confusion. The performance of multiple complementary imaging studies too often results in discordant data and frequently leads to the cascade effect, previously mentioned, whereby one test leads to another, and a chain of uncontrolled events is unleashed. Another serious problem is delay in obtaining the appropriate study, usually after the patient is started on antibiotic therapy. This can have serious consequences for the sensitivity and specificity of studies, in particular scintigraphy.

The relative advantages and disadvantages of ultrasound, CT, and scintigraphy have been thoroughly discussed in an excellent review (12). Table 8.4.4, taken from this paper presents a detailed comparison of ultrasound, CT, gallium-67, and indium-111 WBC imaging in abdominal abscess diagnosis, whereas Table 8.4.5 describes the typical appearance of abscess on ultrasound, CT, and scintigraphy (12). Altmeier, Neff, Mintz, and others (1, 11, 13) give helpful guidelines for imaging,

Table 8.4.4. Comparison of Techniques for Abdominal Abscess Detection

Technique	Advantages	Disadvantages
US	Portable Immediate results No ionizing radiation Excellent visualization of right upper quadrant, kidneys, pelvis Excellent for detection of fluid collections Can provide guidance for needle aspiration or percutaneous drainage Least expensive	Highly dependent on operator skill and persistence Visualization of left upper quadrant, mid-abdomen often limited by bowel gas Poor visualization of retroperitoneum Does not visualize spine or paraspinous soft tissues Cannot always distinguish infected and uninfected fluid
CT	Immediate results Excellent anatomic resolution (especially if IV contrast used) Excellent for detection of fluid collections Evaluates bowel, interloop areas (if oral contrast administered) Evaluates retroperitoneum, spine, body wall, thighs, lung bases in addition to abdominal cavity Can provide guidance for needle aspiration or percutaneous drainage	Suboptimal contrast opacification of bowel may limit interpretation Metal clips or devices can obscure surrounding anatomy due to streak artifact Cannot always distinguish infected and uninfected fluid Most expensive
Ga-67 Imaging	Sensitive detection of infection Whole body imaging Can distinguish infected and uninfected fluid	Results only after 24 hours or more Physiologic activity in liver, spleen, bowel may limit interpretation Activity in neoplasms, non-infected inflammatory processes may mimic infection Cannot be directly used to guide needle aspiration or drainage
In-111-WBC imaging	Sensitive detection of infection Highly specific for infection Whole body imaging	Results at 24 hours Physiologic liver and spleen activity may limit interpretation Activity occasionally seen in tumors, other noninfectious processes

Reprinted by permission from *Seminars in Nuclear Medicine* (1988;XV(4):322).

Table 8.4.5. Abdominal Abscess: Typical Appearance

Technique	Appearance
Ultrasound	Mass of variable echogenicity with acoustic enhancement (increased through transmission) and refractive artifact indicative of fluid nature of mass "Dirty shadowing" and "ring down" artifact (indicating gas) may be present Fluid-debris interface may be seen
CT	Low density mass that does not enhance centrally after IV contrast administration (rim may enhance) Round or oval in shape if within solid organ parenchyma Conforms to surrounding structures if extraparenchymal
Ga-67 imaging	Intense, focal activity unchanging in distribution on follow-up images
In-111-WBC imaging	Intense, focal activity

Reprinted by permission from *Seminars in Nuclear Medicine* (1988;XV(4):322).

occasionally marked by a preference for an algorithmic schema. Their approach, based on location of disease and medical status of the patient, has the unmistakable merits of logic and common sense.

ULTRASONOGRAPHY

Returning to Table 8.4.4 we note that ultrasonography gives poor visualization of the left upper quadrant, midabdomen, retroperitoneum, and paraspinous region. Conversely, excellent imaging is obtained of the right upper quadrant, kidneys, and pelvis. In a classic study of 540 abdominal abscesses in 501 patients 36% were shown to be intraperitoneal (most commonly right lower quadrant), 38% were retroperitoneal, and 26% visceral (1). Patients with no previous surgery usually had abscesses in the pelvis. On this basis we might estimate that only 30–50% of unselected abdominal abscesses might be accessible to ultrasonography, a reasonable assumption, though difficult to verify. However, because of its speed, ease, and availability, ultrasonography in most cases is the preferred first procedure.

CT

CT has high sensitivity and specificity for detection of abdominal collections because of its excellent anatomical resolution. This also holds true for detection of adjacent lung and body wall septic masses, which may mimic intraabdominal disease. For this reason, CT is thought by most to be the best single procedure for abdominal abscess detection and localization in the noncritical patient. Furthermore, like sonography, CT has the simultaneous advantage of providing guidance for percutaneous aspiration or drainage. Yet CT also has disadvantages. For certain locations the sensitivity of abscess detection may be quite poor, for example, as low as 60% in the interloop areas (13, 14). Furthermore, CT, unlike radionuclide studies, cannot reliably distinguish infected from uninfected collections, nor can the method provide adequate information in patients unable to receive oral or intravenous contrast. CT, of course, is eliminated in the critically ill patient unable to be moved from the intensive care unit.

RADIONUCLIDE PROCEDURES

Gallium-67 citrate and indium-111-WBC scintigraphy have been used with considerable success in the detection of abscesses (15–17). General sensitivity is high, but with gallium specificity in the abdomen is low because of normal bowel uptake of the radiopharmaceutical, which can make interpretation extremely difficult. Indium-111-labeled WBCs are almost always preferable in the search for abdominal abscesses compared to gallium (though the two radiopharmaceutical agents are generally equivalent in detecting infection elsewhere in the body). However, minor problems may occur, for example, from focal activity in uninfected incision and drain sites, areas of bleeding, and particularly in swallowed indium-111-WBC activity from nasogastric and endotracheal tubes, pneumonia and sinusitis, among other sources.

The preparation of indium-111-labeled autologous WBCs poses technical problems in imaging children, because 35–50 ml blood have to be withdrawn from the patient. Preparation problems are also complex and expensive. Furthermore, indium-111-labeled WBCs are of limited value in patients with low WBC counts, e.g. those who are immunocompromised, such as patients on chemotherapy or with AIDS. The greatest advantage of scintigraphy rests on its ability to detect sepsis outside as well as inside the abdomen, because unlike CT and ultrasound, the entire body is visualized.

Two papers report the serendipitous discovery of other causes of fever in 16% of patients (16, 18). Radionuclide studies are probably most useful in the patient in whom localizing signs are absent. Many of these patients will have low-grade peritonitis or collections too small or inaccessible for CT or ultrasound (19).

Oates (20) has written an extremely useful paper on the diagnosis of infection with radionuclides. She also summarizes the comparative clinical and radiopharmaceutical considerations of indium-111 WBCs vs. gallium-67 for the diagnosis of sepsis and inflammation in Tables 8.4.6 and 8.4.7, taken from her superb paper.

THE CRITICALLY ILL PATIENT

Ultrasound examination of the critically ill patient has been made possible with the advent of excellent portable machines suitable for the intensive care unit. With good portable equipment the desperately ill patient need not be subjected to the very real perils of transport to and from the imaging department. Often the diagnosis can be made and percutaneous drainage or aspiration performed immediately at the bedside. Only when ultrasonography is nondiagnostic and clinical suspicion remains high is CT or scintigraphy required in the intensive care patient.

Summary of the Diagnostic Approach to Intraabdominal Abscess or Collection

Surgeons must be very careful
When they take the knife!
Underneath their fine incisions
Stirs a Culprit-life!

Emily Dickinson
The Complete Poems

1. Always suspect and examine for a wound infection or abscess before assuming the patient has an intraabdominal collection. Even if clinical features are nondiagnostic, always use ultrasound to examine the incision or wound site and subjacent abdominal wall before proceeding.

2. In the presence or absence of localizing signs, generally start with ultrasound to survey the right upper quadrant, subhepatic space, kidneys, and pelvis. Ultrasonography frequently suffices for diagnosis in these regions.

3. In patients with nondiagnostic ultrasound, and particularly in those with suspected disease in the left subphrenic space, spleen, midabdomen and lesser sac, always proceed to CT.

4. If both CT and ultrasound are nondiagnostic, proceed to indium-111-WBC scintigraphy.

5. In patients with fever but without localizing signs and negative ultrasound, scintigraphic study with indium-111 WBCs usually should be done first to exclude peritonitis or extraabdominal sepsis. In the event that focal disease is seen abdominally, the finding can be followed up with CT for more precise localization and possible percutaneous drainage.

6. MRI is not at present competitive with CT or ultrasound in the search for intraabdominal sepsis and therefore is not generally recommended.

Table 8.4.6. Comparative Clinical Indicators

Clinical problem	Ga-67 citrate	In-111-WBCs
Occult sepsis	−	*
Abscess		
Acute	−	*
Chronic	*	−
Pyogenic	−	*
Nonpyogenic	*	−
Abdominal site	−	*
Renal	−	*
Inflammatory bowel disease	−	*
HIV-positive status		
Pulmonary infection	*	−
Nonpulmonary infection	−	*
Lymphadenitis	*	−
Bone and joint infection		
Acute	−	*
Chronic	(*)	*
Complicated	−	*
Prosthesis	−	*
Prosthetic cardiovascular grafts/catheters	−	*
Granulomatous diseases		
Sarcoid	*	−
Occult malignancy	*	−

Reprinted by permission from *Applied Radiology* (1992;22(1):48–53).
*Preferred radiopharmaceutical.

Table 8.4.7. Comparative Radiopharmaceutical Considerations

	Ga-67 Citrate	In-111 WBCs
Physical properties	Cyclotron-produced T 1/2 = 78 hrs	Cyclotron-produced T 1/2 = 67 hrs
Imaging photons	93 keV (38%)	173 keV (89%)
(% abundance)	184 keV (24%)	247 keV (94%)
	300 keV (16%)	
Preparation and route of administration	Ready for intravenous injection	In vitro labeling of isolated WBCs with In-111 oxine for intravenous injection
Normal biodistribution	Liver, skeleton, spleen, nose/salivary/ lacrimal glands, breasts, genitalia	Spleen, liver, bone marrow
Routes of excretion	Renal (24 hrs), gastrointestinal	None
Dose (adult)	3-5 mCi	0.5 mCi
Dosimetry	<1.0 rad/mCi colon	13 rad/mCi spleen
	<0.5 rad/mCi body	<0.5 rad/mCi body
Cost	$35 per dose	$135 in house
		$350 commercial
Limitations for use	None	IV access (19 g)
		Leukopenia
		Impaired chemotaxis
		Abnormal WBCs
		Children

Reprinted by permission from *Applied Radiology* (1992;21(1):48–53).

REFERENCES

1. Altemeier WA, Culbertson WR, Fullen WD, Shook CD. Intraabdominal abscesses. Am J Surg 1973; 125(1):70–79.
2. Doberneck RC, Mittelman J. Reappraisal of the problems of intra-abdominal abscess. Surg Gynecol Obstet 1982;154(1):875–879.
3. Pitcher WD, Musher DM. Critical importance of early diagnosis and treatment of intra-abdominal infection. Arch Surg 1982;117(3):328–333.
4. Fry DE, Garrison RN, Heitsch RC, Calhoun K, Polk Jr HC. Determinants of death in patients with intraabdominal abscess. Surgery 1980;88(4):517–523.
5. Lundstedt C, Hederstrom E, Brismar J, et al. Prospective investigation of radiologic methods in the diagnosis of intraabdominal abscesses. Acta Radiol Diagn 1986;27(1):49–54.
6. Rutkow IM. Socioeconomics of Surgery. 1st ed. St. Louis: C. V. Mosby Company, 1988:16–29.
7. Ghahremani GG. Internal abdominal hernias. Surg Clin North Am 1984;64(2):393–406.
8. Ghahremani GG, Jimenez MA, Rosenfeld M, Rochester D. CT diagnosis of occult incisional hernias. AJR 1987;148(1):139–142.
9. Ghaharemani GG, Meyers MA, Hietala SO, et al. Hemorrhage complicating gastrointestinal surgery. In: Meyers MA, Ghahremani GG, eds. Iatrogenic Gastrointestinal Complications. New York: Springer-Verlag, 1981:235–253.
10. Ghaharemani GG, Gore RM. CT diagnosis of postoperative abdominal complications. Radiol Clin North Am 1989;27(4):787–804.
11. Neff CC, Simeone JE, Ferrucci Jr JT, Mueller PR, Wittenberg J. The occurrence of fluid collections following routine abdominal surgical procedures: sonographic survey in asymptomatic postoperative patients. Radiology 1983;146(2):463–466.
12. Gagliardi PD, Hoffer PB, Rosenfield AT. Correlative imaging in abdominal infection: an algorithmic approach using nuclear medicine, ultrasound, and computed tomography. Semin Nucl Med 1988; XVIII(4):320–334.
13. Mintz MC, Arger PH, Kressel HY. An algorithmic approach to the radiologic evaluation of a suspected abdominal abscess. Semin Ultrasound 1983;4:80–90.
14. Dobrin PB, Gully PH, Greenlee HB, et al. Radiologic diagnosis of an intra-abdominal abscess: Do multiple tests help? Arch Surg 1986;121(1):41–46.
15. Hoffer PB, Bekerman C, Henkin RE. Gallium-67 Imaging. New York: Wiley, 1978:90.
16. Seabold JE, Wilson DG, Lieberman LM, Boyd CM. Unsuspected extra-abdominal sites of infection: scintigraphic detection with Indium-111 labeled leukocytes. Radiology 1984;151(1):213–217.
17. Knochel JQ, Koehler PR, Lee TG, Welch DM. Diagnosis of abdominal abscesses with computed tomography, ultrasound and 111-In leukocyte scans. Radiology 1980;137(2):425–432.
18. Moir C, Robins RE. Role of ultrasonography, gallium scanning, and computer tomography in the diagnosis of intraabdominal abscess. Am J Surg 1982;143(5):582–585.
19. McNeil BJ, Sanders R, Alderson PO, et al. A prospective study of computed tomography, ultrasound and gallium imaging in patients with fever. Radiology 1981;139(3):647–653.
20. Oates E. Scintigraphic diagnosis of infection and inflammation. Appl Radiol 1992;21(1):48–53.

9

Cancer Diagnosis and the Metastatic Work-Up

While there are several chronic diseases more destructive to life than cancer, none is more feared.

Charles H. Mayo

The term *work-up*, so fashionable in medical speech, somehow seems unfortunate because of its connotation of schematic orthodoxy. A fastidious formalism is hardly a substitute for common sense and in fact violates the pragmatic basis of clinical practice. Although algorithms have their uses, rule-bound formulae for the diagnosis or treatment of cancer, chest pain, "gas," or any condition, lead inevitably to mindless or defensive medicine in which all bases are covered but few hits are made.

Persuasive examples of the diagnostically doctrinaire include various species of the time-honored work-up, the cardiac, the GI, the neurological—one for each specialty, disease, or condition. It reminds one of the remark by Moarji Desai: "An expert seldom gives an objective view. He gives his own view." Metastatic work-up is the modern-day paradigm for the laboratory investigation of cancer patients in which the search for disease spread follows a methodical, predictable routine, often unrelated to the type of malignancy or its clinical behavior. Thus, we have vast numbers of cancer patients undergoing endoscopy, CT, MRI, or scintigraphy of organs that are rarely the site of metastasis for a given tumor. Moreover, untold patients with far-advanced disease are subjected to diagnostic studies, the results of which will have no implications for their treatment, let alone their longevity. It does not seem heretical to suggest more effective strategies for detecting cancer dissemination at the time of initial treatment, *when such strategies offer a realistic chance of improving patient management or quality of life*. Before discussing the various types of malignancies, a word about the imaging approach to cancer diagnosis itself seems appropriate.

Does Medical Imaging Help in the Diagnosis of Cancer?

A man once was asked if he had trouble making up his mind. His response was the same as the answer to the above question: "Yes and no." A diagnosis of cancer, like all diagnoses, first must be invoked from suspicion based on clinical findings. The choice and sequence of imaging studies should be guided by the results of the medical history and physical examination. *Diagnostic imaging, as always, should be signs-and-symptoms oriented.* Imaging, of course, can suggest a diagnosis of cancer, but only tissue biopsy can confirm it.

When should the diagnosis of a malignant condition be anticipated with reasonable probability? This may seem an ingenuous question, but it bears examination. There should be little argument about the high probability of cancer in the presence of a solitary pulmonary nodule in a 65-year-old smoker. Nor is a diagnosis of malignancy unlikely in the woman with a fixed breast mass, the patient with extensive unexplained cervical and supraclavicular adenopathy, and the middle-aged individual with dysphagia or a change in bowel habits, anemia, and weight loss. In such patients a search for a diagnosis of malignancy is mandatory and already anatomically oriented. While awaiting the results of mammography or biopsy, a search for metastatic disease indeed may be justified.

However, in the patient with protean, ill-defined symptoms *unaccompanied by any other clinical clues on history, examination, or routine laboratory tests,* an aimless search for cancer is almost invariably nonproductive. Fatigue, weakness, anorexia, or weight loss, the latter often difficult to verify, are frequent initiators of failed fishing expeditions for malignancy using a battery of imaging and other diagnostic studies. This practice is ill advised and usually futile. Despite occasional cases of early asymptomatic malignancy, for example, lymphoma or pancreatic cancer, patients, particularly elderly individuals, who often have ill-defined complaints and no findings, rarely turn out to have cancer. The most common causes of weight loss, anorexia, and fatigue in such individuals include stress, poor or distorted eating habits due to factors such as loss of spouse, diet fads, alcoholism, institutionalization, poor fitting dentures, and, most important, depression, dementia, and aging itself (1, 2).

Sometimes none of these causes can be verified, despite searching history and physical examination. When the patient proves to have normal routine blood studies, urinalysis, and chest radiographs, including perhaps prostate-specific antigen or other "marker" (generally nonspecific) antibodies, and if suspicion of cancer lingers, we are stranded in a wilderness of uncertainty. In the absence of any clinical clues, logic would suggest the search begin with the most likely cancers in the general population. Table 9.1 gives estimated numbers of new cancer cases and percentages by site in the United States for 1990 (3). Figure 9.1, prepared by the American Cancer Society, shows 1992 estimated cancer incidence and deaths by site and sex (4). Table 9.2 reproduces the second part of Table 9.1, listing male and female cancer deaths in order of frequency by site. A study of the charts makes clear the problems associated with undirected or blind diagnostic testing. If we are to embark on a voyage to diagnose the most likely cancers, where are we to start? For example, how does one go about diagnosing lung cancer in the face of a negative radiograph, or breast, prostate cancer, or lymphoma with a negative physical examination and blood findings? One may make a case for mammographic screening in females, CT of the chest in smokers, and sonography of the upper abdomen and upper and lower GI barium studies to help exclude pancreatic, stomach, or colon malignancy. But again, a study of the actual incidence rates of cancer in the general population indicates the poor PPV of any study because of the low prior probability of disease. One therefore would have to reject the blind use of imaging in detecting a possible malignancy. What indeed is the designation *cancer suspect* but our solemn invocation of the unknown in the forest of the obscure? Obscure, because in the absence of some clinical indicators, such as bowel complaints, a breast mass, anemia, a positive chest radiograph, or elevated prostate-specific antigen, there is simply no logical place to begin.

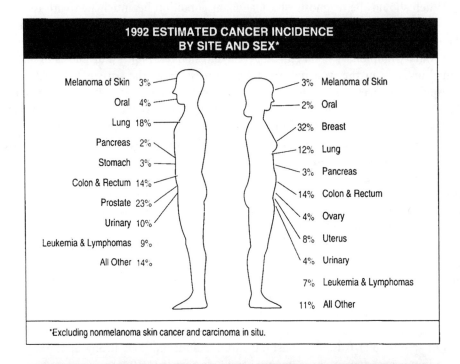

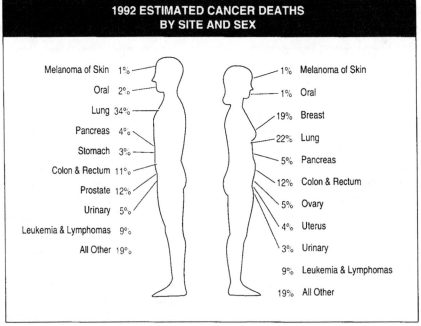

Figure 9.1. 1992 Estimated cancer incidence and death by site and sex. Reprinted by permission from *CA* (1992;42:21).

Table 9.1. Estimated Number of New Cancer Cases in the United States in the Year 1990 by Site

Cancer site	Number	Percentage
Lung	157,000	15
Colon and rectum	155,000	15
Breast	150,900	15
Prostate	106,000	10
Bladder	49,000	5
Non-Hodgkin's lymphoma	35,600	3
Uterus (endometrium)	33,000	3
Oral cavity and pharynx	30,500	3
Pancreas	28,100	3
Leukemia	27,800	3
Melanoma	27,600	3
Kidney	24,000	2
Stomach	23,200	2
Ovary	20,500	2
Brain and other nervous system	15,600	2
Cervix	13,500	1
Liver	13,100	1
Larynx	12,300	1
Thyroid	12,100	1
Multiple myeloma	11,800	1
Esophagus	10,600	1
Hodgkin's disease	7,400	<1
Testis	5,900	<1
All other sites[a]	69,500	7
Total	1,040,000	100

Reprinted by permission from Henderson E, Ross RK, Pike MC. Toward the primary prevention of cancer. *Science* (1991;254:31–38). Projections for 1990 were obtained for the American Cancer Society based on the incidence of cancer for 1984–1986 applied to the 1990 estimated total U.S. population.
[a]The number of new cases of Kaposi's sarcoma has been increasing as a sequelae of HIV infection. These nonepithelial cancers of the skin were not separately estimated in this report. However, the actual number of cases in 1990 may exceed the number of testis cancer cases.

Table 9.2. 1992 Estimated Cancer Deaths by Site and Sex, Listed in Order of Frequency

	Males	Percentage	Females	Percentage
1.	Lung	34	Lung	22
2.	Colon/rectum	11	Breast	19
3.	Prostate	12	Colon/rectum	12
4.	Leukemia/lymphoma	9	Leukemia/lymphoma	9
5.	Urinary	5	Ovary	5
6.	Pancreas	4	Pancreas	5
7.	Stomach	3	Uterus	4
8.	Melanoma (skin)	2	Urinary	3
9.	Oral	2	Oral	1
10.	All other	19	Melanoma (skin)	1
11.			All Other	19
Total		100		100

Adapted from Boring et al. (4).

Imaging of Metastatic Disease in the Cancer Patient

In taking a pragmatic approach, preferring to emphasize common vs. rare conditions, we will discuss only the major malignancies. Thus, no attempt is made to be exhaustive, but, rather, the discussion is condensed. The principal aim is to outline a general imaging approach to cancer spread in both the initial and late stages of disease, *given a known site of tumor origin and the known frequency of associated regional and distant organ involvement.* The discussion of diagnostic methods is limited to the major indirect imaging modalities. This excludes endoscopic and other direct invasive methods, which might be useful for making the initial diagnosis of malignancy *when there are clear clinical indications for their use.* For example, upper EGD is never a substitute for the upper GI series as a first test in suspected stomach cancer any more than bronchoscopy precedes the chest radiograph or CT in lung malignancy. Except for the chest X-ray, none of these procedures, in point of fact, are screening tests. Even if they were, screening for cancer in a population at low risk already has been shown to be self defeating.

This may change one day, however. Newer imaging techniques include radioimmunoscintigraphy, an evolving scintigraphic method using radiolabeled immune-specific tumor markers, such as monoclonal antibodies, to image malignant tumors. Because this technique is presently in a state of research and development and not generally available, it will be omitted from further discussion. Use of such radiolabeled antibody markers one day may revolutionize diagnostic imaging of malignant disease, but these compounds are still of unproven effectiveness, their advent is some years away, and moreover their use will almost certainly be limited to diagnosis of tumor spread, not the primary diagnosis of malignancy. In addition, certain seldom-used imaging methods also have been omitted from discussion, for example, radionuclide lymphoscintigraphy, the imaging of regional lymph nodes with intracutaneous or rectus sheath injection of radioactive-labeled colloid. This technique, especially useful for identifying internal mammary and pelvic nodes before radiation therapy, never has gained significant clinical acceptance. Furthermore, the diagnosis of cancer already has been suspected by the presence of a regional mass. Conventional lymphangiography, a much more difficult technique of lymph node visualization and of limited clinical value, has been discussed briefly in Chapter 2.

Principles and Purposes of the Cancer Staging Process

The official cancer staging schemes now reflect the orthodoxies of the "splitters" rather than the "lumpers." We now have a profusion of exquisitely detailed categories which depend on criteria sometimes difficult, if not impossible, to validate. The most widely used staging method promises an admirable framework on which to base a clinical approach to malignancy. In this system, adopted by both the International Union against Cancer and the American Joint Committee on Cancer (AJJC), classification is based on the logical premise that cancers of similar histology or site of origin share similar patterns of growth and spread. This so-called TNM system uses the elegant and simple formulation, "the size of the untreated primary tumor (T) increases progressively, and at some point in time regional lymph node involvement (N) and, finally, distant metastases (M) occur" (5). Thus, staging is based on the initial size, extent and invasiveness of the primary tumor, as in "T1, T2, ..." etc. Lymph node spread is based on extent and group of nodes involved, "N1, N2, ..."

etc., and finally distant metastases are designated as "M1," sometimes "M1a, M1b," etc. The various stages, 0, I, II, III, and IV, are derived from combinations and permutations of Ts, Ns, and Ms, differing for each tumor of origin. Stage 0 and I cancers are the earliest, smallest, and most localized, progressing to stage IV, the most invasive and far-advanced, usually with distant spread. For example, a stage IIIA breast cancer might be represented as T1, N2, or M0. Other designations, however, should be noted, because they are of fundamental importance and indicate, respectively, "*no evidence* of primary tumor, lymph node extension, or metastases" (T0, N0, or M0) and "evidence of primary tumor, lymph node, or distant metastasis *cannot be assessed*" (TX, NX, or MX), etc. (5) (emphasis added). These commonly used categories are an acknowledgment of the frequent undecidability of cancer staging.

Thus, cancer staging classification schemes suffer a fatal flaw in that they depend on ascertaining three frequently unascertainable facts about cancer: extent of primary tumor, the presence or absence of lymph node involvement, and distant spread. Before we follow a patient for a few months, years, or until death, or even after we subject the patient to surgery, staging in many cases becomes, at best, an exercise in begging the question, at worst, a retrospective clinical guess. No matter how involved or simple these schema become, the clinician often is faced with the basic enigma: can one determine with any precision how far a cancer has progressed at the time of its discovery? For some malignancies, in particular those with good responses to surgery, radiation, or chemotherapy, the accuracy of staging may be proven only retrospectively. In some malignancies such as colon cancer, staging at operation is useful at least prognostically. But where survival is poor, as in cancers of the lung, pancreas, stomach, esophagus, and ovary, the staging process is usually imprecise and therefore of dubious clinical value. An unrelated yet important problem is the attempt to correlate tumor stages with clinical response to chemotherapeutic drugs in various investigative drug trials. Considering only the patient accrual problem, for breast cancer alone there are more than 3460 permutations of Ts, Ns, and Ms. An interesting article gives cogent practical reasons for abandoning the TNM staging of (at least) breast cancer (6). Obtaining properly matched controls based on cancer staging for chemotherapeutic and combined chemoradiation therapy trials is the most difficult problem in accurately assessing results of treatment protocols.

Sites of Malignant Metastatic Disease

A classic and oft-quoted paper by Abrams et al. (7) gives invaluable statistical information about the spread of various malignant conditions to specific organs based on 1000 autopsies of cancer patients. As the authors were aware, the study suffers the obvious drawbacks of any autopsy analysis that attempts to quantify findings in specific conditions. The numbers are derived from results in dead subjects, not living patients. At the very least the clinical stage of disease at the time of death and the cause of death would have to be taken into account for any valid estimate of the likely or "true" incidence of organ metastases in given tumors during life.

However, we can be confident that the percentages listed in this and other studies represent an upper limit for metastatic organ involvement. For example, the maximum numbers of living patients with lung cancer having bone metastases hardly would be expected to exceed the percentages reported in autopsy figures. Table 9.3 summarizes the autopsy incidence of bone metastases in several malignancies from various series, whereas Table 9.4 relates a positive bone scan to clinical stages of

Table 9.3. Incidence of Bone Metastases at Autopsy in Several Malignant Diseases: General Overview

Site of primary	Percent involvement
Common tumors of adulthood	
Bladder	12–25
Breast	50–85
Hodgkin's	50–70
Kidney	30–50
Lung	30–50
Melanoma	30–40
Prostate	50–70
Thyroid	40
Common tumors of childhood	
Ewing's	60
Neuroblastoma	80
Osteosarcoma	25
Wilms	1–10

Reprinted by permission from *Seminars in Nuclear Medicine* (1984;XIV(4):277–286).

Table 9.4. Yield of Positive Bone Scans According to Clinical Stage

	True positive scans
Clinical stage I	6/307 (2%)
Clinical stage II	14/215 (2.3%)
Clinical stage III	36/193 (18.6%)

Reprinted by permission from *Seminars in Nuclear Medicine* (1984;XIV(4):277–286).

Table 9.5. Incidence of Liver Metastases Reported at Autopsy in 1000 Malignant Tumors (6)

Site of primary	Percent with liver involvement
Colon	65
Pancreas	63
Ovary	52
Breast	61
Rectum	47
Stomach	45
Lung	40
Kidney	27

Adapted from Barr and Baum (6).

breast cancer (8). Table 9.5 shows the frequency of liver metastases at autopsy in various neoplasms in Abrams et al.'s series (7). Despite the shortcomings of this and other autopsy studies, the authors and investigators preceding them have performed a priceless service to clinicians and cancer researchers alike. Because the autopsy will probably never again regain its preeminent place in the study of disease, we are fortunate to have had this invaluable information compiled and captured for us more than 40 years ago.

Why is this knowledge so important for present-day clinicians? By carefully noting the frequency of organ involvement in various tumors, we can choose the most efficient methods for imaging tumor dissemination. Furthermore, we obtain a much deeper insight into the most striking and discouraging aspect of cancer, its relentless spread throughout the organism. Even though this data on the biological nature of

Table 9.6. Incidence of Metastatic Involvement in 1000 Consecutively Autopsied Cases of Carcinoma

Site, metastasis	Frequency of involvement	Percent Involvement
Abdom. nodes	495	49.5
Liver	494	49.4
Lungs	465	46.5
Mediast. nodes	421	42.1
Pleura	277	27.7
Bone	272	27.2
Adrenal	270	27.0
Peritoneum	269	26.9
GI tract[a]	204	20.4
Diaphragm	183	18.3
Pericardium	131	13.1
Kidney	126	12.6
Pancreas	116	11.6
Ovary	111	11.1
Spleen	90	9.0
Cervical nodes	89	8.9
Axillary nodes	63	6.3
Uterus	59	5.9
Gallbladder	58	5.8
Breast	50	5.0
Skin	44	4.4
Ureter	43	4.3
Heart	38	3.8
Bladder	36	3.6
Esophagus	31	3.1
Inguinal nodes	20	2.0
Thyroid	19	1.9
Fallopian tubes	19	1.9
Pituitary	18	1.8
Common bile duct	12	1.2
Vagina	11	1.1
Prostate	7	0.7
Trachea	6	0.6
Pineal gland	4	0.4
Cervix	3	0.3
Testes	3	0.3
Epiglottis	2	0.2
Parotid gland	2	0.2
Pharynx	1	0.1
Tongue	1	0.1
Salivary glands	1	0.1
Brain[b] (cerebral)	43	17.6
(dural)	24	9.8
Spinal cord[c] (dural)	4	7.7

Reprinted by permission from *Cancer* (1950;3:74–85).
[a]The majority of these were serosal.
[b]These figures are based on 244 examinations of the brain.
[c]These figures are based on 52 examinations of the spinal cord.

malignancy is disheartening, it enables us to draw some helpful, if sobering, clinical conclusions.

In Table 9.6 the incidence of metastatic involvement by organ is listed for all of Abrams et al.'s 1000 cases (7). This table, of course, reflects the frequency distribution of cancers seen at necropsy, the resultant of both incidence and mortality rates in the general population at the time of the study. Although some of these respective rates, particularly breast, colon, Hodgkin, uterine, and testicular, have changed somewhat over the years, they have not done so sufficiently to alter our interpretation of the data. From these rates of organ involvement, we note the following:

In 42–50% of all cases, metastases were found in four sites: *abdominal and mediastinal nodes, liver, and lung.* In more than 25% of cases, four other principal sites were involved: *pleura, bone, peritoneum, and adrenal.*

Even with CT and MRI, our methods of tumor detection are relatively insensitive for five of these most common sites: lung, thoracic and abdominal nodes, pleura, and peritoneum. For two of the remaining sites, liver and bone, our techniques are reasonably good, but the importance of the adrenal, for which we have available good scintigraphic methods, is rarely acknowledged in the metastatic survey. For the fastest growing tumors, those with such appalling survival rates—lung, esophagus, stomach, and pancreas again come to mind—it is probable that the figures of tumor spread at the time of diagnosis begin to resemble autopsy statistics, i.e. those patients harboring malignancies with the worst prognoses almost certainly have undetectable metastases at diagnosis.

LUNG METASTASES

One of the most frequent cryptogenic sites of cancer spread may well be the lung. The 50% figure in Abrams et al.'s series may *seem* high (7), but pulmonary microemboli occur much more frequently than clinicians realize, because, as Kvale observes (9), the lungs are the first downstream capillary sieve from the systemic venous circulation. In an important study, Winterbauer and colleagues (10) reviewed 366 autopsies of patients with five types of tumors and found that pulmonary tumor embolism occurred in 26%, including 17% in breast cancer. The lung is an organ where metastases, if present, are rarely detected during life unless they are extremely widespread. The problem of dyspnea in cancer patients is a common one. Pneumonia usually can be diagnosed by the presence of cough, fever, leukocytosis, and findings on physical examination and the chest radiograph, whereas pulmonary embolism, known to be increased in cancer patients, usually can be diagnosed by clinical findings plus ventilation-perfusion lung scintigraphy. To these two causes now must be added a third, tumor embolization, the true frequency of which can only be guessed at. Most of these patients will have abnormal, usually "intermediate," probability lung scans for typical pulmonary embolism but with a characteristic appearance called "contour mapping" (11), normal chest X-rays, and *normal pulmonary angiograms.* The imaging findings in 24 cases are summarized in Table 9.7 (12).

What should be done when scintigraphy shows this characteristic pattern of tumor involvement in cancer patients with dyspnea? Certainly, one should avoid angiographic studies, because little can be done to help these patients. This is a complex problem which is thoroughly discussed in the important editorial referred to above (9). We bring it up only to suggest that the presence of undetectable pulmonary metastatic disease may be one of the most important reasons for inaccurate tumor staging. That the duration of symptoms before death was so short in these recorded cases indicates that lung metastases (tumor emboli) must have been present for some time before presentation, by which time lung involvement was obviously widespread. Certainly, we need no reminders of our frequent failure to appreciate the already advanced state of many malignancies.

Table 9.7. Summary of Results of Imaging Studies in 24 Cases of Microscopic Pulmonary Tumor Embolism

Type of cancer	Av duration of pulmonary symptoms (wk)	Clear lung fields on CXR	Perfusion defects (mult. seg)	Emboli on angio
Breast (16)	3	12/16	11/14	0/8
Adenoca (2)	5	2/2	2/2	1/2
Hepatoma (2)	5	2/2	2/2	1/2
Prostatic (1)		1/1		0/1
Gastric (1)		1/1	1/1	
Pancreatic (1)	20	1/1	1/1	0/1
Bladder (1)	>1	1/1	1/1	0/1
		20/22	18/21	2/15

Adapted with permission from Schriner et al. (11).

Approaches to Cancer Diagnosis, Prognosis, and Treatment

In the following sections we will address the important question, given a patient with a primary malignancy of site A, how do we best determine the extent of tumor spread to sites B, C, D, and E, in order to make the best initial treatment decisions? Aside from prognostic information, therapeutic considerations are the only justifiable reason for the cancer work-up. In the past, treatment for most tumors was only a matter of the appropriate operation, sometimes preceded or followed by radiation therapy. Today, the question of chemotherapy for virtually every cancer—no matter at what cost (or benefit) to the patient—continues to generate quiet if surreptitious controversy in some quarters. Therapeutic drug trials, of course, will and should continue full speed. Moreover, no one can question the enormous effectiveness of chemotherapy and the resulting improved survival seen in Hodgkin lymphoma and cancers of the breast, testis, and other organs. But if there are lingering questions about therapeutic results in some malignancies, inevitably there will be questions of means. The selling of unproven chemotherapy has had secondary effects. This is because therapy *drives* diagnosis. Therapeutic effectiveness has to be validated, not promoted with unfounded claims, otherwise diagnosis, as well as therapy, become deceptive and expensive games and sometimes dangerous clinical preoccupations.

For example, in pancreatic cancer the average survival is 14 weeks, and fewer than 10% of patients are alive 1 year after diagnosis (13). This figure has not changed appreciably over the past 22 years. Chemotherapy is of doubtful help. "Trivial differences may exist between regimens, but the vast majority of patients are not benefited" (14).

The litany continues; from 1973 to 1983 the average 5-year survival rate of esophageal carcinoma was 5%. Again, according to the authoritative 1989 edition of the classic text on cancer, "Without . . . proof (of survival advantage for prospectively randomized patient trials using various therapies), *chemotherapy will join surgery and radiation as another toxic, inadequate therapy for primary cancer of the esophagus*" (15) (emphasis added).

In gastric cancer, like other malignancies, various clinical trials continue to face study design problems when investigators attempt to assess the results of chemotherapy. In any chemotherapeutic trial, the patients most likely to "respond" obviously will be those with limited disease; those least likely to respond will be those with dissemination. Unfortunately, at the outset of a prospective trial it is frequently impossible to stratify or stage such patients accurately. For nonprotocol gastric cancer patients, in using radiation plus chemotherapy, "It should be emphasized that there are no combined modality regimens that are dramatically successful, and there is continued need for active investigation in the use of combined radiation plus chemotherapy" (16).

In combined treatment with radiation and chemotherapy of nonsmall cell carcinoma of the lung with curative intent, "... *there remains no convincing evidence that chemotherapy (plus) ... high-dose radiation therapy reproducibly and significantly increases the median survival ...*" (17) (our emphasis). Furthermore, in patients having either "curative" surgery or marginal resection of more advanced disease, "... there seems to be *no role* at this time for routine chemoradiation therapy after resection of nonsmall cell cancer ..." (17). One hopeful sign on the horizon is the development of various novel chemotherapeutic agents. In renal cancer a promising new biological treatment with lymphokine-activated cells plus interleukin-2 is now being pioneered by Rosenberg and colleagues at the Surgical Branch of the National Cancer Institute (18).

For the present, however, it is clear that chemotherapy of many malignancies is still investigational and associated with significant toxicity with resultant mortality. Remission, when it can be demonstrated, is often measured in weeks, and lengthened survival is often difficult to demonstrate convincingly. Quality of life is rarely improved and often degraded. In patients not enrolled in therapeutic drug trials there are important implications for pursuing a diagnosis or staging a tumor at all cost. This approach makes for a depressing fatalism, but for the far-advanced patient, and some not so far-advanced, there may be meager benefits. We, and no doubt others, see patients after surgery and radiation with advanced lung and esophageal cancer who were subjected to needlessly repeated endoscopies, CTs, MRIs, and bone scintiscans in vain attempts to *visualize* the reason for continued uncontrollable thoracic pain so that further "palliative chemo" could be given. Many such patients already have been on continuous narcotics and had presumed invasion of the spinal roots or thoracic plexuses but no evidence on imaging. Many physicians continue to receive requests for multiple imaging studies of patients with documented, widespread metastatic disease — for whom therapy is largely hopeless. It is impossible to estimate how many patients with advanced malignancies have had needless and futile diagnostic imaging studies.

BREAST CANCER

Table 9.8 (7) indicates the autopsy site of metastases in 167 consecutive cases of breast cancer. Notable is the extremely high incidence of lung, pleural, bone, liver and mediastinal node, adrenal, and other distant involvement at death. Fortunately, widespread metastatic disease is exceedingly unusual in the newly discovered case of breast cancer. This is because breast cancer is among the more slowly growing tumors, and the natural history of breast malignancy is characterized by a long duration often measured in years or decades. Even though some patients have an aggressive form of the disease and do poorly, "an equal number have such indolent disease that it is difficult to demonstrate that therapy has *any effect at all* on survival" (19).

Combined studies previously shown in Table 9.4 indicate that in stage I or II disease, the yield of true-positive bone scans is only 2% and even in stage III less than

Table 9.8. Metastases of 167 Consecutive Autopsied Cases of Carcinoma of the Breast

Site, metastasis	No. with metastases	Percent
1. Lung	129	77.2
2. Bone	122	73.1
3. Mediast. nodes	111	66.5
4. Pleura	108	64.7
5. Liver	102	61.1
6. Adrenal	90	53.9
7. Abdom. nodes	74	44.3
8. Pericardium	59	35.3
9. Axillary nodes[a]	55	32.9
10. Peritoneum	41	24.6
11. Diaphragm	41	24.6
12. Ovary	39	23.4
13. Breast	36	21.6
14. Skin	31	18.6
15. Spleen	28	16.8
16. Cervical nodes	25	15.0
17. GI tract[b]	24	14.4
18. Pancreas	23	13.8
19. Kidney	21	12.6
20. Pituitary	15	9.0
21. Heart	14	8.4
22. Uterus	14	8.4
23. Ureter	13	7.8
24. Gallbladder	11	6.6
25. Thyroid	9	5.4
26. Esophagus	7	4.2
27. Fallopian tubes	6	3.6
28. Pineal gland	4	2.4
29. Inguinal nodes	4	2.4
30. Bladder	4	2.4
31. Common bile duct	3	1.8
32. Vagina	2	1.2
33. Trachea	1	—
34. Parotid gland	1	—
35. Brain[c] (cerebral)	13	28.8
(dural)	15	33.3
36. Spinal cord[d]	3	—

Reprinted by permission from *Cancer* (1950;3:74–85).
[a]This is not an accurate figure, since many of the patients had had axillary-node dissections.
[b]The majority of these were serosal.
[c]These figures are based on 45 examinations of the brain.
[d]These figures are based on eleven examinations of the spinal cord.

20% (8). Even with a PPV of 50%, however, if systemic or adjunctive chemotherapy is decided on, bone scintigraphy should be performed before therapy is initiated. If surgery alone with or without radiation is chosen, there is no compelling reason for initial bone scintigraphy.

Liver involvement is only rarely found in the usual patient with breast cancer. Despite 40% of patients with hepatic metastases found at autopsy, the number diagnosed during life using hepatic scintigraphy, CT, or ultrasound is vanishingly small. In three series quoted by Harbert (20) totaling 400 patients, the false-positive rates for liver scintigraphy were double the number of true-positive rates, 3% vs. 1.5.%. In one of these series of 234 patients with routine preoperative liver scintigraphy the true-positive rate was only 1%. Almost all patients with positive imaging studies will be far advanced and have hepatomegaly and significant abnormalities of liver function. Three patterns may be seen in these patients: a hepatocellular picture due to hepatic metastases, an obstructive picture secondary to involved nodes at the porta hepatis, and a combination of the two.

CT and MRI of the brain are extremely sensitive for the detection of brain metastases, but brain secondaries are almost never diagnosed antemortem in breast cancer except in the far-advanced patient, and then usually with accompanying neurological signs. The yield of these studies is therefore so low their use in the neurologically intact patient rarely can be justified.

Bilateral mammograms should be done in all patients before biopsy of a suspicious breast mass. This is necessary in order to detect any occult lesion in the ipsilateral or contralateral breast that also should be biopsied. Of course, *negative mammography in the presence of a suspicious breast mass is never a justification to avoid biopsy.* The discovery of additional lesions in the ipsilateral or contralateral breast obviously will have important implications for management.

There is no indication for the use of breast CT or MRI in primary breast tumor diagnosis at the present time. Neither of these modalities have been shown superior to plain mammography, and both are inferior in detecting calcification. New developments in MRI imaging of the breast, however, may change this in the future. Ultrasound study of the breast and its use alone or in combination with mammography already has been discussed. This modality is of most help in the younger patient with a breast mass, when cystic changes are a possibility, or in the older patient with recurrent benign cystic masses and equivocal mammography.

All breast cancers must be removed, regardless of their size and extent, otherwise they will cause local invasion and ultimately lead to open, draining exophytic tumors. Because staging cannot be completed before definitive surgery, which usually includes axillary node removal, the following procedure is advised.

Initial or Presurgical Assessment of the Breast Cancer Patient

1. Routine chest radiographs and bilateral mammography should be done before biopsy or definitive surgery in all breast cancer suspects.

2. Bone scintigraphy need not be done preoperatively but should be performed before adjunctive or systemic chemotherapy or within the first year after initial surgical/radiation therapy.

3. CT, MRI, and scintigraphy are not indicated in the preoperative assessment of these patients. Specifically, *liver scintigraphy should not be performed initially.*

Assessment of Advanced Breast Cancer

1. In all patients with stage III or IV disease or in the presence of unexplained musculoskeletal pain, bone scintigraphy should be performed.

2. If metastatic bone disease is discovered in any patient with breast cancer, serial bone scintigraphy should be performed at 4 to 8-month intervals to assess the progress of osseous disease and the response and need for further chemoradiation therapy.

3. All patients with osseous metastases in danger of pathological fracture of the long bones or threatened with vertebral collapse and imminent damage to the spinal cord should have much more frequent serial bone scintigrams, plain radiography, and/or CT. These studies should be used in appropriate combination and frequency,

particularly scintigraphy and CT, to determine progress of disease and the need for radiation treatment or to assess the response to radiation.

4. In the presence of unexplained hepatomegaly or hepatic dysfunction in advanced breast cancer, CT of the liver is the best indicator of metastases. Liver scintigraphy, preferably with the SPECT technique, however, may be substituted for CT in this setting without significant loss of sensitivity. In the case of an obstructive picture, hepatobiliary scintigraphy may be required along with CT to distinguish diffuse metastatic liver disease from involved nodes at the porta.

5. The development of any neurological signs or symptoms always raises the possibility of metastatic disease of the brain and calls for CT or MRI.

LUNG CANCER

Once the diagnosis of lung cancer has been made, the only important management decision is whether or not to attempt curative resection. This is a therapeutic issue only in patients with nonsmall cell tumors, about 80% of cases. In individuals, with small cell tumors surgery is not an option except in the rare patient with a localized peripheral tumor. In view of the extremely unfavorable prognosis of lung cancer, which has an average 5-year survival rate of 13% (21), we can only assume that the great majority, perhaps 75–80% of patients with nonsmall cell cancers have regional or distant spread at the time of diagnosis. This is borne out by various statistics on CT/MRI, and other imaging, which already have been reviewed in Chapter 8 (22–28). The purpose of preoperative imaging, therefore, is to identify those few patients likely to benefit from resection and save the remainder from futile and possibly fatal thoracotomy. Unfortunately, if CT is negative for regional adenopathy, 20–35% of patients still will be discovered to have micro- or macroscopic mediastinal or hilar involvement at surgery (22, 23). This means if CT is relied on to exclude regional spread (and frequently even if gallium is used), up to one-third of patients will still have futile thoracotomies.

The best staging results in lung cancer only can be obtained with multiple imaging studies that have as their purpose the detection of both regional and distant spread. If any cancer deserves a work-up for metastasis, lung cancer is the most important candidate. Because asymptomatic distant tumor spread to the brain, bone, liver, adrenals, or soft tissue may be seen in another 20–25% of patients (22, 28), and gallium scintigraphy has an important place in detection of primary and metastatic lung cancer (29–32), the following schema are based on the presumption that tumor dissemination, if present, is detectable in a sizable number of these cases.

Summary of Imaging Studies to be Used to Establish Operability in Patients with Nonsmall Cell Lung Cancer

1. Perform CT of the thorax. If positive for mediastinal node involvement, stop.

2. If CT is negative, proceed with total body gallium-67 scintigraphy to exclude mediastinal involvement in CT negative patients, and simultaneously to help exclude distant spread to brain, bone, adrenal, etc. If significant gallium uptake is seen in the lung lesion and also in the mediastinum or peripherally, the uptake can be assumed with more than 90–95% certainty to be in metastic foci.

3. If the gallium study is negative, the absence of metastatic disease still cannot be assumed. All such patients should undergo brain and upper abdominal CT, the latter to include liver, kidneys, and adrenal.

4. Total body bone scintigraphy should be performed if 1, 2, and 3 are negative.

5. Because of the high percentage of adrenal adenomas in the population, there is a distinct place for NP-59 adrenal scintigraphy in patients with positive CT for adrenal masses (see Chapter 8). This is because an adrenal mass found on CT without other evidence of metastasis in a patient with known cancer is *not necessarily metastatic.* Localization of NP-59 to the side opposite the CT abnormality (discordance) indicates the mass on CT is metastatic. Concordant uptake indicates benign adenoma. These findings are almost 100% specific. In lung cancer patients with an adrenal mass on CT and bilateral uptake with NP-59, the possibility of metastatic adrenal cancer is about 50% on the side of the CT abnormality, and the patient should have an adrenal biopsy before being subjected to thoracotomy.

6. *Only in the event that 1, 2, 3, and 4 (and, if indicated, 5) are negative should thoracotomy be performed.* This sounds very involved and could cost thousands of dollars in "preop" lung cancer work-ups. But compared to the cost and potential toll of unnecessary thoracotomy, the price is small indeed.

COLON AND RECTUM

> *Cancer's a funny thing:*
> *I wish I had the voice of Homer*
> *To sing of rectal carcinoma,*
> *Which kills a lot more chaps, in fact,*
> *Than were bumped off when Troy*
> *was sacked . . .*
>
> *J. B. S. Haldane*
> *Written while mortally ill with cancer.*

The management of colorectal cancer, unlike lung, is similar to that of breast and most other malignancies. Surgery may or may not be curative, but *in all cases it must be performed.* Otherwise, local extension, obstruction, or bleeding will ensue. It follows, therefore, that because the results will not influence therapy, preoperative imaging studies are largely unnecessary in colorectal carcinoma. Liver CT and scintigraphy, intraluminal ultrasound, lymphangiography, and lymphoscintigraphy all have been used for staging, but they have little to offer preoperatively, and neither positive nor negative findings have any implications for management compared to more definitive staging, which can only be done at surgery.

The only exception to this rule would be the use of liver imaging in the patient with advanced rectal cancer. CT at present is clearly preferable to MRI and more sensitive than scintigraphy in demonstrating hepatic metastases (28). In the presence of such metastases, the surgeon might well limit the extent of attempted primary resection. However, though CT has an overall sensitivity of 84%, it is only 50% sensitive in detecting liver metastases less than 1 cm in size.

In Table 9.9 (7) is listed the frequency of various organ metastases at autopsy in colon carcinoma. Autopsy findings in subjects with cancer, as we have already indicated, represent the upper limit of expected organ dissemination in the living patient. The table shows, as expected, that most metastases at death are found in intraabdominal organs, liver, nodes, serosa, etc., and in *lung*, but rarely in bone (9%). Thus, colon cancer metastatic to bone is so unusual that bone scintigraphy has little or no

Table 9.9. Metastases of 118 Consecutive Autopsied Cases of Carcinoma of the Colon

Site of metastasis	Total no. of cases	Percent metas.
Liver	77	65.3
Abdom. nodes	70	59.3
Lung	44	37.3
Peritoneum	33	30.0
Gastroint. tract[a]	32	27.1
Mediast. nodes	18	15.3
Adrenal	17	14.4
Ovary	16	13.6
Pleura	16	13.6
Diaphragm	13	11.0
Bone	11	9.3
Kidney	9	7.6

Reprinted by permission from *Cancer* (1950;3:74–85).

place in this malignancy, except in extremely rare cases with compelling local findings such as bone pain.

Summary of Preoperative Imaging in Colorectal Cancer

We assume that complete colonoscopy/barium enema always has been performed to establish the diagnosis and exclude the presence of synchronous colonic tumors, which may be present in 3–5% of cases (33, 34). Beyond this and the routine chest radiograph, which always should be done preoperatively in cancer surgery, it is rarely productive to perform any other routine preoperative imaging studies in cases of colorectal cancer (35). The only exception would be the use of liver CT to exclude metastasis when, in the opinion of the surgeon, this knowledge would influence the extent of attempted surgical resection.

Table 9.10 is from Cohen's, Shank's, and Friedman's recommendations for follow-up of patients after potentially curative surgical treatment (36). They do not recommend routine postoperative imaging other than regular colonoscopy and yearly chest radiography. (We would add yearly barium enema and make colonoscopy less frequent, depending on the circumstances.) According to the authors, chest, abdominal, or pelvic CT, and abdominal, renal, or pelvic ultrasonography should be performed only if indicated by elevated carcinoembryonic antigen levels or clinical findings. The question of routine yearly CT for liver metastases would seem to depend on figures documenting efficacy of chemotherapy in this tumor.

Imaging in Other Malignancies
ESOPHAGUS, GASTRIC, AND PANCREATIC CANCER

It is more often appropriate to stop rather than to continue imaging patients who have been diagnosed with any of these malignancies. Beyond the use of chest radiography CT, esophagoscopy, esophagogram, and the upper GI, the attempt to stage esophageal, gastric, or pancreatic cancers preoperatively is usually an exercise in futility and in any event has little or no implication for management. It is lamentable that these particular cancers have such dismal prognoses. Their respective 5-year survival rates have improved slightly between 1960–1963 and 1981–1985, from 4% to 7.5% for esophagus, 10% to 14.7% for stomach, and 1% to 2.7% for pancreas (4, 37). However, when mortality is corrected for changes in incidence, the true survival rates

Table 9.10.   General Guidelines for Follow-Up of Patients After Potentially Curative Surgery

Procedure/test	Frequency	Comment
History/examination	Every 3–4 mo for 3 yr, then every 6 mo for 2 yr	Detects ⅓ of recurrences
Fecal occult blood	Same	
Sigmoidoscopy	Same	Only if anastomosis in pelvis
Colonoscopy	Preoperatively or 4–6 mo postoperatively, then every 6–36 mo	Every 3 yr once free of polyps
Chest x-ray	Yearly	
CEA	Every 2-4 mo	
Liver chemistries		
Chest CT		
Abdominal CT		
Pelvic CT	As indicated by findings on history, examination, or elevated CEA levels	
Liver–spleen scan		
Liver US		
IVP		
Bone scan		

Reprinted by permission from DeVita Jr VT, Hellman S, Rosenberg SA, eds. *Cancer. Principles and Practice of Oncology.* 3rd ed. Philadelphia: J. B. Lippincott Co. (1989:945).

for cancers of esophagus and pancreas have actually decreased; only stomach cancer has improved slightly (Sturman, M. F., Pilipski, M., manuscript in preparation). These figures suggest that 25 years of cancer therapy have done little to alter the outlook of patients with these three malignancies.

Esophageal cancer may not be operable at the time of initial diagnosis because of extent of disease or for purely medical reasons, such as the presence of chronic obstructive lung disease or cardiac conditions. Gastric cancer usually requires an initial operation even though the patient may subsequently prove to be unresectable at surgery. (Obviously, both esophageal and gastric cancers will be diagnosed by EGD after radiographic and clinical indications.) In pancreatic cancer, CT imaging or occasionally laparoscopy at the time of diagnosis often helps avoid unnecessary surgery by demonstrating the presence of extensive and inoperable disease.

Clinical or imaging evidence of distant metastases is extremely unusual in esophageal carcinoma, but autopsy studies demonstrate that dissemination is almost always present before death (38, 39). At the time of diagnosis most of these metastatic deposits probably are already present subclinically in multiple sites, including lung, pleura, stomach, peritoneum, adrenal gland, brain, liver, and bone. Even if metastases could be imaged, it is of no practical help in management. In one study, *94% of patients had residual tumors locally at postmortem;* 9% had only local tumors, and 85% had associated metastases (40). Synchronous malignancies of the upper respiratory or digestive tract occur 5–12% of the time with esophageal and lung cancers (41–43). Thus, associated tumors of the oral cavity, pharynx, head, and neck are seen in a significant number of esophageal cancers. Associated laryngeal cancer is more often seen in association with lung tumors. This indicates that all patients with esophageal cancer should have thorough examination of the head, neck, and oropharynx, and laryngoscopic screening to exclude coexistent malignancy. Assuming the patient can withstand a thoracotomy with or without laparotomy and regardless of the presence of tumor spread, palliative surgical resection should be attempted, followed by radiation therapy. Thus, preoperative imaging for distant metastases is generally unrewarding, because it will not influence management. The use of CT, scintigraphy, and other imaging studies in the patient with *advanced* esophageal cancer is also unrewarding and almost never of any practical value. The same dictum holds for advanced pancreatic and gastric malignancy. Neither liver-spleen nor bone scintigraphy is indicated on a routine basis in any of these cancers at the time of diagnosis because of the extreme rarity of detectable hepatic and osseous metastases (8, 20).

In gastric, pancreatic, and other biliary tract cancers with hepatocellular dysfunction, it is important to distinguish between metastatic involvement of the liver with or without the presence of extrahepatic obstruction due to direct extension or involved nodes at the porta. When these malignancies are associated with laboratory or clinical evidence of liver involvement, *CT of the liver and hepatobiliary scintigraphy always should be performed before any invasive procedures are contemplated.* If obstruction is demonstrated, the choice for palliative stent insertion lies between transhepatic and endoscopic placement. This is a *therapeutic, not a diagnostic,* decision.

Summary

1. Routine imaging procedures are not needed preoperatively in patients with esophageal, gastric, or pancreatic malignancies other than the usual preoperative chest radiograph, upper GI series and esophagogram, EGD, and CT of the chest or abdomen.

2. In advanced malignancies of these sites, routine liver-spleen and bone scintigraphy are of no demonstrable value. In the presence of jaundice or other signs of hepatic dysfunction, CT followed by hepatobiliary scintigraphy should be done to detect the presence of intra or extrahepatic obstruction.

3. ERCP or transhepatic cholangiography should be considered *only as therapeutic procedures and then only when functionally significant extrahepatic obstruction is demonstrated by hepatobiliary scintigraphy.*

GU TRACT CANCERS
Renal Cancer

We have already stressed the infrequent occurrence of cancer among unselected renal masses. In Lang's series (44), previously quoted, only 5.5% of such masses were malignant neoplasms. The IVP would be helpful in the presence of painless hematuria, unexplained pain, fever, or weight loss in a kidney tumor suspect, especially because of the possibility of detecting a mass anywhere in the GU tract. Otherwise, however, a better initial renal imaging study would be sonography. Recall the frequent finding of renal masses in asymptomatic patients, 90–95% of which prove to be benign cysts on ultrasonography. Most renal malignancies will first be suspected sonographically because of their solid appearance, and confirmed by CT followed with biopsy.

Renal and other GU malignancies are similar to colorectal and breast cancer in requiring primary surgical treatment at the time of initial diagnosis, regardless of extent of disease. In this sense, the purpose of diagnostic imaging is primarily to guide the surgeon and help him avoid surprises at the operating table. In order to discuss which studies are most valuable for this purpose, a summary of renal cancer staging and prognosis is helpful.

The most popular staging system for renal malignancy avoids the complexities of the standard American Joint Committee on Cancer method and is in use by most urologists in this country. This is the Robson modification of the system of Flocks and Kadesky (45). Stage I renal carcinoma is confined to the kidney; stage II extends through the renal capsule; and stage III involves the renal vein or inferior vena cava (IIIA) or the renal hilar nodes (IIIB). In stage IV the tumor has spread to adjacent organs or to distant sites. Five- and 10-year survival rates were reported in 1986: stage I, 88% and 66%; stage II, 67% and 35%; stage III, 40% and 15%; and stage IV, 2% and 0 (46).

In most tumors, CT with contrast suffices for visualizing tumor extent, local extension, and renal vein and nodal involvement. In a study of 111 patients CT correctly identified perirenal extension in 79%, lymph node involvement in 87%, renal vein involvement in 91%, and local infiltration into adjacent organs in 96% (47). Ancillary diagnostic studies of tumor extent include conventional or color Doppler ultrasonography and occasionally intravenous urography. In a minority of cases invasive imaging modalities also may be required to provide adequate information. In studying vascular anatomy of large renal tumors preoperatively, and the small indeterminate renal mass lesion, digital subtraction angiography combined with CT is a much safer technique than arteriography and generally should replace it (48). Inferior venacavography is sometimes performed rather than digital subtraction angiography in the presence of large tumors when there is a question of extension into the cava despite negative findings on CT and sonography. The addition of invasive studies to CT, MRI, and sonography is sometimes a matter of personal preference of the individual surgeon, who may insist on precise delineation of renal arterial anatomy preoperatively.

Approximately 45% of patients have localized renal disease at the time of presentation; 25% have locally advanced disease; and 30% present with metastatic disease, the most frequent sites being lung, 75%, soft tissue, 36%, bone 20%, and liver, 18% (49). Of these, however, only 1.5–3.5% present with solitary metastases. In this tiny subset of patients, resection of a "single" metastasis may be of therapeutic benefit. The problem remains to verify *single* vs. multiple metastases, a formidable challenge given the nature of tumor dissemination and our limited ability to detect it. According to Lineham et al. (50), patients presenting with an initially *solitary* metastatic lesion have a 30–40% chance of surviving for 5 years. This is to be contrasted with the 0–20% survival rate of patients with nonsolitary metastatic disease (50–52). If we assume some of these patients will benefit from excisional surgery and radiation, then in addition to chest radiography, chest, abdominal, and brain CT, and bone scintigraphy should be performed in all patients after initial surgery. "In patients presenting with a solitary metastasis to the lung, spine, or brain, initial or de novo surgery should be considered, usually followed by postoperative irradiation" (53). This issue still must be considered controversial, however, because of the difficulty in identifying a metastasis as truly solitary. If we accept the top figure of 3.5% of patients initially having solitary metastases, and assume very high sensitivities for imaging procedures, we can show the exceedingly low PPV of bone scintigraphy, as well as lung, brain, and liver CT in excluding additional secondaries. Given either a positive or negative bone scintiscan or lung, brain, or liver CT, the predictive values for the presence of a solitary metastasis are so low as to be virtually useless.

All of this suggests that the search for metastatic disease in renal malignancy has little if any implications for immediate therapy unless the patient is to be assigned to an investigative chemotherapy protocol. The most important determinant of prognosis remains the extent of local disease shown by CT or MRI at the time of presentation and, finally, at initial surgery.

Summary of Work-Up for Renal Cell Cancer

1. Once the diagnosis of renal malignancy has been made or suspected, CT or MRI should be done. No additional preoperative studies are generally indicated except in the following instances:

a. Large tumors, including those in which the surgeon requires specific information about vascular anatomy; and
b. The rare, indeterminate small mass lesion.

Both a and b will require invasive studies, either digital subtraction angiography, inferior venacavography, or, rarely, renal arteriography. Liver-spleen, bone, and other scintigraphy, brain CT and MRI, and other imaging studies are not indicated in the initial investigation of renal cancer patients unless there are specific indications. For example, bone scintigraphy would be appropriate in the presence of bone pain or an elevated alkaline phosphatase, brain CT or MRI with focal neurological findings, etc.

2. Serial chest radiographs and lung CT are the only ways to detect lung metastases from renal cell carcinoma. Whether this will have any implications for therapy depends on the outcome of further investigative drug trials.

Bladder Cancer

Although bladder cancer is localized in about 90% of all patients at the time of initial diagnosis, up to 80% will develop recurrences (54). Staging via cystoscopy and histological examination of transurethrally resected tumor is therefore extremely important in the management of early bladder carcinoma. In stage 0 (in situ) and superficial tumors, including stage T1 (A) (invasion into the lamina propria but not beyond—sometimes a difficult call), treatment is local resection. Despite the high recurrence rates, fewer than 25% of these patients will progress to invasive disease (53). Once the presence of localized disease is confirmed, diagnostic imaging such as pelvic CT or bone scintigraphy is unnecessary and therefore makes little sense unless the patient complains of pelvic or bone pain.

The difficulty with staging in relatively early bladder cancer is the discordance between clinical and pathological status, estimated as high as 50% in the important subset of patients with muscle-invading tumors (55, 56). Once the diagnosis of advanced or invasive bladder cancer has been made, the feasibility of radical cystectomy as a curative procedure should be considered; the role of segmental resection in transitional cell bladder carcinoma remains controversial. Distant metastases to lung or bone may be present even before urinary symptoms appear and of course are a contraindication to radical surgery. Dissemination, therefore, must be ruled out with chest radiography and bone scintigraphy before radical treatment is contemplated.

Two series report bone metastases at postmortem in 25% of bladder cancer patients (7, 57), but these are obviously patients in advanced stages of disease. Other studies report low incidence of osseous secondaries in stage I or II disease (only 5%), and only 15% with stage III or IV disease (58). Liver scintigraphy is probably worse than useless in bladder cancer. In a metaanalysis of four series totaling 166 patients collected by Harbert (20) only 1 true-positive and 9 false-positive scans were reported. Whether CT is helpful would depend on a high pretest likelihood of hepatic involvement, suggested by hepatomegaly or abnormal liver function tests. These figures are difficult to estimate from the autopsy figures in bladder cancer of 18% for liver-lung metastases and 14% for liver metastases only (59).

Summary

1. In the presence of documented early bladder cancer, i.e. in situ, superficial, and stage 1 (A) disease, no imaging studies other than the routine chest radiograph are indicated.

2. When invasive bladder carcinoma is diagnosed, radionuclide bone scintiscan and, if liver function tests are abnormal, CT of the liver should be performed before any radical bladder surgery is undertaken. The low predictive values of these studies, however, should be kept in mind when assessing the prognosis of patients about to undergo radical operation.

3. Before radiotherapy and any type of bladder cancer resection, CT or MRI of the pelvis is necessary in order to assess the extent and nodal spread of disease.

4. In addition, preoperative renal ultrasonography, IVP, or radionuclide renal scintigraphy is essential before bladder resection and/or radiotherapy. This is necessary to detect the presence of renal functional impairment and particularly lower tract urinary obstruction before treatment.

PROSTATE CANCER

Cancer of the prostate is the most common malignancy in men, with greater than 22% incidence, exceeding lung. It is estimated that this malignancy will cause 12% of all male cancer deaths in 1991. Many treatment choices and protocols exist for prostatic cancer depending on the extent of disease: different types of surgery, hormones, lymph node dissection, interstitial radionuclide therapy, and radiation. However, staging of this cancer presents many problems. Pelvic lymphangiography, for example, results in a high incidence of false-negative results, 22–40% according to several studies (60–62). CT likewise has many limitations, having an accuracy of 70% for assessing lymph node status and only 47% for determining tumor extent (63). For this reason the place of radical prostatectomy, like that of radical cystectomy, remains uncertain despite the development of potency-sparing operations.

Several authors have stressed the importance of bone scintigraphy in the staging of patients with clinically localized prostatic cancer in whom radiation or surgery is planned (64, 65). Prognostically this also is important because of the more favorable outlook with negative scintigraphy. Bone scintigraphy by identifying symptomatic bone metastases also has important implications for systemic and local therapy for osseous disease. Chest radiography is important, of course, in surveillance for lung secondaries. But here, the advantage would seem to be limited to prognostic and not therapeutic considerations.

ENDOMETRIAL, CERVICAL, AND OVARIAN CANCER

Gynecological malignancies represent 12% of all cancers in women and account for 9% of all female cancer deaths (4). Patients with advanced cervical and uterine malignancies do not as a rule die of distant visceral disease, though bone involvement occasionally complicates cervical cancer. Rather, these patients usually succumb to localized intraabdominal disease or locally invasive tumor and renal failure resulting from lower tract urinary obstruction. This development along with other complications may be an unfortunate result of local radiation therapy, an established treatment modality in these types of cancer. Patients with ovarian cancer in addition die of generalized abdominal metastatic disease, particularly that involving liver, peritoneum, mesentery, intestines, and other visceral structures.

Staging and, therefore, treatment approaches are beyond the scope of this section. However, the initial imaging approach to gynecological tumors is fairly limited, though it helps to keep certain facts in mind when considering them. In stage 0 cervical cancer, carcinoma in situ, and stages 1 (limited to the cervix) and II A (extension beyond cervix but not involving the parametrium), the outlook is good with average 5-year survival rates when treated by radiotherapy or radical hysterectomy of 70–80% (66). Survival rates, like those of other malignancies, decline precipitously with more advanced stages. In stage IIIB 5-year survival is 25–48% (66).

Because there is a significant lack of correlation between clinical and surgical staging in patients with all stages of cervical cancer (67), pretreatment imaging studies such as CT and MRI are of doubtful or limited value in these patients, though they probably should be performed. Pelvic ultrasound is likewise extremely limited in estimating tumor spread or extension, but it is the most effective screening test for the gamut of ovarian, uterine, and adnexal disease. Ultrasonography therefore should be used routinely before surgery or radiation therapy to alert the physician to coexisting conditions that may alter timing of treatment and choice of management.

Patterns of metastasis in gynecological tumors do not generally favor the use of scintigraphy in these patients. Moreover, as pointed out, most patients dying of these malignancies do so as a result of local, not distant, disease. Several studies quoted by Harbert (20) concluded that liver scintigraphy was of little or no value as screening in uterine, cervical, or ovarian cancer. Experiences reported in other studies indicate that bone and liver scintigraphy are of limited value in patients with more advanced gynecological cancers unless there are laboratory or clinical indications of hepatic or bone involvement (8, 68, 69). In early endometrial, cervical, and ovarian cancer, the yield of positive studies was close to 0, whereas even in advanced endometrial and ovarian cancers the percentages of positive scans were only 15% and 8%, respectively (68–70). Liver and bone scintigraphy in asymptomatic patients with early or advanced gynecological cancers are usually a waste of time and money (71).

We already have remarked on the extremely high percentage of patients with pelvic malignancies developing urinary tract obstructive disease during the courses of their illnesses, and the fact that renal failure is one of the most frequent causes of death. In Katz et al.'s series (71), 43% of their patients with advanced cervical cancer had unilateral or bilateral renal obstruction, but even in stage I and II disease 5% of patients had this complication. Furthermore, as previously mentioned, ureteral edema or trauma is much more frequent postoperatively than is generally appreciated. As a general rule, we advise postoperative or "baseline" as well as follow-up renal imaging studies in all patients with gynecological malignancies. Historically the IVP has been the favored renal imaging method, but in our view this procedure, which still entails some risk, is also distinctly inferior to the nuclear study in following gynecological malignancies. Although the pyelogram offers the advantages of improved anatomical detail, particularly of the collecting system, this is not the type of information that is of any practical help in managing the most important renal complications in these patients. Radionuclide renal scintigraphy has higher sensitivity in detecting minimal degrees of obstruction and renal functional impairment than does the IVP.

Summary

1. Preoperative or preradiation imaging in gynecological malignancies should include the routine chest radiograph, pelvic CT or MRI, ultrasonography, and the renal scintiscan using DTPA. Bone or liver scintigraphic studies are seldom, if ever, indicated.

2. Renal scintigraphy using DTPA is advisable within 4–6 weeks postoperatively to exclude the possibility of early GU problems resulting from inapparent surgical trauma. Obviously, if there are signs of urinary tract problems early in the postoperative period, renal scintigraphy should not be delayed.

3. The possible development of renal dysfunction and urinary obstructive disease should be monitored on a 6-month to yearly basis in all patients with pelvic cancers whether treated initially with radiation, surgery, or combination therapy.

4. If renal problems are encountered, scintigraphy should be performed as often as necessary to follow the progress of obstruction and response to any therapeutic intervention.

5. Bone, liver, and other scintigraphic studies are not helpful even in advanced gynecological malignancies unless clinical or laboratory studies suggest metastases to these sites, i.e. bone pain or development of hepatocellular dysfunction.

6. CT, and to a lesser extent MRI, remain the preferred imaging modalities for monitoring local tumor recurrence, extension, and development of regional nodal involvement.

7. Pelvic ultrasonography is usually of little value as a first study, compared with CT or MRI in monitoring the posttreatment gynecological cancer patient for local recurrence. This is because of its poor visualization of the posthysterectomy pelvis, particularly in imaging the lateral and posterior pelvic structures. However, ultrasound is useful in following the progress of known recurrent disease, especially if it is extensive.

CANCER OF UNKNOWN PRIMARY SITE

From 3–15% of all cases of malignant neoplasms seen in cancer referral centers occur in patients presenting with metastatic cancer arising from unknown primary sites (72). The reason for this variation may be largely due to definition. In some series, all patients presenting with metastases whose primary sites are not found after initial clinical examination are included. In others, eligibility is limited to patients with different cell types or to cases in which the primary sites remain unknown either during life or at autopsy. Management of these cancer patients is a frustrating and difficult problem, because by definition most patients are undiagnosed or undiagnosable. In addition, treatment is limited or virtually nonexistent. When autopsy data are analyzed it is clear that these patients pursue an entirely different clinical course from those whose primary sites are the first manifestation of disease. This leads to the inescapable conclusion that patients first presenting with metastatic malignancy of unknown origin have tumors of unusually aggressive biological behavior. Poor treatment results even in those patients whose primary sites are found underlines the fact that therapy is largely a losing proposition. The prognosis is abysmal, with a median survival of 2–6 months and less than 25% surviving beyond 1 year

Table 9.11. Histological Cell Types in Patients With a Microscopically Confirmed Diagnosis of Cancer of Unknown Primary Site

Cell type	No. of cases	Percent of total
Adenoca	485	38.2
Ca	201	15.8
Squamous cell ca	148	11.6
Neoplasm, malignant	95	7.5
Ca, anaplastic type	88	6.9
Papillary adenoca	40	3.1
Malignant melanoma	37	2.9
Mucinous adenoca	33	2.6
Mucin-producing adenoca	21	1.7
Neuroblastoma	13	1.0
Large cell ca	11	0.9
Sarcoma	10	0.8
Small cell ca	10	0.8
Clear cell adenoca	8	0.6
Amelanotic melanoma	8	0.6
Leiomyosarcoma	6	0.5
Carcinoid tumor	5	0.4
Mesothelioma	4	0.3
Infiltrating duct ca	3	0.2
Chorioca	3	0.2
Fibrosarcoma	3	0.2
Reticulosarcoma	3	0.2
Basal cell ca	3	0.2
Ca undifferentiated type	2	0.15
Malignant lymphoma	2	0.15

Other cell types with a frequency of 1 each include papillary ca, squamous cell ca (spindle cell type), transitional cell ca, cholangioca, signet ring cell ca, chromophobe ca, adenosquamous ca, Nodular melanoma, spindle cell sarcoma, liposarcoma, tumor cells (malignant), malignant tumor (small cell type), malignant tumor (fusiform cell type) rhabdomyosarcoma, mixed tumor (malignant), carcinosarcoma, mesenchymoma (malignant), and lymphosarcoma. Ca, Carcinoma. Reprinted by permission from *Cancer* (1986;57:122).

(73). This has led LeChavalier et al. (72) to conclude that, (because) "The site and number of metastases at the time of presentation have a greater prognostic importance than the knowledge of the primary site, (it) is the main reason that extensive, expensive, and time-consuming workups are both disappointing exercises and probably poor medical care." As the authors point out, "The essential issue remains as to whether the discovery of the primary tumor modifies the outcome of the disease when patients initially present with metastatic disease" (72). The answer to this question has clear implications for pursuing any diagnostic strategy.

In Table 9.11 are listed the histological types in a large retrospective series from Yale (73). It should be noted that by far the largest percentage of cases are adenocarcinoma. In the smaller French series (72) the biopsy results failed to help identify the sites of origin in 80% of 257 cases. (In 123 cases the primary site was suggested by the histological appearance, but was later proven correct in only 50 cases.) In this series, the primary sites were identified during life in 27%, at autopsy in 57%, and remained unidentified in 16%. Survival was identical in all groups.

A large number of diagnostic studies were performed in these patients, including chest radiographs in 302 patients, of which 184 or 61% were abnormal. Of 31% of these thought to be primary cancers, only 10% were confirmed. An upper GI series done in 150 patients showed "tumor-related findings" in 18 patients or 12%, but of these only 6 patients proved to have primary sites confirmed at autopsy, 5 gastric, 1 esophageal, so the positive yield was only 4%. Other multiple studies were performed, including barium enemas, IVPs, mammography, endoscopic examinations, etc.

Despite the depressing conclusions one is apt to draw from the above facts, an approach based on diagnostic and therefore therapeutic nihilism will be unacceptable to most cancer patients and their families. Furthermore, a small number of patients may indeed have treatable tumors, and some palliation may be possible. Important examples of this are the following:

1. The single head and neck lymph node with squamous cancer for which no primary site is found (negative otorhinolaryngology examination). Here, with presumed, but unproven head and neck cancer, radiation therapy produced almost 50% 3-year survival (74).

2. In women with positive undifferentiated cancer in axillary nodes the most likely site is breast, even in the presence of negative mammography. Such patients in whom no extramammary sources can be found should be treated with radiation, chemotherapy, or in most cases simple mastectomy (75).

3. There are always the rare patients whose metastatic lesions were misdiagnosed and in whom lymphomas were noted at autopsy. This was seen in 2 of 12 patients reported from Australia (76). When this happens it is a tragedy of undeniable magnitude. It always implies either mistaken microscopic diagnosis, an inadequate tissue specimen, or faulty communication between clinician and pathologist (77).

4. Embryonal cell carcinomas and certain hormone-sensitive tumors may be detected with new markers, i.e. immunoperoxidases and hormonal and steroid receptor assays (78–80).

5. Never overlook the rare case when the biopsy diagnosis of (primary or metastatic) cancer proves to be in error, and indeed there is no histological evidence of malignancy.

OTHER MALIGNANCIES

If the above discussion, condensed as it is, touches upon diagnostic issues in more than 70% of clinical malignancies, we must be forgiven for what may be regarded as serious omissions. In particular, the diagnostic approach to Hodgkin and non-Hodgkin lymphomas, which comprise about 7% of all malignancies, has not been discussed. These conditions are of great clinical importance and certainly in the case of Hodgkin are often among the most successfully treated. The use of gallium scintigraphy is especially important in staging and following the response to treatment of the Hodgkin lymphomas. The complexities of classification and staging, however, along with controversies surrounding the use of gallium scintigraphy, lymphography, and other techniques, make simplification as well as synthesis a formidable task. The medical imager surrenders here to the oncologist.

REFERENCES

1. Morley JE, Silver AJ, Miller DK, Rubenstein LZ. The anorexia of the elderly. Ann NY Acad Sci 1989; 575:50–59.
2. Olsen-Noll CG, Bosworth MF. Anorexia and weight loss in the elderly. (Causes range from loose dentures to debilitating illness.) Postgrad Med 1989;85(3):140–144.
3. Henderson BE, Ross RK, Pike MC. Toward the primary prevention of cancer. Science 1991;254: 1131–1138.
4. Boring CC, Squires TS, Tong T. Cancer statistics, 1992. CA 1992;42(1):19–20.

5. Beahrs OH, Henson DE, Hutter RVP, Myers MH, eds. Manual for Staging of Cancer Third Ed. American Joint Committee on Cancer. Philadelphia: J. B. Lippincott Co., 1988:3.
6. Barr LC, Baum M. Time to abandon TNM staging of breast cancer? Lancet 1992;339:915–917.
7. Abrams HL, Spiro R, Goldstein N. Metastases in carcinoma. Analysis of 1,000 autopsied cases. Cancer 1950;3:74–85.
8. McNeil BJ. Value of bone scanning in neoplastic disease. Semin Nucl Med 1984;XIV(4):277–286.
9. Kvale PA. The cancer patient with dyspnea: unusual cause [Editorial]. Mayo Clin Proc 1991;66(2):215–218.
10. Winterbauer RH, Elfenbein IB, Ball Jr WC. Incidence and clinical significance of tumor embolization to the lungs. Am J Med 1968;45(2):271–290.
11. Sostman HD, Brown M, Toole A, Bobrow S Gottschalk A. Perfusion scan in pulmonary vascular/lymphangitic carcinomatosis: the segmental contour pattern. AJR 1981;137(5):1072–1074.
12. Schriner RW, Ryu JH, Edwards WD. Microscopic pulmonary tumor embolism causing subacute cor pulmonale: a difficult antemortem diagnosis. Mayo Clin Proc 1991;66(2):143–148.
13. Moertel CG, Reitmeier RJ. Advanced Gastrointestinal Cancer: Clinical Management and Chemotherapy. New York: Harper & Row, 1969.
14. Brennan MF, Kinsella T, Friedman M. Cancer of the pancreas. In: DeVita Jr VT, Hellman S, Rosenberg SA, eds. Cancer. Principles and Practice of Oncology. 3rd ed. Philadelphia: J. B. Lippincott Co., 1989:830.
15. Rosenberg JC, Lichter AS, Leichman LP. Cancer of the esophagus. In: DeVita Jr VT, Hellman S, Rosenberg SA, eds. Cancer. Principles and Practice of Oncology. 3rd ed. Philadelphia: J. B. Lippincott Co., 1989:751.
16. MacDonald JS, Steele Jr G, Gunderson LL. Cancer of the stomach. In: DeVita Jr VT, Hellman S, Rosenberg SA, eds. Cancer. Principles and Practice of Oncology. 3rd ed. Philadelphia: J. B. Lippincott Co., 1989:790.
17. Minna JD, Pass H, Glatstein E, Ihde DC. Cancer of the lung. In: DeVita Jr VT, Hellman S, Rosenberg SA, eds. Cancer. Principles and Practice of Oncology. 3rd ed. Philadelphia: J. B. Lippincott Co., 1989:555.
18. Rosenberg SA, Lotze MT, Muul LM et al. A progress report on the treatment of 157 patients with advanced cancer using lymphokine-activated killer cells and interleukin-2 or high dose interleukin-2 alone. N Engl J Med 1987;316(15):889–897.
19. Henderson IC, Harris JR, Kinne DW, Hellman S. Cancer of the breast. In: DeVita Jr VT, Hellman S, Rosenberg SA, eds. Cancer. Principles and Practice of Oncology. 3rd ed. Philadelphia: J. B. Lippincott Co., 1989:1200.
20. Harbert JC. Efficacy of liver scanning in malignant diseases. Semin Nucl Med 1984;VolXIV(4):287–295.
21. Faber LP. Lung cancer. In: Holleb AI, Fink DJ, Murphy GP, eds. (American Cancer Society) Textbook of Clinical Oncology. Atlanta: The American Cancer society, 1991:194.
22. Sider L, Horejs D. Frequency of extrathoracic metastases from bronchogenic carcinoma in patients with normal-sized hilar and mediastinal lymph nodes on CT. AJR 1988;151(5):893–895.
23. Hirleman MT, Yiu-Chiu VS, Chiu LC, Schapiro RL. The resectability of primary lung carcinoma: a diagnostic staging review. J Comput Tomogr 1980;4(2):146–163.
24. Matthews MJ, Kanhouwa S, Pickren J, Robinette D. Frequency of residual and metastatic tumor in patients undergoing curative surgical resection for lung cancer. Cancer Chemother Rep 1973;4(2):63–67.
25. Aronchichk JM. CT of mediastinal lymph nodes in patients with non-small cell lung carcinoma. Radiol Clin North Am 1990;28(3):573–581.
26. McKenna Jr RJ, Libshitz HI, Mountain C. Roentgenographic evaluation of mediastinal nodes for preoperative assessment in lung cancer. Chest 1985;88(2):206–210.
27. Patterson GA, Ginsberg RJ, Poon PY, et al. A prospective evaluation of magnetic resonance imaging, computed tomography, and mediastinoscopy in the preoperative assessment of mediastinal node status in bronchogenic carcinoma. J Thorac Cardiovasc Surg 1987;94(5):679–684.
28. Sider L, Horejs D. Frequency of extrathoracic metastases from bronchogenic carcinoma in patients with normal-sized hilar and mediastinal lymph nodes on CT. AJR 1988;151(5):893–895.
29. Alazraki NP. Usefulness of gallium imaging in the evaluation of lung cancer. CRC Crit Rev Diagn Imaging 1980;13:249.
30. Alazraki NP, Ramsdell JW, Taylor A, Friedman PJ, Peters RM, Tisi GM. Reliability of gallium scan chest radiography compared with mediastinoscopy for evaluating mediastinal spread in lung cancer. Am Rev Respir Dis 1978;117(3):415–420.

31. DeMeester TR, Golomb HM, Kirchner P, et al. The role of gallium-67 scanning in the clinical staging and preoperative evaluation of patients with carcinoma of the lung. Ann Thorac Surg 1979;28(5): 451–464.

32. Neumann RD, Merino M, Hoffer PB. Gallium-67 in hilar and mediastinal staging of primary lung carcinomas. J Nucl Med 1980;21:32.

33. Enker WE, Dragacevic S. Multiple carcinomas of the large bowel: a natural experiment in etiology and pathogenesis. Ann Surg 1978;187(1):8–11.

34. Langevin JM, Nivatvongs S. The true incidence of synchronous cancer of the large bowel. Am J Surg 1984;147:330–333.

35. Cohen AM, Shank B, Friedman MA. Colorectal cancer In: DeVita Jr VT, Hellman S, Rosenberg SA, eds. Cancer. Principles and Practice of Oncology. 3rd ed. Philadelphia: J. B. Lippincott Co., 1989: 910–911.

36. Cohen AM, Shank B, Friedman MA. Colorectal cancer In: DeVita Jr VT, Hellman S, Rosenberg SA, eds. Cancer. Principles and Practice of Oncology. 3rd ed. Philadelphia: J. B. Lippincott Co., 1989: 945.

37. Cancer Incidence and Mortality in the United States. SEER. 1973–1981. U.S. department of Health and Human Service, U.S. Public Health Service, National Institutes of Health.

38. Mantravadi R, Lad T, Briele H, et al. Carcinoma of the esophagus: sites of failure. Int J Radiat Oncol Biol Phys 1982;8:1897.

39. Mandard AM, Chasle J, Marnay J, et al. Autopsy findings in 111 cases of esophageal cancer. Cancer 1981;48(2):329–335.

40. Anderson I, Lad T. Autopsy findings in squamous cell carcinoma of the esophagus. Cancer 1982;50: 1587.

41. Cahan WG. Multiple primary cancers of the lung, esophagus, and other sites. Cancer 1977;40(suppl 4):1954–1960.

42. Goldstein HM, Zornoza J. Association of squamous cell carcinoma of the head and neck with cancer of the esophagus. Am J Roentgenol 1971;131:791.

43. Shons AR, McQuarrie DG. Multiple primary epidermoid carcinomas of the upper aerodigestive tract. Arch Surg 1985;120(9):1007–1009.

44. Lang EK. Diagnosis of renal and parenchymal tumors. In: Skinner DG, deKernion JB, eds. Genitourinary Cancer. Philadelphia: W. B. Saunders, 1978:42.

45. Robson CJ, Churchill BM, Anderson W. The results of radical nephrectomy for renal cell carcinoma. J Urol 1969;101(3):297–301.

46. Golimbu M, Joshi P, Sperber A, Tessler A, Al-Askari S, Morales P. Renal cell carcinoma: survival and prognostic factors. Urology 1986;27(4):291–301.

47. Jashke W, Kaick GV, Peter S, et al. Accuracy of computed tomography in staging of Kidney tumors. Acta Radiol 1982;23:593–598.

48. Zabbo A, Novick AC, Risius B, Montie JE. Digital subtraction angiography for evaluating patients with renal carcinoma. J Urol 1985;134(2):252–255.

49. Maldazys JD, deKernion JB. Prognostic factors in metastatic renal carcinoma. J Urol 1986;136:376–379.

50. Lineham WM, Shipley WU, Longo DE. Cancer of the kidney and ureter. In: DeVita Jr VT, Hellman S, Rosenberg SA, eds. Cancer. Principles and Practice of Oncology. 3rd ed. Philadelphia: J. B. Lippincott Co., 1989:992.

51. Selli V, Hinshaw WM, Woodard BH, Paulson DF. Stratification of risk factors in renal cell carcinoma. Cancer 1983;52(5):899–903.

52. Bassil B, Dosoretz DE, Prout Jr GR. Validation of the tumor, nodes and metastasis classification of renal cell carcinoma. J Urol 1985;134(3):450–454.

53. Richie JP, Shipley WU, Yagoda A. Cancer of the bladder. In: DeVita Jr VT, Hellman S, Rosenberg SA, eds. Cancer. Principles and Practice of Oncology. 3rd ed. Philadelphia: J. B. Lippincott Co., 1989: 1011.

54. Richie JP, Shipley WU, Yagoda A. Cancer of the bladder. In: DeVita Jr VT, Hellman S, Rosenberg SA, eds. Cancer. Principles and Practice of Oncology. 3rd ed. Philadelphia: J. B. Lippincott Co., 1989: 1008.

55. Whitmore Jr WF, Batata MA, Ghoneim MA, Grabstald H, Unal A. Radical cystectomy with or without prior radiation in the treatment of bladder cancer. J Urol 1977;118(2):184–187.

56. Prout Jr GR. Radiation therapy and cystectomy. Urology 1984;23(suppl 4):104–109.

57. Kishi K, Hirota T, Matsumota K, Kakizoe T, Murase T, Fujita J. Carcinoma of the bladder: a clinical and pathological analysis of 87 autopsy cases. J Urol 1981;125(1):36–39.

58. Davey P, Merrick MV, Duncan W, Redpath AT. Bladder cancer: the value of routine bone scintigraphy. Clin Radiol 1985;36(1):77–79.
59. Gilbert HA, Kagan AR, Hintz BL. Patterns of metastasis. In: Weiss L, Gilbert HA, eds. Liver Metastases. Boston: G. K. Hall Medical Publishers, 1982:19–39.
60. Freiha FS, Pistenma DA, Bagshaw MA. Pelvic lymphadenectomy for staging prostatic carcinoma: is it always necessary? J Urol 1979;122(2):176–177.
61. Paulson DF, Uro-Oncology Research Group. The impact of current staging procedures in assessing disease extent of prostatic adenocarcinoma. J Urol 1979;121(3):300–302.
62. Hilaris BS, Whitmore WF, Batata MA, et al. Behavioral patterns of prostate adenocarcinoma following an I-125 implant and pelvic node dissection. Int J Radiat Oncol Biol Phys 1977;2:631–637.
63. Golimbu M, Morales P, Al-Askari S, Shulman Y. CAT scanning in staging of prostatic cancer. Urology 1981;18(3):305–308.
64. Lund F, Smith PH, Suciu S (EORTC Urological Group). Do bone scans predict prognosis in prostatic cancer? A report of the EORTC protocol 30762. Br J Urol 1984;5691:58–63.
65. Merrick MV, Ding CL, Chisholm GD, Elton RA. Prognostic significance of alkaline and acid phosphatase and skeletal scintigraphy in carcinoma of the prostate. Br J Urol 1985;57(6):715–720.
66. Hoskins WJ, Perez C, Young RC. Gynecologic tumors. In: DeVita Jr VT, Hellman S, Rosenberg SA, eds. Cancer. Principles and Practice of Oncology. 3rd ed. Philadelphia: J. B. Lippincott Co., 1989: 1114–1115.
67. Averette HE, Ford Jr JH, Dudan RC, et al. Staging of cervical cancer. Clin Obstet Gynaecol 1979; 133:814.
68. Kamath CRV, Maruyama Y, DeLand FH, Van Nagell JR. Role of bone scanning for evaluation of carcinoma of the cervix. Gynecol Oncol 1983;15(2):171–185.
69. Mettler Jr FA, Christie JH, Crow Jr NE, et al. Radionuclide bone scan, radiographic bone survey, and alkaline phosphatase. Studies of limited value in asymptomatic patients with ovarian carcinoma. Cancer 1982;50(5):1483–1485.
70. Salazar OM, Feldstein ML, DePapp EW, et al. Endometrial carcinoma. Analysis of failures with special emphasis on the use of initial preoperative external pelvic radiation. Int J Radiat Oncol Biol Phys 1977;2(11–12):1101–1107.
71. Katz Rd, Alderson PO, Rosenshein NB, Bowerman JW, Wagner Jr HN. Utility of bone scanning in detecting occult skeletal metastases from cervical carcinoma. Radiology 1979;133(2):469–472.
72. Le Chevalier T, Cvitkovic E, Caille P, et al. Early metastatic cancer of unknown primary origin at presentation: a clinical study of 302 consecutive autopsied patients. Arch Intern Med 1988;148(9): 2035–2039.
73. Altman E, Cadman E. An analysis of 1539 patients with cancer of unknown primary site. Cancer 1986; 57(1):120–124.
74. Jesse RH, Perez CA, Fletcher GH. Cervical lymph node metastasis: unknown primary cancer. Cancer 1973;31(4):854–859.
75. Copeland EM, McBride CM. Axillary metastases from unknown primary sites. Ann Surg 1973;178(1): 25–27.
76. Stewart JF, Tattersall MHN, Woods RL, Fox RM. Unknown primary adenocarcinoma: incidence of overinvestigation and natural history. Br Med J 1979;1(6177):1530–1533.
77. Moertel CG. Adenocarcinoma of unknown origin [Editorial]. Ann Int Med 1979;91(4):646–647.
78. Ruddon RW. Tumor markers in the recognition and management of poorly differentiated neoplasms and cancers of unknown primary. Semin Oncol 1982;9(4):416–426.
79. Mackay B, Ordone NG. The role of the pathologist in the evaluation of poorly differentiated tumors. Semin Oncol 1982;9(4):396–415.
80. Kiang DT, Kennedy BJ. Estrogen receptor assay in the differential diagnosis of adenocarcinomas. JAMA 1977;238(1):32–34.

10

Imaging in HIV Infection and AIDS

The composer Alban Berg (1885–1935) is said to have refused a blood transfusion in the Vienna Hospital because he was afraid that it might contain the blood of a composer of operettas.

> *He hath a thousand slayn this pestilence,*
> *And, maister, er ye come in his presence,*
> *Me thinketh that it were necessarie*
> *For to be war of swich an adversarie:*
> *Beth redy for to mete him evermore . . .*
>
> Geoffrey Chaucer
> From "The Pardoner's Tale,"
> The Canterbury Tales

Scope of the Problem

Never had death become so real or terrifying a symbol of the end of the world as in the 14th century, when bubonic plague, The Black Death, swept through Europe. Today, despite the appearance of a new if entirely different plague, our collective sense of terror is constantly fed by other concerns, mostly media announcements of the visibly dramatic, natural, and man-made disasters. One only has to view the 6:00 news to receive daily reports of earthquakes, serial killers, tornadoes, air crashes, terrorist bombings, and civil wars. Average people are still only subliminally aware of a medical disaster that kills one person at a time, all the time, because they cannot make the connection between personal and social calamity. Perhaps the public feels too helpless to acknowledge its fears of such a silent, slow form of contagion and prefers the more hopeful combat against high cholesterol.

Acquired immunodeficiency syndrome (AIDS) represents the last stage of advancing immune suppression caused by the human immunodeficiency retrovirus (HIV). Probably all patients infected with this virus ultimately develop AIDS, although some may be asymptomatic carriers for 10 years or longer. Table 10.1 gives the estimated prevalence of HIV and annual incidence of new HIV infections for 1986 and 1989 (1). Figures 10.1 and 10.2 give the prevalence estimates of HIV cases in the United States in various subgroups from 1981–1990 (2). Table 10.2 shows projected numbers of AIDS cases, deaths, and living persons with AIDS by year of diagnosis through 1993, whereas Table 10.3 gives projected numbers of AIDS cases by risk-behavior group (1). The shocking increase in AIDS now has made it the second cause of death in men in the 25- to 44-year age group. From 1981–1990, almost 101,000

Table 10.1. Estimates of the Prevalence of HIV[a] and the Annual Incidence of New HIV Infections, United States, 1986 and 1989

Category	January 1986	July 1989
Prevalence	approx. 750,000[b]	approx. 1,000,000[c]
Annual incidence		
Newborns	NA[d]	1,500-2,000[e]
Adults and adolescents	NA[d]	≥40,000[f]

Source: *MMWR* (1990;39(RR-16)7).
[a]Total current infections, excluding persons who have died.
[b]Based on unadjusted figures of 500,000–650,000 from back-calculation models, adjusted to 650,000–900,000 for the effects of acquired immunodeficiency syndrome (AIDS) underreporting, life-threatening symptomatic HIV infection not meeting the AIDS case definition, and prior deaths.
[c]Based on unadjusted figures of 550,000–1,100,000 from back-calculation models, adjusted to 650,000–1,400,000, and on a range of 800,000–1,200,000, most consistent with preliminary seroprevalence data from CDC's family of surveys.
[d]Not available.
[e]National seroprevalence of 1.5/1,000 in 1989 for childbearing women multiplied by approximately one-third (rate at which infected women transmit HIV perinatally to their infants) times the number of births (approximately 4,000,000).
[f]Assumes that the minimum observed HIV seroconversion rate for active-duty military personnel is equalled or exceeded by the rate for the U.S. population-at-large 15–39 years of age.

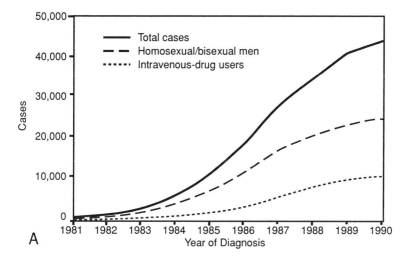

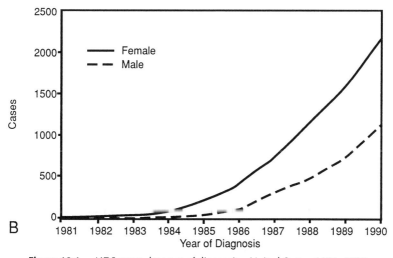

Figure 10.1. AIDS cases, by year of diagnosis—United States, 1981–1990.

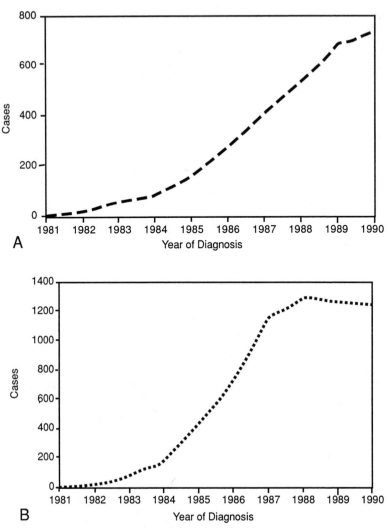

Figure 10.2.   AIDS cases, by year of diagnosis—United States, 1981–1990, continued.

Table 10.2.   Projected Numbers[a] of AIDS Cases, Deaths, and Living Persons with AIDS, United States, January 1989–December 1993

| Year | AIDS cases | | |
	New cases[b]	Alive	Deaths
1989	44,000–50,000	92,000–98,000	31,000–34,000
1990	52,000–57,000	111,000–122,000[c]	37,000–42,000
1991	56,000–71,000	127,000–153,000	43,000–52,000
1992	58,000–85,000	139,000–188,000	49,000–64,000
1993	61,000–98,000	151,000–225,000	53,000–76,000
Cumulative total through 1993[d]	390,000–480,000	—	285,000–340,000

Source: *MMWR* (1990;39(RR-16):12).
[a]Projections are adjusted for unreported diagnoses of AIDS by adding 18% to projections obtained from reported cases (corresponding to 85% of all diagnosed cases being reported: 1/0.85 = 1.18) and rounded to the nearest 1,000.
[b]Number of cases diagnosed in that year.
[c]This number differs from the number (101,000) published in the *MMWR* (1990;39:110-2, 117-9) because of a transcription error.
[d]Rounded to the nearest 5,000. Includes an estimated 120,000 AIDS cases diagnosed through 1988, 48,000 persons alive with AIDS at the end of 1988, and 72,000 deaths among patients diagnosed as having AIDS through 1988.

Table 10.3. Projected Numbers of AIDS Cases, by Risk-Behavior Group, United States, 1989–1993

Year	Homosexual/bisexual men		Heterosexual male and female intravenous drug users	Heterosexual transmission	Perinatal transmission
	Not intravenous drug users	Intravenous drug users			
1989	26,000–28,000	2,600–2,800	11,000	2,600–2,900	1,000–1,100
1990	29,000–31,000	2,700–3,000	13,000–14,000	3,700–4,000	1,300–1,500
1991	30,000–38,000	2,600–3,400	14,000–18,000	4,800–6,100	1,600–2,200
1992	30,000–44,000	2,500–3,600	16,000–23,000	6,100–8,800	2,100–3,100
1993	30,000–48,000	2,400–3,800	17,000–27,000	7,600–12,200	2,600–4,100
Cumulative total through 1993[b]	219,000–262,000	21,000–25,000	95,000–118,000	29,000–38,000	11,000–14,000

Source: *MMWR* (1990;39(RR-16):13).

[a]Projections are adjusted for unreported diagnoses of AIDS by adding 18% to projections obtained from reported cases (corresponding to 85% of all diagnosed cases being reported: 1/0.85 = 1.18) and rounded (to the nearest 1,000 for the first and third groups, and to the nearest 100 for the other three groups).

[b]Rounded to the nearest 1,000. Includes the following numbers of cases estimated to have been diagnosed through 1988: 74,000 among homosexual and bisexual men who are not intravenous drug users (IVDUs); 8,600 among homosexual and bisexual men who are IVDUs; 25,000 among heterosexual male and female IVDUs; 4,200 attributed to heterosexual transmission; and 1,900 attributed to perinatal transmission.

deaths among persons infected with the HIV were reported to the Centers for Disease Control (CDC); almost one-third of these deaths occurred in 1990 alone (3). As of 1991 The World Health Organization (WHO) put the total AIDS cases at 700,000 worldwide and estimated that 6–8 million people have contracted the virus that causes it.

In 1987 WHO asked epidemiologists studying AIDS to give projections for the year 2000. These so-called Delphi predictions suggested there would be 15–20 million human beings infected with HIV by the turn of the century, and an estimated 5–6 million sick with AIDS (4). Some WHO experts now think these numbers will be reached not long after the mid-1990s (5). Some now estimate by the year 2000 there will be 40 million infected with HIV worldwide and about 10 million cases of AIDS. Figure 10.3 shows the total estimated global and U.S. cases through the end of this century. In a striking map, Figure 10.4, the "sobering geography" of AIDS is portrayed, in which global infections by country and incidence by sex are graphically shown.

Unless by some miracle a cure is found, most of the 1 million Americans now infected with HIV will have AIDS by the year 2000. Assuming an average 15 months length of survival and a lifetime cost of treating a person with AIDS to be $75,000 in 1988 dollars, and with an estimated 104,000 new cases in 1993, the CDC has forecast that the lifetime medical care costs of treating all people diagnosed with AIDS will be $7.8 billion in that year (6). This projects to approximately $19 billion in 2001 in 1988 dollars, but the cost easily could double with the effects of inflation and increasing spread of the disease.

What do these dreadful statistics tell us as practicing physicians who, in a few years, may be ordering untold millions, perhaps billions of dollars of laboratory tests on patients with AIDS? The bizarre, multifaceted clinical nature of immunodeficiency disease and its apparent 100% mortality have to be seen against the background of improving survival rates for many people with AIDS. These alarming numbers prefigure profound changes in the character of clinical practice in the com-

AIDS EPIDEMIC
U.S. and Worldwide Cases *

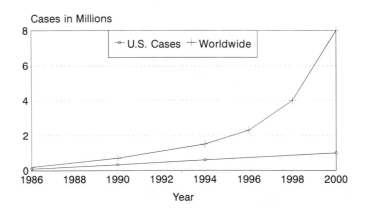

* "Delphi" projections

Figure 10.3. AIDS epidemic: U.S. and worldwide cases.

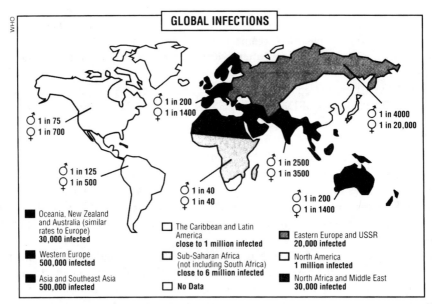

Figure 10.4. Proliferating virus. Although sub-Saharan Africa still has the most infections, other regions appear to be catching up. Incidence by sex is for adults aged 15–49. Reprinted by permission from *Science* (1991;252:372). Copyright 1991 by the AAAS.

ing decades. We can only hope that professional and federal guidelines will somehow be developed as a response to the catastrophic socioeconomic consequences of the AIDS epidemic. This can be achieved only if some consensus evolves on treatment of far-advanced and end-stage patients. The problem has become so politicized, however, one wonders how this will be achieved. Whether or not some imaginative agenda is developed for the AIDS pandemic, of one thing we can be certain: We have entered a grim period when it is no longer possible to pretend we have limitless medical resources. Choices will have to be made over allocation of economic resources among diagnostic, therapeutic, and especially research demands. How much money will be spent on keeping terminal patients with AIDS and cancer in an intensive care setting vs. how much will be spent on AIDS and cancer research? How many dollars for liver and heart transplants, MRI machines, drug rehabilitation, and measles immunization? The list is endless. The choices will be politically and ethically painful and have profound implications not only for people with AIDS, who, though increasing, will still comprise only a small proportion of our total population suffering with chronic and life-threatening conditions.

The Changing Face of HIV Infection and AIDS

Almost 60% of the first 60,000 AIDS patients are reported to have died. In 1987, the median survival time of patients after diagnosis of AIDS was reported to be approximately 12 months, but longer survival times were seen in younger patients, in the white race, among males, and those presenting with Kaposi's sarcoma compared with *Pneumocystis carinii* pneumonia (PCP) (7). In a larger series, 31% of patients were reported dead within 1 year of diagnosis, and 56% and 76% dead in 2 and 3 years, respectively (8). However, reporting of deaths is unreliable. In one series of 147 patients with AIDS who were *not* reported to have died in 3 years, 31% had indeed died, 30% were lost to follow-up, and 39% were alive (9).

An actual cure for HIV is unlikely to be found for some years, if ever, but immunization against it is a much more realistic hope. The probability of HIV-positive individuals remaining AIDS-free for a longer interval continues to improve largely from the development of various new antiretroviral drugs, notably zidovudine (AZT), didanosine (DDI), and dideoxycytodine (DDC). People with AIDS are also experiencing enhanced survival times, the result of new immunorestorative compounds and drugs directed both against the virus itself and the various devastating diseases of immune suppression. In the past 4 years survival has steadily improved, as shown by a large drop in the case fatality rates reported between 1985–1990 (10). A few patients with AIDS are now surviving as long as 4–5 years after diagnosis.

Most of the improvement in overall AIDS survival can be attributed to the prophylaxis and therapy of PCP, still the most common complication of AIDS (though it is becoming less common). Some progress also has been made against other opportunistic infections associated with AIDS, specifically toxoplasmosis and Mycobacterium-avium complex (MAC; also called MAI). Cryptosporidiosis and Cytomegalovirus (CMV), however, are relentless, and survival remains poor. Similarly, treatment of advanced malignant and lymphoproliferative diseases resulting from immune suppression caused by the virus is at present extremely limited and largely ineffective.

Classification Systems for HIV Infection and Case Definitions

The old CDC classification system of HIV infections is shown in Table 10.4 (11). In many ways this system gives a better overall clinical concept of the infection and its complications, though it lacks the merit of being "scientifically based." The four major subgroups are mutually exclusive, but in group IV, virtually all patients with actual AIDS, the five subgroups are not mutually exclusive, that is, many patients can and do have concurrent diagnoses in one or more categories. This older classification is hierarchical in that once a patient is classified in group III or IV, he cannot be reclassified into a prior group even if symptoms of infection or malignancy resolve.

Table 10.4.   CDC Classification of HIV Infections

Group I	Acute HIV infection
Group II	Asymptomatic infection
Group III	Persistent generalized lymphadenopathy[a]
Group IV	Other disease

Subgroup A Constitutional disease
Subgroup B Neurologic disease
Subgroup C Secondary infectious disease
Category C-1 Specified secondary infectious diseases listed in the CDC surveillance for AIDS
Category C-2 Other specified infectious diseases
Subgroup D Secondary cancers[b]
Subgroup E Other conditions (e.g. LIP)

[a]Patients in Groups II and III may be subclassified on the basis of a laboratory evaluation.
[b]Includes those patients whose clinical presentation fulfills the definition of AIDS used by the CDC for national reporting.

These former groupings give a good idea of the progression of HIV infection. Group I patients have an acute, symptomatic, but transient and self-limiting viral or acute mononucleosis-like syndrome, which appears shortly after exposure to HIV but often before seroconversion occurs. It is extremely difficult to determine what proportion of infected patients go through this stage, because the discovery of HIV infection may not occur for months or years afterwards, and transient viral infections are seen in almost all patients, often going unreported. Many experts, however, feel a majority of patients infected will indeed experience this syndrome after exposure, whether or not it is recalled on history.

Group II patients, by far the largest subset, are completely asymptomatic but show continued laboratory evidence of HIV infection.

Group III patients have persistent lymphadenopathy but are otherwise asymptomatic. Most workers feel this is an unfavorable sign and in fact may be a "pre-AIDS" syndrome.

Group IV encompasses patients with AIDS, including most of those now subsumed under the newer CDC classification (vide infra). These are individuals who have diverse HIV-related diseases. This group is broken down into five subgroups:

A. "Wasting syndrome," those with constitutional symptoms, i.e. fever, fatigue, night sweats, weight loss, and persistent diarrhea without an identifiable infectious cause (the old, ill-defined term "AIDS-related complex" (ARC) is no longer used, because it was probably misapplied to some non-Group IV patients);
B. Those with neurological diseases such as dementia, myelopathy, or peripheral neuropathy;
C. Patients with an astounding variety of secondary bacterial, viral, protozoal, fungal, and other infections;
D. Patients with secondary malignancies, specifically Kaposi sarcoma (KS) and a variety of lymphomas; and
E. Patients with a miscellaneous group of conditions including lymphoid interstitial pneumonitis.

Our discussion centers principally on this old Group IV, subgroups C, D, and E. These are patients with full-blown AIDS, i.e. those with previously asymptomatic HIV infections for months or years finally showing the results of prolonged immune

Table 10.5. 1992 Revised Classification System for HIV Infection and Expanded AIDS Surveillance
Case Definition for Adolescents and Adults

	Clinical Categories		
CD4⁺ cell categories	(A) Asymptomatic or PGL	(B) Symptomatic, not (A) or (C) conditions	(C) AIDS-indicator conditions
(1) >500/mm³	A1	B1	**C1**
(2) 200-499/mm³	A2	B2	**C2**
(3) <200/mm³ AIDS-indicator cell count	**A3**	**B3**	**C3**

The bold-face values illustrate the expansion of the AIDS surveillance case definition. People with AIDS-indicator
conditions (category C) are currently reportable to the health department in every state and U.S. territory. In addition to
people with clinical category C conditions (categories C1, C2, and C3), persons with CD4⁺ lymphocyte counts of less
than 200/mm³ (categories A3 or B3) also will be reportable as AIDS cases.

suppression with development of some opportunistic infection, malignancy, or both.
A few patients thought to have HIV encephalopathy (subgroup B) may in fact be
suffering from other treatable CNS complications of AIDS. Obviously, these patients
should not be denied appropriate investigation.

The new CDC classification of HIV infection, based on the $CD4^+$ cell count,
is shown in Table 10.5. This has the unmistakable merit of relating the results of a
laboratory test to the various clinical categories and specific complications. A fairly
reliable relationship exists between the $CD4^+$ cell count and the appearance of
specific indicator diseases and disease susceptibility shown in Figure 10.5, which
depicts this link and also plots $CD4^+$ counts against time. There are problems
with this latest classification scheme, however, not the least of which is the difficulty of performing the $CD4^+$ test reliably in the average laboratory. Furthermore, many authorities are still arguing over the merits of using "relative" (meaning the ratio to the total lymphocyte count) vs. the "absolute" $CD4^+$ count. A
certain percentage of patients will have an initial low total lymphocyte count due
to preexisting conditions (hepatitis, hypersplenism, or chronic infection) *unrelated
to* HIV, so that estimates of CD4:total lymphocyte ratios will be falsely high. The
most important implication of the new classification is that the definition of AIDS
has been considerably widened, a fact with serious financial implications for government and third-party payers.

Imaging in AIDS: General Principles

The assessment of HIV-positive patients for the appropriateness of any clinical
testing requires first and foremost that the patient be classified as having AIDS by the
new CDC criteria, namely the clinical and CD4⁺ cell categories shown in Table
10.5. This occasionally may be more difficult than it seems. For example, a significant group of HIV-positive individuals are symptomatic despite a $CD4^+$ count of
more than 500. These individuals often present with nonspecific complaints of fatigue, frequent minor infections, unexplained muscle aches and rashes, occasional
fever, mental lassitude, or "just not feeling right," but with few if any objective findings on examination. Some of these patients may well be suffering from anxiety or
depression, but it is usually difficult to prove this. In these individuals the T cell
counts by themselves may not be reliable indicators of the presence of AIDS and
therefore the necessity of treatment. Some patients may have the disease with counts
in the 500–600 range, and yet other patients with counts below 200 may be entirely

RELATION OF CLINICAL MANIFESTATIONS TO CD4 COUNT IN HIV INFECTED PATIENTS *

Circulating CD4 Count at Time of Initial Susceptibility	> 900	> 500	500-200	< 200	< 50
Seronegative	X				
Asymptomatic		X			
Kaposi Sarcoma		X			
Fever, Sweats, Weight Loss			X		
Hairy Leukoplakia			X		
Oral/Esophageal Candida			X		
Tuberculosis			X		
Pneumocystosis				X	
Cryptococcosis				X	
Dementia				X	
Toxoplasmosis					X
Mycobacterium A.I.					X
Cytomegalovirus					X
Death					X
Typical Time Course	< 3 months				< 10 years

* Adapted from: Shelhamer JH, et al. Respiratory Disease in the Immunosuppressed Patient. Ann Intern Med;117(5):415-431.

Figure 10.5.   Relation of clinical manifestations to CD4$^+$ count in HIV-infected patients. Adapted from: Shelhamer JH, et al. Respiratory disease in the immunosuppressed patient. *Ann Intern Med* (117(5):415–431).

asymptomatic. The presence of viruses, especially CMV, herpes simplex and zoster, as well as tuberculosis, may occur in the absence of HIV infection and thus may not be T cell dependent. On the other hand, certain index diseases are indeed related to, and may indeed be predictable from, the absolute T cell count as shown in Figure 10.6.

Before assuming that such patients are indeed suffering from the AIDS syndrome, the physician is faced, as in every HIV-positive patient, with a classic dilemma, to assume the worst and test or watch and wait. When faced with the prospect of subjecting these patients to anything more involved than routine blood studies, urinalyses, and a chest radiographs, it is prudent to consider the risks of embarking on undirected ruling-out strategies in anxious HIV patients. Physicians in our hospital's busy HIV/AIDS clinic are faced with this problem almost daily when the decision is usually made to refer the patient at least for gallium scintigraphy if there is any question of AIDS. This makes good sense in most cases, even those with equivocal clinical findings. Any HIV-positive patient who appears clinically ill should have at the very least a chest radiograph and appropriate bacteriological tests. The diagnostic approach, *as in all other conditions*, becomes a matter of clinical judgment. In view of the almost endless number of possibilities, the frequency data for various opportunistic or indicator diseases are extremely helpful in developing some diagnostic tactics. However, these data are constantly changing. The information available in 1991 is

Table 10.6. Ranked AIDS Indicator Diseases Diagnosed during 1990 Adults/Adolescents: Totals Include Definitive and Presumptive Diagnoses

Disease	Distribution (%)
PCP	49
HIV wasting syndrome	17
Candidiasis (esophageal, lungs, and trachea)	15
Kaposi's sarcoma	11
Cytomegalovirus (total)	8
Cryptococcosis, extrapulmonary or disseminated	6
HIV encephalopathy (dementia)	6
Toxoplasmosis of brain	5
Mycobacterium avium or kansasii, disseminated or extrapulmonary	4
Mycobacterium tuberculosis and other mycobacterial disease, disseminated or extrapulmonary	4
Herpes simplex	3
Lymphoma	3
Cryptosporidiosis, chronic intestinal	2
HIV encephalopathy	2
Non-Hodgkin lymphoma	2
Extrapulmonary tuberculosis	1
Disseminated histoplasmosis	
Cytomegalovirus retinitis	
Progressive multifocal leukoencephalopathy	Each <1%
Primary lymphoma of the brain	
Recurrent Salmonella septicemia	
Chronic isosporiasis	
Disseminated coccidioidomycosis	

Adapted from Ref. 9. HIV/AIDS Surveillance Year-End Edition. U.S. Department of Health and Human Services. Public Health Services. Centers for Disease Control. (January 1991:16, Table 11).

displayed in Table 10.6, listing the indicator diseases in adults and adolescents in order of frequency. As noted, the total percentages exceed 100% because many patients have more than one complicating condition.

The figures must be considered *minimum estimates* only, however, and comparative statistics can be taken only as rough approximations. This is because there is substantial underreporting of opportunistic diseases diagnosed after the initial case report to the CDC. Thus, the number of patients with complex MAC has been reported as high as 34% in one series (12) and 15–24% in another (13). This should be compared with the CDC percentage of MAC as of December 1990 of only 4%. The percentage of patients with HIV encephalopathy, CMV, disseminated tuberculosis, and perhaps many if not all the opportunistic diseases will increase substantially with length of survival. For some index diseases such as CMV and MAC the incidence may rise to 60–100% in advanced cases judging by the autopsy figures. These statistics are, of course, not reflected in the CDC table. Another problem with attempting to estimate the prior probability of a specific opportunistic disease is not only the rapidly changing incidence of various conditions with time, but the enormous geographical, racial, and group variability in their occurrence. KS and lymphoma, for example, are considerably more common in homosexual patients, whereas other opportunistic diseases show different attack rates in drug addicts, black people, hemophiliacs, and other groups.

PULMONARY COMPLAINTS

Pulmonary disease is one of the major complications of AIDS. Murray and Mills (14) list 25 such pulmonary complications, viral, fungal, parasitic, bacterial, neoplastic, and a miscellaneous group of conditions. A realistic view, however, must acknowledge that few of these complicating infections are statistically likely in the first bout of pulmonary infection. By far the most common opportunistic infection encountered in patients with AIDS is PCP, but CMV, bacterial, fungal, and tuberculous pneumonias may occur alone or in combination with each other and PCP. PCP rarely occurs with a CD4$^+$ count greater than 250. In 1987 20% of patients with AIDS were reported to develop PCP within 6 months, 50% in 9 months, and 65% within 18 months (15). However, over the past 4 years, PCP is becoming increasingly less frequent. Clinically, these patients may display a spectrum of findings ranging from the classic presentation with fever, dyspnea, mild or nonproductive cough, and dry rales, to a subtle prolonged preclinical course with minimal findings, almost no fever, minimal to absent cough, and a negative chest radiograph.

The most useful initial study is nevertheless the chest radiograph, though as suggested above, a negative film does not exclude the diagnosis. From 15% to perhaps 35% in some series have normal plain X-rays (16). Our experience in a high AIDS population agrees with these findings.

If PCP is suspected and the chest radiograph is negative, atypical, or nondiagnostic, the next step is gallium-67 scintigraphy. This technique has a large sensitivity, up to 100% in one series (17), but a lower specificity. This depends largely on the *pattern of uptake*, because the gallium study usually will be positive in a variety of pulmonary conditions associated with AIDS, including Kaposi's sarcoma (KS), tuberculosis and MAC, CMV, cryptosporidiosis, and other infections. In these patients, the pattern of gallium uptake, however, is usually focal and not diffuse. Radiogallium uptake also is seen in lymphomas and other neoplasms of lung, but again the pattern is usually different from the typical diffuse picture of PCP. In terms of predictive value, because PCP is by far the most common pulmonary complication of AIDS, the value of a positive gallium scintiscan with a negative chest radiograph is unquestioned, especially in the scan showing diffuse bilateral lung uptake. Barron et al.'s findings (18) are confirmatory, and based on their series with an AIDS prevalence of only 49%, if a patient is thought to have AIDS and PCP, but the gallium-67 scan is negative, there is only a 7% chance that PCP is present. On the other hand, any patient with a typically positive scan has a 77% probability of having PCP (18). As the reader already knows, the PPV of an abnormal gallium scan rises significantly with a higher prior probability of disease. In Barron's series (18) the specificity of gallium was 85% primarily because of atypical gallium scintiscans (nondiffuse pattern). It is important to realize that the absence of pulmonary symptoms with a negative chest radiograph essentially excludes the diagnosis of PCP, though a significant number of such patients subjected to bronchoalveolar lavage (BAL) or transbronchial biopsy will have diffuse interstitial pneumonitis (19). In one of Kramer et al.'s series (20) with an unusually high number of KS, when chest X-rays were negative and gallium scans positive, the most common diagnosis was KS. Yet the prior probability of PCP in AIDS pulmonary disease is at present higher by far than any other condition.

With a diffuse pattern of gallium uptake and an abnormal chest radiograph, PCP was still the most common diagnosis (20). PCP occurred more often with heterogeneous diffuse uptake (PPV of 87%) than with homogeneous diffuse gallium uptake, and the operative word here is still *diffuse*. Localized patterns of lung uptake are most commonly due to bacterial pneumonia, less commonly to PCP; ill-defined, perihilar uptake to CMV or PCP; and focal (lymph node) uptake to tuberculosis or lymphoma.

Using Murray et al.'s prevalence of 85% for PCP in patients with AIDS with pulmonary complaints (21) and a sensitivity of 94% for a diffuse picture of uptake on gallium-67 scintigraphy, the PPV of this test probably exceeds 95% even with a negative chest radiography. This probability of PCP in a patient with AIDS with respiratory complaints is not unreasonable, because very few symptomatic opportunistic pulmonary infections other than PCP would produce a negative chest X-ray.

These figures have important implications for the diagnostic problem posed by insistence on parasitological confirmation of the presence of PCP. The difficulty lies with the fact that *Pneumocystis* is rarely found in unprepared sputum samples. This has resulted in the insistence of some authorities that BAL with or without transbronchial or lung biopsy be performed in the majority of these patients. These procedures, besides being exceedingly unpleasant in the unanesthetisized patient, carry some risk in the presence of respiratory insufficiency often seen in acute cases. In addition, biopsy, when performed, carries a small but definite risk of pneumothorax and/or bleeding (22). How many thousands or tens of thousands of these procedures have been performed on AIDS patients is impossible to estimate even from the NCHS data, which lists only total procedures, not procedures by diagnosis. Thus, this diagnostic approach in diagnosing the most common of all AIDS complications is increasingly being questioned. Pozniak et al. (23) have suggested that in a patient with a typical X-ray appearance and history, empirical treatment is justified, with mandatory bronchoscopy only if the patient does not improve within 5 days, as is usual, or deteriorates. Certainly, with the development of effective therapies such as pentamidine and trimethoprim-sulfamethoxazole (Bactrim), the "need to demand a histoligic diagnosis of PCP can be reconsidered" (24). Finally, new sputum examination methods have made bronchoscopy an outdated procedure for diagnosing not only PCP, but cryptosporidiosis, for which the polymerase chain reaction is almost as specific. The old method using a rapid Giemsa-like stain on induced sputum gave a sensitivity for detection of PCP of 77% (25). An impressively higher yield of 92% was obtained with an indirect immunofluorescent stain using monoclonal antibodies directed against *P. carinii* (26). With the present sensitivities and specificities of this method and other methods, rarely is there clinical justification for subjecting PCP suspects to bronchoscopic intervention for a bacteriological diagnosis. (This may not be the case with other opportunistic infections, however, e.g. CMV and herpes.) Fifty years ago, if bacteria could not be cultured or recovered from sputum, one wonders which would have been developed first, bronchoscopy or an improved and better sputum test. This is a typical example of "invasive diagnostic thinking."

Some authors have used indium-111-labeled WBCs in preference to gallium for detecting opportunistic disease in patients with AIDS (27). This approach raises thorny problems, however. In preparing indium-labeled WBCs, 30–50 ml HIV-contaminated blood have to be removed from the patient for labeling of the WBCs. This large quantity of potentially fatal blood is handled by at least six different individuals before it is reinjected into the patient. Furthermore, even the remote possibility of misadministration raises the specter of death for an innocent bystander. The significant risk to medical and other personnel would seem to vastly outweigh any potential benefit to the patient. Furthermore, in the immunocompromised patient, white cell count and function is reduced so that in fact labeled-111-leukocytes are not generally as effective as gallium.

GI TRACT DISEASE

After pulmonary problems, largely PCP, GI diseases account for the second largest group of opportunistic infections associated with AIDS. The most common conditions include Candidiasis, CMV, and Cryptosporidiosis, but Histoplasmosis, Salmonella, and the various mycobacteria are also important pathogens. Furthermore, KS and lymphoma are frequently involved. Probably more than two-thirds of patients have multiple sites of involvement.

Diagnoses are confirmed with microbiological studies, but the esophagogram, GI series with small bowel follow-through, and barium enema remain the most reliable imaging techniques in these patients and should always be used before and, if possible, instead of, upper and lower GI invasive procedures. CT is also helpful, especially in visualizing intraabdominal nodes and bowel wall changes (28). Dysphagia, a common complaint in patients with AIDS, is most often caused by *Candida*, but CMV and herpes account for a significant number of cases. The double-contrast esophagram shows characteristic findings in most cases of *Candida* and CMV infection, though advanced esophageal herpes can be difficult to distinguish from CMV (28). Trials of therapeutic drugs may be more helpful to these patients in the long run than indiscriminate upper GI endoscopy, especially because both candidiasis and herpes, as well as some secondary bacterial infections, are responsive to effective treatment. KS causes the majority of AIDS-related esophageal neoplasms and shows typical findings on X-rays.

AIDS-related lesions of the stomach rarely produce symptoms but are often found incidentally on esophagogram or upper GI studies. The duodenum and small bowel account for the greatest percentage of GI radiographic abnormalities. Thirty to 80% of patients with AIDS suffer diarrhea (29). A significant number of patients with advanced AIDS with chronic diarrhea, the so-called "AIDS enteropathy," have occult enteric infections with negative stool examinations and are subjected to endoscopic biopsies with viral and other cultures. But interestingly, morphological studies of villus and crypt architecture by Greenson et al. (30) did not correlate with the presence of AIDS enteropathy, infection, or diarrhea. These authors found the most common pathogens undetected by routine studies were MAC (MAI) and cryptosporidiosis in equal numbers. Other commonly noted conditions responsible for both enteritis and colitis are CMV, KS, lymphoma, and *treatable* Salmonella and Isospora. A more complete discussion of the radiology of AIDS, including the use of CT for the detection of lymphoma and other index diseases, is covered in Federle et al.'s text (28).

Because of the widespread nature of opportunistic diseases, no part of the GI (or any other body region) is immune from involvement. Physicians taking care of patients with AIDS also see a variety of biliary tract disorders, including acalculous cholecystitis and sclerosing cholangitis secondary to CMV or cryptosporidia (31) and diffuse liver disease or space-occupying hepatic masses. On gall bladder sonography thickening of the gall bladder wall is frequently found with or without ductal dilatation in patients with presumed acalculous cholecystitis or cholangitis. Gall bladder wall thickening by itself, however, is more often a nonspecific finding in sick patients, especially those with liver disease or hypoproteinemic states. The finding of cholelithiasis without ductal dilatation is always troubling in a patient with localizing upper abdominal quadrant findings, but no specific relationship of cholelithiasis development to HIV infection has been described. The frequency of asymptomatic gall stones in the general population always must be taken into account when assessing these individuals. Furthermore, if there is any question of extrahepatic biliary obstruction, the procedures of first choice remain, as in any such patient, abdominal ultrasound followed by the hepatobiliary scintiscan. This latter study is mandatory in these patients if there is any question of either calculous or acalculous cholecystitis. Biliary tract surgery should be avoided in these patients if at all possible (vide infra).

CNS

As time goes on more and more patients are discovered to have CNS complications of AIDS. In 1985, Levy et al. (32) found 39% of 352 AIDS patients with such complaints. Of this group, 10% presented with neurological symptoms before any other manifestations of HIV infection. Autopsy series have shown neuropathological lesions in up to 80% of cases (33).

Probably the most common symptom is progressive dementia, occurring in over half of all patients with AIDS (34). In most cases this is caused by direct infection by HIV. Among other organisms causing CNS disease *Toxoplasma gondii* is the most common followed by *Coccidioides*, CMV, and a variety of other organisms including *Candidiasis*, *Aspergillosis*, Herpes simplex, Mycobacteria, Treponema, and, rarely, bacteria. KS and lymphoma also may involve the CNS. In view of the impossibility of distinguishing these various causes of CNS complaints on clinical grounds alone, most of these patients will require neuroimaging studies. The most common neurological complaints other than changes in mental status include altered level of consciousness, headache, seizures, focal motor or sensory deficits, and cranial nerve palsies. On neuroradiological imaging, usually CT, and occasionally MRI, the findings can be classified into four general groups in decreasing order of frequency:

1. Cerebral atrophy, by far the most common finding;
2. Single or multiple mass lesions secondary to either infection or neoplasm;
3. Focal or diffuse white matter involvement; and
4. Leptomeningeal/ependymal disease.

In patients with dementia, diffuse atrophy and ventricular dilatation, both equally well-detected by both CT and MR, infection with HIV is the usual cause. However, other diffuse infections may be involved, particularly CMV encephalitis, which is seen pathologically in the brains of 25% of patients with AIDS at autopsy (35). Intracranial mass lesions are also common in patients with AIDS, occurring in 23% of 153 patients in the above autopsy study in which almost half had toxoplasmosis and one-quarter had primary CNS lymphoma. Less common causes of cerebral mass lesions include *Candida* abscesses, tuberculomas, *Cryptococcomas*, KS, and bacterial infections, but in fact these complications are exceedingly rare. Because toxoplasmosis followed by herpes simplex, cryptosporidiosis, and tuberculosis are the most common therapeutically responsive intracranial disease in patients with AIDS, it is far better to treat these patients empirically. It is understandable that neurosurgeons almost never wish to perform diagnostic craniotomies on patients with AIDS. Most authors, therefore, advise against biopsy of patients with intracerebral mass lesions (36).

White matter disease in AIDS may occur in various patterns in almost one-third of patients with neurological disease and is best seen on MRI, though CT imaging is usually adequate. The conclusion reached in a series of 365 patients was that the diffuse pattern of involvement was the most common and was best correlated with AIDS dementia (caused by HIV). More focal or patchy patterns were much less common and not seen in AIDS dementia but noted in focal infection or tumor (6 cases of progressive multifocal leukoencephalopathy were seen, less than 2%) (37).

Leptomeningeal and ependymal disease, peripheral neuropathy, and myelopathy also must be considered in AIDS patients with neurological symptoms. In general, contrast-enhanced CT is superior to MRI in demonstrating changes at the bases of the brain or of the ependymal ventricular lining (28). Meningitis is most often caused by fungal, usually *Cryptococcus*, and mycobacterial infection, but *Candida*, *Aspergillus*, *Histoplasmosis*, and *Coccidioidomycosis* are encountered. Not to be overlooked is the *hyper-infection syndrome*, due to organisms previously present in patients from endemic areas such as Puerto Rico or Vietnam, e.g. Strongyloidiasis.

THE KIDNEYS

Renal involvement occurs frequently in people with AIDS. Of the nearly 30% of patients with AIDS who ultimately develop renal failure, less than 3% are reversible (38). Rao et al. (39) have reported 100% mortality in AIDS patients within 6 months after the onset of uremia despite hemodialysis. Untreatable or unresponsive cases are typically considered "HIV-associated nephropathy," but the role of this entity, other infections, preexisting renal disease, and in particular heroin and other toxins in causing interstitial, tubulo-glomerular, and other pathological changes in patients with AIDS remains obscure. Sonographic-pathological correlation has been attempted, but the results remain inconclusive (40). Based on clinical experience various types of renal parenchymal abnormalities, usually nonspecific, are seen in the majority of patients with AIDS sent for renal sonography. Some of these changes are regarded as "characteristic" of AIDS, though in fact we see them along with other abnormalities in non-AIDS patients with the gamut of chronic medical renal diseases. Many, if not most, of these cases in the population with AIDS probably represent examples of heroin nephropathy. There is no way of distinguishing these patients from those with "pure" AIDS, because we almost never see heroin users who are HIV negative. When we observe any of these changes on sonography we merely report medical renal disease. However, in pure chronic medical renal disease, the kidneys often shrink, whereas this is not true in AIDS nephropathy.

The major advantage of ultrasonography in studying the kidneys, not only of patients with AIDS but others as well, is in helping to eliminate the need for other renal imaging studies, in particular IVP. The main distinction (other than stone) in renal disease is between a medical and an obstructive condition, i.e. treatable obstructive vs. predominantly untreatable nonobstructive disease. If there is no obvious hydronephrosis on renal sonography of a patient with AIDS, other renal imaging studies are not indicated. This is critical, in view of the known dangers of contrast material in patients with renal functional impairment. Perhaps it is not surprising in the age group typical of the population with AIDS that so far we have seen only one patient out of several hundred with AIDS who proved on renal ultrasonography to have an obstructive problem.

Imaging in Terminal and Preterminal AIDS

A curious logic suggests that to omit an imaging procedure in a brain-dead victim, let alone a patient with far-advanced Alzheimer's disease, is not the same as depriving a patient with end-stage AIDS of more intensive therapy or yet another diagnostic test. In addition to our universal professional revulsion at death, there may be some unconscious hope that in extending life a few more weeks—even days—some new life-saving treatment may be discovered in the interim, just in time to be rushed to the bedside.

For those of us taking care of patients dying of AIDS, most of whom were only recently in life's prime, there are painful practical and moral decisions to face almost every day. Therapeutically, these decisions determine whether we place patients on dialysis or respirators, transfer them to the intensive care unit, or subject them to major surgery. In view of these Hobsonian choices, diagnostic decisions would seem to assume a subservient role. Prognosis has improved somewhat for advanced PCP patients given intensive care and placed on mechanical ventilation (41–43), yet it is also clear that for most patients with far-advanced and often multiple opportunistic diseases who have already and are presently receiving standard therapy, survival is extremely short term, measured in days or weeks. This is generally true regardless of the relatively temporary expedients noted above. In addition, emergency major surgery on patients with AIDS is attended by an appalling mortality, 70–80% in one small unselected series (44).

When we use the term *end stage* to describe a clinical state, and the patient also has a CD4$^+$ count below the 50–75 range, this is no longer begging the question. It clearly describes a final clinical juncture in the life history of AIDS. This is obviously not the point at which any reasonable therapeutic attempts should necessarily be discontinued, though there comes a time when therapy kills. It does signal a moment when *diagnostic* approaches need to be regarded as medically futile. We have, for example, been requested to perform lung scintigraphy on a respirator-dependent patient with AIDS to "rule out" pulmonary embolism, and gall bladder sonography and abdominal CT on a semicomatose patient to "exclude" cholelithiasis and an intraabdominal abscess. One patient with terminal AIDS died in the nuclear medicine department while having a gallium scan. If the number of fruitless imaging procedures in terminal patients with AIDS is easily documented, to refuse to carry them out is not to be equated with inhumanity. On the contrary, it is a form of decency.

Summary: Diagnostic Imaging in AIDS

Acquired immunodeficiency disease presents the most difficult therapeutic challenge in medicine, because it is a condition of devastating immune failure leading to a cascade of clinical castastrophes, few of which are effectively treated and all of which are eventually fatal. AIDS is not 1 condition, but more than 150 different infectious and neoplastic diseases, which alone or in combination may involve virtually any organ system in the body. In this section, we have attempted to synopsize a large body of information, which would easily fill a separate text. The purpose is merely to provide rough guides for the clinician. The known effectiveness of therapy for a given condition is the best guide for the intensity of its diagnostic pursuit. The principal organ system involvement is again summarized. In the following guidelines, no assumption is made except that the patient is known to be HIV positive and a CD4$^+$ count has been performed.

PULMONARY SYMPTOMS

1. Any pulmonary symptoms in a patient with AIDS lasting more than a few days to 1 week, even the mildest, require chest radiographic examination. The clinical spectrum includes anything from a minimal cough without fever to severe, nonproductive cough, fever, dyspnea, and dry rales. The longer symptoms persist and the more severe, the more likely the presence of opportunistic lung disease. A common initial site of involvement in AIDS is the lungs, and by far the most common index disease is PCP.

2. If the radiograph is positive and shows diffuse disease, the most likely disease is PCP, and, if available, special sputum examination for *Pneumocystis* should be carried out for confirmation (25, 26). If these tests are positive, treat for PCP.

3. If the sputum tests are not available or are negative, gallium scanning should be performed. If, like the X-ray, gallium studies show a diffusely abnormal pattern, PCP is almost certainly present, and therapy should be commenced. If there is no significant improvement in 5 days, BAL, bronchial biopsy, and, rarely, lung biopsy for organisms may be necessary.

4. If the radiograph is negative in the presence of pulmonary symptoms, PCP still has a probability of 15–30%, and special sputum studies still should be done. If sputum studies are negative in the presence of a diffusely positive gallium study, proceed as in 3, first with a 5-day therapeutic trial for PCP.

5. Any pulmonary symptoms with or without abnormal chest radiographs call for sputum studies for *Pneumocystis*. Any negative sputum examination requires gallium scintigraphy. Even if the gallium pattern is atypical or focal, PCP with or without another organism cannot be excluded, and BAL may be required.

6. Depending on the location of radiographic and gallium abnormalities, in the presence of negative studies for *Pneumocystis*, the most likely diagnoses are typical and atypical tuberculosis (MAI), cryptosporidiosis, CMV, bacterial infection, and, less commonly, KS and lymphoma.

7. If sputum studies, the radiograph, and gallium scan are all negative, the likelihood of PCP or other opportunistic infection is almost nil. Of those patients with persistent pulmonary symptoms, however, many will have interstitial pneumonitis, an essentially untreatable condition.

8. If either radiographs or gallium scans are abnormal but atypical, and if sputum and possibly bronchoscopic studies fail to identify any organism, CT studies of the mediastinal structures may be helpful in excluding KS or lymphoma.

GI SYMPTOMS

1. GI symptoms, in particular dysphagia, diarrhea, and malabsorption, are extremely common in patients with AIDS. In the case of the upper GI symptoms, dysphagia and odynophagia, the most common causes are esophageal candidiasis, CMV, and, least likely, herpes. In most cases these can be diagnosed by double contrast esophagogram; rarely is esophagoscopy indicated to distinguish herpes from CMV.

2. The cause of chronic diarrhea in the patient with AIDS often can be diagnosed on stool cultures, with the most common organisms causing enterocolitis being *Cryptosporidiosis*, various mycobacteria, especially MAC, followed by CMV, *Candida*, and, less frequently, *Salmonella* and *Histoplasmosis*. However, KS and lymphoma remain possible causes.

3. In some patients without positive stool cultures, upper GI series with barium follow-through and barium enemas with or without CT may help establish a likely etiology, especially in the case of neoplasm, gastric, or small bowel lymphoma or KS. These studies are occasionally helpful in some cases of herpes, MAC, *Candida*, and CMV when characteristic findings are demonstrated.

4. When a definite etiology cannot be established in patients with chronic diarrhea or malabsorption, despite bacteriological and radiographic studies, the diagnosis of HIV enteropathy is often made. In order to exclude a treatable infection, diagnostic large or small bowel samples sometimes have to be obtained in order to get adequate culture material. However, histological changes in the intestinal crypts or mucosa are unlikely to yield any helpful information (30).

CNS SYMPTOMS

1. CT is generally preferable to MRI in neuroimaging in patients with AIDS. However, MRI may offer some advantages over CT in white matter disease.

2. Progressive dementia is the most common CNS symptom seen in patients with AIDS. Other common symptoms and findings run the gamut from headache, altered level of consciousness, seizures, focal motor or sensory deficits, and cranial nerve palsies. Dementia is most commonly caused by infection of brain tissue with HIV. Most of these patients show diffuse cerebral atrophy and ventricular dilatation on CT.

3. In some patients CMV may produce a similar picture, but because there is no specific treatment for either HIV or CMV, the etiological distinction is academic only.

4. Intracranial mass lesions have a variety of etiologies. In practical terms, toxoplasma is involved in half the cases and is the most therapeutically responsive condition. Even herpes simplex, cryptosporidiosis, and MAC may respond to treatment, however, and any of these possible conditions should be treated on an empirical basis rather than subject the patient to brain biopsy. About 25% of patients will have lymphoma, which is poorly responsive to treatment.

5. White matter disease, like cerebral atrophy, is most commonly caused by HIV, though focal infection, tumor, or progressive multifocal leukoencephalopathy may be the cause. Treatment is largely useless.

6. In the brain, leptomeningeal and ependymal diseases of various etiologies are also poorly responsive to treatment. This is not the case in specific meningitides caused by treatable fungal or bacterial infections such as cryptosporidiosis, coccidioidomycosis, tuberculosis, *Candida*, etc.

RENAL IMAGING IN AIDS

1. Renal involvement probably occurs in most patients with AIDS; 30% ultimately will develop renal failure, of whom less than 3% are reversible; 100% of the remainder will be dead in 6 months whether or not they are on dialysis.

2. Renal imaging is indicated only if there is chemical evidence of functional impairment and should be performed with ultrasonography. Because of the known danger of contrast material in patients with renal functional impairment, do not perform IVP.

3. Most patients with AIDS will show increased echogenicity or nonspecific "medical renal disease" on sonography; virtually none in the young age group characteristic of AIDS will show treatable (obstructive) disease. Intense echogenicity in normal-sized kidneys resulting in loss of the corticomedullary boundaries is characteristic of heroin/AIDS nephropathy. Renal imaging, therefore, has virtually no therapeutic implications for these patients.

4. There may be some favorable prognostic value of negative renal sonography in an HIV-positive patient who is not yet definitely established as having AIDS. But this is conjecture.

IMAGING IN PRETERMINAL OR END-STAGE AIDS

We do not recommend it.

REFERENCES

1. HIV prevalence estimates and AIDS case projections for the United States: report based upon a workshop. MMWR 1990;39(RR-16):7–13.
2. The HIV/AIDS epidemic: the first 10 years. MMWR 1991;40(22):360.
3. Mortality attributable to HIV infection/AIDS—United States, 1981–1990. MMWR 1991;40(3):41–44.
4. Cowley G, Hager M, Marshall R. AIDS, the next ten years. [Quoted] Newsweek 1990; June 26:20–27.
5. Palca J. The sobering geography of AIDS. Science 1991;252(5004):372–373.
6. Hellinger FJ. Updated forecasts of the costs of medical care for persons with AIDS, 1989. Public Health Rep 1990;105(1):1–12.
7. Rothenberg R, Woelfel M, Stonburner R, Milberg J, Parker R, Truman B. Survival with the acquired immunodeficiency syndrome: experience with 5833 cases in New York City. N Engl J Med 1987; 317(21):1297–1302.
8. Lemp GF, Barnhart JL, Rutherford GW, Temelso T, Werdegar D. Predictors of survival for AIDS cases in San Francisco. 115th Annual American Public Health Association Meeting, New Orleans, La, 1987.
9. The Long-Term Survivor Collaborative Study Group, Hardy AM. Characterization of long-term survivors (LTS) of AIDS (Abstract). In: Proceedings and abstracts of the 27th Interscience Conference on Antimicrobial Agents and Chemotherapy, October 4–7, 1987. New York: The American Society of Microbiology, 1987:98.
10. HIV/AIDS Surveillance, Year-End Edition. U.S. Public Health Service Centers for Disease Control, Division HIV/AIDS, Jan 1991.

11. Revision of the CDC surveillance case definition for acquired immunodeficiency syndrome. MMWR 1987;36(Suppl 1S–15S).
12. Agins B, Spicehandler D, Della-Latta P, et al. *M. avium-intracellulare* infection in AIDS. In: Proceedings and abstracts of the 24th Interscience Conference on Antimicrobial Agents and Chemotherapy, October 8–10, 1984. Washington, D.C.: The American Society for Microbiology, 1984:229 (Abstract).
13. Horsburgh Jr CR. *Mycobacterium avium* complex infection in the acquired immunodeficiency syndrome. N Engl J Med 1991;324(19):1332–1338.
14. Murray JF, Mills J. Pulmonary infectious complications of human immunodeficiency virus infection. Part I. Am Rev Respir Dis 1990;141(5, pt 1):1356–1372.
15. Brooke GL, Safran GF, Perlmutter BL, Perez JA, Zatlin GS. HIV disease: a review for the family physician. Part II. Secondary infections, malignancy and experimental therapy. Am Fam Physician 1990;42(5):1299–1308.
16. Golden JA, Sollitto RA. The radiology of pulmonary disease. Chest radiography, computed tomography, and gallium scanning. Clin Chest Med 1988;9:481–495.
17. Tuazon CU, Delaney MD, Simon GL, Witorsch P, Varma VM. Utility of gallium-67 scintigraphy and bronchial washings in the diagnosis and treatment of *Pneumocystis carinii* pneumonia in patients with the acquired immune deficiency syndrome. Am Rev Respir Dis 1985;132(5):1087–1092.
18. Barron TF, Birnbaum NSA, Shane LB, Goldsmith SJ, Rosen MJ. *Pneumocystis carinii* pneumonia studied by gallium-67 scanning. Radiology 1985;154(3):791–793.
19. Ognibene FP, Masur H, Rogers P, et al. Nonspecific interstitial pneumonitis without evidence of *Pneumocystis carinii* in asymptomatic patients infected with human immunodeficiency virus (HIV). Ann Intern Med 1988;109(11):874–879.
20. Kramer EL, Sanger JJ, Garay SM, et al. Gallium-67 scans of the chest in patients with acquired immunodeficiency syndrome. J Nucl Med 1987;28(7):1107–1114.
21. Murray JF, Felton CP, Garay SM, et al. Pulmonary complications of the acquired immune deficiency syndrome: a report of a National Heart, Lung and Blood Workshop. N Engl J Med 1984;310(25):1682–1688.
22. Millar AB. Respiratory manifestations of AIDS. Br J Hosp Med 1988;39(3):204–215.
23. Pozniak AL, Tung KT, Swinburn CR, Tovey S, Semple SJ, Johnson NM. Clinical and bronchoscopic diagnosis of suspected pneumonia related to AIDS. Br Med J 1986;293(6550):797–799.
24. Bekerman C, Bitran J. Gallium-67 scanning in the clinical evaluation of human immunodeficiency virus infection: indications and limitations. Semin Nucl Med 1988;XVIII(4):273–286.
25. Ng VL, Gartner I, Weymouth LA, Goodman CD, Hopewell PC, Hadley WK. The use of mucolysed induced sputum for the identification of pulmonary pathogens associated with human immunodeficiency virus infection. Arch Pathol Lab Med 1989;11395:488–493.
26. Kovacs JA, Ng VL, Masur H, et al. Diagnosis of *Pneumocystis carinii* pneumonia: improved detection in sputum with use of monoclonal antibodies. N Engl J Med 1988;318(10):589–593.
27. Fineman DS, Palestro CJ, Kim CK, et al. Detection of abnormalities in febrile AIDS patients with In-111-labeled leukocyte and GA-67 scintigraphy. Radiology 1989;170(3, pt 1):677–680.
28. Federle MP, Megibow AF, Naidich DP, eds. Radiology of AIDS. New York: Raven Press, 1988.
29. Antony MA, Brandt LJ, Klein RS, Berstein LH. Infectious diarrhea in patients with AIDS. Dig Dis Sci 1988;33(9):1141–1146.
30. Greenson JK, Belitsos PC, Yardley JH, Bartlett JG. AIDS enteropathy: occult enteric infections and duodenal mucosal alterations in chronic diarrhea. Ann Intern Med 1991;114(5):366–372.
31. Kavin H, Jonas RB, Chowdhury L, Kabins S. Acalculous cholecystitis and cytomegalovirus infection in acquired immune deficiency syndrome. Ann Intern Med 1986;104(1):53–54.
32. Levy RM, Bredesen DE, Rosenblum ML. Neurological manifestations of the acquired immunodeficiency syndrome (AIDS):experience at UCSF and review of the literature. J Neurosurg 1985;62(4):475–495.
33. Anders KH, Guerra WF, Tomiyasu U, Verity MA, Vinters HV. The neuropathology of AIDS. UCLA experience and review. Am J Pathol 1986;124(3):537–558.
34. Navia BA, Jordan BD, Price RW. The AIDS dementia complex: 1. Clinical features. Ann Neurol 1986;19(6):517–524.
35. Petito CK, Cho ES, Lemann W, Navia BA, Price RW. Neuropathology of acquired immunodeficiency syndrome (AIDS): an autopsy review. J Neuropathol Exp Neurol 1986;45(6):635–646.
36. Cohn J, McMeeking A, Cohen W, Jacobs J, Holzman R. Response and survival in patients treated for presumed versus proven CNS toxoplasmosis. Presented at the Third International Conference on Acquired Immunodeficiency Syndrome (AIDS), Washington, D.C., 1987.

37. Olsen WL, Longo FM, Mills CM, Norman D. White matter disease in AIDS: findings at MR imaging. Radiology 1988;169(2):445–448.
38. Frazer H. Ultrasound spots reversible kidney failure in AIDS. Diagn Imaging 1990;12(8):16–17.
39. Rao TKS, Filippone EJ, Nicastri AD, et al. Associated focal and segmental glomerulo-sclerosis in the acquired immunodeficiency syndrome. N Engl J Med 1984;310(11):669–673.
40. Hamper UM, Goldblum LE, Hutchins GM, et al. Renal involvement in AIDS: sonographic-pathologic correlation. AJR 1988;150(6):1321–1325.
41. El-Sadr W, Simberkoff MS. Survival and prognostic factors in severe *Pneumocystis carinii* pneumonia requiring mechanical ventilation. Am Rev Respir Dis 1988;137(6):1264–1267.
42. Wachter RW, Luce JM. Intensive care for patients with *Pneumocystis carinii* pneumonia and respiratory failure. Are we prepared for our new success? [Editorial]. Chest 1989;96(4):714–715.
43. Efferen LS, Nadarajah D, Palat DS. Survival following mechanical ventilation for *Pneumocystis carinii* pneumonia in patients with the acquired immunodeficiency syndrome: a different perspective. Am J Med 1989;87(4):401–404.
44. Burack JH, Mandel MS, Bizer LS. Emergency abdominal operations in the patient with acquired immunodeficiency syndrome. Arch Surg March 1989;124(3):285–286.

11

Imaging in Patients with Poor Prognoses, Nursing Home Patients, and Terminally Ill Patients

Life is like going to the dentist; first you think you can't stand it, then suddenly it's all over.

Attributed to Bismarck

Dying
Is an art, like everything else.

Sylvia Plath
"Lady Lazarus"
Shortly before she committed suicide

In times long past before intravenous Lasix and ACE inhibitors were available, but when house calls were still in vogue, I once made a late night visit to a 73-year-old gentleman, a hypertensive diabetic who had suffered three previous heart attacks and was being treated for renal insufficiency and chronic congestive failure. He was obviously in acute pulmonary edema. Rotating tourniquets were applied, and I gave him nasal oxygen and morphine. By the time the ambulance arrived 45 minutes later he was out of danger. At this point, his wife asked, "What's the fee?" In a burst of generosity I replied, "Well, $12?" after which the irascible lady asked, "Jeez, for what, doc?" Quite irritated by this display of ingratitude, I answered, "Only for saving his life," to which the lady responded, "Yeah, but for how long?"

When Hope Is Gone: Terminal, Preterminal, and Dying Patients

Few of the very old can count themselves so fortunate as to have complained as did George Bernard Shaw in his last days—he died at 94—that his vitality was preventing his death. Yet what could be more in character than the last coherent remark of Franz Kafka to his friend and physicians, Robert Klopstock, who had promised him morphine, "Kill me, or else you are a murderer."

Society has entered a new and perilous era, a time when misapplied technology is making a mockery of scientific progress. This is especially true in medicine, where we now confront so many painful and unresolvable clinical dilemmas. Up to 20 years ago death and dying were largely the concern of the patient, his family, and the physician. Today, thanks to the unanticipated ironies of science, how and when life begins and ends has become the province of lawyers, ethicists, insurance companies, churches, legislators, and the courts. Inexorably, the state is steadily arrogating to itself the ultimate clinical decision making process.

This may or may not be desirable, but perhaps it is inevitable, given our passivity. Furthermore, the economic and social consequences of needlessly prolonged death affect the very nature and resources of society itself. More than 13% of our gross national product is now devoted to health care, and costs continue to rise at almost double the rate of inflation. According to Lamm (1), if we extrapolate the present trend, by the year 2060, our entire gross national product will be devoted to health care. How much of this will be accounted for by care of patients who are terminal and hopeless no one can say, but the proportion is rising much more rapidly than overall health care costs. One typical example is the estimated 5,000–10,000 patients in persistent vegetative states now being maintained in medical institutions (2).

An abundance of physicians caring for dying patients seem unable to call it quits. For these patients' families the alternatives often lie between "pulling the plug" and the loss of lifetime savings. "Do not resuscitate" orders often are immaterial once the patient is on a respirator. Decent, well-meaning physicians may face court challenges, or worse, criminal charges. The mindless pursuit of medical futility gives way to even more bizarre and macabre practices, such as Dr. Jack Kevorkian and his suicide machine. In the Nancy Cruzan, Karen Anne Quinlan, and untold other less publicized cases we lurch between farce and obscenity committed in the name of medical ethics masquerading as enlightened mortality. This is because as a culture we are ruthlessly committed to evading decisions about death and dying; our sole obsession is in denying mortality itself, a kind of falsified sentimentality, given our bizarre perceptions about the meaning of life. Apropos to American society, the British psychoanalyst D. W. Winnicott has remarked that, "In sentimentality there is repressed or unconcious hate, and this repression is unhealthy. Sooner or later the hate turns up."

With respirators, dialysis, pacemakers, total parenteral nutrition, and feeding gastrostomies, we are now able to sustain a kind of quasi-existence, often for months or years. To witness this cruel parody of life is to perceive our tragic error in viewing technology as an abstraction divorced from the people, not only who design and employ it, but who suffer from it. This misuse of technology is not the fault of our science but of ourselves. According to the American Hospital Association, 70% of the 6,000 deaths occurring daily in the United States are somehow timed or negotiated. Every year 12,000 of the 80,000 people on renal dialysis voluntarily quit, opting for a quick and permanent way out.

In an age busily denying the reality of death, the physician, to his misfortune, has no choice but to remain the realist, if only because he can never abdicate the accessory role of the committed voyeur. Unlike Woody Allen, he is foreclosed from saying, "I'm not afraid of death; I just don't want to be around when it happens." All of us, therefore, need to establish in our minds and our hearts the arrival of that clinical milestone when hope has departed and testing time is over. The moment has long gone when we can afford to shudder at the thought of death. Terminally ill patients, whether institutionalized or not, deserve to die with decorum and not in some MRI machine or on the operating table.

Imaging in Extreme Old Age: Chronic and Nursing Home Patients

Getting old ain't for sissies.
Bette Davis

Old Age is the most unexpected of all things that can happen to a man.
Lev Davidovich (Bronstein) Trotskii (Leon Trotsky)

A related medical and socioeconomic problem deals with our permanently disabled and chronically ill elderly population requiring care in nursing homes and other long-term care facilities. Epidemiologists project that for persons who reached 65 in 1990, 43% will enter nursing homes at some time before they die. Of those who enter nursing homes, more than half will spend at least 1 year, and one in five will spend 5 years of their remaining life there (3). One-third of Medicare expenditures are for patients in their last year of life. In predicting these costs for the next century, others estimate that by 2040, the average age of a post-World War II baby boomer will be 85 years, and the level of Medicare spending for the population over 65 years old could exceed $200 billion in 1987 dollars. Yet this does not include the majority of long-term care, which is not covered under the present Medicare entitlement. Nursing home costs are expected to rise to as high as $139 billion in 2040. By that date there may be two to three times as many individuals over 85 years old in nursing homes as there are people over 65 years old in nursing homes today (4).

The reader is entitled to ask what these meditations and statistics on aging, death, and dying have to do with diagnostic medical imaging. Yet for anyone having ventured this far in the text, the answer should be obvious. In no other arena of medicine are we called upon to render *economic* decisions along with consistently wise and humane clinical judgments. And in no other area are we so often faced with nagging self-doubts and the fear of criticism. "Have I done enough? Is there anything else I can offer this patient?," we ask ourselves endlessly, knowing all the while our guilt and insecurity arises from a sense of helplessness.

Diagnosis is the parent of therapy, not its offspring. If diagnosis determines treatment, then the extent to which medical intervention is useless is the measure of diagnostic futility. Aside from economic considerations, we continue to stress the inescapable logic underlying all diagnostic testing: *Will the establishment of a diagnosis guide or alter therapy, and if so, will any clinical benefit ensure?* If the considered answer to this question is "no," we may experience profound disappointment or sadness, but we need not feel guilt-ridden if the diagnosis is not pursued.

Almost every day in our clinical practice we face problems exemplified by the following: Will the diagnosis of osteomyelitis with bone scintigraphy alter the management of an 85-year-old nursing home patient with a 3-year draining sacral decubitus already on antibiotics for months? Will a positive brain CT mean anything therapeutically for this patient with advanced Alzheimer's disease with seizure onset or a CVA? Will a lung scintiscan and the possible diagnosis of pulmonary embolism have any implications for survival of this respirator-dependent patient with terminal AIDS? Among other examples of "diagnostic malpractice" gleaned from our clinical education, are the following: abdominal and pelvic CT for pain and a pelvic mass (one patient had urinary retention, another a fecal impaction); IVP for recurrent UTI; upper EGD for typical ulcer symptoms due to nonsteroidal antiinflammatory drugs; repeat air contrast barium enema and colonoscopy for known uncomplicated bleeding hemorrhoids; bone scintigraphy for peripheral edema and a typical varicose ulcer; brain MRI for "new" headaches associated with a change in medication; indium-111 WBC scintigraphy, CT of the abdomen, pelvis, and chest, 10 blood cultures, and sonography of the gall bladder, pancreas, and kidneys for fever of unknown origin, which proved to be drug fever, etc.

Note that in each case, the indications would have been inappropriate in *any patient* presenting with the above complaints or findings. In every example given, competent clinical skill could have saved enormous trouble and countless dollars. In this sense, the chronic elderly patient is no different from any other patient. On the other hand, it should be obvious on established medical principles that it is indefensible to deny studies which might benefit these or any patients. Examples would include urine, sputum, or wound cultures and chest radiographs in antibiotic unresponsive infections, sonography and hepatobiliary scintigraphy in suspected acute cholecystitis, and brain CT in suspected subdural hematoma. Common sense, and not fear of missing something, remains the only reliable clinical guide for all patients, young and old—common sense, that is, and human kindness guided by reasonable clinical judgment. In an observation long since relegated to the dustbin of medical history by the technology worshipers of today, the great clinician Trudeau summed it up: "Physicians heal rarely, alleviate often, and comfort always."

One of the most memorable testaments to the twin ironies of vibrant young life and the tragedy of old age was written by an old woman who died in obscurity in an Irish geriatric ward. She left nothing of value but the following poem, found by a nurse among her few possessions. The quality of the old lady's only bequest to posterity so impressed the staff that copies of it were reproduced and distributed to every nurse in the hospital. It has since appeared in the *Beacon House Bulletin* of the Northern Ireland Association for Mental Health and other publications.

A Crabbit Old Woman Wrote This

What do you see, nurses, what do you see?
What are you thinking when you are looking at me—
A crabbit old woman, not very wise
Uncertain of habit, with far away eyes.
Who dribbles her food and makes no reply
When you say in a loud voice—"I do wish you'd try."
Who seems not to notice the things that you do.
And forever is losing a stocking or shoe.
Who unresisting or not, lets you do as you will,
With bathing and feeding, the long day to fill.
Is that what you are thinking—is that what you see?
Then open your eyes, nurse, you're not looking at me.
I'll tell you who I am as I sit here so still;
As I do your bidding, as I follow your will,
I'm a small child of ten with a father and mother,
Brothers and sisters, who love one another.

A young girl of sixteen with wings on her feet,
Dreaming that soon now a lover she'll meet,
A bride soon at twenty—my heart gives a leap,
Remembering the vows that I promised to keep:
At twenty-five now I have young of my own,
Who need me to build a secure, happy home;
A woman of thirty, my young now grow fast,
Bound to each other with ties that should last;
At forty, my young sons have grown and are gone,
But my man's beside me to see I don't mourn.
At fifty, once more babies play round my knee,
Again we know children, my loved one and me.
Dark days are upon me, my husband is dead,
I look at the future, I shudder with dread,
For my young are all rearing young of their own,
And I think of the years and the love that I've known.

I'm an old woman now and nature is cruel—
'Tis her jest to make old age look like a fool.
The body it crumbles, grace and vigour depart,
There is now a stone where I once had a heart,
But inside this old carcass a young girl still dwells,
And now and again my battered heart swells.
I remember the joys, I remember the pain,
And I'm loving and living life over again.
I think of the years all too few—gone too fast,
And accept the stark fact that nothing can last.
So open your eyes, nurses, open and see
Not a crabbit old woman, look closer—see ME!

REFERENCES

1. Lamm RD, Mehlman IH, Caldwell RA. Hard Choices. Denver: The Center for Public Policy and Contemporary Issues, 1988.
2. Cranford RE. The persistent vegetative state: the medical reality (getting the facts straight.) Hastings Cent Rep 1988;18:27–32.
3. Kemper P, Murtaugh CM. Lifetime use of nursing home care. N Engl J Med 1991;324(9):595–600.
4. Schneider EL, Guralnik JM. The aging of America. Impact on health care costs. JAMA 1990;263(17): 2335–2340.

12

Reprise and Reflections on the Methods and Purposes of Medical Diagnosis

Skepticism is the chastity of the mind; do not surrender it to the first comer.

Santayana

In medicine, there exists a spectrum of received wisdom, ranging from the established, accepted treatment of, for example, pneumonia or perforated peptic ulcer, to the merely fashionable ideas of the day. One only has to study recent medical history to conclude that the passage of time does not consistently guarantee medical progress. We are barely three generations removed from the universal remedy of phlebotomy. It is less than 35 years since steroids were abandoned as a panacea for rheumatoid arthritis, and even today serious questions are being raised about the indications for laparoscopic surgery, the almost routine use of episiotomy at delivery, and the effectiveness of specific drug prophylaxes in delaying the onset of AIDS in HIV-positive patients.

With the arrival of high-technology imaging, one would have thought the future could not fail us, for after all, are not universal MRI, arteriography, endoscopy, endovascular sonography, and PET scanning the answers to our dreams of diagnostic perfection? But as with treatment, so with diagnosis: *Newer is not necessarily better.* Some readers will be disappointed at what appears in this book to have been a bias in favor of conventional radiography, sonography, and radionuclide procedures, with less emphasis on the more fashionable and complicated procedures enumerated above. Yet, careful study of the epidemiology of signs, symptoms, and conditions discloses that only a very small percentage of patients benefit from these fancy imaging techniques, some of which require contrast and are invasive and occasionally risky, most of which are overrated, and all of which are expensive and overused. A few examples should suffice. As we have seen, it turns out that headache and other pain syndromes, in particular those of the thorax, abdomen, and GU tract, as well as the usual GI complaints, are rarely, if ever, indications for CT, MRI, or invasive endoscopic studies. Yet, there are panels of imaging experts and other specialists declaring it is far better to subject a patient to one of these procedures than to perform a simple plain film, barium study, or ultrasound examination. Almost 100 years ago, Oscar Wilde observed, "Nothing is so dangerous as being too modern; one is apt to grow old-fashioned quite suddenly."

The list of signs and symptoms in Chapter 6 and the subjects covered in the remaining chapters are not, of course, intended to be complete. The selection of topics and conditions for which appropriate imaging is outlined is intended to be representative of perhaps 70–80% of presentations likely to be encountered by the generalist, and of a majority of patients apt to be seen in the major medical and surgical specialties.

There will be inevitable complaints about missing or slighted modalities, but this is not a text about procedures per se, but about conditions for which they may or may not be indicated. In certain settings, new techniques are evolving and invaluable, particularly the use of duplex Doppler sonography for the identification of vascular structures and flow abnormalities. Some cardiologists will question the almost complete neglect of echocardiography, now almost as routine as electrocardiography, in the discussions of heart disease. We make no apologies for these lacunae, which were unavoidable in view of the relative importance accorded various signs, symptoms, and conditions. Allowances should be made by the thoughtful reader who realizes that no text can satisfy every demand.

On Consensus

An insightful editorial (1) discusses the problem of the newest medical growth industry, the proliferation of committees to produce medical guidelines. The NIH, coming under intense pressure from policy makers to provide a formal system of assessing new medical developments, has come up with the NIH Consensus Development Program, which was proposed as a means of allowing "appropriate members of the medical professions, the research community, consumers [sic] and others to join in evaluating a technology" (2). Yet a consensus view may be achieved only by compromise, by selection of an expert panel whose views conform to each other or present day fashions, or by use of convoluted language and bland generalities that conceal latent differences. Finally, if the so-called experts are in apparent agreement, there is an implication that further debate is meaningless. The consensus approach is thus at odds with controversy, research, and innovation. When "medical guidelines," "standards of care," and other consensus positions edge into the establishment of precedents for malpractice ligation, they deserve to be challenged by the non-specialist as well as the expert.

Our viewpoint throughout has been eclectic, that of the generalist. The forces that drive group opinions often represent a collective attempt to coerce, a form of moral blackmail. One must continually maintain respect for the opinions of informed individuals who, unlike the consensus panel, do not mind being held accountable, because they are not afraid to be wrong. Again, it is the vain search and the virtual *demand* for diagnostic perfection—by the public, the legal profession and ourselves—that becomes our professional undoing and by this means threatens to bankrupt the health care system.

On Medical Errors

Analysis of the following case histories may help illustrate various examples of diagnostic errors. Several recurrent themes can easily be recognized.

A 12-year-old girl had a physical examination by the school "sports doctor" in order to be permitted to join the softball team. The physician found a "distended uterus" and immediately referred her for sonographic examination, which proved to be completely normal. When queried later the girl admitted to having a full bladder at the time of the examination by the school physician.

Comment: Not all patients require medical imaging, not even those with masses.

The patient, a gravida-0 34-year-old woman, complained of pain in the lower left abdomen, which was chronic, recurrent, and persistent for more than 2 years. She was a happily married working woman with no children, no previous history of pelvic pain and an unremarkable menstrual history. She had a total hysterectomy and left salpingoophrectomy for "pain due to ovarian cysts," followed by a right salpingoophrectomy 1 year later for "recurrent" ovarian cysts of "moderate" size. The pain recurred and persisted. A CT of the pelvis disclosed a "cystic mass on the right," and a repeat ultrasound confirmed the presence of a 3-cm cystic right-sided mass, which looked suspiciously like a normal ovary (though a lymphocele was considered a possibility). Finally, on careful questioning the patient disclosed that the pain was most acute immediately after urination, and pyuria was noted. Cystoscopy disclosed a chronic interstitial cystitis.

Comment: Here, an obvious diagnosis of lower urinary tract pain was overlooked. Chronic, recurrent pelvic pain was mistakenly attributed to a physiological ovarian cyst rather than to a bladder condition. This led to two unnecessary major pelvic operations resulting in loss of both ovaries, tubes, and uterus in a young woman.

A physician's wife with rectal bleeding, anemia, and mild weight loss had three negative colonoscopies within a year. Barium studies were "not necessary" according to the gastroenterologist. Colon carcinoma was finally diagnosed when a double-contrast barium enema was finally performed 14 months after onset of symptoms. At surgery, the patient was found to have liver metastases from a carcinoma of the cecum.

Comment: Delay in diagnosing a colon carcinoma because of unjustified reliance on imaging procedure probably cost a woman her life. We are not suggesting that colonoscopy lacks sensitivity in diagnosing colon cancer, not that barium enema is necessarily preferable; we merely urge that when strong suspicion of pathology persists, if one procedure is not diagnostic, others may be relevant and should be pursued. Although we have seen many cases of colon carcinoma, especially of the descending colon and cecum, missed by colonoscopy, it is simply because this procedure has, in some hands, replaced the barium enema — completely.

A 62-year-old diabetic man was seen 10 days after coronary bypass surgery when he developed sudden dyspnea associated with fever and WBC of 15,000. A chest radiograph showed a large right pleural effusion, after which lung scintigraphy was ordered. A perfusion/ventilation lung scan showed findings consistent with bibasilar atelectasis or effusion, with a low probability of PE. The following day he was seen by a pulmonary specialist who felt that even though the possibility of PE was "only 10%," he could not "rule out" the diagnosis without a pulmonary angiogram. During the procedure the patient went into shock, coded, and almost died. He was intubated and put on a ventilator. That evening, bacterial pneumonia was diagnosed on the basis of persistent fever and positive sputum and blood cultures.

Comment: Performance of a hazardous, unjustified procedure in a patient with low pretest probability of disease led to a clinical disaster. In this patient, completely unnecessary clinical imaging (and in case 2, unnecessary therapy) were resorted to because of fear of *missing* a diagnosis. It is this type of clinical error we wish to emphasize.

For many years, two common types of errors have been recognized not only in medicine, but in law, business, government, and virtually all human endeavors. Thus, deciding on guilt or innocence in a criminal case is not very different from any other decision-making process with respect to the unavoidable problem of uncertainty. In the explicit rules of criminal justice in this country and Great Britain the operative rules is: "A man is innocent until proven guilty," or, "when in doubt, acquit." This has been expressed in the maxim, "Better a thousand guilty men go free, than one innocent man be convicted." The reader may find this relevant to our familiar problem, discussed at length in Chapter 1: the self-delusion that we can achieve certainty. Although acknowledging the universal problem of uncertainty in human affairs, we still need some rational way to make decisions. This may end up being a mathematical testing of hypotheses, consideration of probabilistic fluctuations, sampling errors, and the like. But in a deeper sense, one has the option of rejecting or accepting statistical or any other evidence on the basis that the techniques themselves were in error. No matter what the evidence, there are two kinds of errors: rejecting a hypothesis that is true, called an "error of the first kind" or a type I error, or accepting a hypothesis that is false, "an error of the second kind" or a type II error (3).

As physicians, we learn early in our training—and it is implied repeatedly in the wards and in textbooks, not to speak of the malpractice statutes—that *it is far worse to dismiss a sick patient than to retain a well one.* Thus, "when in doubt, continue to suspect illness." In other words, far better a type II error, a false presumption of illness, than a type I error, a false presumption of health.

This traditional stance has enormous implications for our attitude toward diagnosis and treatment, and it forms the philosophical underpinnings of medical practice and our fundamental attitude toward the very concepts of health and disease. In an attempt to deal with decision problems, particularly the type II phenomenon in clinical psychiatry, Thomas Szasz (4) has taken the extreme yet intriguing position that "mental illnesses" have not been discovered by psychiatry, they have been invented. Human behavior, he suggests, whether presenting as neurosis, hysteria, malingering (deceit), psychosis, and do forth, "may be regarded as analogous to the manifest diversity among languages. In each case, behind the apparent phenomenological differences there are certain basic similarities" (4). Szasz tends to contrast the situation in psychiatry with bodily or organic "illness." He does not deal with the possibility that such physical or somatic problems might also be regarded, in some sense, nonillness (we-see-this syndrome). Our orientation toward the etiological, deterministic concept of disease-as-name goes hand-in-hand with our preoccupation with making a diagnosis and our obsession with certainty, already discussed at length. We remain impaled on the horns of this philosophical dilemma, much as we are with the ROC curve. *Better to make a 1000 patients sick than miss one cancer* becomes the watchword.

One can indeed make a strong case for preferring type I to type II errors, but without going into the question, it is useful to mention some older studies on errors in diagnostic imaging. More than 30 years ago, Garland (5) summarized his findings in a study of more than 14,700 chest radiographs for signs of tuberculosis. He found there were 1,216 positive readings for tuberculosis that turned out to be negative (type II errors) and only 24 negative readings that turned out to be clinically active (type I errors). As expected, type II errors are also much more common in therapeutic settings (6). We must constantly be aware that errors of imaging interpretation remain prevalent despite our marvelous new technologies. Whether we are dealing with plain radiographs, scintigraphy, ultrasonography, endoscopy, arteriography, or CT and MRI, interpretive and technical errors will continue to be made in the same proportion of cases. Despite reports of test sensitivities and specifications in the .85–.95 range, we must be wary of such claims. Furthermore, we may be certain there will continue to exist more type II than type I errors (more false-positive than false-negative studies.) This is deeply embedded not only in the nature of our society but in ourselves and our profession.

The Cascade Effect

The problem of abnormal or incidental findings leading to an uncontrollable series of unforeseen events—fear of a type I error—sometimes culminating in catastrophe, has been illustrated in many of our clinical examples and alluded to frequently in these pages. The discussion on incidentalomas deals with only one aspect of this problem. These events, usually a series of unnecessary, sometimes risky diagnostic studies initiated after the discovery of some unexplained or trivial finding, may culminate in emotional if not financial and therapeutic disaster. Cascade fiascos and catastrophes are frequently catalyzed by anxiety on the part of the physician and often the patient, but they are becoming increasingly more common in clinical practice because of the introduction of new and ever more pervasive technologies (7).

A new form of the cascade effect, only recently recognized, gives an insight into the dark side of modern technology. Dr. Howard Spiro, writing about narrow-gauge surgery ("lap choly") or laparoscopic cholecysterectomy, reminds us that not all patients with gall stones will be benefited by the procedure. He discusses a tendency on the part of internists and surgeons to ascribe a variety of abdominal complaints to the incidental findings of gall stones on abdominal sonography (8). In the past, the patient could be managed expectantly, because elective cholecystectomy was not be be taken lightly. The imagined ease of lap choly compared to traditional gall bladder surgery is leading to more and more unnecessary operations on the biliary tract, with unforeseen consequences. As Spiro observes, "Once you've had a cholecystectomy, you are a 'gall bladder' patient forever. Not so long ago, patients who had an 'intractable' peptic ulcer went from one operation to another. . . . After four or five operations such patients learned how dangerous it could be to persist in their complaints, and fell silent to find solace in their scars . . ." (8).

High Technology, Specialization, and the Future

The German poet Otto Hartleben was feeling quite ill and consulted a physician who, after a thorough examination, prescribed complete abstention from smoking and drinking. Hartleben picked up his hat and coat and started for the door. The doctor called after him, "My advice, Herr Hartleben, will cost you 3 marks." "But I'm not taking it," retorted Hartleben, and he vanished.

Medicine, dealing with the entire individual, inevitably suffers from the dangers of specialization. *As we increasingly become a civilization of means without ends, we prefigure August Fruge's remark, "The better the technology, the less efficient the human use for it."* But if CT and MRI are immensely overused, it is not to deny they hold a place in the diagnostic pantheon completely unoccupied just a decade or two in the past. Endoscopy, arteriography, and laparoscopic surgery likewise occupy respected and permanent places in the armamentarium of medicine. Yet we must view these procedures and most new technologies and therapies as incremental advances and not necessarily medical revolutions. Development of fourth-generation scanners or cephalosporins does not yet rank with the discovery of X-rays or penicillin. Medical history is riddled with intellectual betrayals and broken promises. The physician's maxim should remain, "be not the first or the last" to embrace a new diagnostic or therapeutic breakthrough. As for the present status of medical progress, we are reminded of Gandhi when asked what he thought of western civilization: "I think," he remarked, "it would be a very good idea."

REFERENCES

1. Guidelines for doctors in the new world [Editorial]. Lancet 1992;339:1197–1198.
2. Perry S. The NIH Consensus Development Program. N Engl J Med 1980;303:169–172.
3. Schneff TJ. Decision rules, types of error, and their consequences in medical diagnosis. Behav Sci 1963;8(2):97–107.
4. Szasz TS. The Myth of Mental Illness. Revised ed. New York: Harper & Row, 1974:13.
5. Garland LH. Studies on the accuracy of diagnostic procedures. Am J Roentgenol, Radium Ther Nuc Med 1959;82(1):25–38.
6. Bakwin H. Pseudocia pediatricia. New Engl J Med 1945;232:691–697.
7. Mold JW, Stein HF. The cascade effect in the clinical care of patients [Editorial]. New Engl J Med 1986;314(8):512–514.
8. Spiro HM. Diagnostic laparoscopic cholecystectomy [Editorial]. Lancet 1992;339:167–168.

APPENDIX A

Probability and Diagnostic Testing

Henry R. Sturman, M.Sc.Eng. (Delft)

The concept of probability and the use of random events for games and gambling are probably as old as human civilization. Man has always had to deal with uncertainty about the weather, illness, food supply, aggression, and survival itself. Probability theory is the mathematical study of uncertainty.

A commonly used method of randomizing in ancient times was the astragalus (the heel bone of a running animal). In creatures such as deer, horse, oxen, and sheep this bone is so formed that it can be used as a four-surfaced die. Well-polished and often engraved examples have been found on the sites of ancient Egypt. Tomb illustrations and scoring boards show that these were used for games of chance (1). By about the year 3500 B.C. such games were apparently highly developed in Egypt and elsewhere (2). Even though games of chance have existed for so many millennia, surprisingly, the development of probability theory began little more than 300 years ago, around 1660. One of its most important founders is considered to be the great French mathematician Blaise Pascal (1623–1662).

Today, probability theory is fundamentally important in the sciences, business, finance, insurance, weather forecasting, the legal system, and indeed in all aspects of contemporary life. One of the difficulties we face in daily life is the attempt to communicate the idea of uncertainty by the use of such terms as *perhaps, usually, often, rarely, likely, probably*, etc. The disadvantage of using words instead of numbers is that words are imprecise and as a rule interpreted differently by different people. One person may consider *unlikely* as a probability of 25%, whereas another may equate it with a probability of 5%. Some people dislike the idea of talking in terms of probability. They would rather assume if they take a plane it is certain to be a safe trip than consider even the tiny probability of a crash. Unfortunately, there is no such thing as absolute safety, and as long as we live in an uncertain world we are stuck with probabilities.

Despite the fact that probability is a common concept in daily experience, and people generally understand *the meaning of a statement such as "the probability (of a certain event) is 80%,"* surprisingly there is no agreement among statisticians, philosophers, and others about the exact meaning of probability. Here, we shall discuss three interpretations of probability that have been proposed: the classical, the frequency, and the subjective interpretation.

The Classical Interpretation

The classical interpretation is based on the concept of physically identical outcomes. For instance, when a perfectly formed cubical die is thrown, the outcome of any one of the six planes landing face up may be considered physically identical to any of the other planes presenting face up. There is no physical difference between the planes. If the outcomes of an experiment are *physically* identical the probability of an event may be defined as the proportion of possible outcomes for which the event takes place. For instance, the probability of throwing a 6 with a perfect die is 1/6, because there are six possible outcomes, and the event of throwing a 6 takes place for one of those outcomes.

Some students of probability theory have based the classical interpretation on the concept of equally likely outcomes instead of physically identical outcomes. Again, probability is then defined as the proportion of possible outcomes favorable for an event. However, the problem with this view is that probability is defined in a circular way. Equally likely presumably means equally probable. So the definition of probability in this case depends on the concept of probability itself.

The classical interpretation may be useful in situations where there are physically identical outcomes, but it does not suggest how to ascribe probabilities to events when this is not the case. Suppose one wants to determine the probability of 6 coming up when a deformed instead of a perfect die is used. Because the areas and forms of the six surfaces of the die are different, the outcomes are not physically identical, so we cannot use the classical interpretation in this case. We may add that a group of Harvard scholars has estimated that the probability of 6 coming up when throwing a certain type of inexpensive die may be about 1/5.6 (3).

The Frequency Interpretation

In the frequency interpretation the probability of an event is taken to mean the relative frequency of an event occurring during an experiment if the experiment is repeated a large number of times. For example, if it is assumed that the probability of throwing a 6 with a certain die is 1/5.6, it means that if the die is thrown n times (with n large) and 6 comes up x times, then x/n will be about 1/5.6. As in the classical interpretation we may also see this as a proportion of favorable outcomes; the probability of 6 coming up is the proportion of a large collection of trials where a 6 comes up.

Two questions arise. First, what constitutes a large number of times? And second, if is assumed the probability of throwing 6 is 1/5.6, then x/n will be close to 1/5.6. How close should the observed proportion be to 1/5.6 before we may say that the probability of throwing 6 is this ratio?

One way to avoid these questions is not to try to define a probability associated with an event itself but only in relation to the experiments that have been done. Suppose we produce a deformed die and then throw it 100 times, out of which 6 comes up 20 times. Now we define the probability of throwing 6 as the proportion of 6s in all throws up until now. In this case it is 1/5. If we throw 100 more times and 6 comes up 10 times, then we say that the probability of throwing 6 with this die has changed from 1/5 to 30/200 = 3/20. Instead of trying to determine a probability of throwing 6 as a characteristic of the die itself, we relate the probability of throwing 6 to the results of a collection of past trials.

Another way to answer the above questions is to say that the number of trials, n, is taken to tend toward infinity and to assume then that the proportion of favorable outcomes for an event converges to a limit which we call the probability of the event. If an experiment is repeated n times, and out of those n times the event E occurs m times, the probability of the event E is defined as:

$$P(E) = \lim_{n \to \infty}^{*} \frac{m}{n}. \tag{1}$$

The notation P(E) means the probability of the event E. A problem with this definition is that the limit does not behave in a way in which mathematicians normally define a limit. Consider the following limit:

$$\lim_{n \to \infty} \frac{1}{n} = 0. \tag{2}$$

This means that the number $1/n$ tends closer and closer to 0 as n gets larger. The function $1/n$ approaches 0 in a consistent and certain manner. We can pick any small number p and be certain that the function $1/n$ is closer to 0 than p after n has become large enough. For instance, if we take p to be 0.1 then we can be sure that $1/n$ is smaller than 0.1 for all n larger than 10. *However, the limit of a relative frequency with which we defined probability does not have this property.* That is why the limit symbol in formula (1) is written with an *, to distinguish it from the kind of limit normally used in mathematics. If a fair coin is thrown a large number of times we cannot guarantee that the relative frequency of heads is between 0.49–0.51 after a certain number of times, because any proportion of heads is possible. What we can do is calculate the number of trials, n, for which there is a probability of, for example, 90% that the relative frequency of heads is between 0.49–0.51. But if we use this kind of a probabilistic limit, then we end up with a circular definition of probability, just as when we attempt to define probability in terms of equally probable events.

However, the limiting definition of probability stated in formula (1) can still be meaningful. Even though it is a different kind of limit than the one normally used in mathematics we can still take it to mean that the probability of an event is the proportion of favorable outcomes in an infinite number of experiments. This is an abstract way of looking at probability, because in practice it is not possible to repeat an experiment an infinite number of times. But does the fact that one cannot actually do an infinite number of experiments mean there is no such thing as an objective probability of an event? Perhaps it only means one cannot measure exactly the probability of an event, even though there is an objective probability of the event. In the same way, we cannot measure exactly the length of an object. But still the length of an object is a real characteristic of the object, which is independent of our subjective belief.

The Subjective Interpretation

There are certain events for which it is difficult to see how the classical or frequency interpretation can define probability. Consider what the probability is that your friend Mr. X will obtain a certain promotion he is hoping for. We cannot calculate this using the classical interpretation, because there is no reason to assume that the probability of Mr. X getting the promotion is the same as the probability of Mr. X not getting the promotion. Certainly these two possibilities cannot be considered physically identical. Also, it is difficult to use the frequency interpretation, because the situation where Mr. X either does or does not get the promotion occurs only once, i.e. we cannot try this experiment more than once. Here the subjective interpretation of probability will be useful. The subjective interpretation holds there is no objective probability associated with an event. Probability is a subjective belief of an individual representing his own degree of partial belief that some trial has a specific outcome. Person A may consider the probability of Mr. X getting his promotion to be 60%, whereas person B may consider it to be 80%.

Probability theorists have used betting situations to define subjective probability. A possible definition is the following: Your subjective probability estimate of event E is equal to m/n if you are indifferent to accepting one of the following two offers:

1. You win a prize if event E occurs and no prize if it does not occur; or

2. There is a jar with n balls all of the same size and weight. Of these n balls m are blue and the rest are white. The balls are well mixed. You are allowed to draw one ball out of the jar without looking. You win the same prize as in 1 if you draw a blue ball and no prize if you draw a white ball.

The Interpretation of Probability for Medicine

In medicine, probability can be used to answer questions such as, given this patient with these signs and symptoms and with these test results, what is the probability he has disease X? The classical interpretation will not be useful here, because there are no physically identical or equally likely outcomes in clinical situations. Both the frequency and the subjective interpretation will be useful in medicine. In fact, we will see that relative frequency figures and subjective probability estimates can be mixed together in the same formulas. Relative frequency figures can be used to answer questions such as, what is the probability that a patient with disease D has test result T when test X is done? If a study has been done where n people with disease D were tested with test X, out of which m had result T, then we can use m/n as the probability figure sought. If a study was not done, or if we do not think the study result is appropriate for our particular situation, we may alternatively use a subjective probability estimate.

Properties of Probability

Some important properties of probability are the following:

1. The probability of an event is *always between 0 and 1* (alternatively the probability of an event may be given as a figure *between 0% and 100%*).

If the probability of event A is P(A) then we have:

$$0 \le P(A) \le 1. \tag{3}$$

2. The probability of an event that is *certain to occur* is *1*.

3. The probability of an event that is *certain not to occur* is *0*.

4. If the probability of event A happening is P(A) and the probability of event B happening is P(B), then the probability of A or B happening is P(A) + P(B) *if A and B are mutually exclusive*.

In formula form: if the events A and B are mutually exclusive then:

$$P(A \text{ or } B) = P(A) + P(B). \tag{4}$$

Two events are called mutually exclusive if they cannot happen at the same time. We shall illustrate property 4 with the example of a perfect die. Let A be the event of throwing a 2 and B the event of throwing a 3. Then P(A) = 1/6 and P(B) = 1/6. Because one cannot at the same time throw a 2 and a 3, A and B are mutually exclusive events. Therefore the probability of throwing a 2 or a 3 is: P(A or B) = P(A) + P(B) = 1/6 + 1/6 = 1/3.

Now let A be the event of throwing a 1 or 2, and let B be the event of throwing a 2 or 3. $P(A) = 1/3$ and $P(B) = 1/3$. If we throw a 2 then the events A and B happen at the same time. So in this case A and B are not mutually exclusive, and formula (4) does not apply. Because three out of the six possible outcomes (1, 2, and 3) are favorable for either event A or B, $P(A \text{ or } B) = 1/2 \neq P(A) + P(B)$.

A similar property is true for more than two events, say the n events $A_1, A_2, \ldots A_n$. If the events A_1 through A_n are mutually exclusive then:

$$P(A_1 \text{ or } A_2 \text{ or } \ldots \text{ or } A_n) = \sum_{i=1}^{n} P(A_i). \tag{5}$$

The notation on the right hand side of (5) means the sum $P(A_1) + P(A_2) + P(A_3) + \ldots + P(A_n)$.

From property 2 and 4 we can derive a fifth property:

5. The probability of an event occurring *plus* the probability of the same event *not occurring* is *1*.

Because the occurrence and the nonoccurrence of event A are mutually exclusive (an event cannot occur and not occur at the same time) we have: $P(A) + P(\text{not } A) = P(A \text{ or not } A)$. But the event A or not A is certain to occur, because we are sure that A will either occur or not occur. So $P(A \text{ or not } A) = 1$. Thus, we have:

$$P(A) + P(\overline{A}) = 1. \tag{6}$$

The notation $\overline{A}$ means the event "not A." This rule means if you estimate the probability of patient X having disease D to be 70%, it would be logical to estimate the probability of patient X not having disease D to be 30%. Intuitively, of course, this is obvious.

A generalization of property 5 is:

6. If one of n events $A_1, A_2, \ldots A_n$ is *certain to occur* and they are *mutually exclusive events* (i.e. one and only one of these events will happen) then the probabilities of the events A_1 through A_n add up to *1*.

For example, suppose you are certain a patient has disease A, disease B, or disease C, and that the patient cannot have two or three of these diseases at the same time. Then $P(\text{disease A}) + P(\text{disease B}) + P(\text{disease C}) = 1$.

An important practical fact about probabilities is:

7. The probability we associate with an event is *dependent on the information we have*.

Let us illustrate this. Suppose you throw a die and see the outcome. Your friend is not yet allowed to know this outcome. If your friend is asked what the probability is that the outcome was a 6 he will answer 1/6. But you may know that the outcome was in fact a 5. So if you are asked the same question you will answer that the probability the outcome was 6 is 0. You both gave the correct answer given the information each of you had. This means there is no single correct probability that can be assigned to an event out of context. The probability that we assign to an event depends on the information we are given in relation to it. This certainly applies to probability in medicine. If you know nothing about a patient except that he has abdominal pain, you may estimate the probability of his having appendicitis as, say, 5%. But if you are given the additional information that the patient has right lower quadrant pain and tenderness, you may estimate the probability of appendicitis as 75%, which is very different indeed from 5%.

Dependent and Independent Events

The two events A and B are called independent if the knowledge of the occurrence of one of these events does not change the probability of the other event. In formula form, the events A and B are independent if:

$$P(A|B) = P(A) \quad \text{or} \quad P(B|A) = P(B). \tag{7}$$

The notation $P(A|B)$ means the probability of A given the information that event B has occurred. Such a probability is called a *conditional probability*. If no condition is mentioned as in $P(A)$, then we speak of an *unconditional probability*. Satisfaction of one of the equations in formula (7) is enough to conclude that the other one holds, i.e. if $P(B|A) = P(B)$, we may automatically conclude that $P(A|B) = P(A)$. The reason is as follows. We shall see that $P(A \text{ and } B) = P(A) P(B|A)$ and also $P(A \text{ and } B) = P(B) P(A|B)$. So we have $P(A) P(B|A) = P(B) P(A|B)$. Now, if $P(B|A) = P(B)$ the equation becomes: $P(A) P(B) = P(B) P(A|B)$. Dividing both sides of this expression by $P(B)$ we get: $P(A) = P(A|B)$.

The two events A and B are called dependent if the knowledge of the occurrence of one of these events does change the probability of the other event, i.e. $P(A|B) \neq P(A)$ or $P(B|A) \neq P(B)$.

To illustrate: suppose we throw a fair coin and a perfect die. Event A is heads for the coin and event B is 6 for the die. $P(A) = P(A|B) = 1/2$, because the probability of getting heads on the coin is 1/2 regardless of whether we know that we threw a 6 with the die. We may assume that what we throw with the die has no influence on the chances of getting heads with the coin. Therefore in this case A and B are independent.

Now suppose event A is throwing a 6 with the die, and event B is the outcome of an even number for the same throw. Here $P(A) = 1/6$ but $P(A|B) = 1/3$, because if we know we threw an even number then we know we threw either a 2, a 4, or a 6, so there is a probability of 1/3 that it is a 6. In this case A and B are dependent.

In medical practice a test is often done to help diagnose a patient. If a test is done to help determine the presence of disease D, the event of the patient having disease D and the event of getting test result T are dependent events: $P(D|T)$ is not equal to $P(D)$. Otherwise it would be of no use to do the test. If the probability of D is 70% before the test and 70% after the test, then the test gives us no new information. We hope that a test will alter the probability of D, for example, to 5% or 95%, so that we can be more certain whether or not disease D is present in the patient. An important problem is: given a pretest probability of a certain disease $P(D)$, what then is the posttest probability $P(D|T)$ after doing a test that gives test result T? In the next section we shall discuss a method to answer these types of questions.

Bayes' Theorem

In this section we shall show how $P(D|T)$ can be calculated from the probabilities $P(D)$, $P(T|D)$, and $P(T|\overline{D})$. This means that we shall be able to calculate the posttest probability of a disease if we know the pretest probability of the disease and the probability of the test result both in patients with and without the disease.

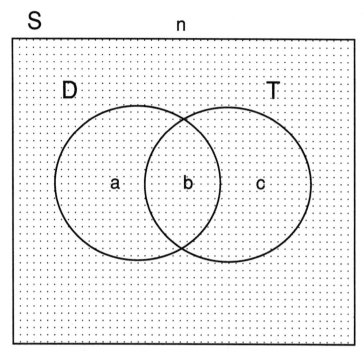

Figure A.1.   Venn diagram for disease D and test result T.

The following equation holds:

$$P(D \text{ and } T) = P(D)P(T|D). \qquad (8)$$

We can reconcile this equation with the frequency interpretation of probability. Suppose we have a large population of patients, some of whom have the disease D and some of whom do not. All of these patients are tested, and some have test result T and some do not have the test result T. In Figure A.1 the situation is depicted in what is called a *Venn diagram*.

In the figure the patients are classified according to whether or not they have disease D and whether or not they have test result T. The *dots* symbolize patients. The *complete square* S includes all patients of the population. The *circle* D includes all patients who have the disease D. Those *outside* this circle do not have disease D. The *circle* T includes all patients who have test result T. Those *outside* this circle do not have test result T (not T). The *overlap* of both circles includes those patients who have both disease D and test result T. Suppose the total population consists of n patients. Of those, *a* have disease D and test result not T; *b* have disease D and test result T; and *c* have test result T and not disease D. The rest of the patients do not have test result T and do not have disease D (not T and not D).

Now P(T|D) is the fraction of patients with disease D who have test result T:

$$P(T|D) = \frac{b}{a+b}. \qquad (9)$$

We will see that this is equal to the fraction of all patients who have both disease D and test result T divided by the fraction of all patients who have disease D. P(D and T) = b/n and P(D) = (a+b)/n. So we have:

$$\frac{P(D \text{ and } T)}{P(D)} = \frac{\frac{b}{n}}{\frac{a + b}{n}} = \frac{b}{a+b}. \tag{10}$$

Combining (9) and (10) we get:

$$P(T|D) = \frac{P(D \text{ and } T)}{P(D)}. \tag{11}$$

This is equivalent to (8). Similarly we have:

$$P(D \text{ and } T) = P(T)P(D|T). \tag{12}$$

The general form for any two events A and B is:

$$P(A \text{ and } B) = P(A)P(B|A). \tag{13}$$

If A and B are independent this becomes:

$$P(A \text{ and } B) = P(A)P(B). \tag{14}$$

Combining (8) and (12) we have:

$$P(T)P(D|T) = P(D)P(T|D). \tag{15}$$

Rearranging we get:

$$P(D|T) = \frac{P(D)P(T|D)}{P(T)}. \tag{16}$$

Using property 4 of probability we have:

$$P((T \text{ and } D) \text{ or } (T \text{ and } \overline{D})) = P(T \text{ and } D) + P(T \text{ and } \overline{D}). \tag{17}$$

But the event $((T \text{ and } D) \text{ or } (T \text{ and } \overline{D}))$ is the same as the event T. So we have:

$$P(T) = P(T \text{ and } D) + P(T \text{ and } \overline{D}). \tag{18}$$

For P(T and D) we may substitute the right side of formula (8). For $P(T \text{ and } \overline{D})$ we may substitute $P(\overline{D})P(T|\overline{D})$ by application of formula (13), and this is equal to $(1 - P(D))P(T|\overline{D})$. So rewriting formula (18) we have:

$$P(T) = P(D)P(T|D) + (1 - P(D))P(T|\overline{D}). \tag{19}$$

Substituting expression (19) in formula (16) we get the formula we were looking for:

$$P(D|T) = \frac{P(D)P(T|D)}{P(D)P(T|D) + (1 - P(D))P(T|\overline{D})}. \tag{20}$$

This formula is known as Bayes' Theorem and is named after the English clergyman Thomas Bayes (1702–1761). With it one can calculate the posttest probability of a disease if one knows the pretest probability of the disease and the probability of the test result for patients with and without the disease. In general, the probability of an event before we have a certain piece of information is called the *prior probability*, and the probability of an event after we have modified the prior probability with Bayes' formula based on a new piece of information is called the *posterior probability*. For

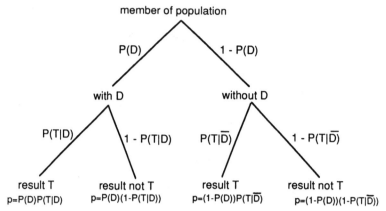

Figure A.2.   Tree structure for combinations of disease presence and test result.

medical testing pretest and prior probability may be used as synonyms, as may post-test and posterior probability.

An alternative way to arrive at Bayes' theorem is based on the tree structure depicted in Figure A.2.

In Figure A.2 we start out with any member of the population considered. We then have two possibilities: the person either has disease D or does not have disease D. The probability of the person having D is P(D), and the probability of the person not having D is $1 - P(D)$. Then a person with D can either have test result T with probability P(T|D) or not have test result T with probability $1 - P(T|D)$. And a person without D can either have test result T with probability P(T|$\overline{D}$) or not have test result T with probability $1 - P(T|\overline{D})$. Figure A.2 shows the probability, p, of ending up at any terminal node of the tree. Let us find the probability of test result T. Two of the four possible routes through the tree give test result T: the routes ending at the *first* and *third end node* from the *left*. We add the probabilities of ending up at one of these two end nodes and find the probability of having test result T to be P(D)P(T|D) + $(1 - P(D))$P(T|$\overline{D}$). We want to find P(D|T). This will be the fraction of the people with test result T who also have disease D. This fraction is equal to the fraction of people who have T and D divided by the fraction of people having T. This is P(D)P(T|D) divided by P(D)P(T|D) + $(1 - P(D))$P(T|$\overline{D}$), which results in formula (20).

Although Bayes' formula is discussed here for its application in calculating the posterior probability of a disease for a certain test result, it can be used to modify the probability of a disease based on any information. It can, for example, also be used to modify the probability of a disease based on the knowledge that the patient has a certain symptom S. One may substitute the symbol S for T in formula (20) in that case.

If we know that a patient has one and only one of the diseases D_1, D_2, ... D_n then we can use the general form of Bayes' Theorem to calculate the probability of a disease D_x given a test result T:

$$P(D_x|T) = \frac{P(D_x)P(T|D_x)}{\sum_{i=1}^{n} P(D_i)P(T|D_i)}. \tag{21}$$

For some of the tables in the main text this formula has been used to calculate the posterior probability of a disease for a certain test result. The calculation is based on knowledge of the prior probabilities of all diseases and the probability of the test result for each disease.

Sensitivity, Nonspecificity, Prevalence, and Predictive Values

Sensitivity and nonspecificity are two indices that characterize a diagnostic test that can have only two results: positive or negative. They determine how well a test can distinguish between patients with and without a certain disease. Their definitions are as follows:

> The *sensitivity* of a test for a disease D is the probability of a positive test result for a patient who has disease D.
> The *nonspecificity* of a test for a disease D is the probability of a positive test result for a patient who does not have disease D.
> A term that is more often used than the nonspecificity is the *specificity*.
> The *specificity* of a test for a disease D is the probability of a negative test result for a patient who does not have disease D.

Since the probability of a negative test result for a patient without disease D is 1 − the probability of a positive test result for a patient without disease D, we have the following relation between the nonspecificity and the specificity:

$$\text{specificity} = 1 - \text{nonspecificity}. \tag{22}$$

In this discussion we shall use the term nonspecificity instead of specificity because we feel it is a less confusing term.

The probability of a negative test for a patient with disease D is 1 − the sensitivity.

Other definitions follow:

> The *prevalence* of a disease is the probability that a patient from a specified population has the disease. In this text prevalence is generally used to mean the pretest probability of a disease in a population of patients with a certain complaint.
> The *positive predictive value* (PPV) of a certain test is a term used for the posttest probability of a disease when the test yields a positive result. If we call the pretest probability of disease D, prevalence (prev), the posttest probability of disease D, PPV and substitute the term sensitivity (sens) for $P(T|D)$ and the term nonspecificity (nonspec) for $P(T|\overline{D})$ then Bayes' formula (20) becomes:

$$\text{PPV} = \frac{\text{prev} \cdot \text{sens}}{\text{prev} \cdot \text{sens} + (1 - \text{prev})\,\text{nonspec}}. \tag{23}$$

The *negative predictive value* (NPV) of a certain test is a term used for the posttest probability of not disease D when the test yields a negative result. We find the figure $1 - NPV$ an easier figure to interpret. This figure is the posttest probability of disease D when the test yields a negative result. We can express $1 - NPV$ again in terms of the prevalence, sensitivity, and nonspecificity. For a negative test result T we have: $P(T|D) = 1 - \text{sensitivity}$ and $P(T|\overline{D}) = 1 - \text{nonspecificity}$. Bayes' formula (20) now becomes:

$$1 - \text{NPV} = \frac{\text{prev}(1 - \text{sens})}{\text{prev}(1 - \text{sens}) + (1 - \text{prev})(1 - \text{nonspec})}. \tag{24}$$

In some texts a distinction is made between the PPV and the posterior probability of a disease. The distinction is that the PPV is based on a standard pretest probability from a study population, whereas the posterior probability may be based on any subjective estimate of the prior probability of disease. In this text we will not make this distinction.

Dependency of Prevalence, Sensitivity, and Nonspecificity on the Population

The prevalence of a disease depends on the group of people or population that is considered. For example, if the population considered is the general public, then the prevalence of a disease X may be low. However, if the population considered is the group of patients presenting at a hospital with a complaint associated with disease X, then the prevalence of disease X will be much higher. Most prevalences listed in the tables of this book are meant to refer to the population of patients with a certain complaint or condition presenting to a physician or hospital. Sometimes more subcategories of such a population are considered. Different prevalences may be given for different age and sex groups.

It is not necessary to use the listed prevalence as the pretest probability of disease. As mentioned before, the probability we associate with an event depends on the information available. So if you have additional information about a patient, such as presence or absence of specific symptoms and signs, you may choose to use a higher or lower figure for P(D) than the prevalence listed. You then consider the prior probability of disease as a subjective estimate. Appendix B has tables with which you can calculate a posttest probability of disease with any prior probability, sensitivity, and nonspecificity. *It is important to realize that your original estimate of prior probability should be based on clinical findings and assumes you have no prior knowledge of any test results used to calculate the posterior probability.*

Not only the prevalence of a disease but also the sensitivity and nonspecificity of a test for a disease depend on the patient or population considered. For example, the sensitivity of a test may be higher for a group of very sick patients with the disease than for a group of less sick patients with the disease. The nonspecificity of a test also may depend on the population considered. For example, the nonspecificity of a test may be lower in a nondiseased population than in a population without the specific disease but with a disease that may be confused with it. Many of the tables in the main text of this book refer to a given population of patients, i.e. those with a specific sign or symptom who therefore are likely to have one of a certain set of diseases. Here, the nonspecificity of a test for disease X refers to the probability of a positive test result for a patient without disease X, i.e. having one of the other diseases in the group.

A Calculation Method for Nonspecificity

Many tables in the main text refer to patients who are assumed to have one and only one of the diseases in the list. Thus, the different diseases in these lists can be considered mutually exclusive events. Some of the estimates for nonspecificity have been calculated based on sensitivity estimates. The method is as follows. Suppose that there are n diseases in the list: $D_1, D_2, \ldots D_n$. We want to determine the nonspecificity for test A and disease D_1. First the sensitivities for test A and the diseases D_2 through D_n are estimated. These are called $sens_2$, through $sens_n$. The estimates are made regardless of whether or not test A would be appropriate for diagnosis of any of these other diseases. Also, sensitivity should refer to exactly the same positive result that is considered as a result favorable to diagnosis of disease D_1. The following formula is used to calculated the nonspecificity for test A and disease D_1:

$$\text{nonspec} = \frac{\sum\limits_{i=2}^{n} P(D_i)\, sens_i}{1 - P(D_1)}. \tag{25}$$

This expression can be derived as follows. Using formula (13) we have:

$$P(\overline{D}_1 \text{ and } T) = P(\overline{D}_1)P(T|\overline{D}_1). \tag{26}$$

Here T refers to a positive test. Rearranging and substituting $1 - P(D_1)$ for $P(\overline{D}_1)$ we get:

$$P(T|\overline{D}_1) = \frac{P(T \text{ and } \overline{D}_1)}{1 - P(D_1)}. \tag{27}$$

The event $(T \text{ and } \overline{D}_1)$ is the same event as $((T \text{ and } D_2) \text{ or } (T \text{ and } D_3) \text{ or } (T \text{ and } D_n))$. So we have:

$$P(T \text{ and } \overline{D}_1) = P((T \text{ and } D_2) \text{ or } (T \text{ and } D_3) \text{ or } \ldots \text{ or } (T \text{ and } D_n)). \tag{28}$$

But because $(T \text{ and } D_2)$, $(T \text{ and } D_3)$, $\ldots$ $(T \text{ and } D_n)$ are mutually exclusive events, we may write:

$$P(T \text{ and } \overline{D}_1) = \sum_{i=2}^{n} P(T \text{ and } D_i). \tag{29}$$

We rewrite (29) as:

$$P(T \text{ and } \overline{D}_1) = \sum_{i=2}^{n} P(D_i)P(T|D_i). \tag{30}$$

Substitution of expression (30) in (27) yields:

$$P(T|\overline{D}_1) = \frac{\sum\limits_{i=2}^{n} P(D_i)P(T|D_i)}{1 - P(D_1)}. \tag{31}$$

This is equivalent to (25).

It must be noted that the nonspecificity according to this calculation depends not only on the sensitivities for the diseases other than the one considered, but also on the ratios between the prior probabilities of these other diseases. This means if you feel you should use another prior probability of disease than the one listed in a table, the quality of the nonspecificity estimate is, in general, inferior. The reason is that a different prior probability of a disease also may alter the ratios between the prior probability estimates of the other diseases to a certain extent. That means a different nonspecificity would have been calculated with formula (25) if this were taken into account. The nonspecificity of a test is independent of the prior probability of the disease in case the probability of a positive test is the same for all the other diseases. In that case the nonspecificity of the test for that disease is the same as its sensitivity for the other diseases.

The Receiver Operator Characteristic Curve

Up to now we have considered tests that have finite numbers of possible results. In particular, we have discussed tests that have only two possible outcomes: positive and negative. However, many tests assumed to have binary, i.e. positive or negative, outcomes actually have ranges of possible results. Some cutoff value is used so that all test results on one side of this value are called positive and all test results on the other side of this value are called negative. Figure A.3 shows an example of the distribution of test results for patients with and without disease D.

This graph means that for patients with disease D a proportion of 0.01 has a test result x between 21 and 22, a proportion of 0.03 has a test result x between 22 and 23, etc. All these proportions add up to 1. The graph for patients without disease D has a similar interpretation.

Suppose we choose a cutoff value of 25 as shown in the figure. This means we call all test results x below 25 negative and all above 25 positive. We can now calculate the sensitivity and nonspecificity. The sensitivity is the probability of a positive test result for a patient with disease D, which is equal to the proportion of patients with disease D who have a positive test result. So the sensitivity = 0.17 + 0.20 + 0.17 + 0.12 + 0.07 + 0.03 + 0.01 = 0.77. Likewise, the nonspecificity is the probability of a positive test result for a patient without disease D, which is equal to the proportion of patients without disease D who have a positive test result. So the nonspecificity = 0.07 + 0.03 + 0.01 = 0.11.

What happens if we lower the cutoff point to 24 in order to increase the sensitivity of the test? Then we have: sensitivity = 0.12 + 0.17 + 0.20 + 0.17 + 0.12 + 0.07 + 0.03 + 0.01 = 0.89. And: nonspecificity = 0.12 + 0.07 + 0.03 + 0.01 = 0.23. This example illustrates the ROC curve principle: *An increase of the sensitivity by changing the cutoff value of a test also increases the nonspecificity.*

ROC stands for receiver operator characteristic. A perfect test has a sensitivity of 1 and a nonspecificity of 0. With such a test one could conclude with certainty that a positive test means the disease is present, because patients without the disease never have a positive test result. Also one could conclude with certainty that a negative test result means the disease is not present, because patients with the disease never have a negative test result. In real life such perfect tests do not exist, but one would like to have as high a sensitivity as possible and as low a nonspecificity as possible. The higher the sensitivity and the lower the nonspecificity the higher is PPV and the lower is 1-NPV, and so the better one is able to distinguish between patients with

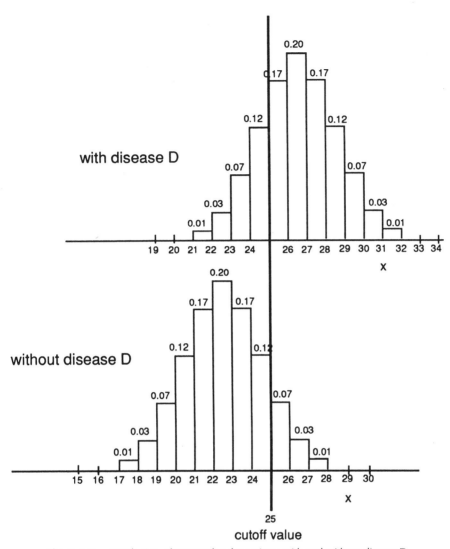

Figure A.3.   Distribution of test result x for patients with and without disease D.

and without the disease. However, the ROC curve principle states that there is a trade-off between higher sensitivity and lower nonspecificity. The sensitivity of a test cannot be increased without an increase in the nonspecificity. A plot of the nonspecificity against the sensitivity is called an ROC curve. An example of this is shown in Figure A.4. Different points on the curve correspond to different values of the cutoff value.

When a test has a range of possible test results, and one uses only the positive or negative result for a calculation of the posttest probability of a disease by introducing a cutoff point, one is throwing away information. A better estimate of the posttest probability of a disease can be calculated if one takes into account the actual test value figure. Let us illustrate this with the example of Figure A.3. First we will rearrange Bayes' formula (20). We divide the numerator and the denominator by $P(T|D)$:

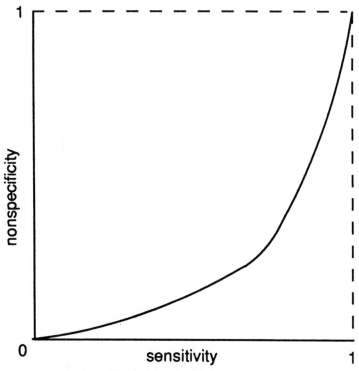

Figure A.4. The ROC curve.

$$P(D|T) = \frac{P(D)}{P(D) + (1-P(D))\frac{P(T|\overline{D})}{P(T|D)}}. \tag{32}$$

The ratio between the probability of test result T in a patient with disease D and the probability of test result T in a patient without disease D is called the *likelihood ratio* (L). In formula form:

$$L = \frac{P(T|D)}{P(T|\overline{D})}. \tag{33}$$

Rewriting formula (32) in terms of the likelihood ratio we get:

$$P(D|T) = \frac{P(D)}{P(D) + \frac{1-P(D)}{L}}. \tag{34}$$

Alternatively we may write this as:

$$P(D|T) = \frac{LP(D)}{LP(D) + (1-P(D))}. \tag{35}$$

Returning to the example of Figure A.3, suppose we use the cutoff value of 25 indicated in the figure. We already calculated in that case the sensitivity is 0.77 and the nonspecificity is 0.11. Let us assume a pretest probability of disease D of 0.7. We can calculate the PPV with equation (20) or (23). But we may use instead equation (35). For a positive test the likelihood ratio is the sensitivity (= probability of a positive test result given the disease) divided by the nonspecificity ($=$ probability of a positive test result given not the disease). For a negative test the likelihood ratio is $(1-\text{sensitivity})$ ($=$ probability of a negative test result given the disease) divided by $(1-\text{nonspecificity})$ ($=$ probability of a negative test result given not the disease). For a positive test we have: $L = 0.77/0.11 = 7$. Filling in formula (35) gives us the PPV:

$$\text{PPV} = \frac{7 \times 0.7}{7 \times 0.7 + 0.3} = 0.94.$$

Now suppose we know not only that the test result was positive, but that the test result x was 25.5. Based on this information we can calculate the PPV with formula (35). The probability of a test result x between 25 and 26 is 0.17 for a patient with disease D (see Figure A.3). The probability of test result x between 25 and 26 is 0.07 for a patient without disease D. So for this test result where x is between 25 and 26 the likelihood ratio L is $0.17/0.07 = 2.43$. Using (35) we now have:

$$\text{PPV} = \frac{2.43 \times 0.7}{2.43 \times 0.7 + 0.3} = 0.85.$$

This is a lower figure for the PPV than the one we calculated based only on the knowledge that the test was positive. Now let us suppose that the test result x was 27.5. The likelihood ratio L is now $0.17/0.01 = 17$. So we have:

$$\text{PPV} = \frac{17 \times 0.7}{17 \times 0.7 + 0.3} = 0.975.$$

This is a higher figure for the PPV than the one we calculated based only on the knowledge that the test was positive. Similar variations in $1-\text{NPV}$ occur in case of different values of x below the cutoff value.

If for a test with a range of possible results we calculate PPV and $1-\text{NPV}$ based only on knowledge of the result being positive or negative, we may state the following two rules. These rules relate such a calculation to one based on the actual test result figure:

If a test result is close to the cutoff value, the *PPV is overestimated* and *1 – NPV is underestimated.*

If a test result is far from the cutoff value the *PPV is underestimated* and *1 – NPV is overestimated.*

If the distributions of test results are known, we advocate using the test result figure instead of only the positive or negative result to calculate the posttest probability of the disease. This will give a better estimate of the posttest probability of the disease.

The Continuous Version of Bayes' Theorem

In this section we shall present the formula to calculate the posttest probability of a disease if the distribution of test results is not given in the histogram form of Figure A.3 but instead in the form of a probability distribution. Figure A.5 depicts the probability distributions of a test result x. The function f(x) is the distribution of test results for patients with disease D and the function g(x) is the distribution of test results for patients without disease D.

A probability distribution, say of variable x, is defined so that the probability of x being between two values x_1 and x_2 is equal to the area under the curve between x_1

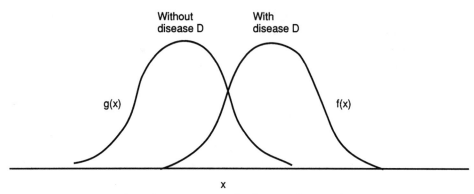

Figure A.5.   Continuous distributions of test result x.

and x_2. Because the probability that x has some value is 1, the total area under a probability distribution curve must be 1.

If we know the distributions of test results f(x) and g(x) then we can use the following form of Bayes' Theorem to calculate the probability of a disease given test result x:

$$P(D|x) = \frac{P(D)f(x)}{P(D)f(x) + (1 - P(D))g(x)}. \tag{36}$$

This equation has the same form as equation (20) with f(x) instead of P(T|D) and g(x) instead of P(T|$\overline{D}$). If here we define the likelihood ratio L as f(x)/g(x), then equation (36) becomes the expression (35). So in order to calculate the posttest probability of a disease you may calculate L = f(x)/g(x) for the test value x and then use formula (35).

Calculation of the Posterior Probability of a Disease Based on More Than One Test Result

In this section we shall discuss how to calculate the posterior probability of a disease if more than one test has been done. One way to do this is by repeated application of Bayes' Theorem for each test result. Every posterior probability of the disease then becomes the prior probability of the disease for the next application of Bayes' Theorem.

An equivalent method will be described here whereby we can do the calculation in only one application of Bayes' Theorem. To do this we shall use formula (35). In this formula we have to fill in P(D)—the prior probability of disease before doing the tests—and L. L was defined as the ratio of P(T|D) and P(T|$\overline{D}$). We can use this formula if we interpret T as standing for the combination of all test results instead of just one test result. The formula then relates the probability of disease D given the combination of test results to the pretest probability of disease D and the probability of the combination of test results both for patients with disease D and patients without disease D. If we have the combination of test results T formed by the n test results T_1, T_2, ... T_n, then P(T|D) is given by:

$$P(T|D) = P(T_1|D)P(T_2|D \text{ and } T_2)P(T_3|D \text{ and } T_1 \text{ and } T_2) \ldots$$
$$P(T_n|D \text{ and } T_1 \text{ and } T_2 \text{ and } \ldots T_{n-1}). \tag{37}$$

If $T_x|D$ and $T_y|D$ are independent, i.e. $P(T_x|D \text{ and } T_y) = P(T_x|D)$ for any x, y, then this reduces to:

$$P(T|D) = P(T_1|D)P(T_2|D) \ldots P(T_n|D). \tag{38}$$

If $T_x|\overline{D}$ and $T_y|\overline{D}$ are independent for any x, y, then we also have:

$$P(T|\overline{D}) = P(T_1|\overline{D})P(T_2|\overline{D}) \ldots P(T_n|\overline{D}). \tag{39}$$

We may write (38) and (39) in the form of:

$$P(T|D) = \prod_{i=1}^{n} P(T_i|D). \tag{40}$$

$$P(T|\overline{D}) = \prod_{i=1}^{n} P(T_i|\overline{D}). \tag{41}$$

We have then for the likelihood ratio of the combination of test results T:

$$L = \frac{\displaystyle\prod_{i=1}^{n} P(T_i|D)}{\displaystyle\prod_{i=1}^{n} P(T_i|\overline{D})} = \prod_{i=1}^{n} \left(\frac{P(T_i|D)}{P(T_i|\overline{D})}\right). \tag{42}$$

If L_i is the likelihood ratio for test result T_i we also can write this as:

$$L = \prod_{i=1}^{n} L_i. \tag{43}$$

So if we assume the test results given D and the test results given $\overline{D}$ are independent, then we can calculate the likelihood ratio, L, of the combination of test results simply as the product of all the separate likelihood ratios. The posterior probability of disease follows then by substituting L and P(D) in formula (35).

We will introduce here a transform of L, which makes the combining of test results even easier. We will call the new figure the *discriminant code* or "d code." This code determines how well a test result or combination of test results distinguishes between patients with and without a disease. The definition is:

$$d = 20\log L. \tag{44}$$

The coefficient 20 is chosen only so the d codes can be rounded off as integers without significant loss of precision. L as a function of d is then given by:

$$L = 10^{\frac{d}{20}}. \tag{45}$$

Here log refers to the logarithm with base 10. The use of a logarithm permits us to add the d codes of separate test results in order to find the d code of the combination of test results. Let us call the d codes of test results T_1 through T_n d_1, d_2, $\ldots d_n$.

Then we can calculate the d code for the combination of test results with the following expression:

$$d = \sum_{i=1}^{n} d_i. \tag{46}$$

That this expression holds is shown in the following derivation:

$$d = 20 \log L = 20 \log \left(\prod_{i=1}^{n} L_i \right) = 20 \sum_{i=1}^{n} (\log L_i) = \sum_{i=1}^{n} (20 \log L_i) = \sum_{i=1}^{n} d_i.$$

We may rewrite expression (35) in terms of the d code, by substituting expression (45) in (35):

$$P(D|T) = \frac{10^{\frac{d}{20}} P(D)}{10^{\frac{d}{20}} P(D) + (1 - P(D))}. \tag{47}$$

We can use this formula to calculate the posterior probability of a disease based on one or several test results. If we have only one test result then we use for d the d code for that test result. If we have several test results we use for d the sum of the d codes of all test results.

Let us summarize here the formulas to calculate the d code for a test result:

$$d \text{ code for test result } T = 20 \log \left(\frac{P(T|D)}{P(T|\overline{D})} \right). \tag{48}$$

$$d \text{ code for positive test} = 20 \log \left(\frac{\text{sensitivity}}{\text{nonspecificity}} \right). \tag{49}$$

$$d \text{ code for negative test} = 20 \log \left(\frac{1 - \text{sensitivity}}{1 - \text{nonspecificity}} \right). \tag{50}$$

As mentioned, this analysis for taking into account a combination of test results is based on the assumption of independency of test results given either the considered disease or its absence. This type of independency is called *conditional independency*. It means that test results are independent *given* the patient has the disease, and also that test results are independent *given* the patient does not have the disease. This is usually not as strong a condition as *general independency*. Test results often may be dependent in general, whereas they are conditionally independent. Suppose test result A and test result B are conditionally independent, i.e. given the patient has disease D the probability of test A positive does not change with knowledge of test result B, etc. Suppose further that test A and test B both tend to be positive with presence of disease D and negative without its presence. Now, if test A is positive the patient is likely to have disease D, so the patient is also likely to get a positive test result for test B (more likely than if we do not know the result of test A). So in general, without separation of patients with and without the disease D, test result B does depend on test result A, even though test result A and test result B may be conditionally independent.

It is not always correct to assume conditional independency. In particular, it will not be true for two different tests that deal with the same aspect of a disease. If test 1 and test 2 test for the same thing, then knowing test 1 was positive means one can assume test 2 probably will be positive as well (both for patients with and without the considered disease). But in that case, test 2 does not give much new information, and adding its result with Bayes' formula will cause an unjustifiable increase in the calculated PPV.

In this appendix we have discussed various ways to calculate the probability of a disease being present in a patient. This is only a first step in the process of medical decision making. The actual use of probabilities is to help in reducing uncertainties in patient management, i.e. what further tests and treatment are required, if any. How probabilities help the physician in answering such questions is part of the subject of medical decision making. An excellent treatment of the subject is presented in the text by Sox et al. (4).

REFERENCES

1. Hacking I. The Emergence of Probability, London: Cambridge University Press, 1975:1–2.
2. DeGroot MH. Probability and Statistics, 2nd ed. Reading: Addison-Wesley Publishing Company, 1986:1.
3. Shafer G. A Mathematical Theory of Evidence. Princeton: Princeton University Press, 1976:10.
4. Sox HC, Blatt MA, Higgens MC, Marton KI. Medical Decision Making. Stoneham: Butterworth Publishers, 1988.

APPENDIX B

Tables for the Posterior Probability of a Disease

Henry R. Sturman, M.Sc.Eng. (Delft)

Using the Tables

This section consists of tables that indicate the posterior probability of a disease based on one or more test results and a prior probability of disease. Table B.1 lists what we have already referred to above as the *d* code. These codes are listed, as will be described, opposite the sensitivity and nonspecificity (1 − specificity) of a test with a positive or negative result. Table B.2 relates this d code and a prior probability of a disease to a posttest probability of a disease. A positive d code indicates an increase and a negative d code a decrease in the probability of disease.

To find the d code for a positive test, look up in Table B.1 sensitivity in the top row and nonspecificity in the far left column (both labeled +). To find the d code for a negative test use the second row from the top and the second column from the left (both labeled −). After finding the d code, use Table B.2 to find the posttest probability of the considered disease opposite the d code and the prior probability.

Example: Let us assume a patient has suspected gall bladder disease to which you assign a pretest probability of, say, 0.1. The abdominal sonogram has a sensitivity of 0.9 for detection of gall stones and a nonspecificity of 0.05. In Table B.1 we find the d code for a positive test is +25. In Table B.2, we find the posttest probability of gall bladder disease for a positive test in the intersection of the row of prior probability (0.1) and the column for d code (+25), which is 0.66. Returning to Table B.1, we find that the d code for a negative test with a sensitivity of 0.9 and a nonspecificity of 0.05 is −20. Thus, the posttest probability of gall bladder disease with a negative abdominal sonogram from Table B.2 is 0.01.

Table B.1 also can be used to find the d code for the result of a test that has any number of possible outcomes. The probabilities of such test outcomes listed in some tables in the main text were clinical estimates, because they were not available in the literature for nonbinary outcomes. (Recall that the terms *sensitivity* and *nonspecificity* are defined in terms of only binary outcomes.) Thus, let $P(T|D)$ refer to the estimated probability of a specific test result T, given disease D, and $P(T|\overline{D})$ refer to the estimated probability of test result T given not disease D. In Table B.1 one looks up $P(T|D)$ in the top row (labeled *sensitivity* and +) and $P(T|\overline{D})$ in the far left column (labeled *nonspecificity* and +). The intersection gives the d code for test result T, which can be used to find the posterior probability of disease in Table B.2.

Example: If $P(T|D)$, the probability of a certain test result T other than positive or negative, given disease D, is estimated to be 0.8, and $P(T|\overline{D})$, the probability of test result T given not D is estimated to be 0.03, then the d code for test result T is +29, from Table B.1.

If there is more than one test result, one can add the d codes of the successive test results to find the total d code to be used in Table B.2 for finding the posttest probability. Adding d codes is only appropriate if it is reasonable to assume conditional independency, i.e. the test results for a patient with the disease are independent of one another, and also the test results for a patient without the disease are independent of one another.

Example: Suppose you, the physician, suspects a patient has either gall bladder disease or some form of hepatitis (viral, alcoholic, or other drug induced). You assign a prior probability estimate of 0.5 to gall bladder disease and also a prior probability estimate of 0.5 to hepatitis. You perform both an abdominal sonogram for detection of gall stones and a liver chemical profile, including hepatitis testing. Suppose both sets of tests are negative. Now let us calculate the posterior probability of gall bladder disease. As in the first example, for a patient with gall bladder disease, the abdominal sonogram has a sensitivity of 0.9 for detection of gall stones and a nonspecificity of 0.05. The d code for a negative abdominal sonogram is −20, from Table B.1. The sensitivity for detection of some form of hepatitis with chemical and antigen/antibody tests for a patient with hepatitis is, let us assume, 0.95, and the nonspecificity is 0.01. If we are considering hepatitis (hepatocellular disease), this means a d code of −26 for a negative test (from Table B.1). However, we want to calculate the probability of gall bladder disease. To find the d code for gall bladder disease with negative liver function/antibody tests, note that the probability of a positive test result is 0.01 for a patient with gall bladder disease (the nonspecificity of chemical testing for hepatitis). So we say that the sensitivity of the hepatitis chemistry/antibody tests for gall bladder disease is 0.01. Likewise, the probability of a positive test result given not gall disease is 0.95 (the probability of a positive test result given hepatitis — we are assuming that if the patient does not have gall bladder disease he has some form of hepatitis). So for gall bladder disease the nonspecificity of hepatitis testing is 0.95. From Table B.1, the d code of a negative test with sensitivity 0.01 and nonspecificity 0.95 is +26. So a negative test result for a hepatitis antibody test means a d code of −26 for hepatitis and a d code of +26 for gall bladder disease. For gall bladder disease we already calculated a d code of −20 for the negative abdominal sonogram. Taking into account both negative tests, this gives us a total d code of +26 − 20 = +6 for gall bladder disease. With a prior probability of 0.5 for gall bladder disease this gives us, from Table B.2, a posterior probability of 0.67 for gall bladder disease (and thus the posterior probability of some form of hepatitis must be 0.33).

An alternative way to do this calculation is to use the posttest probability of gall bladder disease after the first test as a pretest probability of gall bladder disease for the second test (again, this is only appropriate because we are assuming the abdominal sonogram and the hepatitis chemistry/antibody test results are conditionally independent). The negative abdominal sonogram gave a d code of −20 for gall bladder disease. With a pretest probability of 0.5 this results in a posttest probability of 0.09 for gall bladder disease (from Table B.2). The negative hepatitis chemical testing gave a d code of +26 for gall bladder disease. Using 0.09 (rounded off to 0.10) as the pretest probability this gives a posterior probability of 0.69 for gall bladder disease (from Table B.2). This is a bit higher than the 0.67 we found before because of round off errors. The result is not significantly different, however.

Tables of d Codes

TABLE B.1. D CODE

(+) positive test	(−) negative test					sensitivity						
(+)	nonspec. (−)	(+) 0.01 (−) 0.99	0.02 0.98	0.03 0.97	0.04 0.96	0.05 0.95	0.07 0.93	0.08 0.92	0.10 0.90	0.12 0.88	0.15 0.85	0.20 0.80
0.01	0.99	0	+6	+10	+12	+14	+17	+18	+20	+22	+24	+26
0.02	0.98	−6	0	+4	+6	+8	+11	+12	+14	+16	+18	+20
0.03	0.97	−10	−4	0	+2	+4	+7	+9	+10	+12	+14	+16
0.04	0.96	−12	−6	−2	0	+2	+5	+6	+8	+10	+11	+14
0.05	0.95	−14	−8	−4	−2	0	+3	+4	+6	+8	+10	+12
0.07	0.93	−17	−11	−7	−5	−3	0	+1	+3	+5	+7	+9
0.08	0.92	−18	−12	−9	−6	−4	−1	0	+2	+4	+5	+8
0.10	0.90	−20	−14	−10	−8	−6	−3	−2	0	+2	+4	+6
0.12	0.88	−22	−16	−12	−10	−8	−5	−4	−2	0	+2	+4
0.15	0.85	−24	−18	−14	−11	−10	−7	−5	−4	−2	0	+2
0.20	0.80	−26	−20	−16	−14	−12	−9	−8	−6	−4	−2	0
0.25	0.75	−28	−22	−18	−16	−14	−11	−10	−8	−6	−4	−2
0.30	0.70	−30	−24	−20	−18	−16	−13	−11	−10	−8	−6	−4
0.35	0.65	−31	−25	−21	−19	−17	−14	−13	−11	−9	−7	−5
0.40	0.60	−32	−26	−22	−20	−18	−15	−14	−12	−10	−9	−6
0.45	0.55	−33	−27	−24	−21	−19	−16	−15	−13	−11	−10	−7
0.50	0.50	−34	−28	−24	−22	−20	−17	−16	−14	−12	−10	−8
0.55	0.45	−35	−29	−25	−23	−21	−18	−17	−15	−13	−11	−9
0.60	0.40	−36	−30	−26	−24	−22	−19	−18	−16	−14	−12	−10
0.65	0.35	−36	−30	−26	−24	−22	−19	−18	−16	−15	−13	−10
0.70	0.30	−37	−31	−27	−25	−23	−20	−19	−17	−15	−13	−11
0.75	0.25	−38	−31	−27	−25	−24	−21	−19	−18	−16	−14	−11
0.80	0.20	−38	−32	−28	−26	−24	−21	−20	−18	−16	−15	−12
0.85	0.15	−39	−33	−29	−27	−25	−22	−21	−19	−17	−15	−13
0.88	0.12	−39	−33	−29	−27	−25	−22	−21	−19	−17	−16	−13
0.90	0.10	−39	−33	−29	−27	−25	−22	−21	−19	−18	−16	−13
0.92	0.08	−39	−33	−30	−27	−25	−22	−21	−19	−18	−16	−13
0.93	0.07	−39	−33	−30	−27	−26	−23	−21	−19	−18	−16	−13
0.95	0.05	−40	−34	−30	−28	−26	−23	−22	−20	−18	−16	−14
0.96	0.04	−40	−34	−30	−28	−26	−23	−22	−20	−18	−16	−14
0.97	0.03	−40	−34	−30	−28	−26	−23	−22	−20	−18	−16	−14
0.98	0.02	−40	−34	−30	−28	−26	−23	−22	−20	−18	−16	−14
0.99	0.01	−40	−34	−30	−28	−26	−23	−22	−20	−18	−16	−14

Tables of d Codes—*continued*

TABLE B.1. D CODE - CONTINUED

nonspec. (−)	(+)	sensitivity 0.75 / neg 0.25	0.70 / 0.30	0.65 / 0.35	0.60 / 0.40	0.55 / 0.45	0.50 / 0.50	0.45 / 0.55	0.40 / 0.60	0.35 / 0.65	0.30 / 0.70	0.25 / 0.75
0.99	0.01	+38	+37	+36	+36	+35	+34	+33	+32	+31	+30	+28
0.98	0.02	+31	+31	+30	+30	+29	+28	+27	+26	+25	+24	+22
0.97	0.03	+28	+27	+27	+26	+25	+24	+24	+22	+21	+20	+18
0.96	0.04	+25	+25	+24	+24	+23	+22	+21	+20	+19	+18	+16
0.95	0.05	+24	+23	+22	+22	+21	+20	+19	+18	+17	+16	+14
0.93	0.07	+21	+20	+19	+19	+18	+17	+16	+15	+14	+13	+11
0.92	0.08	+19	+19	+18	+18	+17	+16	+15	+14	+13	+11	+10
0.90	0.10	+18	+17	+16	+16	+15	+14	+13	+12	+11	+10	+8
0.88	0.12	+16	+15	+15	+14	+13	+12	+11	+10	+9	+8	+6
0.85	0.15	+14	+13	+13	+12	+11	+10	+10	+9	+7	+6	+4
0.80	0.20	+11	+11	+10	+10	+9	+8	+7	+6	+5	+4	+2
0.75	0.25	+10	+9	+8	+8	+7	+6	+5	+4	+3	+2	0
0.70	0.30	+8	+7	+5	+6	+5	+4	+4	+2	+1	0	−2
0.65	0.35	+7	+6	+5	+5	+4	+3	+2	+1	0	−1	−3
0.60	0.40	+5	+5	+4	+4	+3	+2	+1	0	−1	−2	−4
0.55	0.45	+4	+4	+3	+2	+2	+1	+1	−1	−2	−4	−5
0.50	0.50	+4	+3	+2	+2	+1	+1	0	−1	−3	−4	−6
0.45	0.55	+3	+2	+1	+1	+1	0	−1	−2	−4	−5	−7
0.40	0.60	+2	+1	+1	0	0	−1	−2	−3	−5	−6	−8
0.35	0.65	+1	+1	0	−1	−1	−2	−2	−4	−5	−7	−8
0.30	0.70	+1	0	−1	−1	−1	−2	−3	−4	−6	−7	−9
0.25	0.75	0	−1	−1	−2	−2	−3	−4	−5	−7	−8	−10
0.20	0.80	−1	−1	−2	−2	−3	−4	−5	−5	−7	−9	−10
0.15	0.85	−1	−2	−2	−3	−3	−5	−6	−6	−8	−9	−11
0.12	0.88	−1	−2	−3	−3	−4	−5	−6	−7	−8	−9	−11
0.10	0.90	−2	−2	−3	−3	−4	−5	−6	−7	−8	−10	−11
0.08	0.92	−2	−2	−3	−4	−4	−6	−6	−7	−8	−10	−11
0.07	0.93	−2	−2	−3	−4	−5	−6	−6	−7	−9	−10	−12
0.05	0.95	−2	−3	−3	−4	−5	−6	−7	−8	−9	−10	−12
0.04	0.96	−2	−3	−3	−4	−5	−6	−7	−8	−9	−10	−12
0.03	0.97	−2	−3	−3	−4	−5	−6	−7	−8	−9	−10	−12
0.02	0.98	−2	−3	−4	−4	−5	−6	−7	−8	−9	−10	−12
0.01	0.99	−2	−3	−4	−4	−5	−6	−7	−8	−9	−10	−12

(+) positive test   (−) negative test

Tables of d Codes—*continued*

TABLE B.1. D CODE - CONTINUED

nonspec. (-)	(+)	(+) 0.99 / (-) 0.01	0.98 / 0.02	0.97 / 0.03	0.96 / 0.04	0.95 / 0.05	0.93 / 0.07	0.92 / 0.08	0.90 / 0.10	0.88 / 0.12	0.85 / 0.15	0.80 / 0.20
0.99	0.01	+40	+40	+40	+40	+40	+39	+39	+39	+39	+39	+38
0.98	0.02	+34	+34	+34	+34	+34	+33	+33	+33	+33	+33	+32
0.97	0.03	+30	+30	+30	+30	+30	+30	+30	+30	+29	+29	+29
0.96	0.04	+28	+28	+28	+28	+28	+27	+27	+27	+27	+27	+26
0.95	0.05	+26	+26	+26	+26	+26	+25	+25	+25	+25	+25	+24
0.93	0.07	+23	+23	+23	+23	+23	+22	+22	+22	+22	+22	+21
0.92	0.08	+22	+22	+22	+22	+21	+21	+21	+21	+21	+21	+20
0.90	0.10	+20	+20	+20	+20	+20	+19	+19	+19	+19	+19	+18
0.88	0.12	+18	+18	+18	+18	+18	+18	+18	+18	+17	+17	+16
0.85	0.15	+16	+16	+16	+16	+16	+16	+16	+16	+15	+15	+15
0.80	0.20	+14	+14	+14	+14	+14	+13	+13	+13	+13	+13	+12
0.75	0.25	+12	+12	+12	+12	+12	+11	+11	+11	+11	+11	+10
0.70	0.30	+10	+10	+10	+10	+10	+10	+10	+10	+9	+9	+9
0.65	0.35	+9	+9	+9	+9	+9	+8	+8	+8	+8	+8	+7
0.60	0.40	+8	+8	+8	+8	+8	+7	+7	+7	+7	+7	+6
0.55	0.45	+7	+7	+7	+7	+6	+6	+6	+6	+6	+6	+5
0.50	0.50	+6	+6	+6	+6	+6	+5	+5	+5	+5	+5	+4
0.45	0.55	+5	+5	+5	+5	+5	+5	+4	+4	+4	+4	+3
0.40	0.60	+4	+4	+4	+4	+4	+4	+4	+4	+3	+3	+2
0.35	0.65	+4	+4	+3	+3	+3	+3	+3	+3	+3	+2	+2
0.30	0.70	+3	+3	+3	+3	+3	+2	+2	+2	+2	+2	+1
0.25	0.75	+2	+2	+2	+2	+2	+2	+2	+2	+1	+1	+1
0.20	0.80	+2	+2	+2	+2	+2	+1	+1	+1	+1	+1	0
0.15	0.85	+1	+1	+1	+1	+1	+1	+1	0	0	0	-1
0.12	0.88	+1	+1	+1	+1	+1	0	0	0	0	0	-1
0.10	0.90	+1	+1	+1	+1	+1	0	0	0	0	-1	-1
0.08	0.92	+1	+1	+1	0	0	0	0	0	0	-1	-1
0.07	0.93	0	0	0	0	0	0	0	0	0	-1	-1
0.05	0.95	0	0	0	0	0	0	0	0	-1	-1	-1
0.04	0.96	0	0	0	0	0	0	0	-1	-1	-1	-2
0.03	0.97	0	0	0	0	0	0	-1	-1	-1	-1	-2
0.02	0.98	0	0	0	0	0	0	-1	-1	-1	-1	-2
0.01	0.99	0	0	0	0	0	-1	-1	-1	-1	-1	-2

(+) positive test   (-) negative test   sensitivity

Tables of Posterior Probabilities

TABLE B.2.   POSTERIOR PROBABILITY

prior prob.	0	+1	+2	+3	+4	+5	+6 (d code)	+7	+8	+9	+10	+11	+12
0.01	0.01	0.01	0.01	0.01	0.02	0.02	0.02	0.02	0.02	0.03	0.03	0.03	0.04
0.02	0.02	0.02	0.03	0.03	0.03	0.04	0.04	0.04	0.05	0.05	0.06	0.07	0.08
0.03	0.03	0.03	0.04	0.04	0.05	0.05	0.06	0.06	0.07	0.08	0.09	0.10	0.11
0.04	0.04	0.04	0.05	0.06	0.06	0.07	0.08	0.09	0.09	0.11	0.12	0.13	0.14
0.05	0.05	0.06	0.06	0.07	0.08	0.09	0.10	0.11	0.12	0.13	0.14	0.16	0.17
0.07	0.07	0.08	0.09	0.10	0.11	0.12	0.13	0.14	0.16	0.18	0.19	0.21	0.23
0.08	0.08	0.09	0.10	0.11	0.12	0.13	0.15	0.16	0.18	0.20	0.22	0.24	0.26
0.10	0.10	0.11	0.12	0.14	0.15	0.16	0.18	0.19	0.22	0.24	0.26	0.28	0.31
0.12	0.12	0.13	0.15	0.16	0.18	0.20	0.21	0.23	0.26	0.28	0.30	0.33	0.35
0.15	0.15	0.17	0.18	0.20	0.22	0.24	0.26	0.28	0.31	0.33	0.36	0.39	0.41
0.20	0.20	0.22	0.24	0.26	0.28	0.31	0.33	0.36	0.39	0.41	0.44	0.47	0.50
0.25	0.25	0.27	0.30	0.32	0.35	0.37	0.40	0.43	0.46	0.48	0.51	0.54	0.57
0.30	0.30	0.32	0.35	0.38	0.40	0.43	0.46	0.49	0.52	0.55	0.58	0.60	0.63
0.35	0.35	0.38	0.40	0.43	0.46	0.49	0.52	0.55	0.57	0.60	0.63	0.66	0.68
0.40	0.40	0.43	0.46	0.48	0.51	0.54	0.57	0.60	0.63	0.65	0.68	0.70	0.73
0.45	0.45	0.48	0.51	0.54	0.56	0.59	0.62	0.65	0.67	0.70	0.72	0.74	0.77
0.50	0.50	0.53	0.56	0.59	0.61	0.64	0.67	0.69	0.72	0.74	0.76	0.78	0.80
0.55	0.55	0.58	0.61	0.63	0.66	0.68	0.71	0.73	0.75	0.78	0.79	0.81	0.83
0.60	0.60	0.63	0.65	0.68	0.70	0.73	0.75	0.77	0.79	0.81	0.83	0.84	0.86
0.65	0.65	0.68	0.70	0.72	0.75	0.77	0.79	0.81	0.82	0.84	0.85	0.87	0.88
0.70	0.70	0.72	0.75	0.77	0.79	0.81	0.82	0.84	0.85	0.87	0.88	0.89	0.90
0.75	0.75	0.77	0.79	0.81	0.83	0.84	0.86	0.87	0.88	0.89	0.90	0.91	0.92
0.80	0.80	0.82	0.83	0.85	0.86	0.88	0.89	0.90	0.91	0.92	0.93	0.93	0.94
0.85	0.85	0.86	0.88	0.89	0.90	0.91	0.92	0.93	0.93	0.94	0.95	0.95	0.96
0.88	0.88	0.89	0.90	0.91	0.92	0.93	0.94	0.94	0.95	0.95	0.96	0.96	0.97
0.90	0.90	0.91	0.92	0.93	0.93	0.94	0.95	0.95	0.96	0.96	0.97	0.97	0.97
0.92	0.92	0.93	0.94	0.94	0.95	0.95	0.96	0.96	0.97	0.97	0.97	0.98	0.98
0.93	0.93	0.94	0.94	0.95	0.95	0.96	0.96	0.97	0.97	0.98	0.98	0.98	0.98
0.95	0.95	0.96	0.96	0.96	0.97	0.97	0.97	0.98	0.98	0.98	0.98	0.99	0.99
0.96	0.96	0.96	0.97	0.97	0.97	0.98	0.98	0.98	0.98	0.99	0.99	0.99	0.99
0.97	0.97	0.97	0.98	0.98	0.98	0.98	0.98	0.99	0.99	0.99	0.99	0.99	0.99
0.98	0.98	0.98	0.98	0.99	0.99	0.99	0.99	0.99	0.99	0.99	0.99	1.00	0.99
0.99	0.99	0.99	0.99	0.99	0.99	0.99	0.99	1.00	1.00	1.00	1.00	1.00	1.00

Tables of Posterior Probabilities—*continued*

TABLE B.2. POSTERIOR PROBABILITY - CONTINUED

prior prob.	d code +13	+14	+15	+16	+17	+18	+19	+20	+21	+22	+23	+24	+25
0.01	0.04	0.05	0.05	0.06	0.07	0.07	0.08	0.09	0.10	0.11	0.12	0.14	0.15
0.02	0.08	0.09	0.10	0.11	0.13	0.14	0.15	0.17	0.19	0.20	0.22	0.24	0.27
0.03	0.12	0.13	0.15	0.16	0.18	0.20	0.22	0.24	0.26	0.28	0.30	0.33	0.35
0.04	0.16	0.17	0.19	0.21	0.23	0.25	0.27	0.29	0.32	0.34	0.37	0.40	0.43
0.05	0.19	0.21	0.23	0.25	0.27	0.29	0.32	0.34	0.37	0.40	0.43	0.45	0.48
0.07	0.25	0.27	0.30	0.32	0.35	0.37	0.40	0.43	0.46	0.49	0.52	0.54	0.57
0.08	0.28	0.30	0.33	0.35	0.38	0.41	0.44	0.47	0.49	0.52	0.55	0.58	0.61
0.10	0.33	0.36	0.38	0.41	0.44	0.47	0.50	0.53	0.55	0.58	0.61	0.64	0.66
0.12	0.38	0.41	0.43	0.46	0.49	0.52	0.55	0.58	0.60	0.63	0.66	0.68	0.71
0.15	0.44	0.47	0.50	0.53	0.56	0.58	0.61	0.64	0.66	0.69	0.71	0.74	0.76
0.20	0.53	0.56	0.58	0.61	0.64	0.67	0.69	0.71	0.74	0.76	0.78	0.80	0.82
0.25	0.60	0.63	0.65	0.68	0.70	0.73	0.75	0.77	0.79	0.81	0.82	0.84	0.86
0.30	0.66	0.68	0.71	0.73	0.75	0.77	0.79	0.81	0.83	0.84	0.86	0.87	0.88
0.35	0.71	0.73	0.75	0.77	0.79	0.81	0.83	0.84	0.86	0.87	0.88	0.90	0.91
0.40	0.75	0.77	0.79	0.81	0.83	0.84	0.86	0.87	0.88	0.89	0.90	0.91	0.92
0.45	0.79	0.80	0.82	0.84	0.85	0.87	0.88	0.89	0.90	0.91	0.92	0.93	0.94
0.50	0.82	0.83	0.85	0.86	0.88	0.89	0.90	0.91	0.92	0.93	0.93	0.94	0.95
0.55	0.85	0.86	0.87	0.89	0.90	0.91	0.92	0.92	0.93	0.94	0.95	0.95	0.96
0.60	0.87	0.88	0.89	0.90	0.91	0.92	0.93	0.94	0.94	0.95	0.95	0.96	0.96
0.65	0.89	0.90	0.91	0.92	0.93	0.94	0.94	0.95	0.95	0.96	0.96	0.97	0.97
0.70	0.91	0.92	0.93	0.94	0.94	0.95	0.95	0.96	0.96	0.97	0.97	0.97	0.98
0.75	0.93	0.94	0.94	0.95	0.96	0.96	0.96	0.97	0.97	0.97	0.98	0.98	0.98
0.80	0.95	0.95	0.96	0.96	0.97	0.97	0.97	0.98	0.98	0.98	0.98	0.98	0.99
0.85	0.96	0.97	0.97	0.97	0.98	0.98	0.98	0.98	0.98	0.99	0.99	0.99	0.99
0.88	0.97	0.97	0.98	0.98	0.98	0.98	0.99	0.99	0.99	0.99	0.99	0.99	0.99
0.90	0.98	0.98	0.98	0.98	0.99	0.99	0.99	0.99	0.99	0.99	0.99	0.99	0.99
0.92	0.98	0.98	0.98	0.99	0.99	0.99	0.99	0.99	0.99	0.99	0.99	1.00	1.00
0.93	0.98	0.99	0.99	0.99	0.99	0.99	0.99	0.99	0.99	1.00	1.00	1.00	1.00
0.95	0.99	0.99	0.99	0.99	0.99	0.99	0.99	0.99	1.00	1.00	1.00	1.00	1.00
0.96	0.99	0.99	0.99	0.99	0.99	0.99	0.99	1.00	1.00	1.00	1.00	1.00	1.00
0.97	0.99	0.99	1.00	1.00	1.00	1.00	1.00	1.00	1.00	1.00	1.00	1.00	1.00
0.98	1.00	1.00	1.00	1.00	1.00	1.00	1.00	1.00	1.00	1.00	1.00	1.00	1.00
0.99	1.00	1.00	1.00	1.00	1.00	1.00	1.00	1.00	1.00	1.00	1.00	1.00	1.00

Tables of Posterior Probabilities—*continued*

TABLE B.2. POSTERIOR PROBABILITY – CONTINUED

prior prob.	d code +26	+27	+28	+29	+30	+31	+32	+33	+34	+35	+36	+37	+38
0.01	0.17	0.18	0.20	0.22	0.24	0.26	0.29	0.31	0.34	0.36	0.39	0.42	0.45
0.02	0.29	0.31	0.34	0.37	0.39	0.42	0.45	0.48	0.51	0.53	0.56	0.59	0.62
0.03	0.38	0.41	0.44	0.47	0.49	0.52	0.55	0.58	0.61	0.63	0.66	0.69	0.71
0.04	0.45	0.48	0.51	0.54	0.57	0.60	0.62	0.65	0.68	0.70	0.72	0.75	0.77
0.05	0.51	0.54	0.57	0.60	0.62	0.65	0.68	0.70	0.73	0.75	0.77	0.79	0.81
0.07	0.60	0.63	0.65	0.68	0.70	0.73	0.75	0.77	0.79	0.81	0.83	0.84	0.86
0.08	0.63	0.66	0.69	0.71	0.73	0.76	0.78	0.80	0.81	0.83	0.85	0.86	0.87
0.10	0.69	0.71	0.74	0.76	0.78	0.80	0.82	0.83	0.85	0.86	0.88	0.89	0.90
0.12	0.73	0.75	0.77	0.79	0.81	0.83	0.84	0.86	0.87	0.88	0.90	0.91	0.92
0.15	0.78	0.80	0.82	0.83	0.85	0.86	0.88	0.89	0.90	0.91	0.92	0.93	0.93
0.20	0.83	0.85	0.86	0.88	0.89	0.90	0.91	0.92	0.93	0.93	0.94	0.95	0.95
0.25	0.87	0.88	0.89	0.90	0.91	0.92	0.93	0.94	0.94	0.95	0.95	0.96	0.96
0.30	0.90	0.91	0.92	0.92	0.93	0.94	0.94	0.95	0.96	0.96	0.96	0.97	0.97
0.35	0.91	0.92	0.93	0.94	0.94	0.95	0.96	0.96	0.96	0.97	0.97	0.97	0.98
0.40	0.93	0.94	0.94	0.95	0.95	0.96	0.96	0.97	0.97	0.97	0.98	0.98	0.98
0.45	0.94	0.95	0.95	0.96	0.96	0.97	0.97	0.97	0.98	0.98	0.98	0.98	0.99
0.50	0.95	0.96	0.96	0.97	0.97	0.97	0.98	0.98	0.98	0.98	0.99	0.99	0.99
0.55	0.96	0.96	0.97	0.97	0.97	0.98	0.98	0.98	0.99	0.99	0.99	0.99	0.99
0.60	0.97	0.97	0.97	0.98	0.98	0.98	0.98	0.99	0.99	0.99	0.99	0.99	0.99
0.65	0.97	0.98	0.98	0.98	0.98	0.99	0.99	0.99	0.99	0.99	0.99	0.99	0.99
0.70	0.98	0.98	0.98	0.99	0.99	0.99	0.99	0.99	0.99	0.99	1.00	1.00	1.00
0.75	0.98	0.98	0.99	0.99	0.99	0.99	0.99	0.99	1.00	1.00	1.00	1.00	1.00
0.80	0.99	0.99	0.99	0.99	0.99	0.99	1.00	1.00	1.00	1.00	1.00	1.00	1.00
0.85	0.99	0.99	0.99	0.99	0.99	0.99	1.00	1.00	1.00	1.00	1.00	1.00	1.00
0.88	0.99	0.99	0.99	1.00	1.00	0.99	1.00	1.00	1.00	1.00	1.00	1.00	1.00
0.90	0.99	1.00	1.00	1.00	1.00	1.00	1.00	1.00	1.00	1.00	1.00	1.00	1.00
0.92	1.00	1.00	1.00	1.00	1.00	1.00	1.00	1.00	1.00	1.00	1.00	1.00	1.00

Tables of Posterior Probabilities—*continued*

TABLE B.2 POSTERIOR PROBABILITY - CONTINUED

prior prob.	+39	+40	+41	+42	+43	+44	+45	+46	+47	+48	+49	+50	+51
0.01	0.47	0.50	0.53	0.56	0.59	0.62	0.64	0.67	0.69	0.72	0.74	0.76	0.78
0.02	0.65	0.67	0.70	0.72	0.74	0.76	0.78	0.80	0.82	0.84	0.85	0.87	0.88
0.03	0.73	0.76	0.78	0.80	0.81	0.83	0.85	0.86	0.87	0.89	0.90	0.91	0.92
0.04	0.79	0.81	0.82	0.84	0.85	0.87	0.88	0.89	0.90	0.91	0.92	0.93	0.94
0.05	0.82	0.84	0.86	0.87	0.88	0.89	0.90	0.91	0.92	0.93	0.94	0.94	0.95
0.07	0.87	0.88	0.89	0.90	0.91	0.92	0.93	0.94	0.94	0.95	0.95	0.96	0.96
0.08	0.89	0.90	0.91	0.92	0.92	0.93	0.94	0.95	0.95	0.96	0.96	0.96	0.97
0.10	0.91	0.92	0.93	0.93	0.94	0.95	0.95	0.96	0.96	0.97	0.97	0.97	0.97
0.12	0.92	0.93	0.94	0.94	0.95	0.96	0.96	0.96	0.97	0.97	0.97	0.98	0.98
0.15	0.94	0.95	0.95	0.96	0.96	0.97	0.97	0.97	0.98	0.98	0.98	0.98	0.98
0.20	0.96	0.96	0.97	0.97	0.97	0.98	0.98	0.98	0.98	0.98	0.99	0.99	0.98
0.25	0.97	0.97	0.97	0.98	0.98	0.98	0.98	0.99	0.99	0.99	0.99	0.99	0.99
0.30	0.97	0.98	0.98	0.98	0.98	0.99	0.99	0.99	0.99	0.99	0.99	0.99	0.99
0.35	0.98	0.98	0.98	0.99	0.99	0.99	0.99	0.99	0.99	0.99	0.99	0.99	0.99
0.40	0.98	0.99	0.99	0.99	0.99	0.99	0.99	0.99	0.99	0.99	0.99	1.00	0.99
0.45	0.99	0.99	0.99	0.99	0.99	0.99	0.99	0.99	0.99	1.00	1.00	1.00	1.00
0.50	0.99	0.99	0.99	0.99	0.99	0.99	0.99	0.99	1.00	1.00	1.00	1.00	1.00
0.55	0.99	0.99	0.99	0.99	0.99	0.99	1.00	1.00	1.00	1.00	1.00	1.00	1.00
0.60	0.99	0.99	0.99	0.99	1.00	1.00	1.00	1.00	1.00	1.00	1.00	1.00	1.00
0.65	0.99	0.99	1.00	1.00	1.00	1.00	1.00	1.00	1.00	1.00	1.00	1.00	1.00
0.70	1.00	1.00	1.00	1.00	1.00	1.00	1.00	1.00	1.00	1.00	1.00	1.00	1.00

d code

>

Tables of Posterior Probabilities—*continued*

TABLE B.2. POSTERIOR PROBABILITY - CONTINUED

prior prob.	+52	+53	+54	+55	+56	+57	d code +58	+59	+60	+61	+62	+63	+64
0.01	0.80	0.82	0.84	0.85	0.86	0.88	0.89	0.90	0.91	0.92	0.93	0.93	0.94
0.02	0.89	0.90	0.91	0.92	0.93	0.94	0.94	0.95	0.95	0.96	0.96	0.97	0.97
0.03	0.92	0.93	0.94	0.95	0.95	0.96	0.96	0.96	0.97	0.97	0.97	0.98	0.98
0.04	0.94	0.95	0.95	0.96	0.96	0.97	0.97	0.97	0.98	0.98	0.98	0.98	0.99
0.05	0.95	0.96	0.96	0.97	0.97	0.97	0.98	0.98	0.98	0.99	0.99	0.99	0.99
0.06	0.97	0.97	0.97	0.98	0.98	0.98	0.98	0.99	0.99	0.99	0.99	0.99	0.99
0.07	0.97	0.97	0.98	0.98	0.98	0.99	0.99	0.99	0.99	0.99	0.99	0.99	0.99
0.08	0.98	0.98	0.98	0.98	0.99	0.99	0.99	0.99	0.99	0.99	0.99	0.99	0.99
0.10	0.98	0.98	0.99	0.99	0.99	0.99	0.99	0.99	0.99	0.99	0.99	0.99	1.00
0.12	0.99	0.99	0.99	0.99	0.99	0.99	1.00	1.00	1.00	1.00	1.00	1.00	1.00
0.15	0.99	0.99	0.99	0.99	1.00	1.00	1.00	1.00	1.00	1.00	1.00	1.00	1.00
0.20	0.99	0.99	0.99	1.00	1.00	1.00	1.00	1.00	1.00	1.00	1.00	1.00	1.00
0.25	0.99	0.99	1.00	1.00	1.00	1.00	1.00	1.00	1.00	1.00	1.00	1.00	1.00
0.30	0.99	0.99	1.00	1.00	1.00	1.00	1.00	1.00	1.00	1.00	1.00	1.00	1.00
0.35	1.00	1.00	1.00	1.00	1.00	1.00	1.00	1.00	1.00	1.00	1.00	1.00	1.00

Tables of Posterior Probabilities—*continued*

TABLE B.2 POSTERIOR PROBABILITY – CONTINUED

prior prob.	d code												
	-1	-2	-3	-4	-5	-6	-7	-8	-9	-10	-11	-12	-13
0.01	0.01	0.01	0.01	0.01	0.01	0.01	0.00	0.00	0.00	0.00	0.00	0.00	0.00
0.02	0.02	0.02	0.01	0.01	0.01	0.01	0.01	0.01	0.01	0.01	0.01	0.01	0.00
0.03	0.03	0.02	0.02	0.02	0.02	0.02	0.01	0.01	0.01	0.01	0.01	0.01	0.01
0.04	0.04	0.03	0.03	0.03	0.02	0.02	0.02	0.02	0.01	0.01	0.01	0.01	0.01
0.05	0.04	0.04	0.04	0.03	0.03	0.03	0.02	0.02	0.02	0.02	0.01	0.01	0.01
0.07	0.06	0.06	0.05	0.05	0.04	0.04	0.03	0.03	0.03	0.02	0.02	0.02	0.01
0.08	0.07	0.06	0.06	0.05	0.05	0.04	0.04	0.03	0.03	0.03	0.03	0.02	0.02
0.10	0.09	0.08	0.07	0.07	0.06	0.05	0.05	0.04	0.04	0.03	0.03	0.03	0.02
0.12	0.11	0.10	0.09	0.08	0.07	0.06	0.06	0.05	0.05	0.04	0.04	0.03	0.02
0.15	0.14	0.12	0.11	0.10	0.09	0.08	0.07	0.07	0.06	0.05	0.05	0.04	0.03
0.20	0.18	0.17	0.15	0.14	0.12	0.11	0.10	0.09	0.08	0.07	0.07	0.06	0.04
0.25	0.23	0.21	0.19	0.17	0.16	0.14	0.13	0.12	0.11	0.10	0.09	0.08	0.05
0.30	0.28	0.25	0.23	0.21	0.19	0.18	0.16	0.15	0.13	0.12	0.11	0.10	0.07
0.35	0.32	0.30	0.28	0.25	0.23	0.21	0.19	0.18	0.16	0.15	0.13	0.12	0.09
0.40	0.37	0.35	0.32	0.30	0.27	0.25	0.23	0.21	0.19	0.17	0.16	0.14	0.11
0.45	0.42	0.39	0.37	0.34	0.32	0.29	0.27	0.25	0.22	0.20	0.19	0.17	0.13
0.50	0.47	0.44	0.41	0.39	0.36	0.33	0.31	0.28	0.26	0.24	0.22	0.20	0.15
0.55	0.52	0.49	0.46	0.44	0.41	0.38	0.35	0.33	0.30	0.28	0.26	0.23	0.18
0.60	0.57	0.54	0.52	0.49	0.46	0.43	0.40	0.37	0.35	0.32	0.30	0.27	0.21
0.65	0.62	0.60	0.57	0.54	0.51	0.48	0.45	0.43	0.40	0.37	0.34	0.32	0.25
0.70	0.68	0.65	0.62	0.60	0.57	0.54	0.51	0.48	0.45	0.42	0.40	0.37	0.29
0.75	0.73	0.70	0.68	0.65	0.63	0.60	0.57	0.54	0.52	0.49	0.46	0.43	0.34
0.80	0.78	0.76	0.74	0.72	0.69	0.67	0.64	0.61	0.59	0.56	0.53	0.50	0.40
0.85	0.83	0.82	0.80	0.78	0.76	0.74	0.72	0.69	0.67	0.64	0.61	0.59	0.47
0.88	0.87	0.85	0.84	0.82	0.80	0.79	0.77	0.74	0.72	0.70	0.67	0.65	0.56
0.90	0.89	0.88	0.86	0.85	0.84	0.82	0.80	0.78	0.76	0.74	0.72	0.69	0.62
0.92	0.91	0.90	0.89	0.88	0.87	0.85	0.84	0.82	0.80	0.78	0.76	0.74	0.67
0.93	0.92	0.91	0.90	0.89	0.88	0.87	0.86	0.84	0.82	0.81	0.79	0.77	0.72
0.95	0.94	0.94	0.93	0.92	0.91	0.90	0.89	0.88	0.87	0.86	0.84	0.83	0.75
0.96	0.96	0.95	0.94	0.94	0.93	0.92	0.91	0.91	0.89	0.88	0.87	0.86	0.84
0.97	0.97	0.96	0.96	0.95	0.95	0.94	0.94	0.93	0.92	0.91	0.90	0.89	0.88
0.98	0.98	0.97	0.97	0.97	0.96	0.96	0.96	0.95	0.95	0.94	0.93	0.92	0.92
0.99	0.99	0.99	0.99	0.98	0.98	0.98	0.98	0.98	0.97	0.97	0.97	0.96	0.96

Tables of Posterior Probabilities—*continued*

TABLE B.2. POSTERIOR PROBABILITY - CONTINUED

prior prob.	\-14	\-15	\-16	\-17	\-18	\-19	\-20	\-21	\-22	\-23	\-24	\-25	\-26
0.01	0.00	0.00	0.00	0.00	0.00	0.00	0.00	0.00	0.00	0.00	0.00	0.00	0.00
0.02	0.00	0.00	0.00	0.00	0.00	0.00	0.00	0.00	0.00	0.00	0.00	0.00	0.00
0.03	0.01	0.01	0.00	0.00	0.00	0.00	0.00	0.00	0.00	0.00	0.00	0.00	0.00
0.04	0.01	0.01	0.01	0.01	0.01	0.00	0.00	0.00	0.00	0.00	0.00	0.00	0.00
0.05	0.01	0.01	0.01	0.01	0.01	0.01	0.00	0.00	0.00	0.00	0.00	0.00	0.00
0.06	0.01	0.01	0.01	0.01	0.01	0.01	0.01	0.01	0.01	0.01	0.00	0.00	0.00
0.07	0.01	0.02	0.01	0.01	0.01	0.01	0.01	0.01	0.01	0.01	0.01	0.00	0.00
0.08	0.02	0.02	0.02	0.02	0.01	0.01	0.01	0.01	0.01	0.01	0.01	0.01	0.01
0.10	0.02	0.02	0.02	0.02	0.02	0.02	0.01	0.01	0.01	0.01	0.01	0.01	0.01
0.12	0.03	0.03	0.03	0.02	0.02	0.02	0.01	0.02	0.02	0.01	0.01	0.01	0.01
0.15	0.03	0.03	0.03	0.03	0.02	0.02	0.02	0.02	0.02	0.02	0.02	0.01	0.01
0.20	0.05	0.04	0.04	0.04	0.03	0.03	0.02	0.03	0.03	0.02	0.02	0.02	0.02
0.25	0.06	0.06	0.05	0.05	0.04	0.04	0.03	0.04	0.03	0.03	0.03	0.02	0.02
0.30	0.08	0.07	0.06	0.06	0.05	0.05	0.04	0.04	0.04	0.04	0.03	0.03	0.03
0.35	0.10	0.09	0.08	0.07	0.06	0.06	0.05	0.05	0.05	0.04	0.03	0.03	0.03
0.40	0.12	0.11	0.10	0.09	0.08	0.07	0.06	0.06	0.05	0.05	0.04	0.04	0.04
0.45	0.14	0.13	0.11	0.10	0.09	0.08	0.08	0.07	0.06	0.06	0.05	0.04	0.04
0.50	0.17	0.15	0.14	0.12	0.11	0.10	0.09	0.08	0.07	0.07	0.06	0.05	0.05
0.55	0.20	0.18	0.16	0.15	0.13	0.12	0.11	0.10	0.09	0.08	0.07	0.06	0.06
0.60	0.23	0.21	0.19	0.17	0.16	0.14	0.13	0.12	0.11	0.10	0.09	0.08	0.07
0.65	0.27	0.25	0.23	0.21	0.19	0.17	0.16	0.14	0.13	0.12	0.10	0.09	0.09
0.70	0.32	0.29	0.27	0.25	0.23	0.21	0.19	0.17	0.16	0.14	0.13	0.12	0.10
0.75	0.37	0.35	0.32	0.30	0.27	0.25	0.23	0.21	0.19	0.18	0.16	0.14	0.13
0.80	0.44	0.42	0.39	0.36	0.33	0.31	0.29	0.26	0.24	0.22	0.20	0.18	0.17
0.85	0.53	0.50	0.47	0.44	0.42	0.39	0.36	0.34	0.31	0.29	0.26	0.24	0.22
0.88	0.59	0.57	0.54	0.51	0.48	0.45	0.42	0.40	0.37	0.34	0.32	0.29	0.27
0.90	0.64	0.62	0.59	0.56	0.53	0.50	0.47	0.45	0.42	0.39	0.36	0.34	0.31
0.92	0.70	0.67	0.65	0.62	0.59	0.56	0.53	0.51	0.48	0.45	0.42	0.39	0.37
0.93	0.73	0.70	0.68	0.65	0.63	0.60	0.57	0.54	0.51	0.49	0.46	0.43	0.40
0.95	0.79	0.77	0.75	0.73	0.71	0.68	0.66	0.63	0.60	0.57	0.55	0.52	0.49
0.96	0.83	0.81	0.79	0.77	0.75	0.73	0.71	0.68	0.66	0.63	0.60	0.57	0.55
0.97	0.87	0.85	0.84	0.82	0.80	0.78	0.76	0.74	0.72	0.70	0.67	0.65	0.62
0.98	0.91	0.90	0.89	0.87	0.86	0.85	0.83	0.81	0.80	0.78	0.76	0.73	0.71
0.99	0.95	0.95	0.94	0.93	0.93	0.92	0.91	0.90	0.89	0.88	0.86	0.85	0.83

Tables of Posterior Probabilities—*continued*

TABLE B.2 POSTERIOR PROBABILITY – CONTINUED

prior prob.	d code -27	-28	-29	-30	-31	-32	-33	-34	-35	-36	-37	-38	-39
0.10	0.00	0.00	0.00	0.00	0.00	0.00	0.00	0.00	0.00	0.00	0.00	0.00	0.00
0.12	0.01	0.01	0.00	0.00	0.00	0.00	0.00	0.00	0.00	0.00	0.00	0.00	0.00
0.15	0.01	0.01	0.01	0.01	0.00	0.00	0.00	0.00	0.00	0.00	0.00	0.00	0.00
0.20	0.01	0.01	0.01	0.01	0.01	0.01	0.01	0.01	0.01	0.00	0.00	0.00	0.00
0.25	0.01	0.01	0.01	0.01	0.01	0.01	0.01	0.01	0.01	0.01	0.01	0.01	0.00
0.30	0.02	0.02	0.01	0.01	0.01	0.01	0.01	0.01	0.01	0.01	0.01	0.01	0.00
0.35	0.02	0.02	0.02	0.02	0.01	0.01	0.01	0.01	0.01	0.01	0.01	0.01	0.01
0.40	0.03	0.03	0.02	0.02	0.02	0.02	0.02	0.02	0.01	0.01	0.01	0.01	0.01
0.45	0.04	0.03	0.03	0.03	0.02	0.02	0.02	0.02	0.02	0.01	0.01	0.01	0.01
0.50	0.04	0.04	0.03	0.03	0.03	0.02	0.02	0.02	0.02	0.02	0.01	0.01	0.01
0.55	0.05	0.05	0.04	0.04	0.03	0.03	0.03	0.03	0.03	0.02	0.02	0.02	0.01
0.60	0.06	0.06	0.05	0.05	0.04	0.04	0.03	0.03	0.03	0.02	0.02	0.02	0.02
0.65	0.08	0.07	0.06	0.06	0.05	0.04	0.04	0.04	0.04	0.03	0.03	0.02	0.02
0.70	0.09	0.08	0.08	0.07	0.06	0.06	0.05	0.04	0.04	0.03	0.03	0.03	0.03
0.75	0.12	0.11	0.10	0.09	0.08	0.07	0.06	0.06	0.05	0.05	0.04	0.03	0.03
0.80	0.15	0.14	0.12	0.11	0.10	0.09	0.08	0.07	0.06	0.06	0.05	0.04	0.04
0.85	0.20	0.18	0.17	0.15	0.14	0.12	0.11	0.10	0.09	0.08	0.07	0.06	0.06
0.88	0.25	0.23	0.21	0.19	0.17	0.16	0.14	0.13	0.12	0.10	0.09	0.08	0.08
0.90	0.29	0.26	0.24	0.22	0.20	0.18	0.17	0.15	0.14	0.12	0.11	0.10	0.09
0.92	0.34	0.31	0.29	0.27	0.24	0.22	0.20	0.19	0.17	0.15	0.14	0.13	0.11
0.93	0.37	0.35	0.32	0.30	0.27	0.25	0.23	0.21	0.19	0.18	0.16	0.14	0.13
0.95	0.46	0.43	0.40	0.38	0.35	0.32	0.30	0.27	0.25	0.23	0.21	0.19	0.18
0.96	0.52	0.49	0.46	0.43	0.40	0.38	0.35	0.32	0.30	0.28	0.25	0.23	0.21
0.97	0.59	0.56	0.53	0.51	0.48	0.45	0.42	0.39	0.37	0.34	0.31	0.29	0.27
0.98	0.69	0.66	0.63	0.61	0.58	0.55	0.52	0.49	0.47	0.44	0.41	0.38	0.35
0.99	0.82	0.80	0.78	0.76	0.74	0.71	0.69	0.66	0.64	0.61	0.58	0.55	0.53

Tables of Posterior Probabilities—*continued*

TABLE B.2. POSTERIOR PROBABILITY - CONTINUED

prior prob.	d code -40	-41	-42	-43	-44	-45	-46	-47	-48	-49	-50	-51	-52
0.30	0.00	0.00	0.00	0.00	0.00	0.00	0.00	0.00	0.00	0.00	0.00	0.00	0.00
0.35	0.01	0.00	0.00	0.00	0.00	0.00	0.00	0.00	0.00	0.00	0.00	0.00	0.00
0.40	0.01	0.01	0.01	0.00	0.00	0.00	0.00	0.00	0.00	0.00	0.00	0.00	0.00
0.45	0.01	0.01	0.01	0.01	0.01	0.00	0.00	0.00	0.00	0.00	0.00	0.00	0.00
0.50	0.01	0.01	0.01	0.01	0.01	0.01	0.00	0.00	0.00	0.00	0.00	0.00	0.00
0.55	0.01	0.01	0.01	0.01	0.01	0.01	0.01	0.01	0.01	0.01	0.01	0.00	0.00
0.60	0.01	0.01	0.01	0.01	0.01	0.01	0.01	0.01	0.01	0.01	0.01	0.01	0.00
0.65	0.02	0.02	0.01	0.01	0.01	0.01	0.01	0.01	0.01	0.01	0.01	0.01	0.01
0.70	0.02	0.02	0.02	0.02	0.01	0.01	0.01	0.01	0.01	0.01	0.01	0.01	0.01
0.75	0.03	0.03	0.02	0.02	0.02	0.02	0.01	0.01	0.01	0.01	0.01	0.01	0.01
0.80	0.04	0.03	0.03	0.03	0.02	0.02	0.02	0.02	0.02	0.02	0.02	0.02	0.01
0.85	0.05	0.05	0.04	0.04	0.03	0.03	0.03	0.02	0.02	0.02	0.02	0.02	0.02
0.88	0.07	0.06	0.06	0.05	0.04	0.04	0.04	0.03	0.03	0.03	0.03	0.02	0.02
0.90	0.08	0.07	0.07	0.06	0.05	0.04	0.04	0.04	0.04	0.03	0.03	0.03	0.02
0.92	0.10	0.09	0.08	0.08	0.07	0.06	0.05	0.05	0.04	0.04	0.04	0.03	0.03
0.93	0.12	0.11	0.10	0.09	0.08	0.07	0.06	0.06	0.05	0.05	0.04	0.04	0.03
0.95	0.16	0.14	0.13	0.12	0.11	0.10	0.09	0.08	0.07	0.06	0.06	0.05	0.05
0.96	0.19	0.18	0.16	0.15	0.13	0.12	0.11	0.10	0.09	0.08	0.07	0.06	0.06
0.97	0.24	0.22	0.20	0.19	0.17	0.15	0.14	0.13	0.11	0.10	0.09	0.08	0.08
0.98	0.33	0.30	0.28	0.26	0.24	0.22	0.20	0.18	0.16	0.15	0.13	0.12	0.11
0.99	0.50	0.47	0.44	0.41	0.38	0.36	0.33	0.31	0.28	0.26	0.24	0.22	0.20

Tables of Posterior Probabilities—*continued*

TABLE B.2. POSTERIOR PROBABILITY - CONTINUED

prior prob.	d code												
	-53	-54	-55	-56	-57	-58	-59	-60	-61	-62	-63	-64	-65
0.65	0.00	0.00	0.00	0.00	0.00	0.00	0.00	0.00	0.00	0.00	0.00	0.00	0.00
0.70	0.01	0.00	0.00	0.00	0.00	0.00	0.00	0.00	0.00	0.00	0.00	0.00	0.00
0.75	0.01	0.01	0.01	0.00	0.00	0.00	0.00	0.00	0.00	0.00	0.00	0.00	0.00
0.80	0.01	0.01	0.01	0.01	0.01	0.01	0.00	0.00	0.00	0.00	0.00	0.00	0.00
0.85	0.01	0.01	0.01	0.01	0.01	0.01	0.01	0.01	0.01	0.01	0.01	0.00	0.00
0.88	0.02	0.01	0.01	0.01	0.01	0.01	0.01	0.01	0.01	0.01	0.01	0.01	0.01
0.90	0.02	0.02	0.02	0.01	0.01	0.01	0.01	0.01	0.01	0.01	0.01	0.01	0.01
0.92	0.03	0.02	0.02	0.02	0.02	0.01	0.01	0.01	0.01	0.01	0.01	0.01	0.01
0.93	0.03	0.03	0.02	0.02	0.02	0.02	0.02	0.01	0.01	0.01	0.01	0.01	0.01
0.95	0.04	0.04	0.03	0.03	0.03	0.02	0.02	0.02	0.02	0.02	0.02	0.01	0.01
0.96	0.05	0.05	0.04	0.04	0.04	0.03	0.03	0.02	0.03	0.02	0.02	0.02	0.02
0.97	0.07	0.06	0.05	0.05	0.04	0.04	0.04	0.03	0.03	0.03	0.03	0.02	0.02
0.98	0.10	0.09	0.08	0.07	0.06	0.06	0.05	0.05	0.04	0.04	0.03	0.03	0.03
0.99	0.18	0.16	0.15	0.14	0.12	0.11	0.10	0.09	0.08	0.07	0.07	0.06	0.05

Index

Page numbers followed by "f" indicate figures; those followed by a "t" indicate tables.